Introduction

Raising a child is one of the most rewarding experiences you'll likely ever have. There is perhaps nothing more special than the lifelong bond that forms between a parent and a child. That said, it is hard work! My hope is that you can have fun and feel supported along the way.

Mayo Clinic Guide to Your Baby's First Years is an easy-to-use yet comprehensive how-to manual for caring for your child, from newborn days all the way to toddlerhood. From chapters on month-by-month development to ones on health and safety, this book covers what you need to know. There's also a wealth of tips for coping with the many changes to daily life that come with parenthood. Where evidence-based information is available, it's provided. Still, there is a lot of room for parents to decide what works best for their family, and some of these choices are discussed as well.

The pages that follow will provide you with a lot of helpful information. But you're the one who makes it all happen. A positive attitude, a good support system and plenty of love can go a long way in making the years ahead truly enjoyable.

A project of this scope requires the teamwork of many individuals. A special thanks to all my colleagues who lent their expertise to this book, and to my own family, who encourage and challenge me to be the best parent I can be.

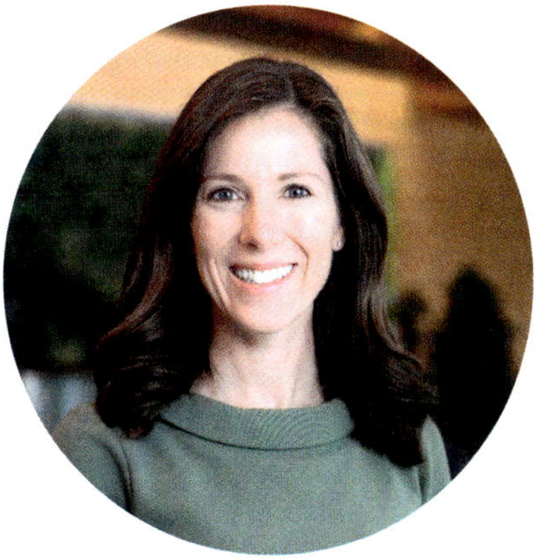

Kelsey M. Klaas, M.D.,
is a pediatrician in the Division of General Pediatric and Adolescent Medicine at Mayo Clinic Children's Center in Rochester, Minnesota. As the mother of two children, she brings both a medical and a parent's perspective to the book.

How to use this book

To help you easily find what you're looking for, *Mayo Clinic Guide to Your Baby's First Years* is divided into six sections.

PART 1: CARING FOR YOUR CHILD

From how to feed your newborn to helping toddlers develop good sleep habits, you'll find basic baby- and toddler-care tips in this detailed section. You'll also find strategies for comforting a crying baby and handling tantrums, as well as tips for toilet training and managing toddler screen time.

PART 2: HEALTH AND SAFETY

Part 2 covers all the key elements to preventing and dealing with injury and illness. You'll read about checkups and vaccinations, as well as suggestions for childproofing your home.

PART 3: GROWTH AND DEVELOPMENT

This section provides monthly insights into your baby's growth and development. It covers a range of topics including toys and games, separation anxiety, and preschool readiness. It also covers developmental milestones such as walking, learning new words and connecting with family members.

Mayo Clinic Guide to Your Baby's First Years

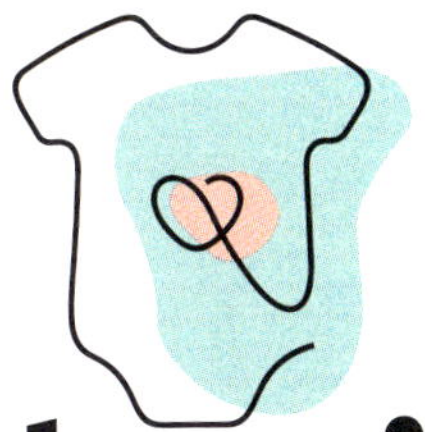

Clear Answers and Expert Advice for Every Phase With Your Infant and Toddler

MAYO CLINIC | Press

Medical Editor
Kelsey M. Klaas, M.D.

Contributing Editors
Nusheen Ameenuddin, M.D., M.P.H., Katelyn R. Anderson, M.D., Wentiirim B. Annankra, M.D., Meghan R. Cain, M.D., Jessica M. Davis, M.D., Asmaa Ferdjallah, M.D., M.P.H., Seth W. Gregory, M.D., Julie L. Hanson, M.D., Sara Hassan, M.D., Jay H. Homme, M.D., Flora R. Howie, M.D., Robert M. Jacobson, M.D., Anna E. Kellund, M.D., Robin M. Lloyd, M.D., Margaret E. Long, M.D., Theresa Madigan, M.D., Chetna Mangat, M.D., Stephanie C. Mavis, M.D., M.H.P.E., Jenny M. Montejo, M.D., Khaled S. Mohammed, M.B., B.Ch., Ann M. Murray, M.D., Paige I. Partain, M.D., Sophia M. Pillai, M.D., Luke C. Radel, M.D., Magdalena Romanowicz, M.D.

Additional contributions from
Rath Indexing

Cover concept by Josh Baker

MAYO CLINIC PRESS
200 First St. SW
Rochester, MN 55905
MCPress.MayoClinic.org

ISBN: 9798887701622 (paperback)
ISBN: 9798887701639 (ebook)

Library of Congress Control Number:
2024032031

Library of Congress Cataloging-in-Publication Data is available upon request.

Printed in United States
Third printing: 2026

PART 4: COMMON ILLNESSES AND CONCERNS

Here you'll find helpful tips for managing conditions that commonly affect young children, such as fevers, colds, ear infections, pink eye, RSV and others. You'll also learn when medication may be appropriate and when it may be best to avoid it.

PART 5: MANAGING AND ENJOYING PARENTHOOD

Caring for a young child can be nerve-racking and exhausting. The information in Part 5 can help you get through the first three years with reassurance and confidence.

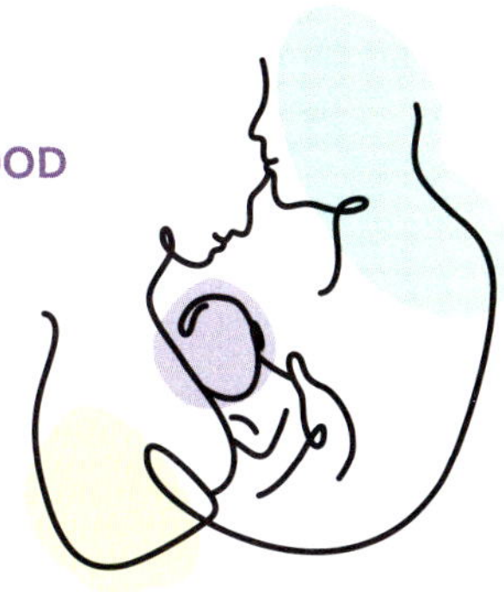

PART 6: SPECIAL CIRCUMSTANCES

Some situations require special care. This section includes information tailored to parents of adopted children, premature babies and multiples. Autism spectrum disorder and developmental delays are also discussed here.

Contents

PART 1

Caring for your child

CHAPTER 1

Welcome to parenthood!

Congratulations! You are now entering one of the greatest phases of your life — parenthood. There is perhaps nothing in life more special than the bond that forms between a parent and a child. It's a relationship that will bring endless years of joy, laughter, admiration and satisfaction. The time you spend raising your child will be time that you will cherish forever. In the years to come, you'll learn more about attachment, love and protectiveness than you ever thought possible.

But not every day in your parenthood journey will be grand and glorious. As in everything else in life, there will be ups and downs. You may find that some of the more stressful and exhausting days of being a parent will come early on, when you first bring your newborn home.

Bringing a baby into your house can turn your life upside down. The routine you once knew — having time to yourself, getting together with friends, going out for a relaxing dinner or spending the day indulging in your favorite hobby — has been put on hold. In its place is a reality that may feel totally foreign to you. That's because children don't arrive with instruction manuals, and parenting is somewhat of a trial-by-fire experience. If you've never had to care for a young child before, you may feel nervous, unsure of yourself and a bit lost. That's to be expected — and is perfectly normal.

PARENTING 101

Many parents describe their first year with a new baby as a roller-coaster ride. As one new parent put it, "One minute you're laughing and joking; the next minute you're crying, not really knowing why." You may go from adoring your baby and marveling at tiny fingers and toes to grieving your loss of independence and worrying about your ability to care for a newborn, all in the space of a single diaper change.

Given all these changes, the first few weeks after you bring your baby home are likely to be one of the most challenging times of your life. The changes in the daily rhythms of your life can feel chaotic, but you will learn to adapt. It may take months or even longer, but you'll get there — in your own way, in your own time, and with your own missteps and triumphs.

Relish the time

As chaotic as it may seem, this is a special time in your life. Appreciate the joy your child brings, and try to let go of your worries. Baby days won't last long. Step back and appreciate the moment. For all the strain associated with these first years, parenthood brings an incredible richness to daily living. Nothing can quite compare to the joy of meeting a newborn's gaze or accompanying the wobbly first steps of a toddler.

Trust your instincts

Caring for a child may be totally new territory for you, but have confidence in yourself. You'll quickly learn the things you need to know to take great care of your child. Also realize that you aren't expected to know it all. It's OK to ask questions and seek guidance from friends, family and healthcare professionals. If you get unsolicited advice, take the advice that fits with your parenting style and feel free to forget the rest.

Check your expectations

Many new parents start out with unrealistic expectations — that life won't be much different from before, that parenting is going to be fun every minute of the day, that the new baby will mostly eat and sleep, that they'll be able to manage everything perfectly. The gap between expectations and reality can lead to stress and disappointment. Throw out any preconceived notions about what life with a little one should be like, and be realistic about the increased demands on your time. That cute little 8-pound addition to your household can create a lot of extra work.

Be patient

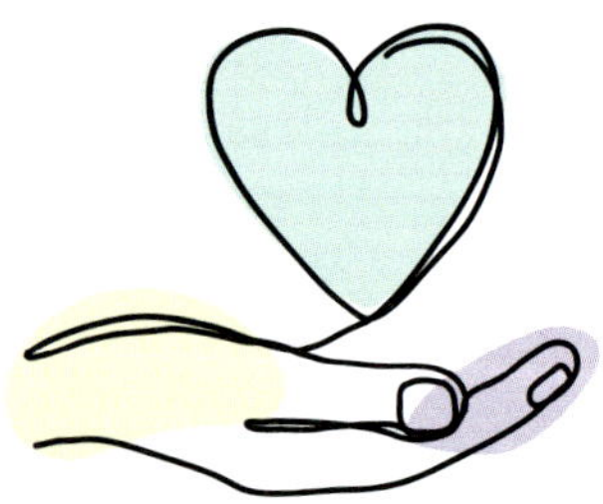

For the first few weeks, your life may seem limited to round-the-clock feeding, bathing, diapering and soothing — all on shortened spans of sleep. You may find it difficult to fit in a shower and do a load of laundry, let alone make dinner. You may fear this is what your life is going to be like forever! It won't be. Soon your baby will be a toddler, and increased mobility, conversation and independence will bring new adventures. Over time you'll adjust to each new phase, revive old routines and create new ones. As your child grows older, you'll find you have a little more time for yourself.

Take care of yourself

Childhood care also extends to parents. Taking good care of your child includes taking good care of yourself. The better you feel, the better able you'll be to care for and enjoy your child. Get as much rest as you can, eat well and fit in some exercise. Most of all, don't be afraid to ask for help when you need it.

An important part of this is giving yourself grace. While these early childhood years are full of wonder and joy for parents, they also can be difficult and exhausting. When you're in a moment that feels particularly hard, remember that it's likely just a hard moment — not a reflection on you. Take a breath and keep going.

Cherish relationships

Children, while wonderful, can be hard on other relationships in your life. If you're starting the parenting journey with your spouse or partner, you may miss your life as just a couple. You may also find that you have differences of opinion on issues related to caring for your child. Be patient with yourself and your partner. Take time to admire your partner's relationship with your child, and you will likely find great inspiration, not only as a parent but also as a couple.

THIS BOOK

As you maneuver the ins and outs of parenting, a little guidance and reassurance can be of great help. *Mayo Clinic Guide to Your Baby's First Years* is designed to help you find answers to common questions during the first three years of a child's life. Some questions have clear, evidence-based answers, and some have more than one possible answer, because every child and every family has different needs and circumstances. This book is intended to give evidence-based answers when they are available and to discuss possibilities for others. It also is intended to empower you with reassurance that you're doing well, and that the emotions and concerns you may be experiencing are the same as those of many other parents.

Dig in by whatever manner works best for you. You can turn the page and begin reading, or you can selectively choose those chapters or sections that are most relevant to you right now. Keep the book handy so that you can turn to it whenever a concern arises or prepare yourself for the months and years ahead.

Remember that parenting is an adventure. Enjoy the journey!

CHAPTER 2

Baby's first days

Your baby is finally here. For so long, you've been anticipating the day you could hold your baby and see your child's face. And now everything leading up to baby's arrival is behind you. Now you can enjoy getting to know this precious little person you've been waiting to meet.

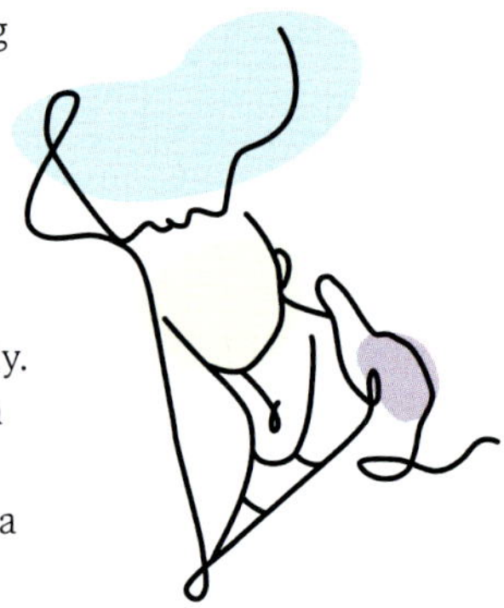

Sometimes the mental picture you've had of your first moments with your baby doesn't exactly match up with reality. Truth is, newborn babies tend to look a bit messy and swollen when they emerge, and you may be exhausted and overwhelmed by the birthing process. Don't worry. Give yourself a moment to take it all in.

In this chapter, you'll learn what to expect during your newborn's first few weeks of life at home — from bonding opportunities to what newborns typically look like. You'll also learn about standard examinations, procedures and screenings, and about some of the common conditions seen in newborns.

BABY BONDING

As soon as they are born, babies are ready to be held, cuddled, stroked, talked to and kissed. These everyday expressions of love and affection promote bonding with the parent. They also help a baby's brain develop. Just as an infant's body needs food to grow, the infant's brain benefits from positive emotional, physical and intellectual experiences. Relationships with other people early in life have a vital influence on a child's development. Some parents feel an immediate connection with their newborn, while for others the bond takes longer to develop. Don't worry or feel guilty if you aren't overcome with a rush of love at the very beginning. Not every parent bonds instantly with a new baby. Your feelings will become stronger with time.

Bonding moments

During the first weeks, most of your time is likely to be spent feeding your baby, changing diapers and helping your baby sleep. These routine tasks present an opportunity to bond. When babies receive warm, responsive care, they're more likely to feel safe and secure. For example, as you change diapers, gaze lovingly into your baby's eyes and speak gently. These simple actions help with bonding and are important for brain development.

Babies also have times when they're quietly alert and ready to engage and learn. These times may last only a few moments, but you'll learn to recognize them. Take advantage of your baby's alert times to get acquainted and play.

Cuddle and touch your baby Newborns are sensitive to changes in pressure and temperature. They love to be held, rocked, caressed, cradled, snuggled, kissed, patted, stroked, massaged and carried.

Don't worry about spoiling your newborn Respond to your child's cues warmly and promptly. Among the signals babies send are the sounds they make, the way they move, their facial expressions, and the way they make or avoid eye contact. Pay close attention to your baby's need for activity as well as quiet times.

Let your baby watch your face Soon after birth, your newborn will become accustomed to seeing you and will begin to focus on your face. Allow your baby to study your features, and provide plenty of smiles.

Play music, dance and sing To add variety to your baby's day, put on some soft music with a beat. Hold your baby's body close to yours and gently sway and move to the tune. Sing with the music or talk to your baby, too.

Establish routines and rituals The first few weeks with your newborn aren't always predictable. But as much as you can, establish small routines and rituals that help you and your baby get to know each other. For example, spend a few minutes cuddling or rocking after a feeding or look out a window together when you get up in the morning. Repeated positive experiences provide children with a sense of security. Be patient with yourself in these first weeks. Caring for a new child can be daunting, discouraging, thrilling and perplexing — all in the same hour! In time, your skills as a parent will grow, and you will come to love this little one far more than you could have imagined.

Serve and return Everyday face-to-face interactions — what some experts call serve-and-return moments, such as when your baby looks at you and you gaze back — are the best way to stimulate and build the nerve connections and pathways in your baby's brain. Evidence suggests that these early connections help a child grow and thrive, even in the midst of stress. Talk, read and sing to your baby, and when they react, respond as if it were a conversation. These early exchanges encourage social and emotional development and provide another opportunity for bonding.

BABY'S LOOKS

Considering what they've been through during childbirth, it's no wonder newborns don't look like the babies often seen on television or on social media. Instead, your newborn may emerge wrinkled and ruddy. Your baby's head may be a bit misshapen and larger than you expected, and the eyelids may be puffy. Your baby's arms and legs may be curled in, and the hands and feet may be bluish, purplish or dusky in color. Newborns also may be somewhat bloody and likely wet and slippery from amniotic fluid.

In addition, most babies will be born with a coating that looks like skin lotion, called vernix. This coating is most noticeable in creases, such as under your baby's arms, behind the ears and in the groin. Most of this vernix will be washed off during your baby's first bath.

Head

At first your baby's head may appear flat, elongated or crooked. This peculiar elongation is one of the common features of a newborn.

A baby's skull consists of several sections of bone that are flexibly joined. This allows the head shape to adjust to the shape of the pelvis as baby moves through the birth canal during childbirth. A long labor usually results in an elongated or tall skull shape at birth. The head of a baby born feet-first, called breech, may have a shorter, broader appearance. If a vacuum extractor was used to assist in the birth, your baby's head may look particularly elongated. Sometimes you can feel ridges on your baby's head where the sections of bone have overlapped.

As your baby's head shape normalizes over the first few days, these ridges will go away and your baby's head will take on a more rounded appearance.

Fontanels When you feel your baby's head, you'll notice two soft areas. These soft spots, called fontanels, are where your baby's skull bones haven't grown together yet.

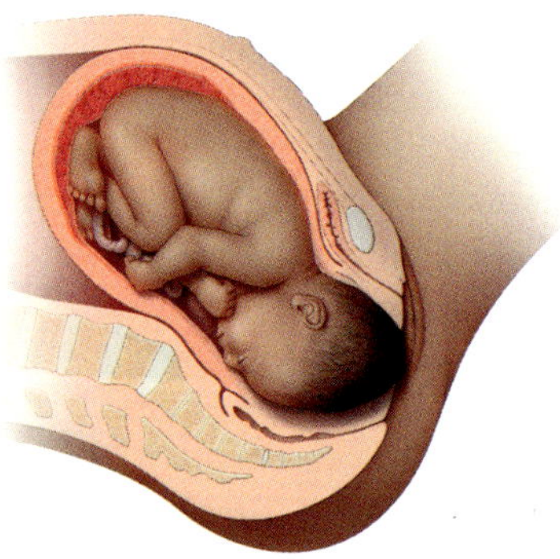

Head elongation

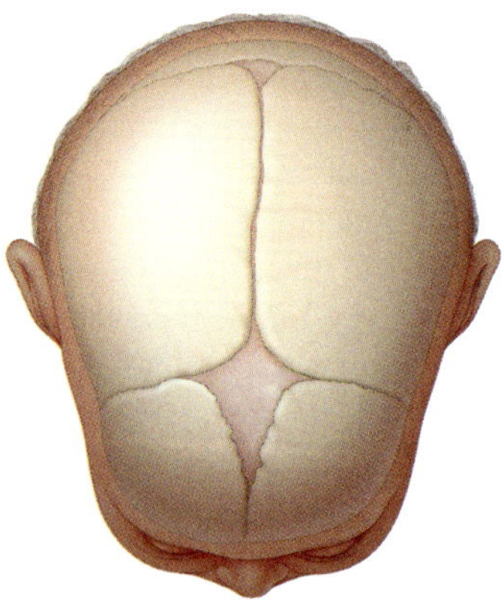

Fontanels

The fontanel toward the front of the scalp is a diamond-shaped spot roughly the size of a quarter. Though it's usually flat, it may bulge when your baby cries or strains. By the time your child is 2 years old, this fontanel will fill in with hard bone. The smaller fontanel at the back of the head is less noticeable. This fontanel is about the size of a dime, and it closes much quicker — around six weeks after birth.

Some parents are anxious about touching baby's soft spots, partly because they don't like the way the soft spots feel. Don't worry. You won't hurt your baby if you do touch a fontanel.

A rounded swelling of the scalp is usually seen on the top and back of the baby's head when a baby is born headfirst. This puffiness disappears within a day or so.

Skin

Most babies are born with some bruising, and skin blotches and blemishes are common.

Pressure from your pelvis during labor can cause a bruise on your baby's head. The bruise may be noticeable for several weeks, and you might feel a small bump that persists for several months. You may also see scrapes or bruises on your baby's face and head if forceps were used during delivery. These bruises and blemishes generally go away within a couple of weeks.

The top layer of a newborn's skin flakes off shortly after birth. You may notice plenty of dry, peeling skin in the first few weeks. In general, this gets better on its own. In the meantime, apply some petroleum jelly to baby's skin.

Evidence suggests that daily moisturizing of a baby's skin during the first six months of life can help prevent the development of eczema. Petroleum jelly is generally the most cost-effective, but other products such as Aquaphor or Vanicream also work well.

There are other common newborn skin conditions, such as milia and baby acne. For pictures and more information on these conditions, see Chapter 7.

Birthmarks

Contrary to their name, birthmarks aren't always present at birth. Some, such as a hemangioma, develop weeks later. And though most are permanent, a few types fade as a child grows. Most birthmarks are harmless, but some may be treated for cosmetic reasons or because of rapid growth or risk of future health problems. See pages 30 and 31 for pictures of common birthmarks.

Salmon patch A salmon patch, sometimes called a stork bite or angel kiss, is a patch of skin that's darker than the surrounding skin, often found just above or below the hairline at the back of the neck. It may appear reddish or pink and will briefly blanch, becoming the color of the surrounding skin, when pressed gently. The medical term is nevus simplex. Salmon patches may also be found on the eyelids, forehead or upper lip. These marks are caused by collections of tiny blood vessels (capillaries) close to the skin. Salmon patches on the forehead, on the eyelids or between the eyes usually fade with time, though they may become more noticeable with increased blood flow to the head, such as when crying or straining. Salmon patches on the nape of the neck may not fade, but they're often covered by hair. Salmon patches don't require any type of treatment.

Slate gray nevus Also called a congenital dermal melanocytosis, this is a typically harmless large brown or dark blue-gray birthmark — darker than the surrounding skin — that's sometimes mistaken for a bruise. It's more common in babies of Asian, African, Hispanic or Native American background and typically appears on the lower back, buttocks or shoulder. This birthmark usually fades later in childhood and doesn't require treatment.

Café au lait spot These birthmarks are flat, oval or round, tan to dark brown

BIRTHMARKS

Café au lait spot

A café au lait spot is tan to brown in color. It is usually present at birth but may develop in the first few years of life. These birthmarks are often oval and can have smooth ("Coast of California") or irregular ("Coast of Maine") borders.

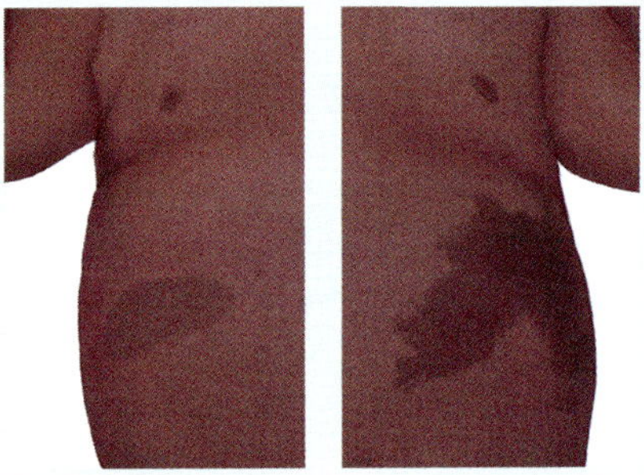

Port-wine stain

A port-wine stain is a birthmark in which swollen blood vessels create a reddish-purplish discoloration of the skin. Early port-wine stains are usually flat and pink in appearance. As the child gets older, the color may deepen to dark red or purplish.

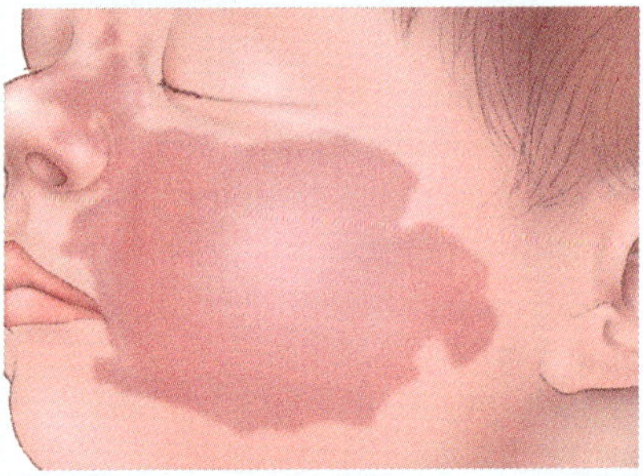

Congenital nevus

A congenital nevus is a dark-colored mole present at birth that may vary in size from small to large. It typically appears on the scalp or trunk but can occur on any part of the body.

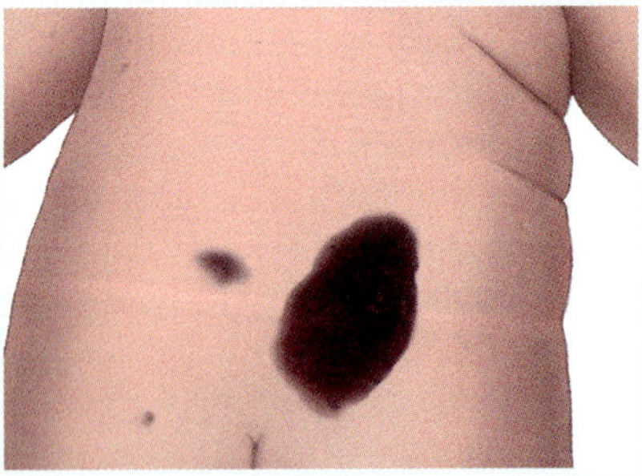

patches. Café au lait birthmarks are very common, and they can occur anywhere on the body. They're usually permanent, but they don't require treatment. However, if your child has more than six café au lait spots, ask your child's healthcare professional whether further evaluation might be warranted.

Hemangioma Hemangiomas are caused by an overgrowth of blood vessels in the top layers of skin. Usually not present at birth, a hemangioma may begin as a small, pale or dusky spot that becomes red in the center. The birthmark enlarges during the baby's first few months and appears as a bright or dark red raised spot. It most often disappears without treatment by school age. Large

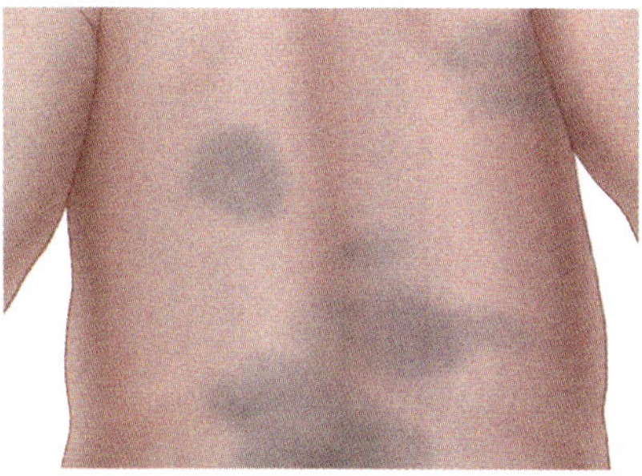

Slate gray nevus

This birthmark often appears on the lower back and ranges in color from deep brown to slate gray or blue-black. It's sometimes mistaken for a bruise. A slate gray nevus usually goes away on its own later in childhood.

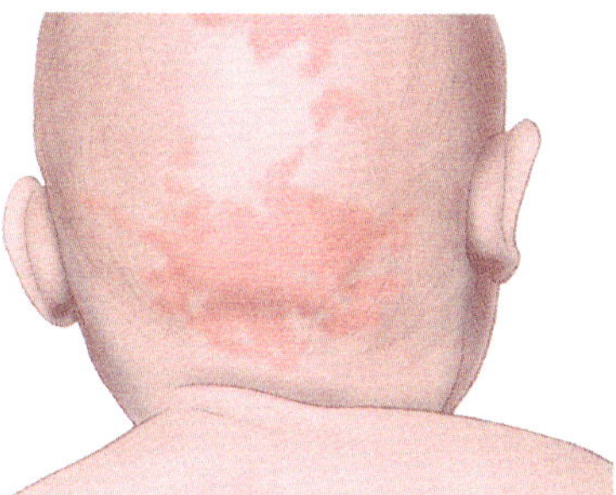

Salmon patch

Also called a stork bite, this mark is caused by tiny blood vessels (capillaries) visible through the skin. Salmon patches are most common on the forehead, eyelids, upper lip and back of the neck.

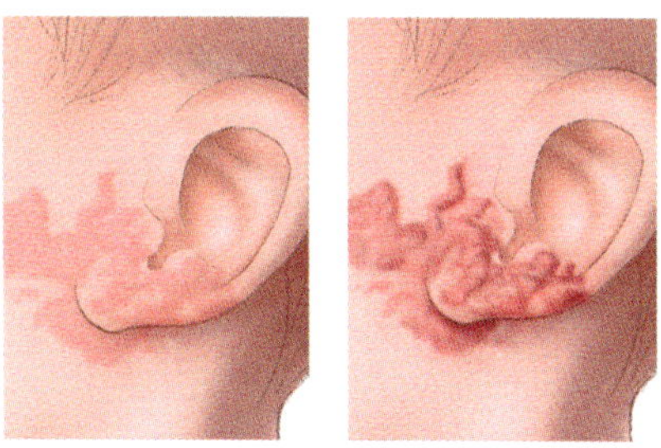

At birth **2 months**

Hemangioma

A hemangioma is an abnormal buildup of blood vessels in the skin. Hemangiomas are usually flat at birth, but they often grow in the first 12 to 15 months and then shrink over the next several years. They typically appear on the neck or facial area.

hemangiomas may cover an entire segment of the face or body. Some fast-growing hemangiomas may require laser treatment or medication. Babies with several hemangiomas or hemangiomas at certain locations may need evaluation for an underlying condition.

Congenital nevus A congenital nevus is a large, dark-colored mole that typically appears on the scalp or trunk of the body. Hair may grow within the birthmark. A congenital nevus can range in size from less than ½ inch to more than 5 inches across, covering large areas. Children with a large congenital nevus are at an increased risk of developing skin cancer as adults. If your child has this type of birthmark, talk with your child's medical professional about checking for skin changes.

Port-wine stain A port-wine stain is a permanent birthmark that can be pink or light brown to deep maroon, often deepening in color as the child gets older. The size of this birthmark will grow proportionately to the child. Most often a port-wine stain appears on the face and neck, but it can affect other areas. The involved skin may thicken and develop an irregular, pebbled surface as the child gets older. Port-wine stains may cause emotional stress and, rarely, may be associated with certain medical problems. The condition is usually treated with laser therapy. Sometimes port-wine stains occur with genetic syndromes, which require regular medical evaluation if present.

Facial appearance

Your baby's nose may seem flattened at first. This is from pressure inside the birth canal. Within a day or two, the nose will take on a more rounded appearance. Your baby's cheeks also may have marks or bruises if forceps were used during the delivery. This, too, will improve in a short time.

Eyes It's perfectly normal for your newborn's eyes to be puffy. Some infants have such puffy eyes that they aren't able to open their eyes wide right away. This will improve within a day or two.

You also may notice that your baby sometimes looks cross-eyed. This, too, is common, and your child will outgrow the condition within several months.

Sometimes babies are born with red spots on the whites of their eyes. These spots result from the breakage of tiny blood vessels during birth. The spots are harmless, and they won't interfere with your baby's sight. They generally disappear in a week to two.

A newborn's eyes give no guarantee of their future color. Although most newborns have dark bluish-brown, blue-black, grayish-blue or slate-colored eyes, permanent eye color may take six months or even longer to appear.

Hair

Your baby may be born bald or with a full head of thick hair — or almost anything in between! Don't fall in love with your baby's hair too quickly. Your baby's hair color at birth may change six months down the road. Blond newborns, for example, may become darker blond as they get older, or their hair may develop a reddish tinge that isn't apparent at birth.

You may be surprised to see that your newborn's head isn't the only place with hair. Downy, fine hair called lanugo covers a baby's body before birth and may temporarily appear on your newborn's back, shoulders, forehead and temples. Most of this hair is shed in the uterus before the baby is born, making lanugo especially common in premature babies. It disappears within a few weeks after birth.

FIRST EXAMINATION

After being born, your baby will be the focus of everyone in the room. Often your healthcare team will ask you about your preferences after delivery. If your baby appears well, your care team may place the baby directly on your chest. Alternatively, the care team may wipe your baby clean, suction your baby's mouth and nose, and check your baby's heart rate. Sometimes babies need to be brought to a warmer in the delivery room for a more thorough examination right after delivery.

All newborns look somewhat bluish-gray for the first several minutes, especially on their lips and tongue. Within 5 to 10 minutes this resolves and they may appear pinker — regardless of race — though baby's hands and feet may still remain bluish. This is typical. Your baby's umbilical cord is clamped with a plastic clamp, and you or your partner may be given the option to cut it.

In the next day or two, your baby's healthcare team will conduct newborn examinations, administer screening tests, and give some injections and preventive treatments designed for newborns.

Apgar score

One of your baby's first examinations will be done to determine an Apgar score. An Apgar score is basically a quick evaluation of a newborn's health. The test is given one minute and five minutes after a baby is born. Developed in 1952 by anesthesiologist Virginia Apgar, this brief examination rates newborns on five criteria: color, heart rate, reflexes, muscle tone and breathing.

Each of these criteria is given an individual score of 0, 1 or 2. The scores are totaled for a maximum possible score of 10. High scores indicate a smoother transition after birth, but don't get too caught up in the numbers. Your baby's healthcare team will tell you how your baby is doing and will keep you updated, especially if your baby needs extra help after delivery.

Other checks and measurements

Soon after birth, your newborn's weight, length and head circumference are measured. Your baby's temperature may be taken, and breathing and heart rate measured. Usually within 12 hours after birth, a thorough physical exam is done to detect any problems or abnormalities.

Treatments and immunizations

The following steps are generally taken shortly after birth to help prevent diseases and conditions that may occur in newborns.

Eye protection To prevent the possibility of an infection being passed from the pregnant person to the baby during birth, all states require that infants' eyes be protected immediately after birth. Gonorrheal eye infections were a leading cause of blindness until early in the 20th century, when treatment of babies' eyes after birth became mandatory. An antibiotic ointment or solution is placed into the baby's eyes. These preparations are gentle to the eyes and cause no pain.

Vitamin K injection In the United States, vitamin K is routinely given to infants shortly after they're born. Vitamin K is necessary for normal blood coagulation, the body's process for stopping bleeding after a cut or bruise. Newborns have low levels of vitamin K in their first few weeks. An injection of vitamin K can help prevent the possibility that a newborn would become so deficient in vitamin K that serious bleeding might develop. This problem is not related to hemophilia.

Hepatitis B vaccination Babies can contract hepatitis B from their parent during pregnancy or the birthing process. Protection against hepatitis B begins with a vaccine given shortly after birth.

Hepatitis B is a viral infection that affects the liver. When infection occurs in infancy, it is more likely to cause even more severe illnesses such as cirrhosis, liver failure or liver cancers.

Respiratory syncytial virus (RSV) antibody injection RSV commonly causes mild cold-like symptoms in healthy older children and adults. However, infants are at increased risk of severe and sometimes life-threatening illness from RSV. (Turn to page 451 for more information.) To help protect babies, one of two forms of immunization is recommended. If a maternal RSV vaccine (Abrysvo) was given during pregnancy, an injection for the baby after birth will likely not be needed. If the vaccine was not given during pregnancy, nirsevimab (Beyfortus) is recommended for all infants younger than 8 months born during or entering their first RSV season. It may be available in the hospital, soon after baby is born, or it may be given during a clinic visit, depending on the season.

NEWBORN ISSUES

Some babies have a bit of trouble adjusting to their new world. Fortunately, most of the problems they experience in the first few hours and days after birth are generally minor and soon resolved.

Low blood sugar

During pregnancy, baby's blood sugar — called glucose — stays at a fairly even level as the placenta continuously provides nutrition. Glucose is the brain's main source of energy. After birth, your baby's body must quickly begin regulating the level of blood glucose on its own.

Some babies don't handle that transition well, and hypoglycemia may occur. Hypoglycemia is a condition in which a person's blood sugar is lower than normal. Too little blood sugar can impair brain function. Severe or prolonged hypoglycemia may result in seizures and serious brain injury.

Babies who are larger or smaller than average and those born to a birthing parent who had certain medical conditions such as diabetes are more likely to have low blood sugar. Some babies with low blood sugar have no symptoms, while others may be more sleepy or jittery than other newborns or won't feed well. Low body temperature and breathing problems are also common symptoms.

A newborn's blood sugar level may be measured within the first few hours after birth. If it's below typical levels, assistance may be given to encourage eating and improve the baby's blood sugar. Treatment may include rubbing a glucose gel inside baby's cheeks or giving glucose through an intravenous (IV) tube.

Breathing difficulties

The lungs are one of the last organs to fully develop during pregnancy. Most newborns have no difficulty breathing, but occasionally breathing problems can occur, especially if an infant is born prematurely.

Transient tachypnea Transient tachypnea of a newborn (TTNB) is a form of respiratory distress that can occur after an uneventful vaginal delivery or cesarean birth. It's due to fluid that remains in the lungs after delivery and is more likely after a rapid vaginal birth or a cesarean birth without labor. Infants with TTNB often have no signs of trouble other than rapid, shallow breathing, though some may have bluish or grayish skin.

Most infants recover within a couple of days. However, rapid breathing makes it more difficult to eat. If baby is breathing too fast to feed well via breast or bottle, they might be given milk via a feeding tube through the nose and into the stomach or via IV fluids. Some babies need extra oxygen through a tube in their nose. Once their breathing becomes more stable, babies with TTNB are more willing to nurse or take a bottle. It usually resolves by the third day of life.

Meconium aspiration Meconium is the first feces, or stool, of a newborn. Normally, meconium isn't passed until after an infant is born. In some cases, though, a baby will pass stool (meconium) while inside the uterus. Once meconium is in the surrounding amniotic fluid, the baby may inhale it. This is called meconium aspiration. The meconium can potentially cause inflammation of the baby's lungs. The infant may work hard to breathe and may have a bluish or grayish skin color.

When a baby is born with meconium in the amniotic fluid, the first step is to suction the mouth. Further treatment is needed only if the baby isn't active and crying immediately after delivery. A tube may be placed in the trachea to suction out the meconium. In more severe cases, a baby may need antibiotics to treat possible infection. Other assistance may be needed for their lungs or oxygen level. However, for most babies there are no long-term health effects.

Respiratory distress syndrome (RDS) Newborns with respiratory distress syndrome have rapid, difficult breathing and perhaps a bluish or grayish skin color (cyanosis). The breathing sound made by a baby with RDS, commonly referred to as "grunting," is often very distinctive. Breathing out may make a noise that sounds like a lamb or a soft cry. Babies with RDS also have to work harder to move air into their lungs.

RDS is caused by the lack of a slippery, protective substance called surfactant, which helps the lungs inflate with air and keeps air sacs from collapsing. RDS is most common in premature infants whose lungs haven't fully developed or produced surfactant. However, giving steroids to a pregnant person at risk for preterm delivery reduces the baby's risk.

Most infants who develop RDS show signs of breathing problems soon after birth. Blood tests and an X-ray of the lungs can help rule out other causes.

A child with RDS is usually cared for in a neonatal intensive care unit (NICU), where vital signs can be constantly monitored. An oxygen tube in the nose and continuous positive airway pressure (CPAP) or other types of breathing assistance may be used. Another option is to give surfactant directly into baby's lungs. Other medications may be given intravenously.

Jaundice

More than half of all newborn babies develop jaundice, which is a yellow tinge to the skin and eyes. Signs generally develop after the first 24 hours and peak about five to seven days after birth. The condition may last several weeks.

A baby develops jaundice when bilirubin, which is produced by the breakdown of red blood cells, accumulates faster than the liver can break it down and pass it from the body. Jaundice may occur for a few reasons:

- Bilirubin is produced more quickly than the liver can handle. This can occur with polycythemia, an uncommon blood disorder in which the bone marrow makes too many red blood cells.
- The baby's developing liver isn't able to remove bilirubin from the blood.
- Too much of the bilirubin is reabsorbed from the intestines before the baby gets rid of it in a bowel movement.

Jaundice treatment All newborns are screened for jaundice, either using a skin sensor or with a blood test. Mild jaundice generally doesn't require treatment, but more severe cases can require a newborn to stay longer in the hospital. Jaundice may be treated in several ways:

- You may be asked to feed the baby more frequently, which increases the amount of bilirubin passed out of the body via bowel movements.
- A healthcare professional may place your baby under a bilirubin light. This treatment, called phototherapy, is quite common. A special lamp helps rid the body of excess bilirubin.
- Rarely, if the bilirubin level becomes extremely high, intravenous (IV) fluids or other specialized treatment may be needed.

Eating problems

Whether you choose to breastfeed or bottle-feed, during the first few days after your baby's birth you may find it hard to interest your newborn in eating. The first feedings can sometimes be difficult. If this is the case, you're not alone. Remember, your baby is learning and so are you. See the next chapter for advice on how to reduce the stress and improve the success of early feedings.

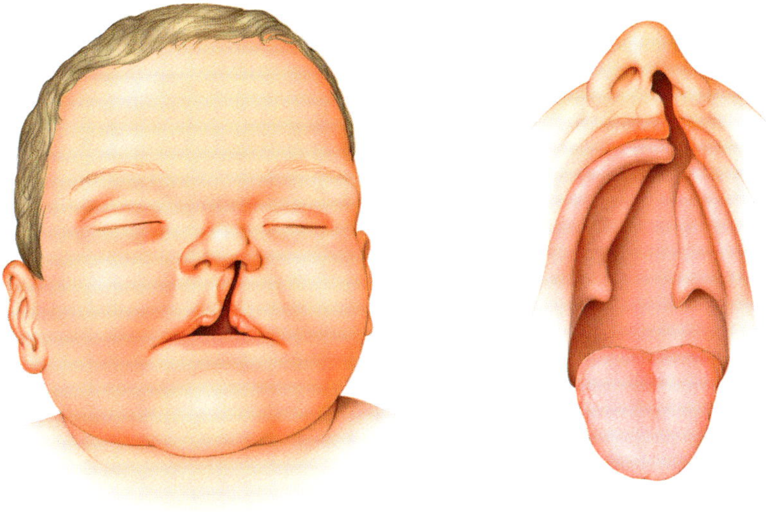

Cleft lip (left) and cleft palate (right)

If things aren't going well or if you're concerned that your baby isn't getting enough nourishment, talk to your baby's healthcare professional. Some babies are slow eaters the first few days, but soon they catch on and breastfeed or bottle-feed with enthusiasm.

Over the first week, a newborn may lose up to 10% of birth weight. But babies typically regain that weight by the end of their second week of life.

Cleft lip and cleft palate Some babies have difficulty feeding because their mouth or lip is formed differently. A cleft is an opening or split in the upper lip, the roof of the mouth (palate) or both. Cleft lip and cleft palate result when facial structures in a developing baby don't completely grow together. This can occur as part of a genetic syndrome or on its own, without other health problems. It is one of the most common birth defects. Screening for this is part of the newborn physical examination, though it may be noted during a prenatal ultrasound exam.

Cleft lip and palate are repaired with surgery. Cleft lip repair is usually done within the first 3 to 6 months of age. Cleft palate repair usually happens between 6 and 12 months. After the initial repair, follow-up surgeries may be recommended to improve speech or change the appearance of the lip and nose.

Meanwhile, medical staff will help you with strategies to feed your baby, such as a special bottle or feeder, if needed.

Infection

A newborn's immune system isn't adequately developed to fight infection. Therefore, any type of infection can be more serious for newborns than for older children or adults.

If things don't seem right — if your newborn seems too fussy or too sleepy — or if your newborn has a fever (a temperature of 100.4 F or higher), don't delay seeking care. This may mean going to the emergency department if the illness occurs in the middle of the night.

Serious bacterial infections, which are uncommon, can invade any organ or the blood, urinary tract or spinal fluid. Prompt treatment with antibiotics is necessary, but even with early diagnosis and treatment, infection in a newborn can be life-threatening.

For this reason, healthcare professionals are often quick to treat a possible or suspected infection. Antibiotics often are given early and stopped only when an infection doesn't seem likely. Although the majority of test results may come back showing no evidence of infection, it's better to err on the side of safety by quickly treating a baby than to risk not treating a baby with an infection soon enough. If the birthing person tested positive for group B streptococcus near the end of pregnancy or was diagnosed with an infection in labor, this may influence the decision to start the baby on antibiotics in the hospital.

Viral infections also can occur in newborns, and some can cause serious illness. Certain newborn viral infections, such as herpes, varicella, HIV and cytomegalovirus, may be treated with antiviral medication.

Hernias

It's not unusual for a baby to be born with a hernia. Hernias can occur either in the groin area (inguinal hernia) or near the bellybutton (umbilical hernia).

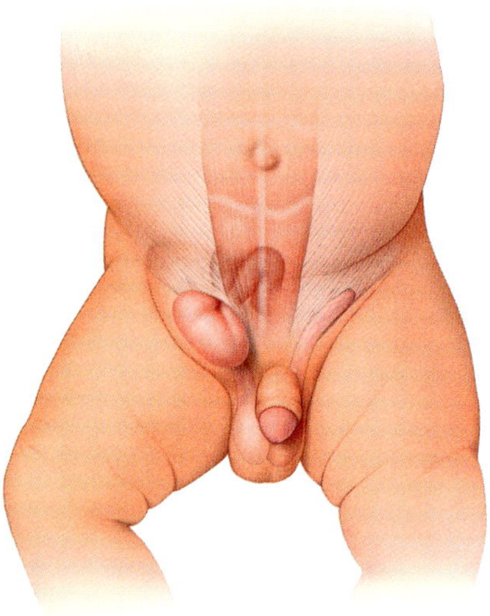

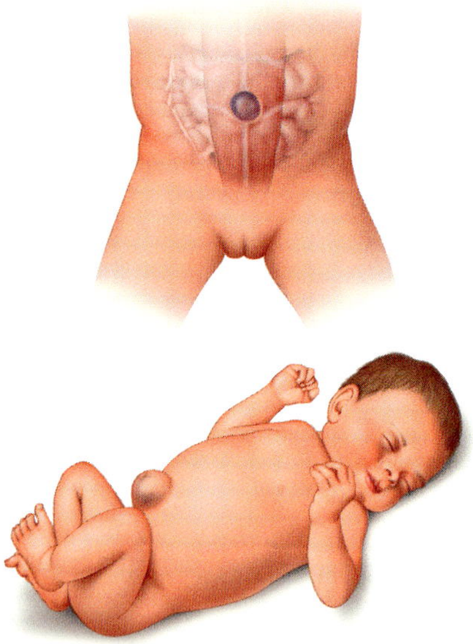

An inguinal hernia (left) results when a portion of the small intestine protrudes through the lower abdominal wall. With an umbilical hernia (right), the small intestine protrudes through an opening in the abdominal wall near the bellybutton.

Inguinal hernia An inguinal hernia is more common in boys than in girls. An inguinal hernia is caused by a weakness in the lower abdominal wall that allows the intestines to bulge outward. The hernia appears as a swelling in the lower abdomen or groin and is generally painless. Sometimes the hernia is visible only when an infant is crying, coughing or straining during a bowel movement.

An inguinal hernia may be small at first, but it tends to gradually enlarge, so an operation is eventually needed to repair the weak spot. An inguinal hernia can cause problems if tissues get stuck in the opening. It won't go away by itself.

Umbilical hernia An umbilical hernia occurs when there is an opening in the upper abdominal muscles near the bellybutton. Part of the intestine, or other abdominal tissues, may protrude. This can be especially evident when an infant cries, causing the baby's bellybutton to bulge.

Most umbilical hernias close on their own by the time a baby reaches 1 year old, though some take longer to go away. Umbilical hernias that don't disappear by age 4 or those that appear later in a person's life may require surgical repair to prevent complications.

Genital conditions

Some birth conditions affect the genitals. These are typically diagnosed on physical examination at birth.

Vaginal discharge Vaginal discharge often occurs in newborn girls. During the first three weeks, you may notice a thick white discharge or a tinge of blood from the baby's vagina. This usually resolves on its own. Vaginal bleeding (a "mini period") is sometimes a newborn girl's response to the falling level of the maternal hormone estrogen after birth.

Hydrocele A hydrocele forms when fluid collects in the thin sac that surrounds a testicle. This results in swelling of the scrotum, the loose bag of skin underneath the penis. Up to 10% of male infants have a hydrocele at birth.

Most hydroceles disappear without treatment within the first year. If a hydrocele doesn't disappear or if it continues to enlarge, it may need to be surgically removed. Sometimes, a hydrocele may recur.

Hypospadias In this condition the opening of the urethra is on the underside of the penis, instead of at the tip. The urethra is the tube through which urine drains from the bladder. In most cases, the opening of the urethra is near the head of the penis. Less often, the opening is at midshaft or at the base of the penis.

Surgery is typically done to reposition the urethral opening and, if necessary, straighten the shaft of the penis. With successful treatment, most boys will be able to stand while urinating and have normal sexual function as adults.

Undescended testicle Testicles form in the abdomen during fetal development and gradually descend into the bag of skin hanging beneath the penis (scrotum). Sometimes the process is stopped or delayed at some stage of development, and the testicle is not where you would expect it to be — it may still be in the abdomen. This is called an undescended testicle — also known as cryptorchidism. It is more common in babies born before 37 weeks.

In most cases, the testicle descends into the scrotum during the first few months on its own. Sometimes, hormones are given to bring the undescended testicle into place. If it hasn't descended by the child's first birthday, it is commonly treated with surgery.

Sometimes, the opening in the abdominal muscles left by an undescended testicle fails to close properly, allowing the intestines to push through (inguinal hernia). If this occurs, the hernia is repaired during the same surgery.

More often, testes descend as they should, but one doesn't remain in the scrotum. This is called a retractile testicle. It may reappear and disappear from the scrotum. It is more likely to appear in the scrotum in a warm bath — something you may be asked about if a testicle isn't felt during a medical exam. This condition usually resolves on its own before puberty.

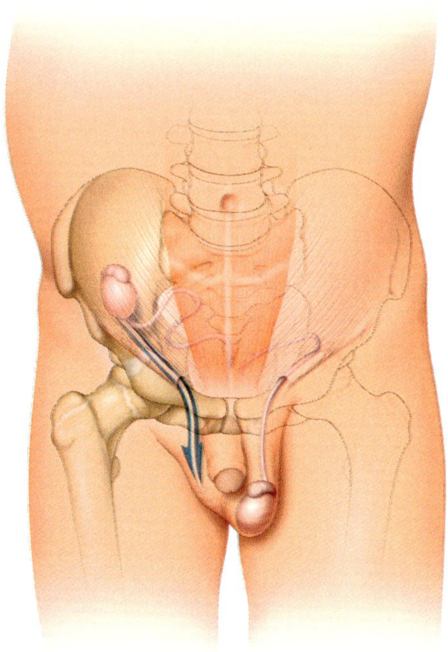

Undescended testicle

CIRCUMCISION

If you have a baby boy, one of the decisions you'll face soon after birth is whether to have him circumcised. Circumcision is an elective surgical procedure done to remove the skin covering the tip of the penis. Knowing about the procedure's potential benefits and risks can help you make an informed decision.

Issues to consider

Although circumcision is common in the United States, it's still somewhat controversial. According to the American Academy of Pediatrics, the medical benefits of circumcision outweigh the risks. However, the benefits may be low for most babies, so it is an elective procedure.

Consider your own cultural, religious and social values in making this decision. For some people, such as those of the Jewish or Islamic faith, circumcision is a religious ritual. For others, it's a matter of personal hygiene or preventive health. Some parents choose circumcision because they don't want their child to look different from family or peers.

As you decide what's best for you and your child, consider these potential health benefits and risks.

Benefits of circumcision Some research suggests that circumcision provides certain benefits. These include:

- *Decreased risk of urinary tract infections.* Although the risk of urinary tract infections in the first year is low in males, studies suggest that such infections may be up to 10 times more common in uncircumcised babies than in those who are circumcised. Uncircumcised babies also are more likely to be admitted to the hospital for a severe urinary tract infection during the first three months of life than are those who are circumcised.
- *Decreased risk of cancer of the penis.* While this type of cancer is very rare, circumcised people show a lower incidence of cancer of the penis than do uncircumcised people.
- *Decreased risk of some sexually transmitted infections.* Studies have shown a lower risk of human immunodeficiency virus (HIV), human papillomavirus (HPV) and herpes simplex virus (HSV) infections in circumcised people. However, safe sexual practices are much more important than circumcision in the prevention of sexually transmitted infections.
- *Prevention of penile problems.* Occasionally the foreskin on an uncircumcised penis may narrow to the point where it's difficult or impossible to retract (phimosis). A narrowed foreskin can also lead to inflammation of the head of the penis (balanitis). While circumcision can help prevent these issues, they can still occur from the remaining foreskin in some circumcised people.
- *Ease of hygiene.* Circumcision makes it easy to wash the penis. But even if the foreskin is intact, it's still quite simple to keep the penis clean. Normally

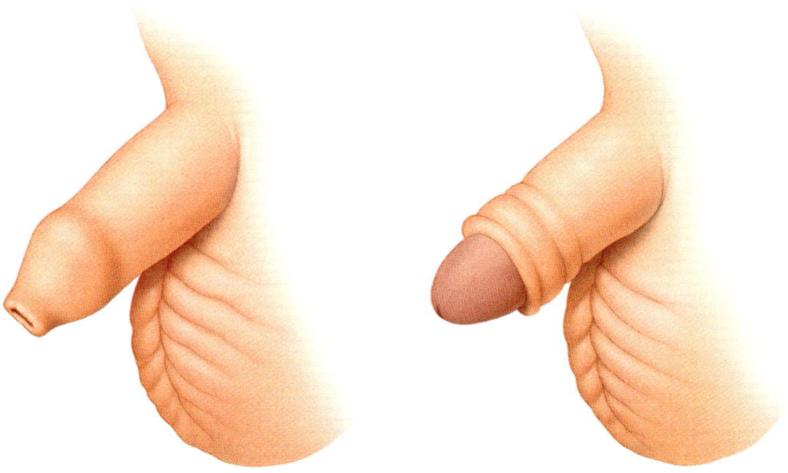

Before circumcision (left), the foreskin of the penis extends over the end of the penis (glans). After the brief operation, the glans is exposed (right).

the foreskin adheres to the end of the penis in a newborn, then gradually stretches back during early childhood.

Risks of circumcision Circumcision is generally considered a safe procedure, but there are some minor risks to consider:

- *Risks of minor surgery.* All surgical procedures, including circumcision, carry certain risks, such as excessive bleeding and infection. There's also the possibility that the foreskin may be cut too short or too long, or that it doesn't heal properly.
- *Pain during the procedure.* Circumcision does cause pain. Typically, a local anesthetic is used to block nerve sensations. Talk to your baby's healthcare professional about the anesthesia process.
- *Cost.* Some insurers don't cover the cost of circumcision. If you're considering circumcision, check whether your insurance company will cover it.
- *Complicating factors.* Sometimes circumcision may need to be postponed, such as if your baby is born prematurely, has severe jaundice or is feeding poorly. It also may not be feasible in certain situations, such as in the rare instance when baby's urethral opening is not at the tip of the penis (hypospadias; see page 39). Other conditions that may prevent circumcision include ambiguous genitalia or a family history of bleeding disorders. Circumcision doesn't affect fertility. There's no evidence to suggest that sexual function or satisfaction is negatively affected by circumcision. Whatever your choice, negative outcomes are rare.

How it's done

If you choose circumcision, your baby's healthcare professional can answer questions about the procedure and help you make arrangements at your hospital or clinic. Usually circumcision is done before you and your baby leave the hospital. At times it's done in an outpatient setting. The procedure itself takes about 10 minutes.

Typically, your baby lies on his back with his arms and legs restrained. After the penis and surrounding area are cleansed, a local anesthetic is injected into the base of the penis. A special clamp or plastic ring is attached to the penis, and the foreskin is cut away. An ointment, such as petroleum jelly, is applied. This protects the penis from adhering to the diaper.If your newborn is fussy as the anesthetic wears off, hold him gently — being careful to avoid putting pressure on the penis. It usually takes about 7 to 10 days for the penis to heal.

Circumcision care

The tip of your baby's penis may seem raw for the first week after the procedure. Or a yellowish mucus or crust may form around the area. This is a normal part of healing. A tiny amount of bleeding may occur in the first day or two.

Clean the diaper area gently, and apply a liberal amount of petroleum jelly to the end of the penis with each diaper change. This will keep the diaper from sticking while the penis heals. If there's a bandage, change it with each diapering. At some hospitals, a plastic ring is used to remove the foreskin. The ring will remain on the end of the penis until the edge of the circumcision has healed, usually within a week. The ring will drop off on its own. It's OK to wash the penis as it's healing. See page 117 for cleansing instructions.

Problems after a circumcision are rare, but call your baby's healthcare professional in the following situations:

- Your baby has trouble urinating 12 to 18 hours after the circumcision.
- Bleeding around the tip of the penis is persistent.
- The penis tip is significantly swollen.
- A foul-smelling discharge comes from the penis tip, or there are crusted sores that contain fluid.
- The ring is still in place two weeks after the circumcision.
- Your baby has a fever.

SCREENING TESTS

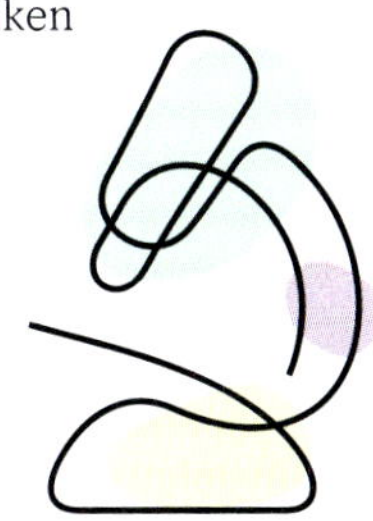

Before your baby leaves the hospital, a small amount of blood will be taken and sent to the state health department or a private laboratory working in collaboration with the state laboratory. This blood sample, which may be taken from a vein in your baby's arm or a tiny prick on the heel, is analyzed to detect the presence of rare but important genetic diseases. This testing is referred to as newborn screening. The purpose of the testing is to identify babies who might be at risk and enable families to access relevant treatment and resources. Results are generally available in one to two weeks.

The conditions that are screened for can have severe effects on health, including developmental delays and seizures, and can even be life-threatening. However, all can be managed when they are diagnosed early, allowing parents to help their child live a longer, healthier life.

Each state independently operates its newborn screening program, resulting in slight differences between the tests offered. Current national recommendations include a panel of tests to check for 35 core disorders and 26 secondary disorders. Some states check for additional conditions.

Occasionally a baby needs to have the test repeated. Don't be alarmed if this happens to your newborn. To ensure that every newborn with any of these conditions is identified, even borderline results are rechecked. Retesting is especially common for premature babies.

You also may request a specific genetic test if you feel your child may be at risk of a certain genetic disorder.

Newborn screening

Following are some of the diseases that can be detected by the screening.

Biotinidase deficiency This involves the lack of an enzyme called biotinidase. Signs and symptoms of the disorder include seizures, developmental delay, eczema and hearing loss. With early diagnosis and treatment, all signs and symptoms can be prevented.

Congenital adrenal hyperplasia (CAH) This group of disorders is caused by a deficiency of certain hormones. Signs and symptoms may include lethargy, vomiting, muscle weakness and dehydration. Infants with mild forms are at risk of reproductive and growth difficulties. Severe cases can cause kidney dysfunction and even death. Lifelong hormone treatment can suppress the condition.

Congenital hypothyroidism About 1 in 3,000 babies has a thyroid hormone deficiency that slows growth and brain development. Left untreated, it can result in intellectual disability and stunted growth. With early detection and treatment, healthy growth and development is expected.

Cystic fibrosis Cystic fibrosis causes the body to produce abnormally thickened mucous secretions in the lungs and digestive system. Signs and symptoms generally include salty-tasting skin, poor weight gain, and, eventually, persistent coughing and shortness of breath. Affected newborns can develop life-threatening lung infections and intestinal obstructions. With early detection and treatment, infants diagnosed with cystic fibrosis now often live longer and in better health than infants diagnosed in the past.

Galactosemia Babies born with galactosemia can't metabolize a sugar (galactose) found in breast milk and most baby formulas. Although newborns with this condition typically appear otherwise healthy, they may develop vomiting, diarrhea, jaundice and liver damage within a few weeks of their first milk feedings. Left untreated, the disorder may result in mental disabilities, blindness, growth failure and, in severe cases, death. Treatment includes avoiding all dairy products.

Homocystinuria Caused by an enzyme deficiency, homocystinuria can lead to eye problems, mental disabilities, skeletal abnormalities and abnormal blood clotting. With early detection and management — including a special diet and dietary supplements — growth and development should be typical.

Maple syrup urine disease (MSUD) This disorder affects the metabolism of amino acids. Newborns with this condition typically appear healthy, but by the first week of life they experience feeding difficulties, lethargy and poor growth. MSUD is treated with a special diet. Left untreated, this disorder can lead to coma or death.

Medium-chain acyl-CoA dehydrogenase (MCAD) deficiency This rare hereditary disease results from the lack of an enzyme required to convert fat to energy. Babies with MCAD deficiency develop serious vomiting, lethargy that can worsen into coma, seizures, liver failure and severely low blood sugar. With early detection and monitoring, the condition can be effectively managed.

Phenylketonuria (PKU) Babies with PKU retain excessive amounts of phenylalanine — an amino acid found in the protein of almost all foods. This disorder is treated with a special diet. Without treatment, PKU can cause mental and motor disabilities, poor growth rate, and seizures. But with early detection and treatment, growth and development should be typical.

Sickle cell disease This inherited disease prevents blood cells from circulating easily throughout the body. Infants with sickle cell disease experience slow growth rates and an increased susceptibility to infection. The disease can cause bouts of pain and damage to vital organs such as the lungs, kidneys and brain. With early treatment, the complications of sickle cell disease can be minimized.

Hearing screening

Your baby may have a hearing test while in the hospital. Although hearing tests are not done routinely at every hospital, newborn hearing screening is becoming widely available. The testing can detect possible hearing loss in the first days of a baby's life. If possible hearing loss is found, further tests may be done to confirm the results.

Two tests are used to screen a newborn's hearing. Both are quick (about 10 minutes) and painless and can be done while your baby sleeps. One test measures how the brain responds to sound. Clicks or tones are played through soft earphones into the baby's ears while electrodes taped on the baby's head measure the brain's response. Another test measures specific responses to sound waves that enter a baby's ear. As clicks or tones are played into a baby's ear, a probe placed inside the ear canal measures the response.

Critical congenital heart defect (CCHD) screening

Before leaving the hospital, your baby also likely will be screened for any heart defects. Ultrasounds can identify many heart defects during a pregnancy. However, some issues may be missed or cannot be detected until after a baby is born.

For this test, an oxygen sensor (pulse oximeter) is placed on your baby's hands or feet. The test is quick and does not cause discomfort to your baby. If the oxygen levels are low or different on the right and left sides, your baby's healthcare professional will most likely recommend additional testing.

CHAPTER 3

Feeding your baby

If it seems like all you do at first is feed your baby, you're right! Newborns don't eat a lot at once, but they eat often. And in those first few weeks with your new baby, much of your life will revolve around satisfying that hunger. Just when you think you have a moment to relax or perhaps fit in a shower, your little one will probably want to eat again.

At first, all these feedings may seem exhausting. For almost every new parent, early days with a newborn can be demanding and sometimes stressful. Both you and your baby are adapting to a new reality, and that typically takes time.

Throughout this adjustment, remember that feeding your newborn is about more than just nourishment. It's a time of cuddling and closeness that helps build the connection between you and your baby. You want to make every feeding a time to bond with your baby. Cherish this time before your baby doesn't need help eating. That time will come soon enough.

BREAST MILK OR FORMULA?

Some families know right from the start what they'll feed their babies — breast milk or formula — while others struggle.

Most child health organizations advocate breastfeeding, and "Breast is best" is a commonly used phrase. There's no doubt that breastfeeding is a wonderful way to nourish a newborn — breast milk provides numerous benefits. Mayo Clinic experts agree.

However, medical professionals also realize that people's life situations differ. Depending on your circumstances, certain factors may lead you to choose infant formula instead of breast milk. Or you may opt for a combination of both breast milk and formula. Exclusive breastfeeding simply does not work for some people.

If you worry that you're not being a good parent or you're not putting the needs of your child first if you don't breastfeed, don't. As the alternate saying goes, "fed is best." Your baby needs nutrients, love and a parent who is not overwhelmed with stress about feeding.

Feeding, regardless of how it's delivered — breast milk or formula, breast or bottle — promotes intimacy.

Know that both options can provide your child the nutrition needed to grow and thrive.

Questions to ask

If you haven't had your baby yet and you're debating between breast milk and formula, you might consider these questions:

- *What does your medical professional suggest?* Your medical professional likely will be very supportive of breastfeeding unless you have health issues — such as a certain disease or disease treatment — that make formula-feeding a better choice.
- *Do you understand both methods?* Many people have misconceptions about breastfeeding. Learn as much as you can about feeding your baby. Seek out expert advice if needed.
- *Do you plan to return to work?* If so, how will that impact breastfeeding? Does your place of work have accommodations available where you can use a breast pump, if that's your plan?
- *How does your partner feel about the decision?* Successful breastfeeding may require a lot of support from your partner, so it's smart to include your partner in the decision process.
- *How have other parents you trust and respect made their decisions?* If they had it to do over again, would they make the same choices?

BREASTFEEDING

Breastfeeding is highly encouraged by experts because it has many known health benefits for babies and nursing parents. The longer you breastfeed, the greater the chances that your baby will experience these benefits, and the more likely those benefits are to last.

Benefits for babies

Breast milk provides babies with:

- *Ideal nutrition.* Breast milk has just the right nutrients, in just the right amounts, to nourish your baby completely. It contains the fats, proteins, carbohydrates, vitamins and minerals that a baby needs for growth, digestion and brain development. Breast milk also is individualized; the composition of your breast milk changes as your baby grows.

- *Protection against disease.* Breast milk provides antibodies that help your baby's immune system fight off common childhood illnesses. Breastfed babies may have fewer colds, ear infections and urinary tract infections than do babies who aren't breastfed. Breastfed babies also may have fewer problems with asthma, food allergies and skin conditions such as eczema. They may be less likely to experience a reduction in the number of red blood cells (anemia). Research suggests that breastfeeding also might help to protect against sudden infant death syndrome (SIDS), and it may offer a slight reduction in the risk of childhood leukemia. Breast milk may even protect against disease in the long term. Studies suggest that adults who were breastfed as infants may have a lowered risk of heart attack and stroke, and may be less likely to develop diabetes.
- *Lower risk of obesity.* Research indicates that babies who are breastfed are less likely to experience obesity. Formula-fed infants generally have a higher calorie intake than do babies fed breast milk. And breast milk itself appears to have components that help control hunger and energy balance.
- *Easy digestion.* Breast milk is easier for babies to digest than is formula or cow's milk. Because breast milk doesn't remain in the stomach as long as formula does, breastfed babies spit up less. They have less gas and less constipation. They also have less diarrhea, as breast milk appears to kill some diarrhea-causing germs and helps a baby's digestive system grow and function.

Benefits for nursing parents

For birthing parents who breastfeed, the benefits include:

- *Faster recovery from childbirth.* The baby's suckling triggers your body to release oxytocin, a hormone that causes the uterus to contract. This means that the uterus returns to its pre-pregnancy size more quickly after delivery.
- *Suppressed ovulation.* Breastfeeding delays the return of ovulation and, therefore, menstruation. This may help extend the time between pregnancies. However, breastfeeding is not a guarantee against pregnancy. You can still become pregnant while breastfeeding.
- *Possible long-term health benefits.* Breastfeeding may reduce your risk of getting breast cancer before menopause. Breastfeeding also appears to provide some protection from uterine and ovarian cancers.
- *Convenience.* Many mothers find breastfeeding to be more convenient than bottle-feeding. It can be done anywhere, at any time, whenever your baby shows signs of hunger. Plus, no equipment is necessary. Breast milk is always available — and at the perfect temperature. Because you don't need to prepare a bottle and you can nurse lying down, nighttime feedings may be easier.
- *Cost savings.* Breastfeeding can save money because you don't need to buy formula, and you may not need bottles.

Challenges

Admittedly, breastfeeding also can present some challenges and inconveniences. Drawbacks to breastfeeding for nursing people include:

- *Exclusive feeding duties.* At first, newborns nurse every 2 to 3 hours, day and night. That can be tiring for you, and your partner may feel left out. But you also can express milk with a breast pump, if desired, which can let others take over some feedings.
- *Certain dietary restrictions, including alcohol.* If you're breastfeeding, the general rule is to avoid drinking alcohol before nursing. The alcohol level in breast milk is basically the same as in your bloodstream. One standard drink — such as 5 ounces of wine or 12 ounces of beer — takes 2 to 3 hours to leave the bloodstream (and therefore breast milk). If you do have a drink, the safest approach is to wait at least a couple of hours before breastfeeding. "Pumping and dumping" — pumping after drinking alcohol and discarding the breast milk — isn't necessary. The level of alcohol in your milk, as in your blood, goes down with time. See also "What goes in, comes out" below.
- *Sore nipples.* Some nursing people may experience sore nipples and, at times, breast infections. These may be avoided with the right positioning and technique. A lactation consultant or your medical professional can advise you on proper positioning.
- *Other physical side effects.* When you are lactating, your body's hormones may keep your vagina relatively dry. Using a water-based lubricating jelly can help treat this problem. It also may take time for your menstrual cycle to once again establish a regular pattern.

In addition, to help baby learn to breastfeed, you may want to avoid giving a pacifier, unless medically necessary, until breastfeeding is well established.

WHAT GOES IN, COMES OUT

While you're breastfeeding, keep in mind that the foods and other items you ingest can be passed on to your baby through your breast milk.

A few things to remember while breastfeeding:

- *Avoid or limit alcohol.* If you do have an occasional drink, keep it to a minimal amount and do it right after breastfeeding (see above).
- *Limit caffeine.* Drink mainly caffeine-free beverages.
- *Check your medications.* Most are safe to take, but consult your baby's medical professional first.

Only rarely do the foods you eat cause your baby to be fussy or gassy. Babies can get fussy for many reasons, and they can experience gas from the air they swallow when they cry or eat. However, if you suspect your child may be intolerant to something you ate, try eliminating the food for a while and see how your baby responds.

Milk production

During pregnancy, your milk-producing (mammary) glands prepare for nursing even before your baby is born. By about the sixth month of pregnancy, your breasts are ready to produce milk.

Your milk supply gradually increases between the third and fifth days after your baby's birth. As the milk-producing glands fill with milk, your breasts will be full and sometimes tender. They may also feel lumpy or hard (engorged).

Milk is released from the glands when your baby nurses. The milk is propelled down milk ducts, which are located just behind the dark circle of tissue that surrounds the nipple (areola). The sucking action of the baby compresses the areola, forcing milk out through tiny openings in the nipple. The baby's sucking stimulates nerve endings in the areola and nipple, sending a message to the brain to release the hormone oxytocin. Oxytocin acts on the milk-producing glands in the breasts, causing the ejection of milk to the nursing baby. This release is called the let-down reflex, which may be accompanied by a tingling sensation.

Although your baby's sucking is the main stimulus for the let-down reflex, other stimuli can have the same effect. For example, hearing a baby cry — or even thoughts of your baby or the sounds of rippling water — may set things in motion. The timing of this reflex can sometimes be inconvenient if you're not ready to breastfeed at the moment.

Regardless of whether your plan is to breastfeed, your body produces milk after childbirth. After that, your milk supply is based on demand. If you decide not to breastfeed, your milk production eventually stops. If you do breastfeed, the more frequently your breasts are emptied, the more milk they produce.

Getting started

The time to begin breastfeeding is right after your baby is born. If possible, put baby to your breast in the delivery room. Early skin-to-skin contact is known to improve breastfeeding outcomes.

Breastfeeding may be a natural process, but that doesn't mean it comes easily, especially the first time around. Nothing can really prepare your nipples for a nursing baby. If this is your first child, you may feel uncertain holding your baby — let alone putting baby to your breast. It may take a few attempts before you and your baby get the hang of it.

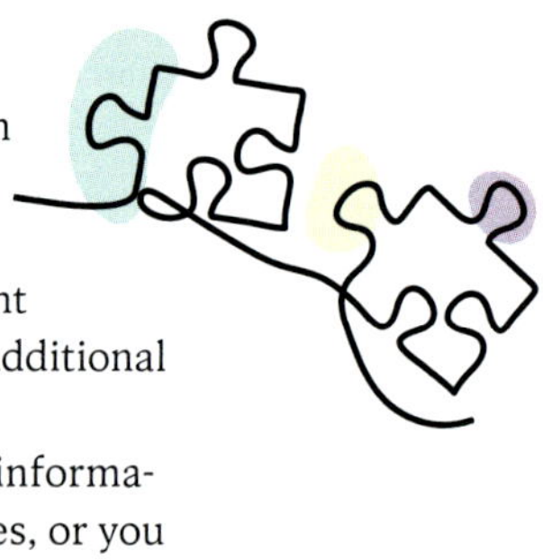

While you're in the hospital, ask a lactation consultant or nurse to assist you. These experts can provide hands-on instruction and helpful hints. After you leave the hospital or birthing center, you might want to arrange for a public health nurse who is knowledgeable about infant feeding or a certified lactation consultant to visit you for additional one-on-one instruction.

It's a good idea to take a class on breastfeeding. Often information on breastfeeding is offered as part of childbirth classes, or you may be able to sign up for a class. Most hospitals and birthing centers offer classes on feeding a newborn.

Supplies to have on hand

If possible, buy a couple of high-quality nursing bras. They provide important support for lactating breasts. What distinguishes nursing bras from regular bras is that both cups open to the front, usually with a simple maneuver that you can manage unobtrusively while you hold your baby.

You also may want nursing pads, which sit inside the bra to absorb milk that leaks from your breasts. Options include disposable pads or washable and reusable versions. Avoid those with plastic shields, which prevent air circulation around the nipples. Nursing pads can be worn continuously or on occasion. Some people don't bother with the pads, but many find them helpful, especially in the first few months.

Get comfortable

When it's feeding time, find a quiet location and take advantage of this time with your baby. Get into a position that's comfortable for both you and baby. If you're taking a seated position, it helps to sit up straight. Put a pillow behind the small of your back and one under your arms for support. A nursing pillow that wraps around your body also can make breastfeeding more comfortable by raising your baby to your breast.

Hold baby across your body. Position your baby's face to your breast, with your baby's mouth near your nipple. Make sure your baby's whole body is facing you — tummy to tummy — with ear, shoulder and hip in a straight line. Place your free hand up under your breast to support it while squeezing lightly to point the nipple straight forward.

Different people find different nursing positions most comfortable. Experiment with the positions on pages 52 and 53 to see which works best for you.

A good latch

When your baby connects or latches well to your breast, your baby can nurse effectively and your breast feels little discomfort. To help your baby get a good latch, hold your baby close and brush your nipple against your baby's cheek to trigger the rooting reflex — the motion your baby makes while searching for your nipple. If your baby is hungry and interested in nursing, their mouth should open, and your baby will turn toward your breast. When this happens, bring your baby's mouth to your nipple. You want your baby to receive as much nipple and areola as possible and your baby's lips to flare out, with chin and cheeks touching your breast.

As your baby starts suckling and your nipple is being stretched in your baby's mouth, you may feel some surging sensations. After a few suckles, those sensations should subside. If they don't, or if you have pain, sandwich the breast more and draw baby's head in more closely.

If it's still painful, gently remove baby from your breast, taking care to release the suction first. To break the suction, gently insert the tip of your finger into the corner of your baby's mouth. Slowly push your finger between your baby's gums until you feel the release. Repeat the latching-on procedure until your baby has latched on properly. You want there to be a firm bond of suction.

FEEDING POSITIONS

Cross-cradle hold

Bring your baby across the front of your body, tummy to tummy. Support your baby with the arm opposite the breast you're feeding with. Use that hand to support the back of baby's head as you position your baby to latch on. With your free hand, support your breast from the underside in a U-shaped hold to align with baby's mouth.

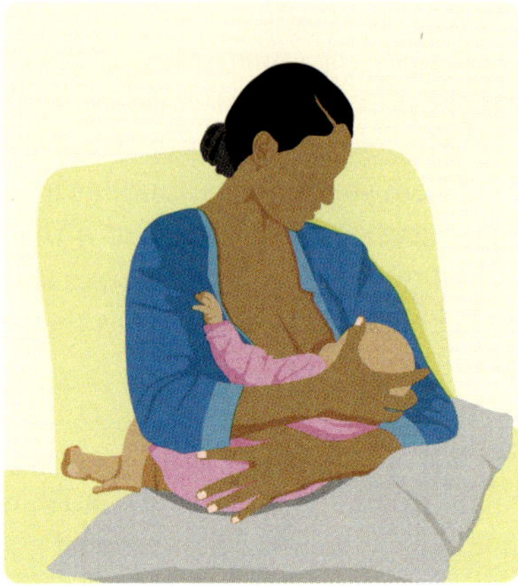

Cradle hold

Cradle your baby in your arm, with your baby's head resting comfortably in the crook of your elbow on the same side as the breast you're feeding with. Your forearm supports your baby's back. Use your free hand to support your breast.

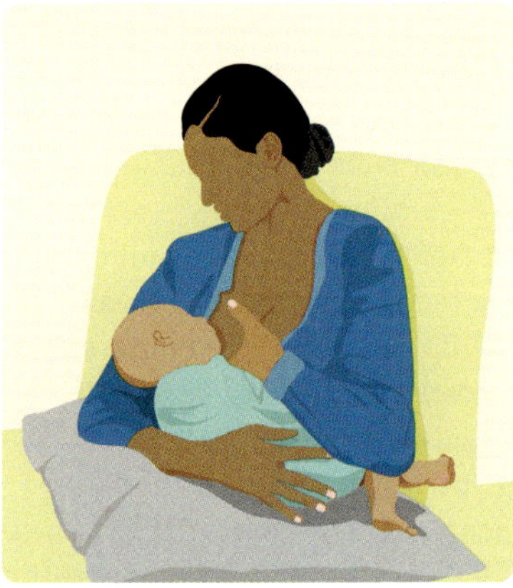

Laid-back nursing

For this position, sit where you can recline at about a 45-degree angle. Place baby's nose to the nipple and allow them to self-attach.

This position may help baby get a good latch, as gravity can help bring the chin and tongue forward a little bit more. It may also be a helpful option if you have an oversupply or a strong let-down.

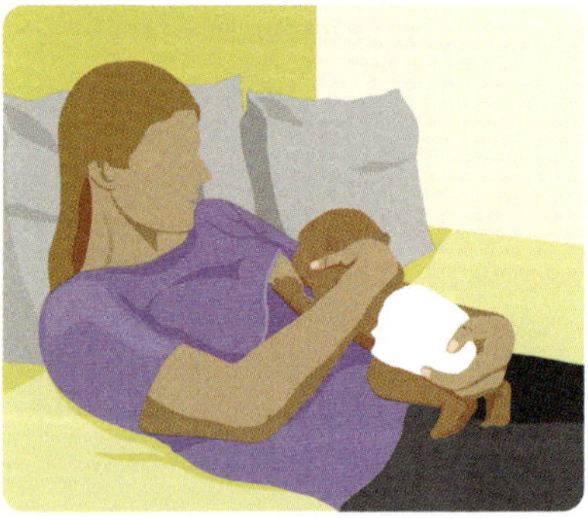

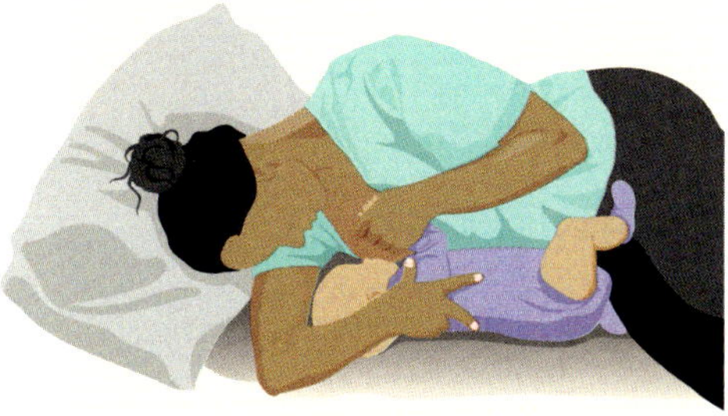

Side-lying hold

Although most people learn to breastfeed in a sitting position, at times you may prefer to nurse while lying down. Use the hand of your lower arm to help keep your baby's head positioned at your breast. With your upper arm and hand, reach across your body and grasp your breast, touching your nipple to your baby's lips. After your baby latches on firmly, you can use your lower arm to support your own head and your upper hand and arm to help support your baby.

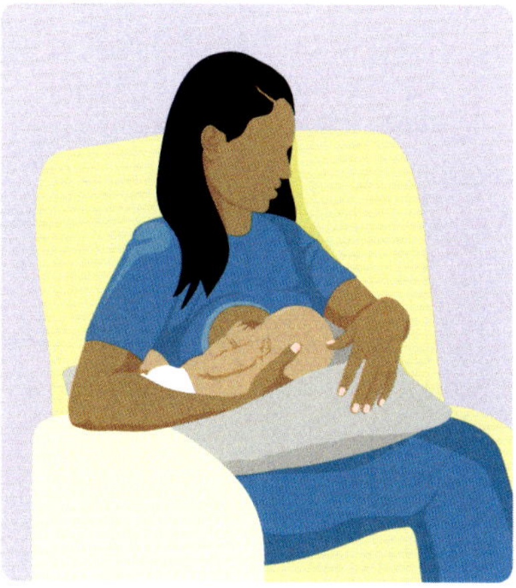

Football (clutch) hold

In this position, you hold your baby like a running back tucks a football under the arm. Hold your baby at your side on one arm, with your elbow bent and your open hand firmly supporting your baby's head face-up at the level of your breast. Your baby's torso will rest on your forearm. Put a pillow at your side to support your arm. A chair with broad, low arms works best.

With your free hand, support your breast from the underside in a C-shaped hold to align with baby's mouth. Because the baby isn't positioned near the abdomen, the football hold is popular among people recovering from C-sections. It's also a frequent choice of those who have large breasts or who are nursing premature or small babies.

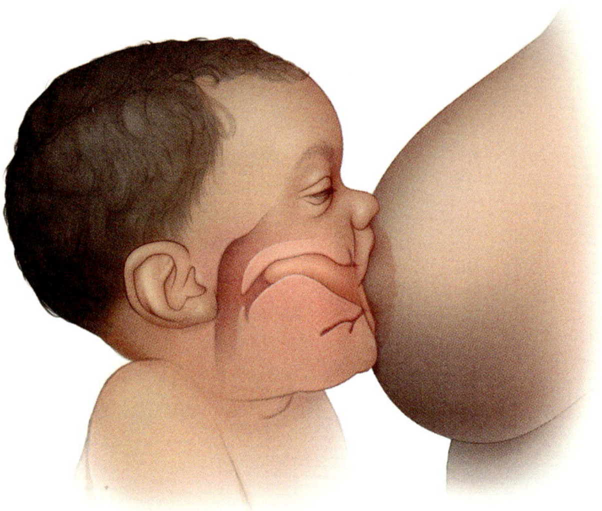

You know your baby has a good latch when you feel little discomfort in your breast, your baby's lips flare out, and your baby's chin and cheeks touch your breast.

You'll know that milk is flowing and your baby is swallowing if there's a strong, steady, rhythmic motion visible in your baby's cheeks. Also, listen for the "k" sound of your baby's swallowing. If your breast is blocking your baby's nose, elevate your baby slightly, or angle baby's head back and in to provide a little breathing room. If your baby attaches and sucks correctly — even if the arrangement feels awkward at first — the position is correct.

Once nursing begins, you can relax the supporting arm and pull your baby's lower body closer to you.

How often should you nurse?

Because breast milk is easily digested, breastfed babies usually are hungry every few hours at first. During those early days, breastfeeding may start to feel like a marathon session!

Most newborns eat 8 to 12 times a day — about every 2 to 3 hours. By 6 to 8 weeks after birth, your baby probably will begin to go longer between feedings. During growth spurts, your baby may take more at each feeding or want to feed more often. Trust your body's ability to keep up with the increased demand.

How long should a nursing session be?

In general, nurse as long as your baby wants. The length of feedings may vary considerably. However, on average, a nursing session may take about half an hour for most babies.

Offer your baby both breasts at each feeding. Allow your baby to end the feeding on the first side. Then, after burping your baby, offer the other side. See burping positions on page 72. Alternate starting sides to equalize the stimulation each breast receives.

You want baby to finish one breast before switching to the other side. This is because the milk that comes first from your breast, called the foremilk, is rich in lactose, a type of sugar, which satisfies baby's thirst. But the longer your baby sucks, the more he or she gets the hindmilk, which is rich in calories and fat, and therefore helps your baby gain weight and grow. So wait until your baby seems ready to quit before offering your other breast.

Is my baby getting enough?

A baby's need for frequent feeding usually isn't a sign that baby isn't getting enough; more likely it reflects the easy digestibility of breast milk. If your baby is satisfied after feeding and is growing, you can be confident that you're doing well.

If you're concerned that baby may not be getting enough milk, ask yourself:

- *Is baby gaining weight?* Steady weight gain is often the most reliable sign that a baby is getting enough to eat. Although most babies lose weight soon after birth, it's typically regained — and then some — within 10 days to two weeks. An average weight gain is about 1 ounce per day for the first three months, and then the rate will slow.
- *Can I hear baby swallowing?* Listen carefully and you'll be able to hear your baby swallowing. Also look for a strong, steady, rhythmic motion in your baby's lower jaw, or even a bit of milk dribbling out of your baby's mouth.
- *How do my breasts feel?* When your baby is latched on successfully, you'll feel a gentle pulling sensation on your breast, rather than a pinching or biting sensation on your nipple. Your breasts may feel firm or full before the feeding, and then softer or emptier afterward.
- *What about baby's diapers?* The number of wet diapers will increase daily in the first week of life, to an average of 6 to 8 per day by the end of the first week. Also expect regular bowel movements. The stool will be dark and sticky for the first couple of days, eventually becoming seedy, loose and golden yellow.
- *Does baby seem healthy?* A baby who seems satisfied after feedings and is alert and active at other times is likely getting enough milk.

Breast care

As you start to breastfeed, you may have some occasional problems. Though these can be uncomfortable, they often go away with time or can be easily treated.

Fullness A few days after your baby is born, your breasts may become full, firm and tender, making it challenging for your baby to grasp your nipple. This swelling, called engorgement, also causes congestion within your breasts, which makes your milk flow slower. So even if a latch is possible, your baby may be less than satisfied with the results.

To manage engorgement, express some milk by hand before trying to breastfeed. Support your breast with one hand. With your other hand, gently stroke your breast inward toward your areola. Then place your thumb and forefinger at the top and bottom of the breast just behind the areola. Gently compress the breast between your fingers, and milk should flow or squirt out of the nipple. Taking a warm shower also may result in let-down of milk and provide some relief from engorgement. You can use a breast pump to express some milk, too.

As you release your milk, you'll begin to feel your areola and nipple soften. Once enough milk is released, your baby can comfortably latch on and nurse. Frequent, lengthy nursing sessions are the best means to avoid engorgement.

Nurse your baby regularly and try not to miss a feeding. Wearing a nursing bra both day and night will help support engorged breasts and may make you feel more comfortable.

If your breasts are sore after nursing, apply a cold pack to reduce swelling. Some women find that a warm shower also relieves breast tenderness. Fortu-

VITAMIN D

Talk with your baby's medical professional about vitamin D supplements for your baby. Breast milk likely won't provide enough vitamin D, and infant formula may not, either. Your baby needs vitamin D to absorb calcium and phosphorus. Too little vitamin D can cause rickets, a softening and weakening of bones, as well as low calcium levels, which can cause additional health problems. Not getting enough vitamin D also increases the risk of respiratory infections.

Since sun exposure — an important source of vitamin D — isn't recommended for babies younger than 6 months, supplements are the best way to prevent vitamin D deficiency in infants.

The American Academy of Pediatrics recommends that babies who are breastfed or formula-fed receive 400 international units (IU) of liquid vitamin D a day, starting in the first few days after birth. Continue giving your baby vitamin D as long as you breastfeed. If you're using infant formula, continue giving vitamin D supplements until your baby drinks at least 32 ounces of formula a day.

As your baby gets older and begins to eat solid foods, you can help your baby meet the daily vitamin D requirement. Serve foods that contain vitamin D, such as eggs and fortified foods, although most babies won't consistently eat these foods during their first year. After age 12 months, you also can offer whole cow's milk.

When giving your baby liquid vitamin D, make sure you don't exceed the recommended amount. Carefully read the instructions that come with the supplement and use only the dropper that's provided.

nately, the period of engorgement is usually brief, lasting no more than a few days after delivery.

Nipple discomfort At first you may experience some nipple discomfort as baby latches on. But this discomfort should ease as your baby feeds. For some women, though, breastfeeding can be downright painful. If so, the first step is to check that your baby is latching on correctly.

Sore or cracked nipples are usually caused by incorrect positioning and latching. At each feeding, check that the baby has the areola in the mouth, rather than just the nipple. To avoid pulling at the nipple, make sure that your baby's head and body are in line with each other.

To care for your nipples, express milk onto your nipples and let them air-dry after each feeding. You don't need to wash your nipples after nursing. There are built-in lubricants around the areola that provide a natural salve. Soap and water with daily bathing is fine. Afterward, let your nipples air-dry.

Blocked milk ducts Sometimes milk ducts in the breast become clogged, causing milk to back up. Blocked ducts can be felt through the skin as small, tender lumps or larger areas of hardness. Because blocked ducts can lead to an infection, you should treat the problem right away.

The best way to open up blocked ducts is to let your baby empty the affected breast, offering that breast first at each feeding. If your baby doesn't empty the affected breast, express milk from it by hand or by breast pump. It also may help to apply a warm compress before nursing and to massage the affected breast. If the problem doesn't go away with self-treatment, call a lactation consultant or your medical professional for advice.

Breast infection Infection (mastitis) can occur if some milk remains in your breasts after feedings. Infection also may result when germs gain entry into your milk ducts from cracked nipples and from your baby's mouth. These germs are not harmful to your baby; everyone has them. They just don't belong in your breast tissue.

Mastitis starts with flu-like signs and symptoms such as a fever, chills and body aches. Swelling, tenderness and color change, such as redness or a dusky appearance, then follow. If you develop these symptoms, call your medical professional. You may need antibiotics, in addition to rest and more fluids.

Keep nursing if you're taking antibiotics. Treatment for mastitis doesn't harm your baby, and emptying your breasts during feedings will help to prevent clogged milk ducts, another possible source of mastitis. Applying cold compresses to your breasts after feedings can help soothe swelling. Your medical professional also may recommend taking an over-the-counter pain reliever.

Support

If you're having problems breastfeeding, or if you're worried that baby isn't getting enough milk, ask for help. If you sense something isn't right, or if breastfeeding seems too painful, don't be afraid to contact your baby's medical professional or a lactation consultant.

Many hospitals and clinics have lactation consultants on staff who can answer your questions or help you resolve any problems you may encounter.

Breastfeeding may feel awkward at first, but you'll get the hang of it. Friends who've breastfed may have valuable insights and provide needed support. You also might consider seeking out a lactation consultant in your area. Look for someone with an International Board Certified Lactation Consultant (IBCLC) credential or a Breastfeeding and Lactation Medicine physician specialist.

Weaning

There will come a time when it's best for baby and you to transition away from breastfeeding — weaning. Weaning can mean replacing breast milk with infant formula if your child is younger than 1 year, adding solid foods, or eliminating breast milk from their diet sometime after their first birthday or later.

You may have mixed emotions about weaning. But you can smooth the transition by taking a gradual approach and offering plenty of love and affection. Choose the right time and do what you can to make it a growing experience.

Timing You may wonder when's the best time to start weaning. There really isn't a right or wrong answer. Experts recommend exclusively breastfeeding babies for the first six months and continuing to breastfeed after starting solid foods as long as you and baby want to, till age 2 years or later. Breastfeeding beyond 1 year old may continue to have benefits for both you

GOING BACK TO WORK

With a little planning and preparation, you can do both — breastfeed and return to work. Some people work from home, while some arrange to have their baby brought to them for feedings or they go to the baby. Most, though, rely on the help of a breast pump.

Using a double breast pump is the most effective way to pump. A double breast pump requires about 15 minutes of pumping every three to four hours (plus time to clean and store supplies). If you need to increase your milk supply, nurse and pump more often.

Some people pump primarily at home. You might pump after the morning feeding and after the feeding when you return from work. As long as all of your milk produced in 24 hours is removed either by your baby or from pumping, you'll maintain a good supply.

Many people also pump while at work, storing the milk and saving it for the next day. If you're planning to pump at work, talk to your employer as early as possible. Ask about access to a clean, private space (not a bathroom) with a comfortable chair and an outlet. You'll also need a cooler bag, a refrigerator or freezer in which to store expressed milk and a place to rinse out pump parts. For the most part, employers are becoming more aware of the needs of working parents and are willing to work together to help new parents stay productive.

and baby. Breast milk contains the right balance of nutrients for your baby and boosts your baby's immune system. Still, when to start weaning your child is a personal decision.

It's often easiest to begin weaning when your baby initiates the process — which may be sooner or later than you expect. The process of weaning often begins naturally at 6 months old, when solid foods are typically introduced and feeding sessions start to become less frequent.

Some children begin to gradually turn away from breast milk and seek other forms of nutrition and comfort at around age 1, when they've begun eating a variety of solid foods and may be able to drink from a cup. Other children may not start weaning until their toddler years, when they become less willing to sit still during breastfeeding.

You also may decide when to start the weaning process yourself. This may be more difficult than following your child's lead — but can be done with some extra care and sensitivity.

Resist comparing your situation with that of other families. Also, consider rethinking any deadlines you may have set for weaning when you were pregnant or when your baby was a newborn.

You might consider delaying weaning if your child isn't feeling well or is teething. Children are more likely to handle the transition well if they're in good health.

You also might consider postponing weaning if a major life change has occurred, such as moving to a new home or starting a new job. You don't want to add more stress during a stressful time for you and your child if you can avoid it.

Some research suggests that exclusive breastfeeding for at least four months may have a protective effect for children with a family history of food allergies. If food allergies run in your family, talk to your child's healthcare professional about the potential benefits of delaying weaning.

Method When you start the weaning process, take it slow. Eliminate one breastfeeding session a day every 2 to 3 days. Slowly tapering off the number of times you breastfeed each day will cause your milk supply to gradually diminish and prevent discomfort from engorgement.

Children tend to be more attached to the first and last feedings of the day, when the need for comfort is greater — so it might be helpful to drop a midday breastfeeding session first. You also might choose to wean your baby from breast milk during the day but continue breastfeeding in the evening. It's up to you and your child. When eliminating a breastfeeding session, offer an alternative, such as a book, toy or other fun activity.

Depending on your approach, weaning could take days, weeks or months. Remember, however, that slower is often more successful. Rushing the weaning process may be upsetting for your child and cause engorgement for you.

Ongoing nutrition If you wean your child before age 1, substitute breast milk with iron-fortified formula. Ask your child's medical professional to recommend a formula. Don't give your child cow's milk until after age 1. You can provide formula to your child in a bottle or, if your child seems ready, in a cup.

If you're introducing your child to a bottle for the first time, do so at a time when your child isn't extremely hungry and may have more patience. It also may help if a separate caregiver introduces the bottle, since some children may refuse a bottle when the opportunity to breastfeed is nearby.

Choose a bottle nipple with a slow flow at first. If you use a bottle nipple with a fast flow, your child may become frustrated with the slower flow of milk during breastfeeding (or overwhelmed by the fast flow from the bottle).

PUMPING BREAST MILK

If you're returning to work or would like to share feeding duties with your partner, pumping breast milk is a useful option. It allows your baby to continue receiving your breast milk even when you're not there.

It may help to nurse exclusively during the first few weeks so that you and your baby learn how to breastfeed and so that your milk supply becomes well established. Once you feel confident that the two of you are doing well with

HOW LONG CAN YOU STORE BREAST MILK?

	Room temperature	**Insulated cooler with ice packs**	**Refrigerator (40 F)**	**Freezer (0 F or colder)**
Fresh	Best within 4 hours, especially in warm temperatures; acceptable up to 6 hours	Up to 24 hours	Best within 4 days; acceptable within 8 days if cleanly expressed and stored in back of refrigerator	Best within 9 months; acceptable within 12 months if stored in back of deep freezer
Thawed, previously frozen	1 to 2 hours	—	Up to 24 hours	Never refreeze
Left over from a feeding	Use within 2 hours after feeding			

Sources: Centers for Disease Control and Prevention, American Academy of Pediatrics

breastfeeding, you can introduce your baby to breast milk in a bottle. However, some women begin pumping soon after birth and do just fine.

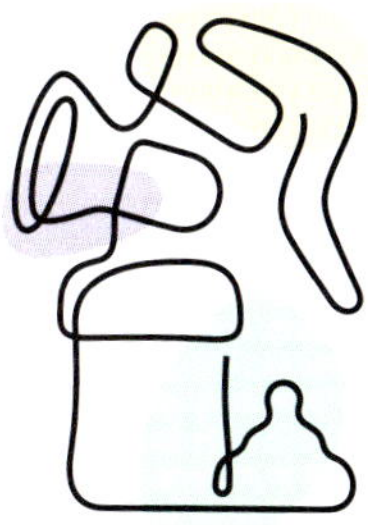

Initially, pump a few times after regular feedings to start building a small stockpile. Consider replacing one or two daytime feedings with a bottle of breast milk. Keep in mind that the feel of a bottle nipple in a baby's mouth is different from that of the breast. The way a baby sucks from a bottle nipple also differs. So it may take some practice to make the switch. It also may help to have someone besides you offer the bottle, since baby is likely to associate your voice and scent with breastfeeding.

Choosing a pump

Most mothers who breastfeed find using a breast pump easier than expressing milk manually. A lactation consultant or your baby's medical professional can help you determine what type of pump is best for you, and offer help and support if problems arise. In deciding on a pump, here are some factors to consider:

- *How often will you use the breast pump?* If you'll be away from the baby only occasionally and your milk supply is well established, a simple hand pump may be all you need. They're small and inexpensive. If you're returning to work full-time, or planning to be away from your baby for more than a few hours a day, you may want to invest in an electric pump.
- *Will you need to pump as quickly as possible?* A typical pumping session lasts about 15 minutes a breast. If you'll be pumping at work or in other time-crunched situations, you'll likely want an electric pump that allows you to pump both breasts at once. If you want to multitask, you may also want a hands-free pumping bra. Certain pumps or accessories can even fit inside a nursing bra for more discreet, faster pumping.
- *How much can you afford to spend?* While manual models generally cost less than $50, electric pumps that include a carrying case and an insulated section for storing milk often cost more than $200. Some hospitals and medical supply stores rent hospital-grade breast pumps. Health insurance plans generally cover the cost of breastfeeding support and supplies. Your insurer may specify what type of breast pump is covered.
- *Is the pump easy to assemble and transport?* If the breast pump is difficult to assemble, take apart or clean, it's bound to be frustrating. This may reduce your enthusiasm for pumping. If you'll be toting the pump to work every day, or traveling with the pump, look for a lightweight model. If you'll need to pump away from a power outlet, look for pumps that can run on batteries. Some breast pumps come in a carrying case with an insulated section for storing expressed milk. Additionally, some electric models are quieter than others. If it's important to be discreet, make sure the noise level is acceptable.
- *Is the suction adjustable?* What's comfortable for some women may not be for others. Choose a pump that allows you to control the degree of suction.

FEEDING TIPS

Over time your baby will gradually need fewer daily feedings and eat more at each feeding. Soon a feeding pattern will begin to emerge. In the meantime, whether you breastfeed or formula-feed, here are a few pointers to keep in mind.

Consider feedings a time to bond

For babies, feeding is as much a social activity as a nutritional one. Your baby's growth and development are based, in part, on the powerful bond that forms during feedings. Take the opportunity to put away your phone or tablet and turn off the television. Hold your baby close during each feeding. Maintain eye contact. Speak with a gentle voice. Don't miss this chance to build your baby's sense of security, trust and comfort.

Feed on cue

Your infant's stomach is very small, about the size of a baby's fist, and the time it takes to become empty varies from 1 to 3 hours. Feeding on cue requires you to watch for signs that baby is ready to eat: your baby makes sucking movements with their mouth or tongue, turns when their cheek is touched (rooting), sucks on their fist, or makes small sounds. Crying is a late cue for hunger. You soon will be able to distinguish between cries for food and those for other reasons, such as pain, fatigue or illness.

When your baby signals hunger, it's important to provide nourishment promptly. This helps your baby learn which kinds of discomfort mean hunger and that hunger can be satisfied by sucking, which brings food. If you don't respond promptly, your baby may become so upset that trying to feed may prove more frustrating than satisfying.

Let baby set the pace

Avoid rushing your baby during a feeding. Let your baby determine how much and how fast to eat. Many babies, like adults, prefer to eat in a relaxed manner. It's normal for an infant to suck, pause, rest, socialize a bit and then return to feeding. Some newborns are speedy, efficient eaters, consistently whizzing through feedings. Other babies are grazers, preferring snack-sized feedings at frequent intervals.

Babies will let you know when they've had enough to eat. A satisfied baby will stop sucking, close the mouth or turn away from the nipple. Your baby may push the nipple out of the mouth with the tongue or arch the back if you try to continue feeding. If, however, your baby needs burping or is in the middle of a bowel movement, your baby might be temporarily distracted. Wait a bit, and then try offering the breast or bottle again.

Feeding a sleepy newborn

Most newborns lose weight in the first few days after birth. Until your newborn regains this lost weight — usually within one week after birth — it's important to feed frequently, even if baby would rather drift off to sleep. You'll no doubt have times when your baby signals hunger, only to doze off once you begin feeding. Try these tips to feed a sleepy baby:

- Watch for and take advantage of your baby's alert stages. Feed at these times.
- If your baby falls asleep while feeding, gently wake baby and encourage eating.
- Give your baby a massage by walking your fingers up the spine.
- Partially undress your baby. Because your baby's skin is sensitive to temperature changes, the coolness may wake baby long enough to eat.
- Stroke a circle around your baby's lips with a fingertip a few times.
- Rock your baby in a sitting position. When a baby is positioned upright, the eyes often open.

Once your baby establishes a pattern of weight gain and reaches the original birth weight, it's generally OK to wait for feedings until baby wakes up.

Be flexible

Don't expect your baby to eat the same amount every day. Babies vary in how much they eat, especially if they're experiencing a growth spurt. At these times, your baby will need and demand more milk and eat more frequently. It may seem like your baby can't get full. During these times, you may need to put your baby to your breast or offer a bottle more often.

Babies often don't eat at precise intervals throughout the day. Most babies bunch (cluster) their feedings at various times of the day and night. It's common for a baby to eat several times within a few hours and then sleep for a few hours.

Stick with breast milk or formula

Don't give your newborn water, juice or other fluids. Introducing these liquids before your baby is 6 months old is unnecessary and can interfere with the desire for breast milk or formula. This may lead to malnourishment and risk potentially dangerous electrolyte imbalances.

Consider supplements

If you're providing iron-fortified formula, your baby is likely getting the recommended amount of iron. If you breastfeed or offer mixed feedings — breast milk and formula — talk to your baby's medical professional about whether to give baby an iron supplement. Your baby may also need a fluoride supplement, depending on your water supply, and a vitamin D supplement (see page 56).

Storing breast milk

Once you start pumping, it's important to know how to safely and properly store your expressed breast milk.

Container Store expressed breast milk in capped glass or plastic containers that have been cleaned in a dishwasher or washed in hot, soapy water and thoroughly rinsed. Consider boiling the containers after washing them if the quality of your water supply is questionable.

You also can use plastic bags designed for milk collection and storage. These can be a space-saving way to freeze milk. However, don't store breast milk in disposable bottle liners or plastic bags designed for general household use. They may spill, leak or become contaminated more easily than hard-sided containers or bags designed for breast milk storage.

Method You can store expressed breast milk in the refrigerator or freezer. Using waterproof labels and ink, label each container with the date and time. Include your baby's name if you're delivering containers to your baby's care provider. Place the containers in the back of the refrigerator or freezer, where the temperature is coldest. Use your earliest milk first.

To minimize waste, fill individual containers with the amount of milk your baby will need for one feeding. Also consider storing smaller portions — 1 to 2 ounces — for unexpected situations or delays in regular feedings. Keep in mind that breast milk expands as it freezes, so don't fill containers to the brim.

You can add freshly expressed breast milk to refrigerated or frozen milk you expressed earlier in the same day. However, cool the freshly expressed breast milk in the refrigerator or a cooler with ice packs for at least one hour before adding it to previously chilled milk. Don't add warm breast milk to frozen breast milk because it will cause the frozen milk to partially thaw. Keep milk expressed on different days in separate containers.

During storage, expressed breast milk will typically separate. The thick, white cream will rise to the top of the container. Before feeding your baby, gently swirl the contents of the container to ensure that the creamy portion of the milk is evenly distributed.

The sooner you use the milk, the better. Some research suggests that the longer you store breast milk — whether in the refrigerator or in the freezer — the greater the loss of vitamin C in the milk. Other studies have shown that refrigeration beyond two days may reduce the bacteria-killing properties of breast milk. Long-term freezer storage also may lower the quality of breast milk's fats (lipids).

Thawing Thaw the oldest milk first. Simply place the frozen container in the refrigerator the night before you plan to use it. Or place the container under warm running water or in a bowl of warm water. Avoid letting the water touch the mouth of the container.

Never thaw frozen breast milk on a counter at room temperature, which enables bacteria to multiply in the milk. Also, don't heat a frozen bottle on the stove or in the microwave. These methods can create an uneven distribution of heat and destroy the milk's antibodies. Use thawed breast milk within

24 hours. Discard any remaining milk. Don't refreeze thawed or partially thawed breast milk.

Thawed breast milk may smell or taste different from freshly expressed milk due to the breakdown of milk fats, but it's still safe for your baby to drink. The milk may separate, so you may need to gently swirl the thawed milk so that it's mixed evenly.

Donor milk

If you've adopted your baby or can't provide your own milk to breastfeed your baby, donor milk may be an option. This is breast milk that has been purchased from a reputable milk bank, ideally a member of the Human Milk Banking Association of North America. Lactating people who are pre-screened for infectious diseases, medications and healthy lifestyle choices provide their milk as a donation. This milk is then pasteurized, tested for bacteria, packaged and sold to private parties or hospitals.

Donor milk is an excellent and safe way to provide the benefits of breast milk in situations where it is otherwise unavailable. It can also be used with babies who are premature or have formula intolerance. It is typically very expensive, however.

Be aware that purchasing breast milk online or through milk-sharing communities is not recommended. These venues have little to no control over the milk collection process, packaging, mailing or screening for infectious diseases. Because of this, the milk may pose risks to your baby's health.

FORMULA-FEEDING

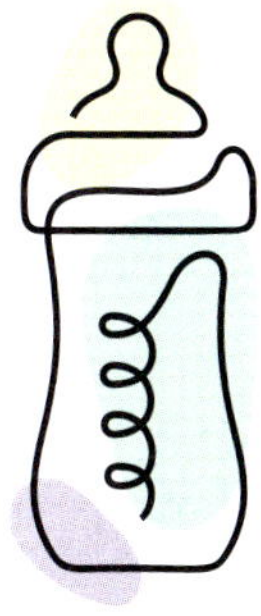

Some parents prefer to feed their infants formula rather than breast milk. This is a personal choice, and there are many reasons parents opt for formula rather than breast milk. In some cases, breastfeeding just isn't possible.

If you choose not to or you aren't able to breastfeed, know that your baby's nutritional needs can be met with the use of infant formula. And your baby still will be happily bonded with you as a parent.

Pros and cons

Parents who formula-feed usually feel the main advantages are:

- *Shared feeding duties.* Using a bottle with formula allows more than one person to feed the baby. For that reason, some nursing mothers feel they have more freedom when they're bottle-feeding. Both parents may like bottle-feeding because it allows them to share more easily in the feeding responsibilities.
- *Convenience.* Some parents feel formula is more portable, especially on outings and in public places. They don't have to find an out-of-the-way location to breastfeed.

Some of the challenges of formula-feeding include:

- *Time-consuming preparation.* Bottles must be prepared for each feeding. You need a steady supply of formula. Bottles and nipples need to be washed. If you go out, you may need to take formula with you.
- *Cost.* Formula is costly, which may be a concern for some parents.

The right supplies

Make sure you have the right supplies on hand. Staff at the hospital or birthing center can provide bottle-feeding equipment and formula the first few days after your baby's birth and show you how to bottle-feed your newborn.

You don't need a ton of equipment for formula-feeding. Generally, it's helpful to have several 4-ounce bottles for the early months, and several 8-ounce bottles as your baby grows and wants more at a time. Some extra nipples, rings and caps, and a bottle brush for cleaning also are nice to have on hand.

In addition to buying the right equipment, consider taking a class on infant feeding, if you haven't taken one already. Often information on feeding a newborn is offered as part of childbirth classes. If you've never bottle-fed a baby before, taking a class will help you feel more comfortable when you bring your baby home.

Bottles Bottles generally come in small and large sizes, ranging from 4 ounces to 8 or 9 ounces. The small bottles come in handy at the beginning when babies don't drink much more than that. The larger bottles should carry you through to weaning once your baby reaches a year old. Bottles may be glass, plastic or plastic with a soft plastic liner. Some bottles have a curved design to try to reduce the amount of air a baby swallows.

Nipples Many types of nipples are on the market. Openings are sized according to a baby's age (newborn, 3 months and so on), a flow rate (slow, medium, fast) or a number (0 to 3).

It's important that formula flows from the nipple at the correct speed. Milk flow that's either too fast or too slow can cause your baby to swallow too much air, leading to stomach discomfort and the need for frequent burping. Test the flow of the nipple by turning the bottle upside down and timing the drops. One drop a second is about right.

Choosing a formula

If you're planning to feed your baby infant formula, you may have many questions. Is one brand of infant formula better than another? Are generic brands OK? Is soy-based formula better than cow's milk formula?

A wide variety of infant formulas are on the market. The majority of them are based on cow's milk. However, never use regular cow's milk as a substitute for formula. In processing formula, the milk has been changed dramatically to make it safe for babies. This processing includes treating the milk by heat to make the protein in it more digestible. More milk sugar (lactose) is added to make the concentration similar to that of breast milk. The fat (butterfat) is removed and replaced with vegetable oils and animal fats that are more easily digested by infants.

Infant formulas aren't just easy to digest. They must contain the right amounts of carbohydrates, fat and protein to meet baby's needs. The Food and Drug Administration (FDA) monitors commercially prepared infant formula. Each manufacturer must test each batch of formula to ensure it has the required nutrients and is free of contaminants.

Infant formula is designed to be an energy-dense food. More than half its calories are from fat. That fat is made up of fatty acids specifically selected because they're similar to those found in breast milk. These fatty acids help in the development of your baby's brain and nervous system, as well as in meeting baby's energy needs.

Types Commercial infant formulas are regulated by the FDA. Three major types are available:

- *Cow's milk formulas.* Most infant formula is made with cow's milk that's been altered to resemble breast milk. This gives the formula the right balance of nutrients — and makes the formula easier to digest. Most babies do well on cow's milk formula. Some babies, however — such as those allergic to the proteins in cow's milk — need other types of infant formula.
- *Soy-based formulas.* Soy-based formulas can be useful if you want to exclude animal proteins from your child's diet. Soy-based formulas also may be an option for babies who are intolerant of or allergic to cow's milk formula or to lactose, a sugar naturally found in cow's milk. However, babies who are allergic to cow's milk also may be allergic to soy milk.
- *Protein hydrolysate formulas.* These are meant for babies who have a milk or soy allergy. Protein hydrolysate formulas are easier to digest and less likely to cause allergic reactions than other types of formula. They're also called hypoallergenic formulas.

In addition to these common types of formula, you can find specialized formulas that are made for premature infants and babies who have specific medical conditions.

Forms Infant formulas typically come in three forms. The best choice depends on your budget and convenience needs:

- *Powdered formula.* Powdered formula is the least expensive. It must be mixed with water.
- *Concentrated liquid formula.* This type of formula also is mixed with water.

LOOK BEFORE YOU BUY

Don't buy or use outdated infant formula. If the expiration date has passed, you can't be sure of the formula's quality.

While checking the expiration date, also inspect the condition of the formula container. Don't buy or use formula from containers with bulges, dents, leaks or rust spots. Formula in a damaged container may be unsafe.

- *Ready-to-use formula.* Ready-to-use formula is the most convenient type of infant formula. It doesn't need to be mixed with water. It's also the most expensive option, and creates the most waste.

Generic vs. brand-name All infant formulas sold in the United States — both generic and brand-name — must meet the nutrient standards set by the FDA. Although manufacturers may vary in their formula recipes, the FDA requires that all formulas contain the minimum recommended amount — and no more than the maximum amount — of nutrients that infants need.

Additional ingredients It's important to buy iron-fortified infant formula. Your baby needs iron to grow and develop, especially during infancy. Using iron-fortified formula, if you're not breastfeeding, is the easiest way to provide this essential nutrient.

Some infant formulas are enhanced with docosahexaenoic acid (DHA) and arachidonic acid (ARA). These are essential fatty acids found in breast milk and certain foods such as fish and eggs. Some studies suggest that including DHA and ARA in infant formula can help infant eyesight and brain development, but other research has shown no benefit.

In addition, in an effort to mimic the immune benefits of breast milk, some infant formulas now include probiotics. These are substances that promote the presence of healthy bacteria in the intestines. The data on probiotic-supplemented formulas is limited and the long-term benefits or complications of these formulas are unknown.

At this point, there's insufficient evidence to recommend the use of enhanced formulas. In addition, they tend to be more expensive than regular formula. If you think your child might benefit from formula supplemented with probiotics or another substance, talk to your baby's medical professional for additional information and guidance.

Preparation

Whatever type and form of formula you choose, proper preparation and storage are essential. This ensures the appropriate amount of nutrition and safeguards your baby's health.

Wash hands and supplies Wash your hands before handling formula or the equipment used to prepare it. All equipment that you use to measure, mix and store formula should be washed with hot, soapy water and then rinsed and dried before every use. Sterilize new bottles, nipples, caps and rings before using them for the first time. Boil the utensils in water for five minutes. Use a pot that's large enough to hold the utensils and cover them completely with water. Remove the utensils from the water using a clean set of tongs. Allow the utensils to air-dry.

After the first use, there's no need to sterilize your utensils as long as you wash and rinse them well. Use a bottle brush to wash bottles. Brush or rub the nipples thoroughly to remove any traces of formula. Rinse well. You also can clean bottles and nipples in the dishwasher.

To help prevent fungal growth, you can rinse nipples daily in equal parts vinegar and water and allow them to air-dry. Also make sure the nipples are open. Hold each nipple upside down and fill it with water, then look for the water to drip slowly out of the nipple.

Mix it up To prepare a bottle of formula, follow carefully the instructions on the label. For ready-to-use formula, shake the container and pour the recommended amount into the bottle. When using powder formula or liquid concentrate, always add the exact amount of water specified on the label. Measurements on bottles may be inaccurate, so pre-measure the water before adding it to the formula. Using too much or too little water isn't good for your baby. If formula is too diluted, your baby won't get enough nutrition to meet growth needs and to satisfy hunger. Formula that's too concentrated strains the baby's digestive system and kidneys, and could dehydrate your baby.

You can use any type of safe, drinkable water — tap or bottled — to prepare liquid concentrate or powdered formula. If you're concerned about the safety of

MILK ALLERGY

A person of any age can have a milk allergy, but it's more common among infants. A milk allergy occurs when the body's immune system mistakenly identifies the protein in milk as something the body should fight off. Some infants have a severe reaction to milk, such as hives, vomiting or trouble breathing, within minutes of or up to two hours after eating milk products. These types of reactions can be life-threatening and should prompt immediate medical attention.

More commonly, babies may have milk protein intolerance. This differs from an allergic reaction but can still cause problems such as bloody stools, diarrhea and possibly reflux. Avoiding milk and milk-based foods — including in your diet if you're breastfeeding — is usually enough to resolve symptoms. Fortunately, most children outgrow milk protein intolerance by age 1 and milk allergy by age 3.

Cow's milk is the usual cause of milk allergy; however, milk from sheep, goats and camels also can cause a reaction. And some children who are allergic to cow's milk are allergic to soy milk, too.

Because most formula is derived from cow's milk, infants who are formula-fed may have a higher risk of developing a milk allergy than those who are breastfed. However, the milk protein in dairy products that triggers the allergic reaction can cross into breast milk and may bother a breastfeeding baby. Researchers don't fully understand why some infants develop a milk allergy and others don't.

If you use formula and your baby has a milk allergy, your baby's medical professional may recommend switching to another type of formula that's less likely to cause an allergic reaction. If you're breastfeeding, restrict the amount of dairy products you eat and drink.

your tap water, bring filtered cold tap water to a rolling boil for one minute only. Then cool the water to room temperature for no more than 30 minutes before using it.

Warm, if needed While warming the formula is not necessary, your baby may prefer warm formula. To safely warm formula:

- Place a filled bottle in a bowl or pan of hot, but not boiling, water and let it stand for a few minutes. Or warm the bottle under running water. You also can use a bottle warmer.
- Shake the bottle after warming it.
- Turn the bottle upside down and allow a drop or two of formula to fall on your wrist or the back of your hand. The formula should feel lukewarm — not hot.
- Don't warm bottles in the microwave. The formula may heat unevenly, creating hot spots that could burn your baby's mouth.

Store safely Store unopened formula containers in a cool, dry place. Don't store formula containers outdoors or in a car or garage, where temperature extremes can affect the quality of the formula.

For ready-to-use formula, cover and refrigerate any leftover formula from a freshly opened container. If you prepare and fill several bottles of liquid concentrate or powdered formula at once:

- Label each bottle with the date that the formula was prepared.
- Refrigerate the extra bottles until you need them — don't freeze them.
- Put the bottles toward the back of the refrigerator, where it's coldest.
- Discard any prepared formula that's been in the refrigerator more than 24 to 48 hours.

Discard any formula that remains in the bottle after a feeding. If you're unsure whether a particular container or bottle of formula is safe, throw it out.

Getting into position

The first step to bottle-feeding is to get comfortable. Find a quiet place where you and your baby can relax and not be distracted.

Cradle your baby in one arm, hold the bottle with the other and settle into a comfortable chair, preferably one with broad, low armrests. You may want to put a pillow on your lap under the baby for support. Pull your baby in toward you snugly but not too tightly, cradled in your arm. Raise your baby's head slightly and rest it in the bend of your elbow. This semi-upright position makes swallowing easier.

Using the bottle nipple or a finger of your hand holding the bottle, gently stroke your baby's cheek near the mouth, on the side nearest you. The touch will cause your baby to turn toward you, often with an open mouth. Then touch the nipple to your baby's lips or the corner of the mouth. Your baby will gradually begin sucking.

When feeding your baby, position the bottle at about a 45-degree angle. This angle keeps the nipple full of milk. Hold the bottle steady as your baby feeds. If your baby falls asleep while bottle-feeding, it may be because your baby has had enough milk, or gas has made your baby full. Take the bottle away, burp your baby (see page 72), then try feeding again.

Always hold your baby while feeding. Never prop a bottle up against your infant. Propping may cause your baby to vomit and may lead to overeating. In addition, never give a bottle when your baby is lying down. This may increase your baby's risk of developing an ear infection.

Although your baby doesn't have teeth yet, they're forming beneath the gums. Avoid making a habit of putting your baby to bed with a bottle. Formula lingers in the mouth of a baby who falls asleep while sucking a bottle. Prolonged contact with the sugars in milk can cause tooth decay.

What's the right amount?

During the first few weeks, your baby will likely drink about 1 to 3 ounces at each feeding. You'll know that your young one is getting enough formula if by the end of the first week there are 6 to 8 wet diapers a day. Your baby also may have one or two bowel movements a day.

Over time, the amount of formula your baby consumes will gradually increase. In general, during the first month, expect 6 to 12 feedings in a 24-hour period — about every 2 to 4 hours. By 6 months, your baby will probably consume 6 to 8 ounces at each of four or five feedings a day.

Transitioning from formula

Infant formula is generally recommended until age 1, followed by whole milk until age 2 — but talk with your child's medical professional for specific guidance. Toddler formulas are often advertised but are not recommended. Reduced-fat or skim milk generally isn't appropriate before age 2 because it doesn't have enough calories or fat to promote early development. Experts recommend weaning your baby from a bottle to a cup by no later than 18 months.

SPITTING UP

Spitting up is a rite of passage for many babies. Although it's messy, you probably don't need to worry. Spitting up rarely signifies a serious problem. As long as your baby seems comfortable and is gaining weight, there's generally little cause for concern. If you keep a burp cloth within reach at all times, you'll be well prepared.

Reflux

Normally a valve between the esophagus and the stomach (lower esophageal sphincter) keeps stomach contents where they belong. Until this valve has time to mature, spitting up may be an issue — especially if your baby eats too much or too quickly. Spitting up tends to peak at age 4 months, and most babies stop spitting up by 12 months.

Minimal spitting up doesn't hurt. It isn't likely to cause coughing, choking or discomfort — even during sleep. Chances are your baby won't even notice the fluid dripping out of the mouth.

BURPING POSITIONS

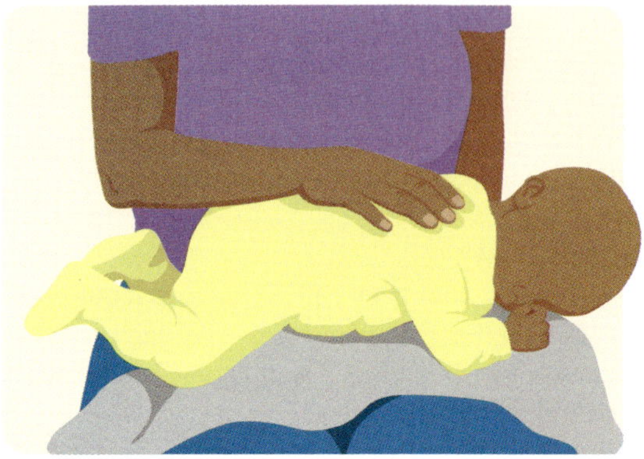

Lay baby facedown across your lap, and gently rub and pat baby's back.

While sitting baby upright and supporting the chin and back, gently rub and pat baby's back.

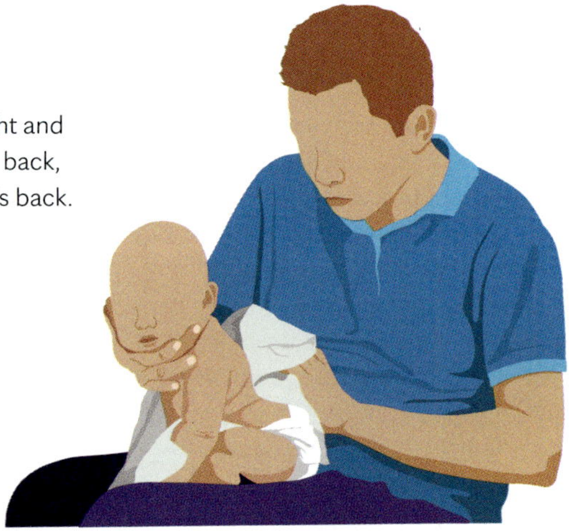

Lay baby facedown across your shoulder, and gently rub and pat baby's back.

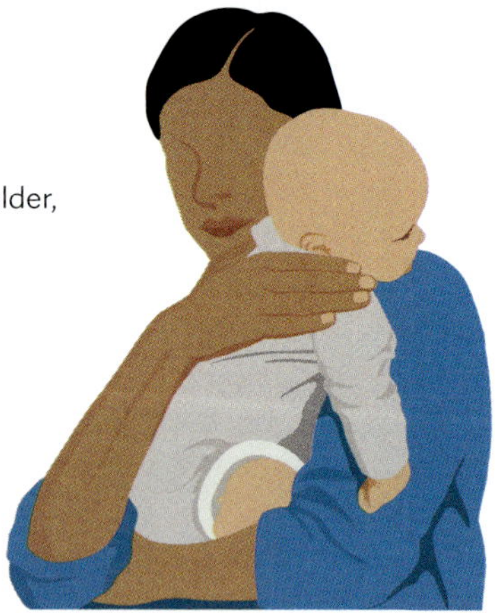

What you can do

To reduce spitting up, consider these tips:

- *Keep your baby upright.* Position baby's head higher than the rest of the body when feeding. Follow each feeding with 15 to 30 minutes in a sitting position. Hold your baby in your arms, or try a front pack, backpack or infant seat. Avoid active play and infant swings while the food is settling.
- *Try smaller, more frequent feedings.* Feeding your baby too much at once can contribute to spitting up. If you're breastfeeding, limit the length of each nursing session. If you're bottle-feeding, offer your baby slightly less than usual.
- *Take time to burp your baby.* Frequent burps during and after each feeding can keep air from building up in your baby's stomach. Sit your baby upright and support your baby's head with one hand while patting the back with your other hand (see opposite page). Babies don't burp after every feeding, though, so you don't need to prolong the burping process.
- *Check the nipple.* If you're using a bottle, make sure the hole in the nipple is the right size. If it's too large, the milk will flow too fast. If it's too small, your baby might get frustrated and gulp air (see page 66).
- *Experiment with your diet.* If you're breastfeeding, your baby's healthcare professional might suggest that you eliminate dairy products or certain other foods from your diet.
- *Pay attention to baby's sleep position.* To reduce the risk of sudden infant death syndrome (SIDS), place your baby to sleep on the back. Placing a baby to sleep on the tummy is rarely recommended to prevent spitting up.

When it's more serious

More severe spitting up may indicate something more serious. Contact your baby's medical professional if your baby:

- Isn't gaining weight
- Spits up so forcefully that stomach contents shoot out of the mouth (vomits)
- Spits up green or yellow fluid, blood, or a material that looks like coffee grounds
- Resists feedings
- Has blood in the stool
- Has other signs of illness, such as fever, diarrhea or difficulty breathing

Some babies experience infant gastroesophageal reflux (see page 449). Special feeding techniques or medication may be helpful.

CHAPTER 4

Solid foods and toddler feeding

When your child is first born, breast milk or formula is the only food that's needed. Eventually, though, your baby will begin to develop the coordination to move solid food from the front of the mouth to the back for swallowing. At the same time, your baby's head control will improve, and your baby will learn to sit with limited support. These are essential skills for eating solid foods.

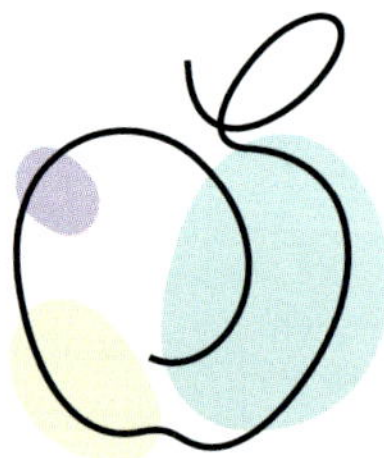

As you expand your child's diet to meet important nutritional needs, you'll also have an early opportunity to encourage healthy eating habits. By setting up a regular schedule for meals and snacks, you'll create a predictable and comfortable routine that your child can rely on. By making family meals a priority, even when your child is young, you'll encourage social skills and togetherness. What's more, you'll be able to model expected mealtime behaviors. You can make the most of these regular family gatherings by keeping mealtimes relaxed and turning off cellphones, televisions and other devices during meals.

These early habits will help your child develop a lifetime appreciation for eating a variety of healthy foods in a safe and comforting setting.

STARTING SOLIDS

So when are babies ready for solid foods? It varies a bit, based on a child's development. Signs that babies might be ready include being able to sit in a high chair or booster chair, hold their heads upright, show an interest in food and open their mouths for a spoon.

The American Academy of Pediatrics (AAP) recommends waiting until a child is at least 4 months old before introducing solid foods to complement breast milk or formula, and preferably holding off until a child is closer to 6 months old. If you have questions about starting solid foods, check with your child's healthcare professional.

First foods

Single-grain baby cereal has traditionally been used as a first food in the United States, and is fortified with iron and vitamins. But there's no one "right" first food. Pureed meats also are a good choice, as they are rich in iron and zinc. These essential nutrients are present at birth but their levels decrease steadily over the first few months (see "The importance of iron" on page 79).

You also can start with pureed vegetables and fruits. Pureed beans and leafy dark green vegetables contain iron, and the vitamin C in many fruits and

BABY-LED FEEDING

One approach to introducing foods to babies is allowing those who are 6 months or older to feed themselves solid foods, to encourage exploration of food and to let them regulate how much food they eat. This approach, called baby-led weaning or feeding, also frees up parents to eat while their child eats, making meals more social. The key part is letting babies guide the food into their own mouths. Several studies suggest that this method may decrease food fussiness while increasing a healthy enjoyment of and openness toward food. There appears to be no difference in weight between self-fed babies and spoon-fed babies. If following this feeding method, take care to offer solid foods of an appropriate texture and size to avoid the risk of choking, and monitor your baby during feeding times. If you'd like to try this approach, consider discussing it with your child's healthcare professional.

The main concern with babies feeding themselves is the risk of choking. But evidence suggests that self-feeding is as safe as being spoon-fed, as long as appropriate precautions are taken.

- To prevent choking while eating, make sure your child is seated in an upright position and is always supervised. Don't leave your baby unattended.
- Offer foods that are easy to pick up and are either mashable in your baby's mouth or easy to gnaw on without breaking up into small pieces that block your child's airway. Think steamed carrots, roasted sweet potato, strips of banana or pear, or other soft fruits cut into pieces about the length of an adult's pinky finger. Avoid coin-shaped pieces. You can also offer cooked ground meat shaped in a similar size and length.
- Avoid foods that are small, coin-shaped, slippery, crunchy, sticky or tough.

vegetables helps iron absorption. Formula or breast milk can be mixed in to thin the puree, if needed. But avoid seasoning your infant's food with added salt or sugar.

Research suggests that infants may be particularly receptive to pureed fruits and vegetables and flavorful foods between the ages of 4 and 9 months, with lasting benefits. Studies show that babies who are introduced to these foods during this window of time are more likely to eat vegetables and fruits later in childhood.

Getting started

Use a small spoon — one that will fit into your baby's mouth — and begin with very small amounts of food. At first your little one may frown, sputter and spit the food out. This isn't necessarily because your baby doesn't like the food. It could be because your baby is not yet familiar with moving the tongue backward. Wait for baby's mouth to open for the spoon — don't force food in. If your baby repeatedly pushes the spoon away with the tongue, uses the tongue to push food out of the mouth, or refuses to open the mouth, this may be a sign that your baby isn't ready for solids yet.

Don't be surprised if your baby puts fingers to mouth to help swallow the food. Your baby also may try to bat away the spoon or hold on to it. Expect it to be a messy experience! To prevent your baby from getting frustrated when very hungry, try feeding with breast milk or formula first and then taking a break for spoonfuls of food. Some parents skip pureed food entirely and let baby lead the learning process by self-feeding appropriate finger foods offered by the parent (see page 75).

Whether starting with purees or appropriate solids, gagging is a normal part of learning to eat. Gagging is distinct from choking. It's a sign that your baby is learning to direct food in the right direction while also reflexively protecting the airway. As long as your baby is able to breathe normally and the gagging stops on its own, stay calm, slow down, and keep feeding if your baby is willing to keep eating.

After getting used to solids, your baby may be ready for a few tablespoons of food a day, including finger foods. By the end of the first year, most children obtain about half of their nutrition from breast milk or formula and half from complementary foods.

Taste and texture

Babies also react to how food feels and tastes in their mouths. While you don't have to follow a particular sequence of food groups, it may help to introduce different tastes and textures gradually. Offer single-ingredient foods at first, and wait three to five days before introducing another new food. If your baby has a reaction to a particular food — such as diarrhea, a rash or vomiting — you'll know the culprit. Spacing out new foods also gives your child a chance to get used to a new taste and texture. It often takes quite a few tries (up to 15 or more!) for a new food to gain acceptance. Don't give up if your baby doesn't like a new food the first few times. Repeated tries can work wonders. In one study, infants who initially rejected a vegetable came to eat it as eagerly as a favored vegetable after being exposed to the rejected food on an average of eight different occasions.

Pureed foods Foods that are soft and runny may be easier for your baby to manage at first. One option is to mix 1 tablespoon of a single-grain, iron-fortified baby cereal with 4 to 5 tablespoons of breast milk or formula. Or add breast milk or formula to pureed meat, vegetables, or fruit to make a similar consistency. Though it will be quite runny, resist the urge to serve it from a bottle. As your baby learns to manage this consistency, serve foods with a thicker pureed consistency. Keep in mind that some babies eat such foods with gusto right from the start. Others are less enthusiastic. Be patient and keep trying.

FOODS FOR BABY

By age 1, your baby should be able to eat most of the foods served to the rest of the family. Just make sure food isn't too hot or a choking hazard, and avoid giving foods that are heavily spiced, salted or sweetened.

If you want to prep food for your baby, use a blender or a food processor to puree the food or cut the food into small, bite-size pieces. For softer foods, you may be able to simply mash them with a fork. Here are some examples of foods to try:

- Apples, peeled and cut in eighths, or in very thin slices with peel after baby has teeth
- Orange sections, peeled and loose membrane removed
- Peaches, ripe, peeled and thinly sliced
- Bananas broken into thirds lengthwise (spears), not coin-shaped pieces
- Egg, boiled, scrambled or poached
- Cheese cut in thin slices, thin spears or cubes
- Soft custards or puddings
- Plain yogurt
- Soft-cooked carrots and other vegetables cut into spears, not coin-shaped pieces
- Well-cooked macaroni, pasta, egg noodles and rice
- Pieces of toast or bagels
- Tender meats — fish, tuna, lamb, chicken, turkey, and some beef and pork
- Spaghetti with meat sauce
- Pancakes and waffles
- Whole-grain crackers and cereals
- Rice
- Soft-cooked beans and lentils
- Soft tofu
- Hummus

Finger foods By about 9 months of age, most babies can handle small portions of finger foods, such as well-steamed vegetables, soft fruits, well-cooked pasta, cheese, graham crackers and tender meats. These foods are usually soft enough to be crushed without teeth or dissolve in baby's mouth. As your baby approaches age 1, mashed or chopped versions of whatever the rest of the family is eating will likely become your baby's main fare. Continue to offer your child breast milk or formula with and between meals.

Juice

Juice, while a popular beverage, is not a recommended part of a baby's diet. Whole fruits, which contain fiber, have more nutritional value than juice.

If you want to give your child fruit juice, wait until after 12 months of age. Be sure to use 100% fruit juice, and limit the amount to 4 ounces a day or less. Too much juice may contribute to tooth decay, digestive issues such as diarrhea, and a preference for very sweet foods that may be associated with excessive weight gain. You also don't want juice to take the place of more nutritious solid foods, breast milk or formula.

What's off-limits for infants

Don't offer cow's milk, honey or corn syrup to your child before 12 months of age. Cow's milk doesn't meet an infant's nutritional needs and contains proteins that infants can't easily digest and process, potentially leading to stress on the kidneys and intestines that may cause significant health problems. It's best to think of cow's milk as part of a balanced diet after age 1, rather than a replacement for formula or breast milk. Honey and corn syrup may contain spores that can cause a serious illness known as infant botulism. Some infants and even toddlers may develop a diaper rash from acidic foods like citrus, so consider dietary causes if this is an issue for your infant.

Choking prevention and first aid

In addition, don't offer your baby foods that could pose a choking hazard. Such foods include:

- Small, slippery, round foods, such as whole grapes, hot dogs or hard candy
- Dry foods that are hard to chew, such as popcorn, raw carrots and nuts
- Sticky or tough foods, such as plain peanut butter or chunks of steak or other meat

If you haven't already, consider taking an infant cardiopulmonary resuscitation (CPR) course. This is strongly recommended for all parents. CPR can be very helpful in case of a choking episode, which can occur whether your child is an infant or a toddler.

You may have seen portable anti-choking suction devices, such as the LifeVac, which are marketed especially for use with children. Based on current evidence, these aren't recommended over back blows and abdominal thrusts, or chest compressions for infants. (See Chapter 17, on home safety, for more information.) To be prepared, it's smart to brush up on these lifesaving techniques.

INTRODUCING PEANUT BUTTER, MILK AND OTHER FOODS

Some foods can cause problems if they're not introduced at appropriate times.

Peanuts and other allergenic foods

To help prevent food allergies, parents were once told to delay feeding infants eggs, fish and peanut butter. But today researchers say postponing the introduction of highly allergenic foods beyond 4 to 6 months of age hasn't been shown to prevent eczema, asthma, allergic rhinitis or food allergy.

In fact, evidence suggests that introducing peanut butter or peanut-containing foods as early as 4 months may help prevent the development of peanut allergy. This is especially true for babies at increased risk of peanut allergies, such as those with eczema, an egg allergy or a family history of food allergies.

If your baby has started eating solid foods already and hasn't shown signs of any food allergies, you can introduce a bit of peanut butter thinned with breast milk, formula or pureed food. It's best to introduce the peanut butter in the morning, and when your baby is healthy. Avoid giving thick peanut butter from the jar or whole nuts, as these are choking hazards. If your baby tolerates it, you

THE IMPORTANCE OF IRON

Iron is a nutrient that's essential to your child's growth and development. Iron helps move oxygen from the lungs to the rest of the body and helps muscles store and use oxygen. Babies are born with iron stored in their bodies, but a steady amount of additional iron is needed to fuel a child's rapid growth and development. Infant formulas are fortified with iron. If you breastfeed, talk to your baby's healthcare professional about starting an iron supplement around 4 to 6 months of age. If your baby was born early, your baby's healthcare professional likely recommended beginning an iron supplement earlier. As your baby grows and begins to eat other foods:

- *Serve iron-rich foods.* When you begin serving your baby solids — typically between ages 4 months and 6 months — choose foods with added iron, such as iron-fortified baby cereal and pureed meats. For older children, good sources of iron include red meat, chicken, fish and tofu.
- *Don't overdo milk.* Once your little one turns a year old and starts drinking milk, don't serve more than 16 to 24 ounces of milk a day. Too much milk can inhibit the body's absorption of iron or even cause iron losses by irritating the lining of the intestine.
- *Enhance iron absorption.* On the other hand, vitamin C helps promote the absorption of dietary iron. You can help your child absorb iron by offering foods rich in vitamin C, such as cantaloupe, strawberries, bell peppers, tomatoes and dark green vegetables.

can gradually increase the amount given. When introducing other allergenic foods, stick to textures your baby eats and likes.

Allergy testing is no longer recommended before introducing allergenic foods. If your baby has eczema or if food allergies run in your family, talk to your baby's healthcare professional.

Cow's milk

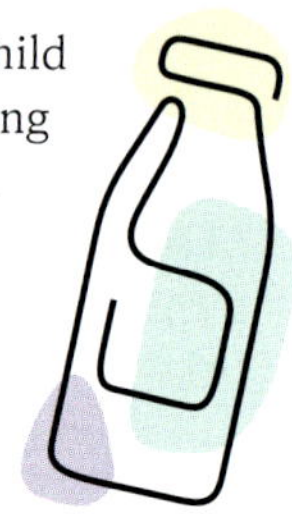

Around your baby's first birthday, you may gradually introduce your child to whole cow's milk. Of course, continue to breastfeed your baby as long as you wish. Cow's milk isn't a replacement for breast milk or formula. As your baby gains nutrients from a wider variety of foods, dairy milk can be an important source of vitamin D, calcium, fat and protein. However, dairy milk is not a necessary part of a child's diet, as these nutrients can be provided by other foods.

If you choose to give dairy milk, the AAP recommends that children be given whole milk until age 2. Low-fat milks — such as 2%, 1% and skim — don't provide enough fat for your child's developing brain. This type of milk shouldn't be given until your child is 2 years old unless specifically recommended by your child's healthcare professional.

Alternative milks — such as soy, nut and other plant-based milks — are typically fortified with vitamin D and calcium, but most have a lower fat content than whole cow's milk. Talk with your child's healthcare professional before

TEETHING AND DENTAL CARE

Your baby's first teeth may erupt by 6 to 7 months. Your baby may be fussy at this time, which may interfere with eating. Teething causes your baby's gums to swell. When your baby makes the effort to suck, more blood rushes into the already swollen gum. This may cause your baby to squirm, whimper and refuse to eat. You may try rubbing your baby's gum before feeding (for more on teething, see page 459).

Once there are teeth, there's the potential for dental decay. Dental cavities typically occur due to prolonged exposure to sugars in foods and drinks. To reduce the risk of dental damage:

- Avoid putting your baby to bed with a bottle of juice or milk. Sugar from milk and juice stays in the mouth longer when a baby drinks from a bottle. This may lead to an increase in dental cavities.
- Wean your baby from a bottle by 18 months.
- Limit sugary foods and drinks to mealtimes. Avoid carbonated, sugared drinks in general. Offer water between meals for toddlers.
- Clean your baby's teeth twice daily by brushing them with a small smear — an amount about the size of a grain of rice — of fluoridated toothpaste.

introducing milk if you have questions and especially if your child was diagnosed with a milk protein intolerance or allergy. Limit your child's milk intake — dairy or non-dairy — to no more than 16 to 24 ounces a day. Too much milk may crowd out other necessary foods.

FAMILY MEALTIMES

Mealtimes are an important part of family life. They offer family members a chance to come together to share not just food but companionship as well. Whenever possible, have your baby eat at the same time as the rest of the family. This helps your baby get used to the process of eating — sitting down, choosing foods to eat, resting between bites and stopping when full — and socializing with others.

These early experiences will help your child learn good eating habits that last a lifetime. Research shows that families that eat together regularly tend to eat more nutritious foods and have healthier eating behaviors, and are less likely to encounter childhood obesity or eating disorders. Some studies also suggest that more frequent family meals are associated with higher academic achievement and well-being, and may reduce risky behaviors in adolescence.

Tips for babies

Consider the following ideas to help mealtimes be a pleasant experience for everyone.

Stay seated At first, you may feed your baby propped on your lap. As soon as your baby can sit easily without support, use a high chair with a broad, stable base. Buckle the safety straps, and keep other children from climbing or hanging on the high chair.

Encourage exploration Your baby is likely to play with food between bites. Although it's messy, this hands-on approach helps fuel your baby's brain development. Placing a drop cloth or washable high-chair mat on the floor can help. Offer your baby new foods to try. To increase the chances of acceptance, offer one new food along with an established favorite. Most babies can and should eat from all food groups as soon as 7 to 8 months of age.

Introduce utensils Offer your baby a spoon to hold while you serve food with another spoon. As your baby's dexterity improves, encourage your baby to dip the spoon in food and use the spoon to eat. Your baby's use of utensils will continue to develop over time. Give your child the chance to practice.

Offer a cup Feeding your baby breast milk or formula from a cup at mealtime can pave the way for weaning from a bottle. At 9 months, your baby may be able to drink from a cup without help. You may want to begin with a non-spill cup, often called a sippy cup, giving your child additional opportunities to practice drinking from an open cup. Drinking through a straw may be another helpful skill to practice.

Dish up individual servings Early on, your baby may eat just a few spoonfuls of food at a time. If you feed your baby directly from a jar or container, bacteria and saliva from the spoon can quickly spoil any leftovers. Instead, place 1 tablespoon of food at a time in a dish, using a clean spoon, and refrigerate the rest. The same goes for finger foods. If your baby finishes the first serving, offer another.

Know when to call it quits When full, your baby may turn away from food or lean backward. Your baby's mouth also might suddenly seal shut. Don't force extra bites, and don't insist on finishing a portion. As long as your baby's growth is on target, you can be confident that your baby is getting enough to eat.

When babies are allowed to decide how much food they want to eat and how fast to eat it, they become fairly adept at it. Doing so allows them to regulate their food intake based on how hungry they are, which contributes to a healthy weight now and later.

FEEDING TODDLERS

As your child moves into toddlerhood, you may notice a drop in appetite. Your child may become fussy about food, run away after a few bites or resist coming to the table at mealtimes. A beloved food may be the number one choice for days on end, and then suddenly your child refuses to eat it at all. These eating habits are common among toddlers — and frustrating for you!

It can be tempting to coax and prod your toddler into eating. But a child's growth rate slows after the first year of life. Fewer calories are needed. Pressuring your child to eat at mealtime may end up doing more harm than good.

Think of it this way: Your job is to provide a selection of healthy and tasty options at regular times for meals and snacks. Your child's job is to choose how much of each food and whether to eat. Navigating mealtime with this balance of limits and flexibility empowers toddlers to trust their internal cues of appetite, hunger and fullness. What's more, it promotes an atmosphere of enjoyment around eating and a positive relationship with food. On the other hand, imposing food rules teaches children to override physical signs of hunger or fullness, and can turn mealtime into a source of tension and struggle rather than pleasure and connection.

Instilling in your child a relaxed, flexible, and accepting relationship with food comes with important benefits. Research suggests that adults who have a positive attitude toward eating and trust their own appetite cues are more likely to maintain a healthy, stable weight and be satisfied with their body weight. They tend to be less picky and more open to new foods, consuming a varied and healthy diet. They're also less likely to engage in disordered eating behaviors.

To encourage healthy eating habits in your growing child, consider these strategies.

Maintain a consistent family meal routine

Offer frequent meals and snacks at predictable times. Aim to provide these eating opportunities no more than two to three hours apart. You want your child to be hungry but not starving and cranky. It's easier for children — and adults — to listen to their internal eating cues when food is reliably provided.

Make the most of family mealtimes by minimizing distractions. Turn off TVs, phones and other electronic devices. This helps your toddler — and everyone else — focus on the meal and each other. Even children who can't speak yet enjoy the back-and-forth communication going on and the feeling of being part of the family. This sort of stimulation is important to your child's development.

Encourage openness to new foods

Try to offer a mix of favored and less favored or less familiar foods. A good rule of thumb is to provide at least one food choice per meal that is familiar and liked by your child. The other choices can be foods that you and other family members enjoy. Stick to one main dish, with at least one side dish that appeals to your child. Being exposed to less familiar foods alongside familiar ones will best equip your child to be a healthy eater in the long run.

Start small Avoid overwhelming your child by loading too much food onto a plate. Portion out a small amount of every food you've prepared — about the size of your child's fist. If your child wants more, offer seconds.

Avoid becoming a short-order cook In the desperation to get their young children to eat, some parents prepare preferred foods as an alternative to

SAMPLE MEALS FOR A 2-YEAR-OLD

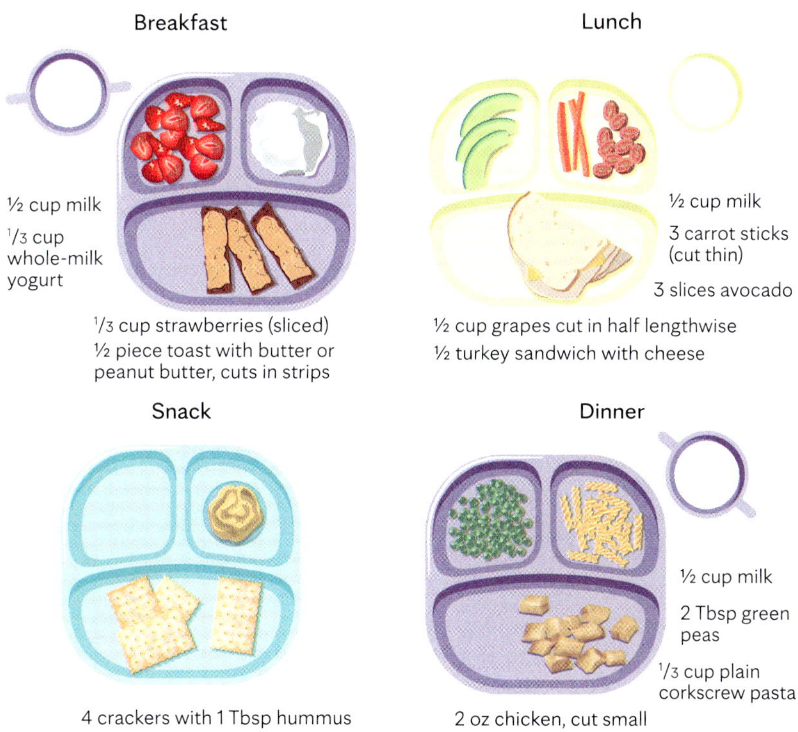

rejected options. They may even plan the family menu around a picky eater's tastes. Research indicates that over-accommodating a child by offering only preferred foods can reinforce food fussiness and strengthen the dislike of unfamiliar or rejected foods. Resist the urge to try pleasing everyone at the table. To promote food acceptance, model a relaxed attitude toward new foods. When you hear the age-old complaint "I don't like that," respond gently but firmly: "You don't have to eat it. Just keep it on your plate."

Strive for neutrality

Mealtime doesn't have to be the site of repeated battles. It can be a source of pleasure and connection.

Avoid power struggles If your child turns away from a certain food, don't push. Simply try again another time. Toddlers often respond to new foods with disgust. Studies show that it can take 8 to 15 exposures for a child to begin accepting a previously rejected food. Approaching food rejection with a combination of patience and persistence — offering a small amount of the same foods with meals over time — will help ensure variety in your child's diet. The harder you push your child to eat, the less likely your child is to comply. Instead, work with your child's healthcare provider to monitor their growth over time. Growth that is on track is the best indication that your child is eating enough.

Avoid using food as a punishment or reward Steer clear of mealtime strategies that involve withholding dessert or other favored foods or using food as a bribe. Research shows that exerting this kind of control at mealtime may backfire. When children learn to choose foods based on parental rules and expectations, they stop listening to their internal signs of hunger and appetite.

Change it up So how can you encourage your child to develop an openness to new foods? One of the best strategies is to walk the walk. Allow your child to see you enjoying nutritious foods. Encourage risk-free exploration by allowing your child to smell, touch or play with an unfamiliar food — without having to eat it. When exposing your child to a previously rejected food, try flavoring it with a different seasoning, sauce, or dressing. It may also help to cut or arrange foods into fun shapes, such as a smiley face, rainbow or heart.

Make mealtimes pleasant Model a positive relationship with food by eating for both sustenance and enjoyment. Showing your child that food can serve as a source of nourishment and pleasure will help to raise a healthier eater.

You can also give your child the freedom to choose how to eat and interact with food. Be flexible with how or whether your child uses utensils. Table etiquette is less pressing during the toddler stage than developing positive feelings about mealtime.

Connect in the kitchen

Meal preparation can be an additional opportunity to expose your toddler to a variety of foods. Consider these suggestions.

Shop together Take your child on some grocery runs, giving permission to feel the shape and texture of foods you put into your cart. This is a low-pressure opportunity for your child to develop an openness to different types of food.

Cook together When possible, involve your child in meal prep. Invite your toddler to help with age-appropriate kitchen activities, such as pouring ingredients into a bowl, stirring and mixing, rinsing produce, or using a pastry brush. To prevent falls at the counter, use an enclosed stool, sometimes called a learning tower. If your child expresses interest in cutting food, choose a dull butter knife or a toy plastic or wood knife, and offer soft foods such as peeled melon, bananas, or cooked and cooled vegetables for them to cut.

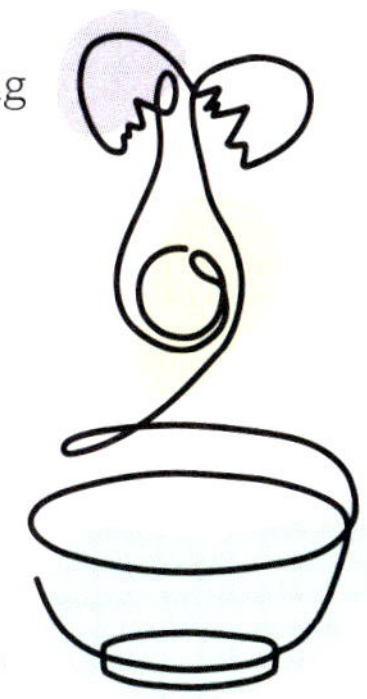

Including your child in these kitchen duties can strengthen fine motor skills and develop interest in the process of making food. What's more, involvement in meal prep conveys the message that making meals is an important part of healthy eating. Studies show that when someone has a habit of preparing meals, they're more likely to make better food choices and eat a varied and healthy diet.

Don't forget cleanup The tasks that come after a meal can also be a family affair. Toddlers can be expected to clear their dishes from the table. This might include rinsing the dish in the sink or placing it in the dishwasher.

Capitalize on your toddler's eagerness to spend time with you and be a helper by establishing helpful habits now. Doing so will make it easier to continue setting those expectations as your child ages.

NOURISHING SNACKS FOR TODDLERS

Like mealtime, snack time can be an opportunity to offer healthy proteins, fruits, veggies and grains. Here are some options:

- Grapes, berries or cherry tomatoes, cut lengthwise
- Bananas, cut lengthwise
- Peas or steamed carrots, green beans, cauliflower or broccoli
- Apples, sliced thin and spread with a thin layer of nut butter or seed butter
- Sliced cheese on whole-wheat crackers
- Cottage cheese mixed with rinsed canned peaches
- Whole-wheat pita triangles dipped in hummus
- Whole-grain quesadilla made with cheese
- Homemade fruit smoothies
- Plain yogurt mixed with smashed berries or rinsed canned fruit

For more ideas, head to trusted sources such as:

- HealthyChildren.org, powered by the American Academy of Pediatrics
- U.S. Office of Disease Prevention and Health Promotion
- U.S. Department of Agriculture (USDA)

INFANT AND TODDLER EATING BEHAVIORS

Children's eating habits are constantly changing as they grow. To help your child enjoy mealtimes and establish healthy eating habits, here are some common behaviors to look for and age-appropriate tips for every stage.

Age	Behaviors	Feeding tips
7 to 12 months	• Grasps food with hands • Takes food from a spoon with lips • Eats soft foods or foods with tiny lumps without gagging	• Offer soft foods such as iron-fortified infant cereal or pureed meat thinned with a bit of liquid • Offer a variety of new foods, one at a time • Don't force-feed
12 to 24 months	• Self-feeds finger foods • Drinks from a sippy cup without help but maybe not without spilling • Appetite decreases as growth slows • May seem uninterested in food for periods of time • May be a cautious, curious or rebellious eater	• Consider weaning from the bottle before 18 months; this avoids risk of overeating and dental decay • Provide safe finger foods • Offer whole milk to drink with meals • Allow exploration of food using all the senses
24 to 36 months	• Appetite is often unpredictable • May shift favorite foods without warning • May eat better than usual at one meal and eat nothing at the next • May struggle to eat independently	• Allow and encourage self-feeding, even if it takes a while • Offer new foods repeatedly • Offer whole milk unless otherwise specified by a healthcare professional • Offer water between meals and snacks

Be intentional about snacks

Many items in the grocery store that are packaged as toddler-friendly foods are ultra-processed. Ultra-processed foods have added colors, sugars, salts and preservatives that contribute no nutritional value. Think crackers, chips, cookies, boxed mac and cheese, frozen pizza, or chicken nuggets. Tasty and convenient as they can be, they may be harmful if consumed frequently. A growing body of evidence points to potential health risks associated with consuming high amounts of ultra-processed foods, including heart disease, type 2 diabetes, certain cancers, and poorer mental health.

Your child's food preferences begin to form in infancy and early childhood. Offering a selection of nutritious foods throughout the week can help shape healthy food tastes. That's not to say parents must rigidly avoid feeding their children all processed foods. Remember, food flexibility and food acceptance are invaluable attitudes to pass down to your child. Packaged snacks can play a role in keeping your child fed — and keeping you sane. Simply be conscious of when and how often you offer ultra-processed snack foods to avoid becoming overly reliant on them.

Don't sweat the picky eater

Picky eating habits are common in the toddler years and through preschool. It helps to keep in mind that these behaviors generally ease with age. You're not responsible for making your child like certain foods. You do play an invaluable role, though, in presenting multiple opportunities to learn about food and try different kinds. Having that in mind will help keep the peace at mealtime and set your child on a path to healthy eating.

CHAPTER 5

Diapers

The average child goes through about 5,000 diaper changes before being toilet trained. There's a lot to look forward to in your baby's first years, but changing diapers may not be at the top of your list. You might wonder: What diapers are best? What should I do about diaper rash? Is it OK that my baby has yellow or green poop?

A bit of prep and info can help make diaper changing a more positive experience. Consider diaper changes as another opportunity to bond with your baby. After all, caring for your child in this way, day after day, offers a moment for you and your baby to pause and connect.

Keep in mind that the routine of diaper changes will only last so long. The next chapter has everything you need to know about toilet training.

FINDING THE RIGHT DIAPER

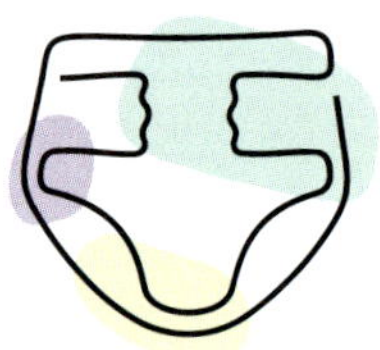

Many types of diapers are available — cloth or disposable, different brands, and countless sizes and styles. Some babies are comfortable in a lot of different types of diapers, while others need a particular kind that works just right for their body. If the diapers you have don't fit your baby well or seem irritating, don't be afraid to try something new.

Disposable

Disposable diapers are highly absorbent and convenient. However, the cost of using them adds up, especially if you have more than one baby.

The materials used in disposables usually keep your baby's skin drier for a longer period of time, compared with cloth.

Disposables are also convenient — you throw them away after each use. However, most disposable diapers aren't biodegradable. At best, they may degrade over a very long period of time. Around the world, an estimated 300,000 diapers every minute are sent to landfills, incinerated or littered. Fortunately, more disposable diaper companies are making efforts to have less of a negative impact on the environment by using different materials, fewer dyes and better packaging.

Compostable diapers are increasingly available, especially through startups via online marketing and ordering. However, if there's no program available in your area for these diapers to be collected and composted, they also go to landfills.

Cloth

Cloth diapers have become increasingly common in recent years, as new brands and styles offer more effective and convenient options. Some parents prefer to have the natural fibers of cloth diapers against their baby's skin, and cloth diapering also saves a lot of money over time. However, cloth diapers are typically less absorbent than disposables, and they require more work.

Cloth diapers typically have two parts. There's an inner layer, which is usually an absorbent material. It may be made from soft cotton, bamboo, hemp or microfiber. An outer cover usually includes a water-resistant layer, such as polyurethane laminate (PUL), or wool or fleece. Some parents like that these materials don't contain chemicals or fragrances that can irritate babies. Today's cloth diapers are usually fastened with snaps or fabric fasteners, not pins. Because cloth diapers usually aren't as absorbent as disposables, they need to be changed quickly after they become dirty to prevent irritation to your baby's skin.

Depending on how many diapers you buy, cloth diapers need to be washed anywhere from a couple of times a week to daily. Some people hire a service to drop off clean diapers and pick up dirty diapers for washing. Some cloth diapers also come with an optional disposable insert, so you can throw away the dirty part of the diaper. There are even some biodegradable disposable inserts that can be composted.

With the rise in cloth diaper use, there also are more accessories to make it easier. These include sprayers that attach to your toilet so that you can rinse off urine and stool from dirty diapers, and special bags (wet bags) to contain the diapers before they're washed.

Sizes

Most disposable diaper packages are labeled with a size that corresponds to your baby's weight. Though the range varies based on the brand, newborn sizes typically go up to 10 pounds, and size 1 is for babies who weigh about 8 to 14 pounds. Preemie diapers are usually for babies who weigh less than 6 pounds. As your baby grows into a toddler, you'll find up to size 7 in most brands.

Some cloth diapers come in different sizes — such as newborn, small, medium and large — while other styles can be adjusted to fit your growing baby.

How many?

If you use disposable diapers, you'll need 6 to 10 per day for the first few months. Older infants typically require fewer. If you plan to buy cloth diapers, the number you'll need depends on how often you plan to wash them. Some people buy enough that the diapers only need to be washed every third day or so, and others buy a smaller quantity and wash daily.

GETTING EQUIPPED

Diaper changes will be easier if you have everything you need on hand.

Changing station

It helps to have one or two places where you always change your baby's diaper. This way, you can keep all your materials in the designated location. If you use a changing table, make sure it has a wide, sturdy base with compartments for storing diaper supplies. Remember to keep one hand on your baby during changes, as there is always a risk of a baby rolling off a high surface. Another option is to change your baby using a changing pad on the floor. You can store supplies in the lower drawer of a crib or in a nearby dresser for easy access.

Diapers

Keep an adequate stock of diapers on hand. If you mostly use disposables, it may help to have some cloth diapers around in case you run out of disposables. If you mainly use cloth, keep a stash of disposables handy for those days when you haven't had a chance to do the wash.

Wipes

You can buy pre-moistened baby wipes, use a moistened cloth or make your own wipes using a homemade solution. If you use pre-moistened baby wipes, choose wipes for sensitive skin that don't contain alcohol or fragrance. This will help prevent irritation. It's not necessary to use wipes with every change. Urine is rarely irritating, so if your baby has only peed, letting the area dry may be enough. Wipes must be thrown away, not flushed. It's best to let baby's bottom dry after wiping before putting the new diaper on.

Diaper pail or wet bag

Diaper pails store dirty diapers and wipes, and wet bags are made to store dirty cloth diapers and reusable wipes before they're washed. There are a variety of types of pails and bags available. Look for one that is convenient, is sanitary and holds in odors.

Ointment or paste

You don't need to apply an ointment or paste unless your baby tends to develop diaper rashes. But it's nice to have a product on hand so that if your baby does develop a rash, you won't have to immediately run out to buy something.

HOMEMADE BABY WIPES

Pre-moistened baby wipes are common in the United States, but they aren't always necessary, and they're often overused. Some pre-moistened wipes contain ingredients that can be irritating to babies' bottoms. One way you can eliminate your baby's exposure to these ingredients, and save money, is to make your own baby wipes.

There are a variety of ways to make homemade wipes, but here are some suggestions to get you started. After reading through the options, decide which approach would work best for you.

Wipes

There are a few different options for wipes. See what you like best:

- Buy rolls of soft paper towels. Cut the rolls in half so that you have two shorter rolls. You'll have a nice size for wipes.
- Buy a stack of reusable wipes, which are often made of flannel or some other form of cotton. Or buy some thin baby washcloths to use as wipes.
- Make your own reusable wipes. Purchase soft flannel, terry cloth or fleece fabric and cut it into 5-inch squares. Then sew the edges so that the fabric won't unravel in the wash.

Moistener

Consider these options:

- Water
- Homemade solution. Here's one recipe:
  - 2 tablespoons baby wash
  - 2 tablespoons olive oil
  - 2 cups water

Container

Use whichever method is easiest for you:

- ***Round plastic storage container.*** Pour your homemade solution in the bottom of the container. Set a half roll of paper towels inside the container and place the cover on the container. The paper towels will absorb the liquid, and then you can tear off each sheet as you need it.
- ***Spray bottle.*** Keep fresh water or your homemade solution in a spray bottle. If you use a solution, wet down your wipes with water first, and then spray each wipe with a couple of squirts of solution.

If you create your own baby-wipe solution, you may want to check with your baby's healthcare professional to ensure that the baby wash or other ingredients in the solution don't contain any potentially harmful or irritating substances. Your baby's skin can absorb these products, so it's important that you're comfortable with the ingredients.

CHANGING DIAPERS

By the time your child is toilet trained, you'll be a diaper-changing pro. In the meantime, the following steps and pointers can help make diaper changing a successful venture for both you and baby.

Mindset

It may help to think of this necessary task as an opportunity for closeness, communication and even playtime with your baby. Your warm words, gentle touches and encouraging smiles help make your baby feel loved and secure. Soon your infant will be responding with gurgles and coos.

Frequency

Because newborns urinate frequently, change your baby's diapers every two or three hours for the first few months. This is especially important if you use cloth diapers. Urine alone doesn't usually irritate a baby's skin. However, the acid in a bowel movement can. Change a messy diaper as soon as your baby awakens.

Preparation

Have your wipes and a new diaper ready and within arm's reach. It may help to pull out or prepare the number of wipes you think you'll need for the job, and open the new diaper to lay it flat. You may want to place it directly under baby's dirty diaper, so it's ready to absorb accidents immediately. Make eye contact and tell your baby that you're going to change the diaper. Gently place your baby face-up on the changing table or pad. If you change the baby anywhere but the floor, remember to keep a hand on your baby at all times.

Remove old diaper

Unfasten the fasteners on the diaper your baby is wearing, and pull down the front side of the diaper. If your baby has had a bowel movement, use the clean inside front of the diaper to pull much of the stool off your baby's skin. Set the diaper off to the side beyond your baby's reach.

THE UMBILICAL CORD

For the first few days that you're changing your baby's diapers, you'll need to work around baby's umbilical cord stump. It's best to expose the stump to air as much as possible as it dries up and eventually falls off. It's also important to keep the umbilical cord stump clean and away from contact with urine and stool. Most newborn diapers are designed with a small cutout so that the diaper sits below the cord and doesn't rub it. If your diapers don't have this feature, fold the top down so that the diaper is positioned below the cord.

Clean baby's bottom

During the cleaning, carefully grasp and hold your baby's legs at the ankles with one hand. Using wipes or a cloth that's been moistened with warm water, clean from baby's front to back. Remember to check and clean out folds, where stool can hide. Place dirty wipes inside the dirty diaper to contain the mess.

Changing baby girls

Remember to wipe from the front side to the back side to avoid getting stool (or more stool) in the vaginal area. Baby girls have more folds and places for poop to hide, so it's important to clean them thoroughly. Girls also often have a white discharge in the folds of the labia, which is not necessary to remove. Too much scrubbing can cause irritation.

Changing baby boys

Baby boys have a tendency to urinate up and out of their diapers, causing leaks and wet clothes. As you put a new diaper on your baby boy, try positioning the penis downward to prevent these leaks. Also, you may want to fold the diaper down and in for extra protection on his front side. And while changing, it's smart to cover the penis with another wipe right away to contain any urine.

Place new diaper

As you lift your baby's legs from the ankles, slide the new diaper underneath the buttocks. The side with tabs should be in the back, underneath your baby. Pull the front of the diaper up between your baby's legs. Place it so that the front side and back side of the diaper will be at about the same level around your baby's body. Then fasten the tape, fabric fastener or snaps so that the diaper fits snugly around your baby's waist. If you're using disposable diapers, make sure that none of the elastic around the legs has folded underneath itself. If you're using cloth, make sure the inner layer is tucked inside the outer layer.

Discard old diaper

If you're using disposables, you can roll up the dirty diaper from the front to the back, with any wipes in the middle of the diaper. Then fasten the tabs around the sides of the rolled-up diaper. Toss the diaper in a diaper pail. If you're using cloth diapers and cleaning them yourself, dump any stool into the toilet, rinse the diaper off and place it in a designated holding spot — such as a wet bag or diaper pail — until you wash your load of diapers. Some families use diaper sprayers, which attach to the toilet. They often can be purchased in a baby store or online.

Wash your hands

When you finish the diaper change and baby is in a safe place, wash your hands with soap and water for at least 20 seconds. Hand-washing is important. It can prevent the spread of bacteria or yeast to other parts of your baby's body, to you or to other children.

PUTTING ON A DISPOSABLE DIAPER

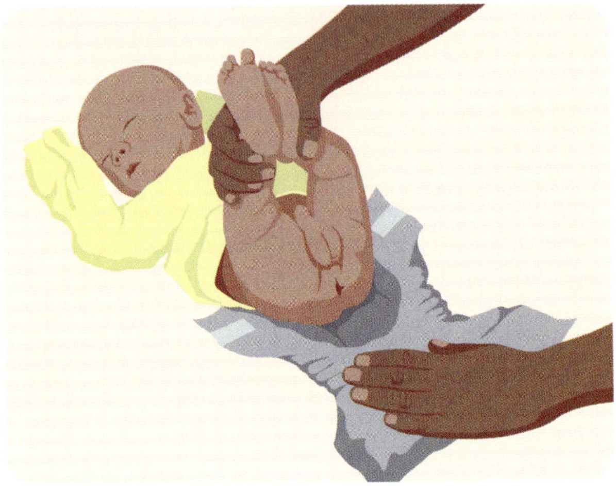

Step 1

When opening the diaper, make sure the tape at the back of the diaper is at the top, or away from you. Slide the diaper under your baby until the top edge (the edge with the tape) lines up with your baby's waist.

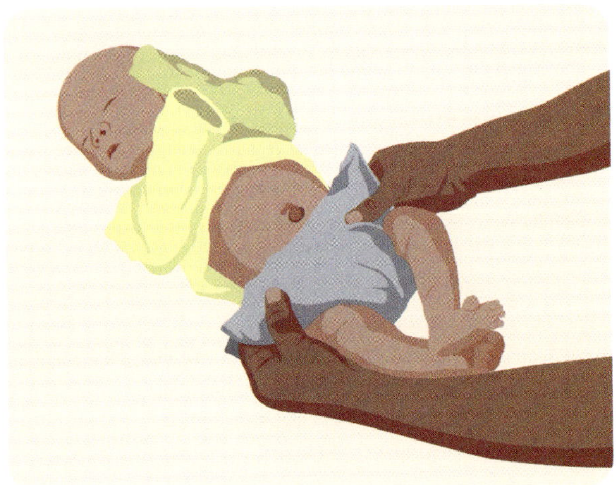

Step 2

Bring the front of the diaper up through the legs, without twisting it to one side.

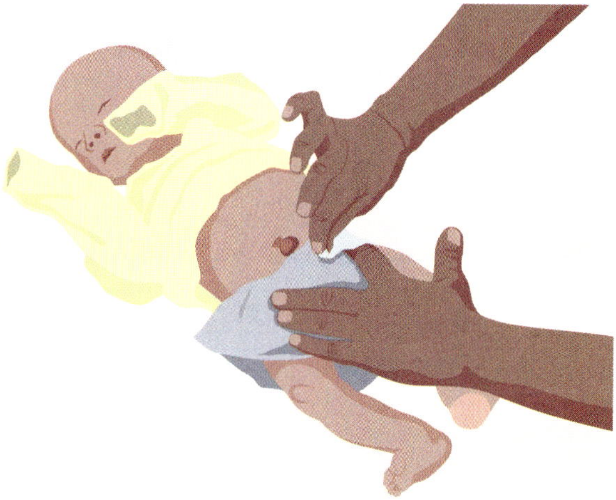

Step 3

Hold one side in position flat against the skin while removing the tab from the tape on the corresponding back side. Pull the tape forward and stick it to the diaper front. Repeat for the other side, making sure the diaper is snug around your baby's legs and not twisted to one side.

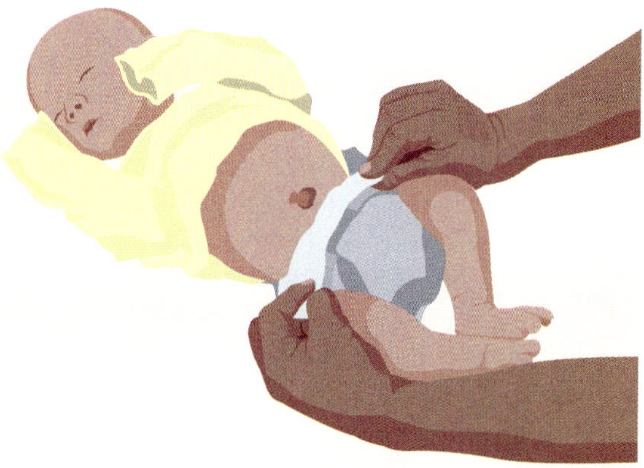

Step 4

For a newborn, fold down the top of the diaper so that it won't rub against the healing umbilical cord. Disposable diapers should fit snugly around the waist, with room enough for only one finger.

WHAT'S TYPICAL

New parents often wonder what's typical when it comes to their baby's urination and bowel movements. For newborns especially, there's a range of what's considered usual for color, consistency and frequency. But there also are guidelines that help you know what to expect and when there's cause for concern.

Urine

In a healthy infant, urine is light to dark yellow in color. Sometimes, as highly concentrated urine dries on the diaper, it creates a chalky, pinkish, red or orangish color, which may be mistaken for blood but is actually urate (uric acid) from the urine. This is common and not a cause for concern. Keep in mind that concentrated urine is different from blood in that it dries to a powder, and it's not as red in color.

By age 3 or 4 days old, your baby should have at least four to six wet diapers a day. Older babies may have a wet diaper with every feeding. As a toddler, your child may urinate less frequently but with a larger volume.

Stools

Your baby's first soiled diaper will probably occur within 48 hours of birth. During the first few days, a newborn's stools often will be thick and sticky — a tar-like, greenish-black substance called meconium. After the meconium is passed, the color, frequency and consistency of your baby's stools will vary depending on how your baby is fed — with breast milk or formula. Once solid foods are introduced, the frequency and consistency of stools will likely change along with their diet.

Color If you're feeding your baby breast milk, your baby's stools likely will resemble light mustard with seed-like particles. They'll be soft and even slightly runny. The stools of a formula-fed infant are usually tan or yellow and firmer than those of a breastfed baby, but no firmer than peanut butter.

Occasional variations in color and consistency are normal. Different colors may indicate how fast the stool moves through the digestive tract or what the baby ate. The stool may be variations of the colors green, yellow, orange and brown.

The color isn't that significant unless the stool has blood — which appears as red or coal-black streaks — or if it is a whitish-gray color instead of closer to yellow-brown. A whitish-gray color could be a sign that the stool is lacking bilirubin, a usual byproduct from the body's breakdown of excess red blood cells. These very pale stools could indicate that your baby's body isn't eliminating waste properly. If you see red or black blood or whitish-gray stools, contact your child's healthcare professional.

Consistency Mild diarrhea is common in newborns. The stools may be watery, frequent and mixed with mucus. Constipation isn't usually a problem for infants. Babies may strain or grunt, or even cry, and their faces might change in color during a bowel movement, but this doesn't necessarily mean they're constipated — even if they don't pass stool with that try. It takes time and practice for infants to learn to coordinate the movements to pass stool. Constipation in infants is defined as hard or firm stools. Constipation may develop in some babies when solid foods are introduced (see page 98) and is fairly common among toddlers, so it's smart to take notice of the consistency after weaning begins and as your child grows.

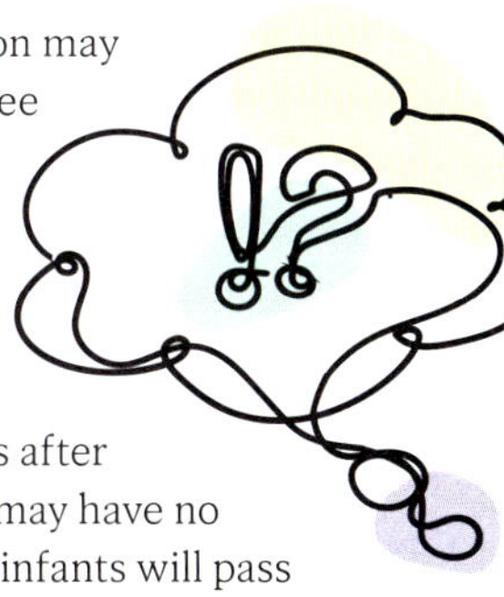

Frequency The range of what's typical is broad and varies from one baby to another, especially for breastfed babies. Babies may have a bowel movement as frequently as after every feeding or as infrequently as once a week. They also may have no consistent pattern. For the first several weeks of life, many infants will pass stool several times per day, often after eating. Around six weeks, some begin to have bowel movements less frequently. More or less frequent stools can be typical, as long as stools are soft and your baby is eating regularly and growing well.

The frequency of stooling will change again when solid foods are introduced, and throughout the process of weaning. Consistency remains important. Hard or very firm stools remain a sign of constipation. Soft stools are usually passed once per day or every other day.

Blood If your child's stools appear to contain blood — whether you see red or coal-black coloring, streaks, flecks or otherwise — contact their healthcare professional and have the problem checked out. Actual blood in stools is always a cause for concern, but don't panic; sometimes the problem isn't serious.

For example, newborns may ingest some blood during delivery, or they may take it in while breastfeeding from cracked or bleeding nipples. Flecks or streaks of blood in stools also may be a sign of an allergy to the protein in cow's milk (which may be found in formula) or breast milk. For older babies and toddlers, red or black in stools could be from certain foods, including tomatoes, beets, spinach, cherries and grape juice. Iron supplements can cause stools to appear very dark as well.

Diarrhea If you notice that your child's stool becomes more watery than usual and your baby is pooping more or more often, contact your child's healthcare professional.

SWIM DIAPERS

Taking your child to the swimming pool can be a fun family activity. For going in the water, infants and toddlers often wear swim diapers or swim pants. These are designed to let fluid pass through but contain solids. Still, it's not clear how well these products contain stool in a pool. Even if the diapers appear to contain everything, some contaminants and germs can leak through. If you take your baby to the pool, change the swim diapers as needed.

Children who are sick or have diarrhea should not go into a pool. Doing so could contaminate the water and make other babies and children sick.

There are many possible causes of diarrhea. Some foods may cause diarrhea. Diarrhea also may be a sign of an illness. And antibiotics are a common cause. Antibiotics wipe out both the good and bad bacteria in the gut.

If antibiotics are the culprit and your child is 6 months or older, you might consider feeding your child foods that contain probiotics, such as yogurt. Probiotics, found in certain fermented foods, are beneficial microorganisms ("good bacteria"). Probiotics may help bring a healthy bacterial balance back to your child's gut and improve digestion.

Probiotics also are available as over-the-counter supplements. However, because not a lot is known about the supplements, and studies with young children are limited, Mayo Clinic pediatricians don't routinely recommend their use. If you have questions about probiotics, talk to your child's healthcare professional.

Constipation Constipation in infants is defined by consistency of stools rather than by frequency. A baby is constipated when bowel movements are hard and perhaps even ball-shaped. Babies may become more prone to constipation once they start eating solid foods regularly, especially if they aren't drinking enough water. If your baby's stools are hard and formed, you can offer a couple of ounces of water in a sippy cup with meals. This water doesn't replace breast milk or formula (which is a meal, not a beverage) but can help give your baby a bit of extra fluid, which can help with constipation.

In toddlers, constipation is defined as fewer than three bowel movements per week, one or more accidents per week after a child is toilet trained, or by consistency (hard or ball shaped stool), which can be painful to pass.

DIAPER SURPRISES

You might occasionally notice a surprising but often harmless substance in your child's diaper.

Gel-like materials

Clear or yellow-tinted beads or particles may come from diaper materials that are overly wet with urine.

Small crystals

A newborn baby's kidneys may make clear crystals if baby is relatively dehydrated. This also can leave a tinted orange or pink stain in the diaper.

Pink stains or small bloodstains

A newborn girl may have some pink stains or small bloodstains in her diapers in the first few weeks. This is generally from exposure to pregnancy hormones right before birth. It isn't usually a problem, and it goes away with time.

Adding more fruits and vegetables to your child's diet can help. Prunes, pears and peaches are frequently used to help soften stools, either as purees or as a small amount of juice. If these changes don't lead to softer stools, talk to your child's healthcare professional about other possible causes and treatments.

DIAPER RASH

Most babies and toddlers get an irritated bottom from time to time, even with frequent diaper changes and careful cleaning. You certainly aren't a bad parent if your baby gets a diaper rash. Usually diaper rash is easily treated and improves within a few days.

Appearance

Diaper rash is marked by red, puffy and tender-looking skin in the diaper area — buttocks, thighs and genitals. The skin may have rashes or just look red and irritated. Your child may seem uncomfortable, especially during diaper changes.

Causes

There are several possible causes of diaper rash.

Irritation from stool Prolonged exposure to a soiled or damp diaper can irritate a baby's sensitive skin. Children may be more prone to diaper rash if they have frequent bowel movements, because feces are more irritating than urine.

Irritation from a new product Disposable wipes, a new brand of disposable diaper, or a detergent, bleach or fabric softener used to launder cloth diapers can irritate your child's delicate skin. Other substances that can add to the problem include ingredients found in some baby lotions, powders and oils.

Introduction of new foods As babies start to eat solid foods, the content of their stool changes, increasing the likelihood of diaper rash. Changes in diet also can increase the frequency of stools, which can lead to diaper rash.

Bacterial or yeast (fungal) infection The area covered by a diaper — buttocks, thighs and genitals — is especially vulnerable because it's warm and moist, making a perfect breeding ground for bacteria and yeast. These rashes generally start hidden within the creases of the skin, and there may be red dots scattered around the edges.

Chafing or rubbing Tight-fitting diapers or clothing that rubs against the skin can lead to a rash.

Use of antibiotics Antibiotics kill bacteria — both bad and good ones. Without the right balance of good bacteria, yeast infections can occur. This can happen when babies take antibiotics or when parents who are breastfeeding their infants take antibiotics. Because antibiotics often cause diarrhea, this also can lead to rashes.

Treatment

The most important factor in treating diaper rash is to keep your child's skin as clean and dry as possible. This often means increasing "diaper-free" time and thoroughly but gently washing the area with water during each diaper change. Avoid washing the affected area with soaps and disposable, scented wipes. Alcohol and fragrances in these products can irritate your child's skin and aggravate or provoke the rash.

If the rash is severe, it might help to clean your baby's bottom with warm water from a squirt bottle instead of using a moistened cloth or wipes, so you won't have to rub the tender skin. It's also important to allow baby's bottom to air-dry completely before putting on a new diaper. If possible:

- Let your child go without a diaper for longer periods of time.
- Avoid using tight-fitting diaper covers.
- Use larger-sized diapers until the rash goes away.

In addition, use a mild ointment such as petroleum jelly or a zinc oxide paste anytime pinkness appears in the diaper area. This can reduce friction and rubbing. It also can block contact with chemical irritants from stools or diaper materials.

Apply the cream in a thin layer to the irritated region several times throughout the day to soothe and protect the baby's skin. You don't have to remove the cream completely at every diaper change if the area is clean — rubbing will only irritate the skin further.

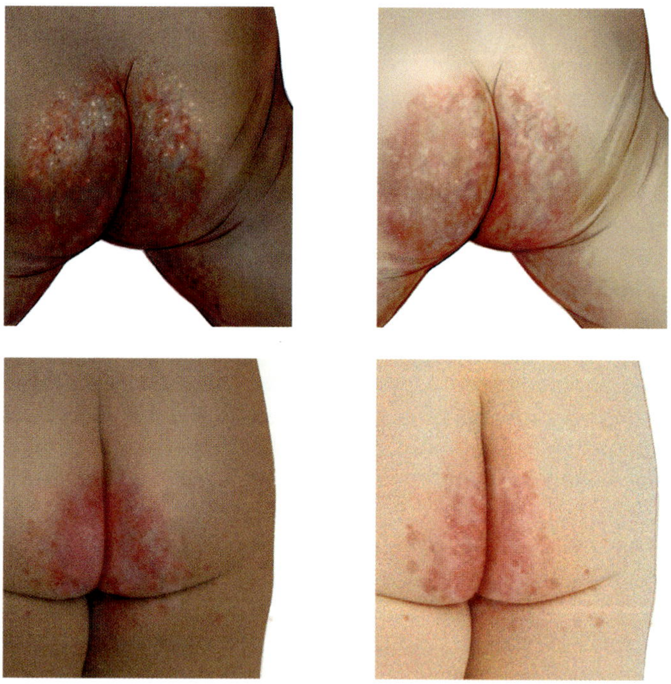

Diaper rash from irritation *(top)* typically results from prolonged contact with urine or stool on the buttocks. A yeast diaper rash *(bottom)* often includes red dots. The dots may be scattered outside the edges of red areas in and near the skin folds.

Many effective creams contain zinc oxide, which helps soothe the skin. Look for a cream that doesn't contain fragrance, preservatives or other ingredients that could cause irritation or allergies, including neomycin. Some substances are absorbed into the body through the skin. And some creams contain ingredients that can be harmful for your child, including boric acid, camphor, phenol, benzocaine and salicylates.

Also avoid creams that have steroids, such as hydrocortisone, in them, unless your baby's healthcare professional specifically recommends such a product. Creams containing steroids can be harmful, and they usually aren't necessary. Also, don't use talcum powder or cornstarch on a child's skin unless recommended by your healthcare professional. A child may inhale talcum powder, which can be very irritating to the lungs. Cornstarch can contribute to a bacterial infection.

When to seek medical treatment

Contact your child's healthcare professional if:

- The rash is accompanied by a fever, especially if your child is less than 2 months old.
- The rash has blisters, boils, discharge or pus-filled sores.
- The rash isn't improving after two to three days of home treatment.
- Your child is taking antibiotics, and the rash is bright red with red spots around the edges. It could be a yeast infection, which needs additional treatment.
- The rash is severe.
- The rash is present on skin outside the diaper area.

Preventing diaper rash

There are a variety of steps you can take to help prevent, or at least reduce the incidence of, diaper rash:

- Change your child's diaper often to limit contact with urine or stools.
- Let your child go diaper free for brief periods once in a while. This will allow their bottom to air out.

PREVENTING RASH: CLOTH OR DISPOSABLE?

When it comes to preventing diaper rash, there's no compelling evidence that cloth diapers are better than disposable diapers or vice versa, though disposables may keep the skin slightly drier. Because there's no one best diaper, use whatever works best for you and your child. If one brand of disposable diaper irritates your child's skin, try another.

Whether it's cloth or disposable, try to change a soiled diaper as soon as you can to keep your child's bottom as clean and dry as possible.

- Avoid using super-absorbent disposable diapers, because they tend to be changed less frequently.
- If you're using cloth diapers, wash and rinse them thoroughly. Prerinse heavily soiled diapers, and use hot water to wash them. Use a mild detergent with no fragrance, and skip fabric softeners and dryer sheets. They can contain fragrances that irritate your baby's skin. Double-rinse the diapers.
- If you use cloth diapers, select snap-on diaper covers, instead of those with elastic bindings, to help improve circulation.
- After changing diapers, wash your hands well to prevent the spread of germs.

CHAPTER 6

Toilet training

Toilet training is a big milestone for kids and parents. Many parents look forward to the day when they no longer deal with changing diapers. Most don't miss the expense, either.

Some parents start very early, during infancy, using a technique called elimination communication. This has been practiced in different areas of the world and involves parents responding sensitively to infant cues and supporting the infant in a secure squatting position for elimination, all done gently and without coercion. Others start later, in the toddler years.

It's important to let your child lead the way. Learning to use the toilet is a natural part of growing up and not much different from learning to drink from a cup, walk, talk or develop any of the other skills that infants and toddlers acquire as they move toward independence. If left to learn how to use the toilet on their own, most children would probably toilet train themselves. As with learning to walk, it would occur in a long series of small successes, each next step happening when the child is ready.

In fact, readiness is the key to successful toilet training. The single most common cause of toilet training problems is that the child isn't ready. Being ready makes toilet training easier and quicker. Patience on the part of parents helps, too.

RECOGNIZING READINESS

Many children show signs of being ready for toilet training between ages 18 and 24 months. However, others might not be ready until they're 3 years old. There's no rush. Rather than relying solely on your child's age — or when peers are being toilet trained — look for your child to show key signs of being ready and interested in using the toilet.

Your child's readiness is related to certain physical, developmental and behavioral milestones. It doesn't have anything to do with intelligence, will or character.

Physical readiness

To use the toilet successfully, a child must have voluntary control over the pelvic muscles. This is something your child grows into with time. You don't have much control over this aspect, and some kids take a little longer than others. Signs of voluntary control usually begin to appear by 18 months or so.

Signs of physical readiness include being able to recognize the urge to urinate or have a bowel movement and sense this urge in time to make it to the toilet or potty chair. Most children achieve this neurological function between 24 and 36 months.

Developmental readiness

A number of motor, language and social skills are important to using the toilet. Look for your child to be able to:

- Walk to and sit on the potty
- Stay dry for up to two hours
- Pull bottom clothes down and back up again
- Follow simple two-step instructions, such as, "Pick up the ball and put it in the toy basket"
- Communicate the need to go potty

Behavioral readiness

You can also look for key indications in your child's behavior, such as:

- Being able to imitate the behaviors of others, such as using the toilet
- The ability to put things where they belong, which helps with understanding that pee and poop go in the toilet
- The ability to say no, which shows a degree of independence from you
- A desire to cooperate and less of a desire to engage in power struggles
- An interest in using the potty and in staying clean and dry

Parent readiness

Your own readiness as a parent is important, too. Expect that toilet training will take some time and patience. It's also likely to get a bit messy.

In general, let your child's motivation, instead of your eagerness, lead the process. Avoid equating toilet training success or difficulty with your child's intelligence or stubbornness.

Also, keep in mind that accidents are inevitable, and punishment has no role in the process. Typically, punishment or criticism tends to make the process take longer. Plan toilet training for when you or another caregiver can devote the time and energy to be consistent on a daily basis for a few months.

ACTIVE TRAINING

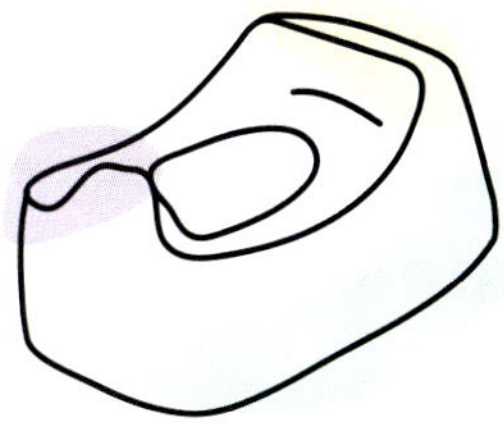

When you think your child might be ready to start using the toilet, go ahead and swing into action. There's no single best way to toilet train. But here are some general suggestions to keep in mind.

Pull out the equipment

Consider purchasing a potty chair, available at most places that sell baby supplies, for the express purpose of toilet training. A potty chair is generally easier to learn on than an over-the-toilet seat and gives your child a more secure footing and better leverage to eliminate. In addition, your child can take ownership of the potty chair by decorating it or drawing on it.

Place the potty chair in the bathroom or, initially, wherever your child spends a lot of time. If you have multiple levels in your home, you might want to put a potty chair on each level where your child spends time.

Encourage your child to sit on the potty chair in clothes to start out. Make sure your child's feet rest on the floor or a stool. If you have the potty chair in the bathroom, take the opportunity to have your child flush the toilet to become accustomed to the noise and motion of the water.

Share the purpose of the potty

Use simple terms to explain what the toilet is for — to catch pee and poop, for example. Use terms consistently and positively. You might dump the contents of a dirty diaper into the potty chair or toilet to show its purpose. Or allow your child to watch you use the toilet.

SETTING THE STAGE FOR SUCCESS

There's not much you can do as a parent to speed up your child's physical readiness for using the toilet. However, as early as your child's first birthday, there are some ways you can begin laying the groundwork for a successful psychological transition from diapers to the toilet.

There are many children's picture books written specifically to interest children in this natural transition. You can read these books with your child. There are also toys, videos and smartphone apps designed to help your toddler get acquainted with the benefits of using the toilet.

Another way to begin building for a successful transition at this early stage is to allow toddlers to watch parents and older brothers or sisters using the toilet. Thus, family members can be role models for a year or more before toilet training actually begins.

Schedule potty breaks

Have your child sit on the potty chair or toilet without a diaper for a few minutes at two-hour intervals, as well as first thing in the morning and right after naps.

Boys can learn to urinate sitting down, and then move to standing up after bowel training is complete.

While your child sits, stay and read a book together. You can also blow bubbles using a bubble wand. This will encourage your child to use the appropriate pelvic muscles to help pass a bowel movement. Even if your child simply sits there, offer praise for trying and explain that they can try again later.

To maintain consistency, consider bringing the potty chair with you on vacation or when you're away from home with your child.

Respond quickly to the "potty dance"

When you notice signs that your child might need to use the toilet — such as squirming, squatting or holding the genital area — respond quickly. Help your child become familiar with these signals. Tell your child to stop any activity and head to the toilet. Give lots of praise when your child tells you about needing to go. This will help reinforce the idea that having to go is a call to quick action. To maximize the chances of success in getting onto the toilet in time, keep your child in loose, easy-to-remove clothing.

Encourage the feeling of comfort

Some parents think that leaving a wet or soiled diaper on will help their children want to use the toilet. But this is generally counterproductive. You want your child to become accustomed to feeling clean and dry. You can help by encouraging your child to come to you when wet or soiled and by changing diapers as soon as needed. At the same time, explain to your child the connection between being clean and dry and using the potty. You can say things such as "If you go in the potty, your diaper (or pants) will stay nice and dry."

DO'S AND DON'TS OF TOILET TRAINING

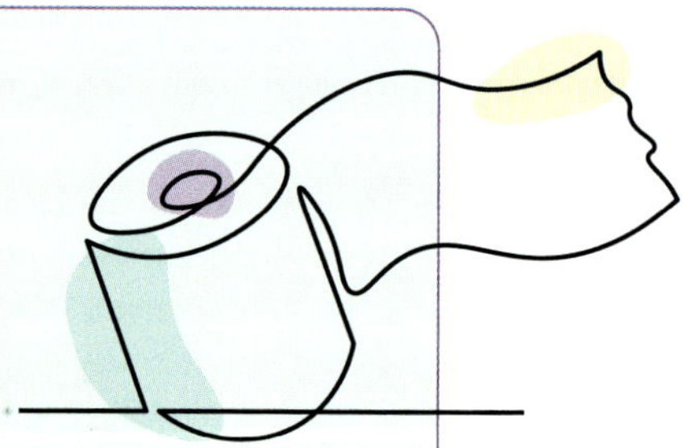

Things to do:

- Make toilet training fun for your child.
- Give lots of praise and encouragement.
- Let your child feel in control.
- Most important, relax.

Things not to do:

- Don't force your child to sit on the potty.
- Don't yell at or punish your child for accidents.
- Most important, don't rush the process.

Explain hygiene

For girls, it's important to wipe carefully from front to back to prevent bringing germs from the rectum to the vagina or bladder. Show your daughter how to spread her legs apart when wiping to make this task easier. Encourage hand-washing after using the toilet.

Ditch the diapers

After a couple of weeks of successful potty breaks and remaining dry during the day, your child might be ready to trade diapers for training pants or underwear. Some experts recommend that children wear regular underwear as opposed to disposable training pants because they feel different from diapers. However, disposable training pants are convenient, especially in child care settings or when away from home. Celebrate your child's transition toward "big-kid" clothes. If your child is unable to remain dry, it's OK to return to diapers and try again at another time.

Praise and reward

Reward your child for listening to body signals, heading toward the bathroom and sitting on the potty. Focus less on mistakes and more on your child's efforts — even minor ones — at using the potty. Your happy voice, hugs and compliments for trying will help reinforce positive steps that build toward your child's success. Consider finding some kind of reward — such as stickers or stars — to offer as additional positive reinforcement, if this helps motivate your child. Reward the behavior the child can control (sitting on the potty), not the outcome (stooling or urinating in the toilet).

Nighttime training

Nap time and nighttime training typically takes longer to achieve. Most children can stay dry at night between ages 5 and 7. In the meantime, use diapers or training pants and mattress covers when your child sleeps.

WHEN TO START AND WHEN TO DELAY TRAINING

If possible, plan toilet training for a time that's relatively stress-free. For instance, if you live in a cold climate, you might plan for toilet training in the warmer months, when layers of clothing aren't so much of an issue.

You may want to delay toilet training if you're anticipating major changes in family life — such as a move to a new home or the arrival of a new sibling. Consider delaying training if the unexpected happens as well — such as a major illness or the death of a family member.

TROUBLESHOOTING

Your child will probably have numerous failures on the way to success. That's OK — it's the nature of learning. There's no need to scold, discipline or shame your child for having an accident. Provide encouragement for behaviors your child can control, such as sitting on the potty. Don't stress about those your child can't control yet, such as urinating only in the potty.

Keep encouraging your child to repeat the learning steps you've already started — knowing when to stop playing and head to the toilet, undressing, sitting on the toilet, dressing and washing hands. Keep a positive attitude and your child will follow suit. And don't worry too much. Your child will get there eventually.

Accidents

Accidents will happen, no doubt about it. Calmly help your child change clothing as soon as you can after an accident. Keep your tone sympathetic. You might say, "You forgot this time. Next time you'll get to the bathroom sooner. You'll get better at this."

In the meantime, be prepared. Keep a change of underwear and clothing handy, especially in the car, on an extended outing or at child care.

In the beginning, many children will urinate or have a bowel movement right after getting off the toilet. This can be frustrating for parents. If this happens frequently, be patient. It takes a while to learn to relax bowel and bladder muscles on command. You might consider holding off on toilet training a bit longer if it leads to anxiety or tension between you and your child.

Lack of interest

If your child isn't interested in using the potty chair or toilet or isn't getting the hang of it within a few weeks, take a break. Chances are your child isn't ready yet. Pushing your child in this situation can lead to a frustrating power struggle. Try again in a few months. Your child's job is ultimately to learn to control the bladder and bowel movements. Your job as a parent is to be patient and support your child's efforts.

Regression

Sometimes a child will lose the willingness to use the toilet or forget certain steps after being toilet trained. This is common, especially if there have been changes in the child's routine. Usually it's just one more step on the way to successful toilet training. Consistent reminders and positive reinforcement while making necessary schedule adjustments are key to keeping your child on track.

Active resistance

Some children are more independent and prefer to do things on their own. As they get older, they might resist "micromanaging" by a parent. They may hold back bowel movements or become constipated. They may even continue to wet and soil themselves.

COORDINATING TOILET TRAINING AND CHILD CARE

Many kids go through toilet training while also attending child care. To keep the process of toilet training going smoothly, communicate closely with child care staff. Tell your child's caregivers about your toilet training efforts so they can continue your efforts at child care or preschool. If you can use similar methods at home and at child care, your child is less likely to become confused and more likely to succeed.

Some advantages of toilet training at a child care center are that staff are often positioned to recognize signs of readiness and can help your child take steps to use the toilet. Being around other kids who use the toilet also may help motivate your child to do the same. Disadvantages may occur if the child care center is understaffed or if there's little communication between staff and parents.

If you've followed the steps described earlier for several months without success and your child is approaching 3 years of age, ask your child's healthcare professional for help. A healthcare professional also can check to see if there's an underlying problem. It may be time to try something new.

Sometimes with older children who enjoy being independent, it can help to step back and let them take responsibility for using the toilet.

Explain that your child is in charge now and that you will no longer remind your child to use the toilet. Tell your child — in the words you've chosen — that the body makes pee or poop every day and that these need to go in the potty. You can say, "I'm sorry I reminded you so much and made you sit on the potty. From now on you don't need my help. You can do it by yourself."

Let your child decide when to go to the bathroom. If your child has an accident, be gentle. Don't punish, criticize, or ask why or how it happened. Simply tell your child to go clean up and change into dry clothes.

When you no longer give your child attention for not going, your child eventually will seek attention for using the toilet correctly. Give plenty of smiles, hugs and praise when your child uses the toilet. Your child soon will embrace these newfound skills.

If you have questions about toilet training or your child is having difficulties, talk to your child's healthcare professional. Also call if your child shows signs of constipation or signs of pain or burning during urination. Treating these problems can help ensure successful toilet training.

CHAPTER 7

Bathing and skin care

Bathing your baby can be a sweet and fun experience. Don't worry if you feel a little awkward at first — it takes practice to get the hang of cleaning a slippery and squirmy baby. And don't be surprised if at first your baby doesn't like being bathed. It's a whole new experience for your baby — and for you, too!

The tips that follow will help make your bath time routine safe and smooth. You'll also learn how to identify and deal with skin conditions that are common in a baby's first years. Sometimes people expect new babies to have flawless skin, but that's rarely the case.

NEWBORN BATHING BASICS

As your child grows, chances are that bath time will be a time for fun. Older babies and toddlers enjoy splashing in the water and playing with bath toys. Newborns, however, don't always like the bath experience. They may not care for getting undressed or the cold feeling that comes with having no clothes on.

Fortunately, infants don't need much bathing. It's not until your child gets older and has more chances to get dirty that baths become more of a regular ritual.

How often?

Generally, babies need only one to three baths a week in the first year, unless otherwise instructed by your baby's healthcare professional.

During your newborn's first couple of weeks, it's OK to give your baby a bath even while the umbilical cord is still attached. Just avoid submerging your baby's belly in water until the cord falls off. If the umbilical cord does get wet, dry the area thoroughly.

In between baths, check your baby's folds — in the thighs, groin, armpits, fists and neck — to see if they need occasional spot cleaning.

Once your baby starts crawling around and eating solid food, bath time may need to happen three days a week.

Sponge bath or full bath?

You don't have to start out with sponge baths, but they're a gentle and easy way to introduce your new baby to bathing. It's a fine alternative to a full bath for the first six weeks or so after your child is born.

A sponge bath basically involves using a warm washcloth to clean your baby. During a sponge bath, provide warmth by covering your baby with a dry towel. Move a piece of the towel aside to clean each area of your baby's body. Once finished, pat that area dry and cover it back up before moving on to another area.

When's the best time?

Find a time for bathing your baby that's convenient for both of you. Many people give their baby a bath before bedtime as a relaxing, sleep-promoting ritual. Others prefer a time when their baby is fully awake. You'll enjoy this time more if you're not in a hurry and aren't likely to be interrupted.

You also may want to wait a bit after your baby eats or drinks to give a bath. This allows the stomach to settle. Waiting briefly also may reduce the chances of your baby peeing or pooping during the bath.

Temperature

For baby's safety, you don't want the water too hot — it could hurt or even burn your baby. You also don't want the water so cool that your baby gets chilled. Generally, a temperature between 95 and 100 F is ideal for a baby's bath.

To start, make sure your home water heater is set at no higher than 120 F. This will prevent dangerously hot water temperatures. Before filling up the tub or basin, test the water temperature with your elbow or wrist. The water should feel warm but not hot. Once you fill the tub or basin, test the temperature again — water temperatures frequently change while the water is running. Never let the bath fill while your baby is sitting in it. Instead, fill the tub or basin and then test the water again.

NO BIG TUB? NO PROBLEM.

If your living space includes only a shower, you still have a number of options for giving your baby and toddler a bath. You might start with a bath cushion in the sink for your newborn. As your baby grows, a child-size tub can be used on the floor of your shower. Some versions even fold up for easy storage.

Attentiveness

It's important to give your baby your full and undivided attention during baths. If the phone rings or someone rings the doorbell, ignore it. Babies can drown in less than an inch of water in an instant, so you don't want to be diverted from the task at hand. They also can roll and fall from high surfaces, or slip and hit their heads, even when they're seated.

During a bath, keep your eyes on your little one at all times. If you forgot something you need for the bath, bring your baby with you to get it, even if the item is just a step away.

BATHING, STEP BY STEP

When you decide it's time to try a full bath, you might start out using a baby bathtub, which you can set inside your regular tub or shower or on the floor or next to the sink. The first few baths should be especially gentle and brief. If your baby doesn't like it, you might stick with sponge baths for a while longer before trying a full bath again. Once your child gets older and is able to sit well without support, baths can happen in a few inches of warm water right in the family bathtub.

Gather supplies

Prepare the bath area with all the items you'll need. Typically this involves:

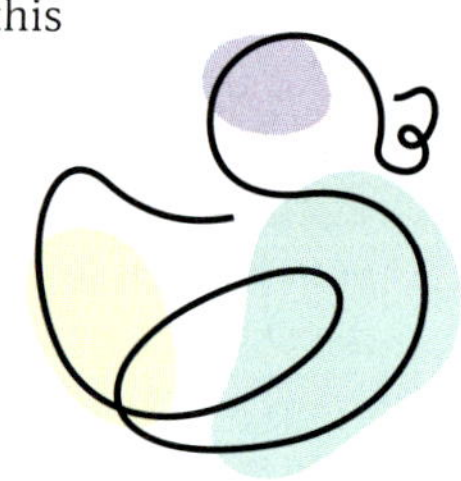

- A couple of clean, soft washcloths.
- A mild fragrance-free baby soap or shampoo. This isn't essential for newborns, as plain water will do just fine. But it becomes more important as baby gets older (and has more chances to get dirty).
- A couple of soft, dry towels. Baby-size ones are easy to manage.
- A fresh diaper and pajamas or clothes.
- Bath toys. These aren't necessary early on, but older babies enjoy having a toy or two to play with in the bath. Make sure the toys stay clean and free of mildew.

Get baby ready

Remove your baby's clothes and diaper. Gently lower your baby into position. Support your baby's head and torso. If baby seems cold or unhappy, you might try draping a warm, wet washcloth or towel over the body to help keep baby warm.

Keep hold

Babies can be slippery and can become suddenly squirmy, so keep a good hold on your baby during bath time. It may help to keep your dominant hand free for reaching and cleaning and use the other hand to keep your baby steady.

Eyes first

Clean the delicate eye area first. Use a cloth dampened with water to wipe from the inside to the outside corner of your baby's eye.

Start at the top

Use a soft cloth to wash your baby's face with water and then pat the face dry. Wash your baby's head with water, too. Tip back your baby's head or cup your hand over your baby's forehead to keep water or soap from running into baby's eyes.

If you give baths several times a week, it's not necessary to shampoo your baby's hair with every bath. Once or twice a week is plenty. If your baby doesn't like having a wet head, save the hair wash for last. You can use a soft washcloth, your fingertips or a baby scrubber to wash the hair and scalp.

Wash and check folds

Wash the rest of your child's body from the top down, including the inside folds of skin and the genital area. For a girl, gently spread the labia to carefully clean the area. For a boy, lift the scrotum to clean underneath. If your son is uncircumcised, don't try to retract the foreskin of the penis. Let your baby lean forward on your arm while you clean the back and bottom, separating the buttocks to clean the anal area.

Towel dry

Once cleaning and rinsing are done, have a towel ready. Carefully pick up your baby — remember, they will be slippery!

One way to dry your baby is to set a towel vertically over your body so that part of it hangs over your shoulder. Bring your baby to your chest and then bring the bottom of the towel up and around your baby. Another option is to spread a towel out on the floor. Place baby on the towel and then wrap the towel around your baby.

Moisturize

Gently pat your baby dry. Patting the skin instead of rubbing it dry will help keep your baby's skin from getting irritated.

After you've dried baby off, moisturize your baby's skin all over with a gentle, fragrance-free moisturizer or petroleum jelly. You might find this easier to do on a changing table or bed than in the bathroom. Some studies show that daily moisturizing can help prevent eczema (atopic dermatitis) in babies, especially those who have a family history of the condition.

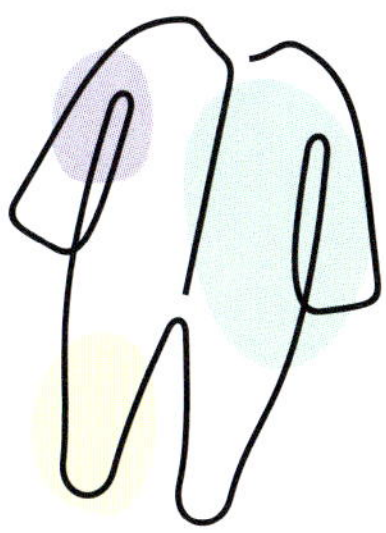

Finishing touches

Place a fresh diaper on your baby, add clothes or pajamas to keep your child warm, and you are done! Enjoy the sweetness.

BABY'S FIRST BATH

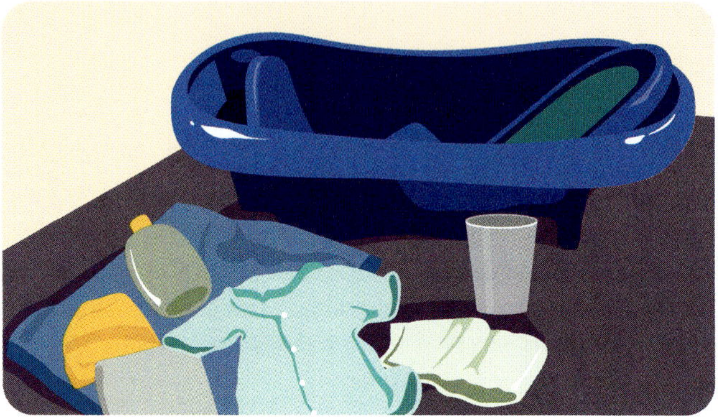

Getting set up

When you're ready to give your baby a tub bath — whether you do so right from the start or you try sponge baths first — you'll have plenty of choices. You can use a free-standing plastic tub designed for newborns, a plain plastic basin or other options designed to fit inside the tub. Lined with a towel or rubber mat, a clean kitchen or bathroom sink might be another option.

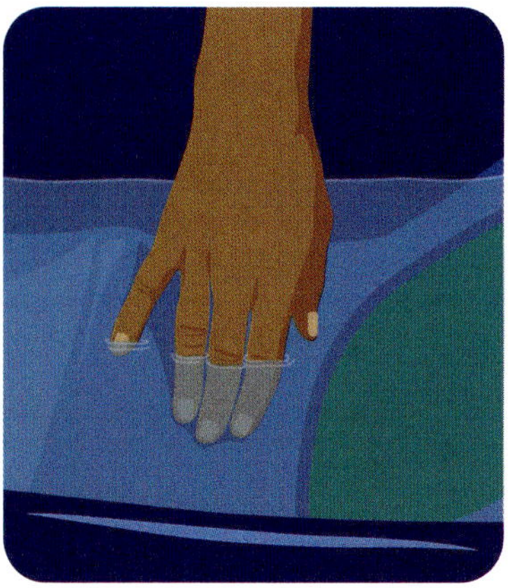

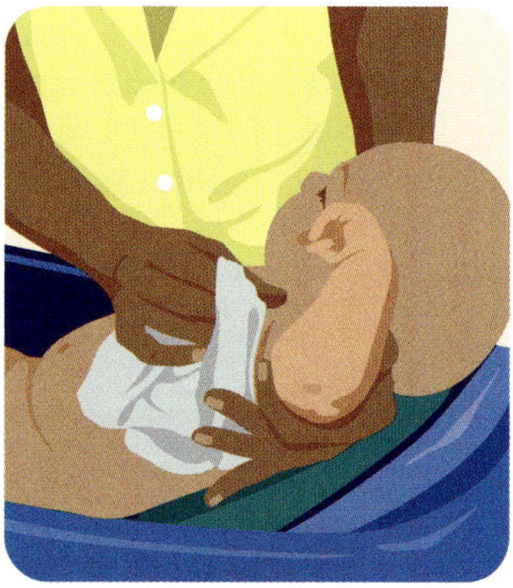

Water temperature

Make sure to check the water temperature before setting baby in the bath. You need only a few inches of warm — not hot — water. A temperature between 95 and 100 F is ideal. To prevent scalding, set your water heater thermostat to below 120 F.

Use a secure hold

A secure hold will help your baby feel comfortable and stay safe in the tub. Use one of your hands to support your baby's head and the other to wash your baby's body.

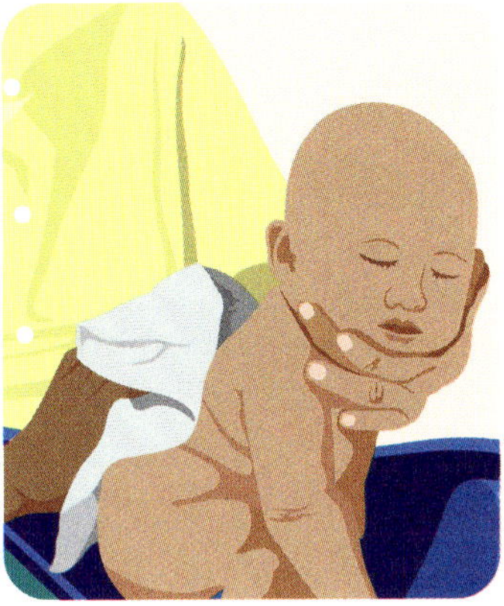

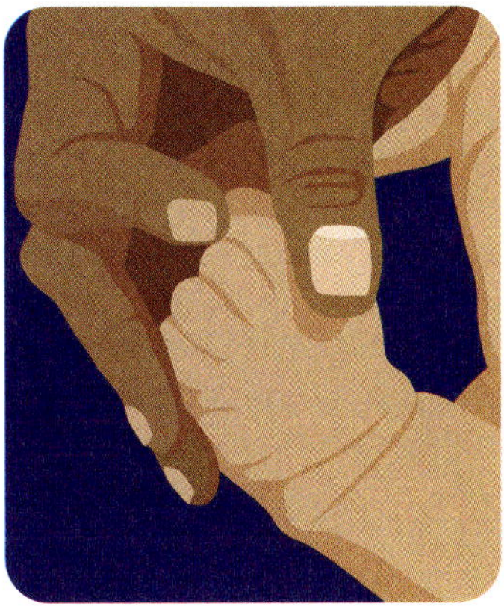

Washing baby's back

To wash the back and buttocks, lean your baby forward on your arm. Continue to grasp your baby under the armpit.

Remember the creases

Pay attention to creases under the arms, behind the ears, around the neck and in the diaper area. Wash between baby's fingers and toes.

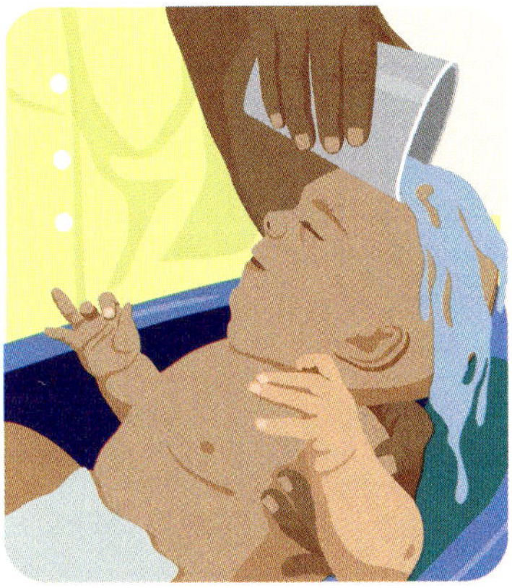

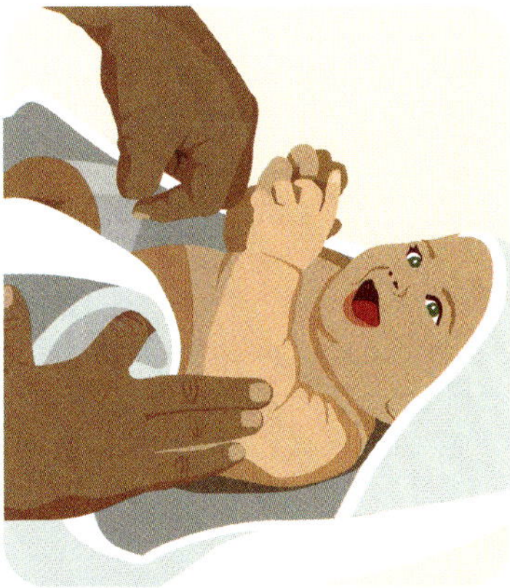

Rinsing baby's hair

When pouring water over the head to rinse, use the other hand to help keep water out of baby's eyes. If bath time is in the sink, you might want to try a football hold under the faucet for washing baby's hair. Support your baby's back with your arm, keeping a firm hold on your baby's head while you rinse.

Drying off

If your baby cries in the tub, stay calm. Try using a warm, wet washcloth over the body for warmth. If that doesn't help, clean what you can and then wrap your baby in a towel. Wait a few days and try again. In the meantime, use sponge baths where needed.

HAPPY IN THE WATER

A bit of water near your baby's eyes and ears is OK — babies can blink to protect their eyes from a little water. If you keep your baby from even the tiniest of splashes, you may end up with a baby who is fearful of water.

As your baby gets older, if bath time is enjoyable, provide extra time to play and splash around. This will help your baby have positive feelings about water and may help reduce anxiety about water later.

UMBILICAL CORD CARE

After your newborn's umbilical cord is cut, all that remains is a small stump. In most cases, the remaining cord will dry up and fall off one to three weeks after birth. Until then, you want to keep the belly area as clean and dry as possible.

Avoid swabbing the cord stump with rubbing alcohol or other antiseptic. Though this practice was recommended in the past, research indicates that doing so may prolong cord separation.

Exposing the cord to air and allowing it to dry at its base will help it naturally separate. To prevent irritation and keep the navel area dry, fold the baby's diaper below the stump. During baths, avoid submerging the belly area in water, and dry the area thoroughly if it becomes wet. In warm weather, dress a newborn in just a diaper and T-shirt to let air circulate and help the drying process.

It's OK to see a bit of crusted discharge or dried blood until the cord falls off. But if your baby's navel looks red or has a foul-smelling discharge, call your baby's healthcare professional. When the stump falls off, you may see a little blood, which is common.

Most babies have no problems with the umbilical cord. But have the area examined by your baby's healthcare professional if you notice any of the following:

- The navel continues to bleed.
- The skin around the base of the cord is red.
- There's a foul-smelling, yellowish discharge from the cord.
- Your baby cries when you touch the cord or the skin near the cord.
- The cord hasn't dried up or fallen off by the time the baby is 2 months old.

Umbilical granuloma

In some cases, the umbilical cord forms a small red mass of scar tissue (granuloma) that remains on the bellybutton even after the cord has fallen off. The granuloma usually drains a light yellow fluid. If you notice these signs, contact your baby's healthcare professional to discuss whether your baby needs to be seen. Typically, an umbilical granuloma resolves on its own after about a week. If it doesn't, your baby's healthcare professional may need to remove the tissue.

Umbilical hernia

If your baby's umbilical cord area or bellybutton protrudes or bulges when your baby cries, strains or sits up, your baby may have an umbilical hernia. In this common condition, part of the abdomen pushes through a hole in the abdominal wall when there's pressure on the area. Umbilical hernias typically resolve on their own and don't need treatment. In rare cases, a baby may need surgery to close the hole. Taping the bulge down or taping a coin over the hernia is a potentially harmful practice and should be avoided.

CIRCUMCISION CARE

If your newborn boy was circumcised, the tip of the penis may seem raw for the first week after the procedure. Or a yellowish mucus or crust may form around the area. This is a normal part of healing. A small amount of bleeding also is common the first day or two.

Clean the area around the penis gently and apply a liberal amount of petroleum jelly to the end of the penis with each diaper change. This will keep the diaper from sticking while the penis heals.

At some hospitals, a plastic ring is used instead of a bandage. The ring will remain on the end of the penis until the edge of the circumcision has healed, usually within a week. The ring will drop off on its own.

Problems after a circumcision are rare, but call your baby's healthcare professional if you notice bleeding, color change that doesn't improve or crusted sores containing fluid around the tip of the penis. Other signs to be aware of are swelling of the penis tip or a foul-smelling drainage coming from the penis tip.

Washing a circumcised penis

It's OK to gently wash the penis as it's healing. And once it's healed, the circumcised penis doesn't need special care. Wash your baby's penis with warm water and mild baby soap, just like you clean the rest of the bottom. Occasionally a small piece of foreskin remains on the penis. If this occurs, gently pull back that skin to make sure the head of the penis is clean.

Caring for an uncircumcised penis

During your baby's first few months, clean the uncircumcised penis with water and a bit of mild baby wash, just like you would clean the rest of the bottom. You don't need to use an antiseptic or cotton swabs. Don't try to pull back or retract the foreskin. Doing so can cause tearing, pain and bleeding. The foreskin will retract on its own, a process that can take months to years.

It's important to watch your uncircumcised baby urinate once in a while. If you notice the urine stream isn't stronger than a trickle, or if your baby seems uncomfortable while urinating, contact your baby's healthcare professional. It's possible that the hole in the foreskin is too small to allow a typical flow of urine.

Because the foreskin separation can take several months or longer, check with your baby's healthcare professional to find out when the separation is complete. Once it is, you can gently retract the foreskin to clean the head of the penis. Then pull the foreskin back over the penis when you're finished.

Once your baby boy is older, it's important to teach him how to properly wash the penis using these three steps:

- Gently pull the foreskin back and away from the head of the penis.
- Use warm water and soap to clean the head of the penis and the fold in the foreskin.
- Pull the foreskin back to its original place over the head of the penis.

NAIL CARE

Your baby's nails are soft, but they're sharp. Newborns can easily scratch their faces — or yours. To prevent scratches, trim or file your baby's fingernails shortly after birth. Then continue to trim your baby's nails a few times a week.

You may be able to carefully peel off the ends with your fingers because baby nails are so soft. Don't worry — you won't rip the whole nail off. You also can

NAIL TRIMMING

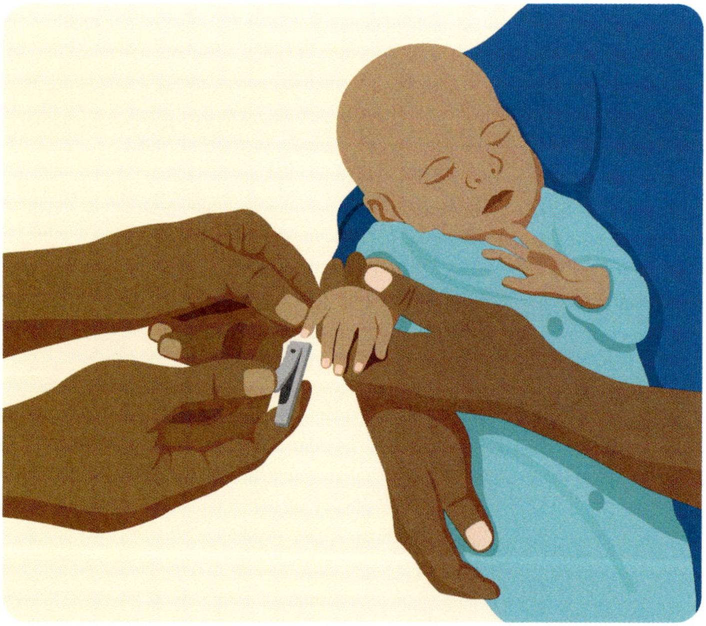

Two hints for making nail trimming easier: Wait until your baby is asleep. Then work in pairs, with one person holding the baby and the other person trimming the nails.

use baby nail clippers or small scissors. Here are some tips to make nail trimming easier for you and your baby:

- Trim the nails after a bath. They'll be softer, making them easier to cut.
- Wait until your baby is asleep.
- Have another person hold your baby while you do nail trimming.
- Trim the nails straight across.

Don't bite your baby's nails as a method of keeping them trimmed — this can cause infection.

Your baby's toenails probably will grow much more slowly than the fingernails. Toenails may need a trim only once or twice a month. Toenails also are softer than fingernails, so they may appear to be ingrown. But unless the skin around the nail looks inflamed, they're probably fine.

COMMON SKIN CONDITIONS

Many parents expect their newborn's skin to be flawless. But most babies are born with some bruising, and skin blotches and blemishes are common. Young infants often have dry, peeling skin, especially on their hands and feet, for the first few weeks. Some blueness of the hands and feet is common and may continue for a few weeks. Rashes also are common, even into the toddler years. Most rashes and skin conditions are treated easily or clear up on their own.

Milia

Milia is the name for tiny white pimples or bumps that appear on the nose, chin and cheeks. Although they appear to be raised, they are nearly flat and smooth to the touch. If your baby has milia, you can wash the face once a day with warm water and a mild baby soap. But avoid using lotion, oils or other products. It's also important to leave the skin alone — never scrub or pinch the bumps. Milia disappear in time, often within a few weeks, and they don't require treatment.

Baby acne

Baby acne (neonatal cephalic pustulosis) refers to small red and white bumps that are seen on the face, neck, upper chest and back of some newborns. The bumps are generally most noticeable within the first few weeks after birth. To care for baby acne, place a soft, clean receiving blanket under baby's head and wash the face gently once a day with mild baby soap. Avoid lotions, oils and other treatments and never scrub, squeeze or pinch the affected skin. The condition typically disappears without treatment within the first couple of months, without scarring. If it doesn't clear up after a few months, talk with your child's healthcare professional.

Erythema toxicum

Erythema toxicum is the medical term for a skin condition that's typically present at birth or appears within the first few days after birth. It's characterized by small white or yellowish bumps surrounded by pink or reddish skin. The

SKIN CONDITIONS

Milia

Many babies are born with tiny white bumps that appear on the nose, chin or cheeks. This condition, called milia, occurs when dead skin cells become trapped near the surface of the baby's skin.

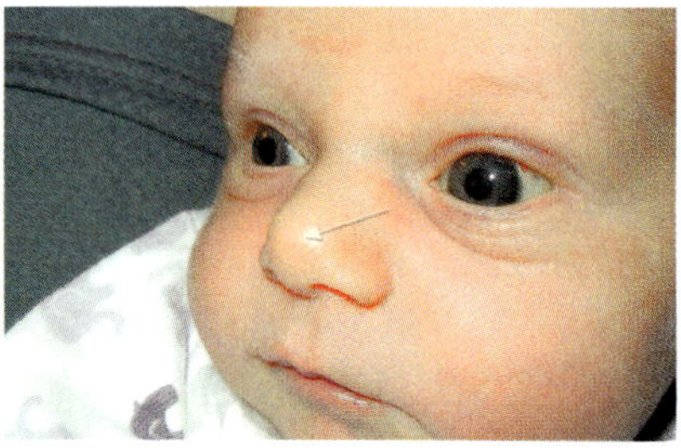

Baby acne (neonatal cephalic pustulosis)

Acne typically appears as red or white bumps on a baby's forehead or cheeks. The condition is related to a normal yeast on the skin called malassezia. It is harmless and will clear up on its own.

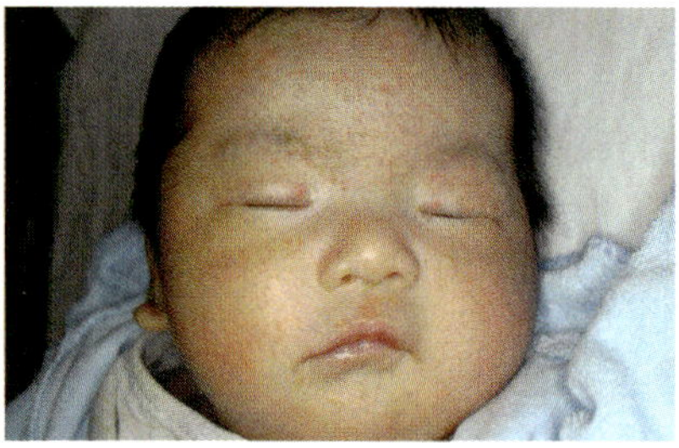

Cradle cap (infant seborrheic dermatitis)

Cradle cap appears as thick, crusty or greasy patches on a baby's scalp. Cradle cap is common in newborns and usually appears within the first few weeks after birth.

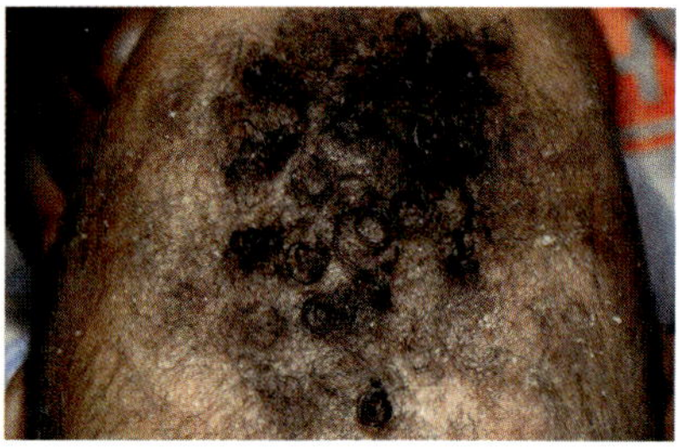

Erythema toxicum

This harmless, temporary newborn rash consists of small, yellow-to-white bumps (papules) surrounded by red skin. There may be a few or many papules.

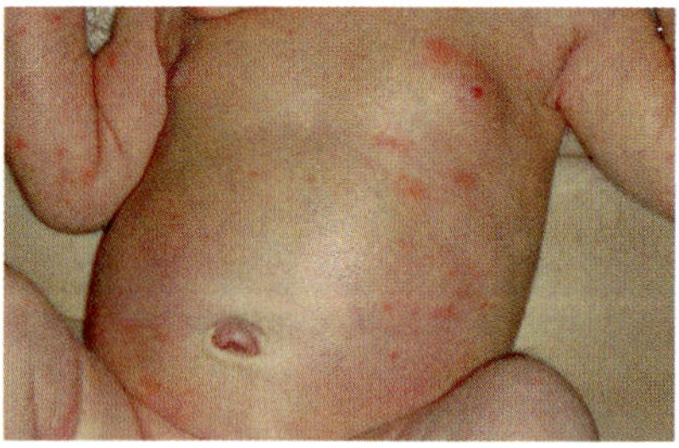

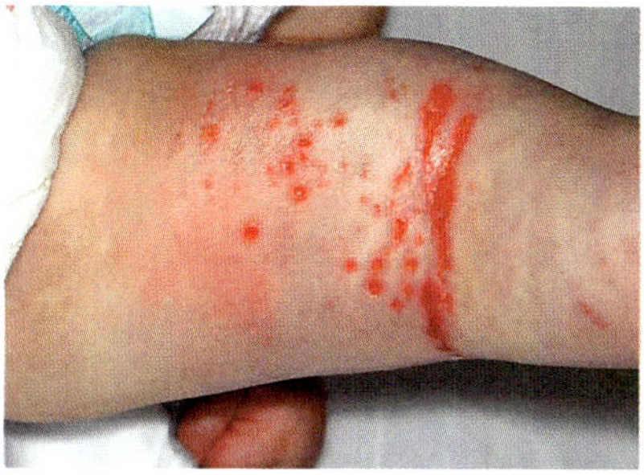

Eczema (atopic dermatitis)

Eczema is a common inflammatory condition characterized by patches of scaly, itchy skin. Occasionally the patches ooze and crust over. Eczema most often appears at the elbows and knees and on the face, arms and legs of infants and toddlers, but it can be anywhere on the body.

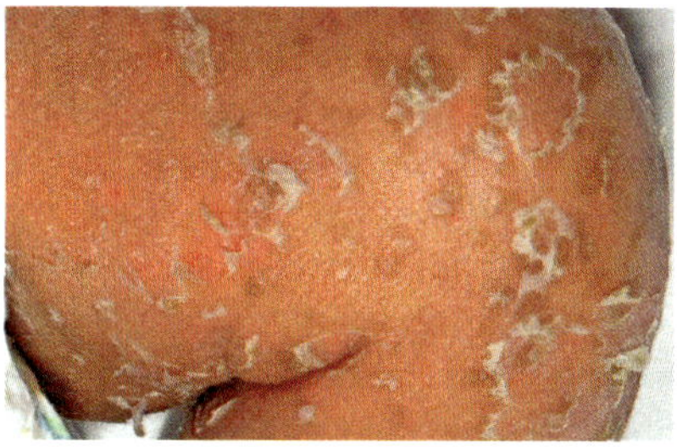

Pustular melanosis

This condition involves small blisters that resemble seeds that dry up and peel away. The blisters leave behind spots, or "freckle" marks, that disappear in weeks to months.

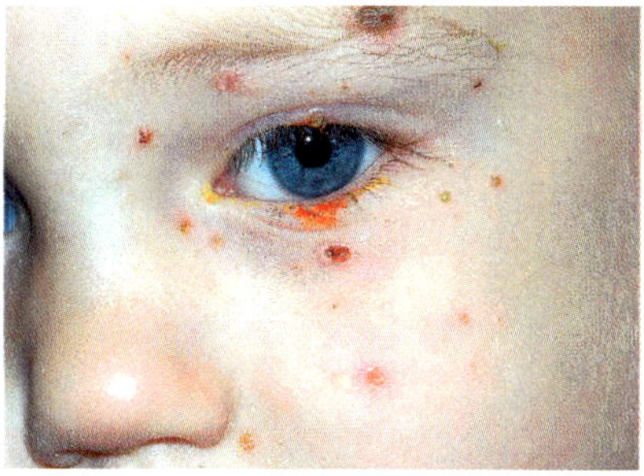

Impetigo

Impetigo is a bacterial infection that starts as a reddish sore that ruptures, oozes for a few days and then forms a honey-colored crust. Sores mainly occur around the nose and mouth and spread to other parts of the face or body.

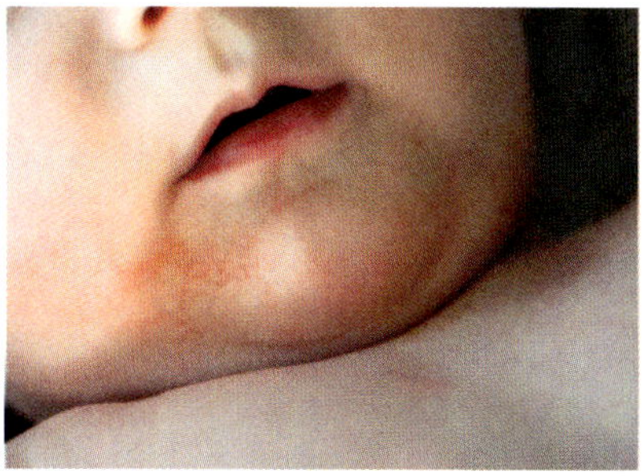

Irritant contact dermatitis (such as drool rash)

This inflammation of the skin is caused by substances, such as drool, sitting on the skin and creating irritation. The resulting rash isn't contagious but may be dry, bumpy, and itchy or uncomfortable.

condition causes no discomfort and isn't infectious. Erythema toxicum disappears in several days, although sometimes it flares and subsides before completely clearing up. Treatment isn't necessary.

Pustular melanosis

These small spots look like yellowish-white sesame seeds that quickly dry and peel off. They may look similar to skin infections (pustules), but pustular melanosis isn't an infection and disappears without treatment. The spots are commonly seen in the folds of the neck and on the shoulders and upper chest. They're more common in babies with darker skin.

Cradle cap

Cradle cap (infant seborrheic dermatitis) refers to a scaliness that develops on a baby's scalp. The cause is unknown. It may be related to overproduction of oil on the scalp. A normal skin yeast called malassezia also may play a role. Cradle cap is common in infants, usually clearing up over a period of weeks or months. It may be mild, with flaky, dry skin that looks like dandruff, or more severe, with thick, oily, yellowish scaling or crusty patches.

Shampooing with a mild baby shampoo can help with cradle cap. Don't be afraid to wash your baby's hair frequently. This, along with soft brushing, will help remove the scales. If the scales don't loosen easily, rub a few drops of mineral oil onto your baby's scalp. Let it soak into the scales for a few minutes, and then brush and shampoo your baby's hair. If you leave the oil in your baby's hair, the scales may accumulate and worsen cradle cap.

If cradle cap persists or spreads to other parts of your child's body, especially in the creases at the elbow or behind the ears, contact your baby's healthcare professional. A medicated shampoo or lotion might be recommended.

Cradle cap isn't usually uncomfortable or itchy for your baby, but sometimes a yeast infection can occur in the affected skin. In this case, the skin will become red or purplish and itchy. If you notice this, mention it to your baby's healthcare professional.

Eczema

Eczema, also known as atopic dermatitis, is marked by dry, itchy, scaly patches of skin that are often found on babies' and toddlers' faces, arms and legs. Sometimes the affected area is small and doesn't bother a baby much, and treatment isn't necessary. Many children outgrow eczema.

In other cases, eczema can cover a lot of skin and be extremely itchy and uncomfortable. In these cases, talk with your child's healthcare professional about whether treatment is needed. You also can try the following methods to prevent eczema from recurring:

- Use fragrance-free baby soaps to wash your child and use laundry detergents that are free of fragrances, dye and deodorants. Even baby soaps labeled as "mild" may have a small amount of fragrance that can irritate sensitive skin.
- Dress your little one in soft cotton clothing, and avoid synthetic fabrics and wool.

- Bathe your baby daily with water, using soap only as necessary on soiled areas.
- Use a fragrance-free moisturizer or ointment such as petroleum jelly right after patting baby dry following a bath. This helps lock moisture from the bath into baby's skin.
- Keep your child away from environmental triggers for eczema, including heat and low humidity.
- Check your child's sleeping conditions and ensure that the area is free of dust and upholstery that may contain dust mites.

Contact dermatitis and "drool rash"

Contact dermatitis is a kind of skin inflammation that occurs when substances touching your skin cause irritation or an allergic reaction. The resulting itchy, dry or bumpy rash isn't contagious or life-threatening, but it can be very uncomfortable. Culprits for young children could include soaps, laundry detergent, rough fabric or even your baby's own drool (with the resulting inflammation sometimes referred to as drool rash).

If you can find the source and keep it away from your child, the contact dermatitis should clear up. Often, using an absorbent bib and changing it frequently can help. You also can apply a barrier cream such as petroleum jelly to the area of irritation. This can prevent the rash from worsening. Contact your child's healthcare professional if the rash is severe or gets worse or if your baby's skin is oozing or extremely itchy.

Impetigo

Impetigo is a highly contagious bacterial skin infection that mainly affects infants and children (see page 441). It usually appears as reddish sores on the face, especially around a child's nose and mouth. The sores may be covered with a yellow-brown scab or crust, or grow into blisters and pimples and ooze pus. Although impetigo commonly occurs when bacteria enter the skin through cuts or insect bites, it also can develop in healthy skin.

Because impetigo can sometimes lead to complications, your child's healthcare professional may choose to treat impetigo with an antibiotic ointment or oral antibiotics.

CHAPTER 8

Sleep and sleep issues

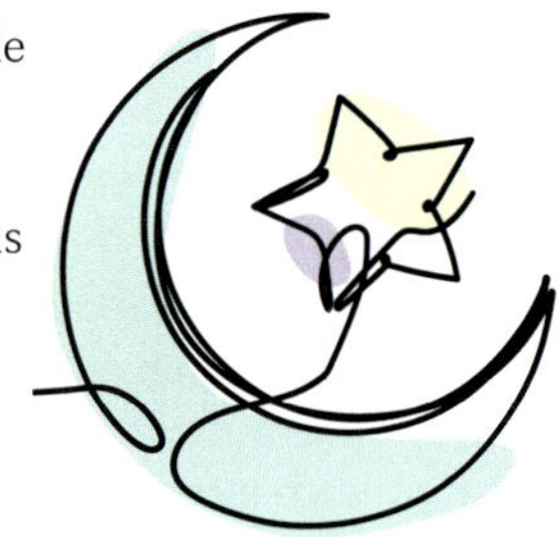

Oh, baby! There's nothing like getting a good night's sleep. While newborns usually sleep up to 16 hours a day, it's frequently for only one or two hours at a time. And as babies grow, it's common for parents to feel like the sleep pattern changes just as you've mastered the previous schedule. Once your child is a toddler, their awareness of everything going on — and the drive to test every limit — can make bedtime a challenge in new ways again.

If you haven't felt well rested since your baby was born, you're not alone. This can truly be one of the hardest parts of parenting in the first few years. But it does get better. Honestly!

Sleep is vital to your child's growth and development. From the time your baby is born, you can encourage good sleep habits. By the end of the first year, your baby likely will do most sleeping at night, usually with a nap or two during the day. These broad sleeping patterns will continue for the next few years.

Every child is different, though. Some seem to be naturally good sleepers. Others don't sleep through the night consistently until they're older.

In general, it's easier to prevent sleep problems than to fix them later. No matter how old your child is, it takes calm, consistent effort and patience to help your child develop healthy sleep habits. This chapter offers tips on sleep schedules, reviews prevention strategies to reduce the risk of sudden infant death syndrome (SIDS) and crib accidents, and outlines steps to help your toddler learn to sleep independently.

Don't beat yourself up if things don't always go as planned. Do your best and eventually everyone will be sleeping through the night.

NEWBORN SLEEP SCHEDULE

It takes a while for newborns to get on any kind of schedule for sleeping. During the first month, they usually sleep and wake around the clock, with relatively equal periods of sleep between feedings.

In addition, newborns don't know the difference between night and day. It takes time for them to develop circadian rhythms — the sleep-wake cycles and other patterns that occur on a 24-hour cycle. As your baby's nervous system gradually matures, so do the phases of sleep and wakefulness.

Fits and spurts

Newborns typically sleep 12 to 16 hours a day, for a few hours or less at a stretch. They may stay awake long enough to feed, or for up to about two hours, before falling asleep again. During the first few days home from the hospital, don't be surprised if you feel exhausted — especially if you're the one who gave birth. Caring for a new baby is nonstop, and you're now adjusting to being up frequently at night.

By the time your baby is 2 weeks old, you'll likely notice that the periods of sleeping and wakefulness are getting longer. By age 3 to 4 months, some babies sleep at least five hours at a time and shift more of their sleep to nighttime. (Hang in there!) By age 6 months, nighttime stretches of nine or more hours are possible for most babies.

NOISY BREATHING

The familiar phrase "sleeping like a baby" conjures up images of a baby lying quietly and breathing ever so softly. But babies — especially newborns — often aren't quiet when they sleep.

Newborns spend about half their time in an active phase of sleep, called rapid eye movement (REM) sleep. During REM sleep, babies may breathe irregularly, grunt and twitch. During deeper sleep, called non-rapid eye movement (NREM) sleep, babies typically sleep more peacefully. As babies get older, they spend more time in NREM sleep and less time in active sleep. So they generally become less noisy.

In addition, newborns are dominantly nose breathers — they breathe through their noses, not their mouths. This is so they can breathe at the same time they nurse. The slightest congestion or mucus in baby's tiny nasal passages as air flows in and out can make a lot of noise. If your baby's breathing sounds a bit stuffy, it might not be due to a cold or allergies.

Noisy breathing in infants can be very worrisome for parents. The noise alone isn't usually a cause for concern. However, if you're concerned that something isn't right, contact your child's medical professional.

Many newborns nap frequently in one-to-two-hour spurts. As baby gets older, nap times may lengthen and become more predictable. With some babies, though, napping remains random, and they never fall into any type of pattern.

Around age 3 months, you may find that your baby falls into a three-naps-a-day schedule: a morning nap, an early afternoon nap and an early evening nap. However, this also varies considerably with each baby.

Syncing days and nights

Some new babies sleep more in the daytime than at night. For parents who are sleep deprived, this can be a stressful time. Generally, though, within a few weeks to a couple of months, days and nights will become more predictable and regular.

One way to help speed up this transition is to limit daytime naps to no more than three or four hours each. In addition, during the day, have baby sleep in a more active area of the house with the lights on and where noises can be heard. In contrast, at night, keep the bedroom dark and quiet.

During nighttime feedings and diaper changes, avoid stimulation. Keep the lights low, use a soft voice, and don't play or talk with your baby. This reinforces the message that nighttime is for sleeping.

SLEEP SAFETY

Sudden infant death syndrome (SIDS) is the unexplained death, usually during sleep, of a seemingly healthy baby. Although the exact cause is still unknown, it appears that sudden infant death syndrome may be associated with problems in the portion of an infant's brain that controls breathing and waking up from

A SAFE SLEEP ENVIRONMENT FOR YOUR BABY

To keep your baby safe during sleep, follow these recommendations from the American Academy of Pediatrics:

- Place your baby on the back to sleep every time.
- Use a firm sleep surface.
- Breastfeed while you can.
- Share your room with your baby, but sleep on separate surfaces.
- Remove soft objects and loose bedding from your baby's sleep area.
- Consider using a pacifier during sleep time.
- Avoid exposing your baby to secondhand smoke, and avoid using alcohol and illicit drugs.
- Avoid sleep situations in which the baby might become overheated.
- Vaccinate your baby.

sleep. Other risk factors include sleeping on the stomach or side, sleeping on a soft surface, bulky bedding or sleeping with parents in the same bed.

SIDS is a scary thing to think about, but there are multiple ways to help reduce your baby's risk of SIDS and put your baby safely to sleep.

"Back" to sleep

Always place your baby to sleep on their back, even for naps. This is the safest sleep position for reducing the risk of SIDS.

Research shows that babies who are put to sleep on their stomachs are much more likely to die of SIDS than babies placed on their backs. Infants who sleep on their sides also are at increased risk, probably because babies in this position can roll onto their stomachs. Since 1992, when the American Academy of Pediatrics (AAP) began recommending the back-sleeping position for infants, the incidence of SIDS in the United States has declined significantly.

The only exceptions to the back sleeping rule are babies who have health problems that require them to sleep on their stomachs because the risk of death is greater if they sleep on their backs. If your baby was born with a birth defect or has a breathing, lung or heart problem, talk to your baby's medical professional about the best sleeping position for your child.

Make sure that everyone who takes care of your baby knows to place baby to sleep on the back. That may include grandparents, child care providers, babysitters, friends and others. Be firm in your instructions. Placing babies on their backs to sleep is based on strong evidence that doing so saves infant lives.

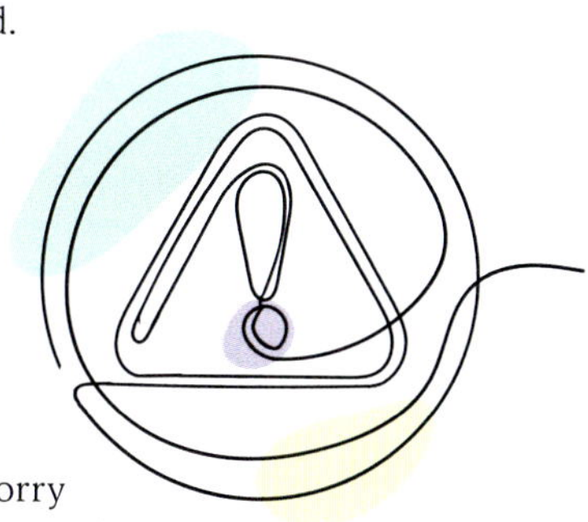

Some babies don't like sleeping on their backs at first, but they get used to it quickly. Many parents worry that their baby will choke if he or she spits up or vomits while sleeping on the back, but researchers have found no increase in choking or similar problems.

A baby who sleeps on the back may develop a flat spot on the back of the head. For the most part, this will improve as your baby spends more time on the tummy and seated. You can help keep your baby's head a typical shape by alternating the direction your baby lies in the crib — head toward one end of the crib for a few nights and then toward the other. This way, the baby won't always sleep on the same side of the head. Frequent tummy time while awake helps, too.

Once baby can successfully roll over from back to stomach and then back again — typically around age 6 months — you can let baby choose the sleep position. Until your baby is at least 12 months old and can move around with no help, keep your baby's bassinet or crib free of loose bedding or stuffed animals. This is to prevent your baby from rolling into them and being unable to roll out.

Share the room, not the bed

Many new parents are tempted to take their baby into bed with them. Often this is because they're tired — understandably so! — and because having baby in bed seems more convenient. For some parents, this is what their parents and grandparents did before them.

But the truth is that bed sharing can increase the risk of harm to your baby. Adult beds generally have softer mattresses than cribs and have lots of blankets and pillows. Though comfortable for adults, these factors can interfere with baby's breathing or make a baby overly warm. In addition, there's a risk of the adult inadvertently rolling over onto the baby during sleep or pushing the baby into bedding and causing suffocation. Falling asleep with your baby on a couch or chair can be even more dangerous because of the cramped quarters.

In addition, if your child learns to sleep well in your bed, it can make transitioning to a separate bed later more difficult and traumatic. As your child gets older, it can be harder to break a bed sharing habit.

Instead of bed sharing, the AAP recommends room sharing during your baby's first year. Rates of SIDS and other sleep-related deaths are highest during the first 4 months of life and decrease after 8 months of age. Room sharing means your baby sleeps in your room with you but in a separate bassinet, crib or other structure designed for infant sleep. Having your baby nearby can put your mind at rest and make it easier to monitor your baby. Evidence suggests that sharing a room with your baby, but not the bed, can decrease your baby's risk of SIDS by as much as half.

A safe sleep space

Make sure your baby is comfortable and safe. If you've made sure the crib and area around it are safe, you won't immediately become concerned about your baby's safety if you hear cries. Follow these safety guidelines.

Avoid old cribs or bassinets Even if an old crib is in good shape, safety standards have improved over the years. It's generally a good idea to buy a new crib if you can; if you do use a hand-me-down crib, make sure that it meets current safety standards. Older cribs with drop sides — the kind that have a side rail that moves up and down — are not considered safe. In addition, some older cribs may have been coated with lead paint, which is a health hazard. A crib should be the one place you feel comfortable leaving your child alone.

Check the slat spacing The crib's slats should be no farther apart than 2 3/8 inches. This applies to bassinets, too. If you can fit a can of soda through the slats, the openings are too large. You're more likely to find this problem in older cribs, but you can't be too safe when it comes to your baby. Check any crib you put your baby in.

Get the right mattress The surface of your baby's mattress should be firm, flat and smooth. Make sure the mattress fits snugly within the frame of the product it's made for, so there's no space for your baby to get trapped.

Remove extraneous items During the first year — or at least until your baby can easily move around the crib without help — remove any extra bedding from the sleep space, such as bumper pads, pillows, cushions and comforters. This prevents your baby from rolling into a potentially suffocating situation. To keep your baby warm, try a sleep sack or other sleep clothing that doesn't require additional covers. Save toys and stuffed animals for when your baby is awake and supervised.

Remove crib mobiles early Crib mobiles typically include string and small attached pieces. Make sure your little one can't reach the mobile and become entangled or pull anything off. When your baby is able to push up on hands and knees, the mobile should be removed from the crib.

Pajama safety

During hot summer months, a sleeper or gown may be all your baby needs while sleeping. During the colder winter months, you may want to put baby in a heavier blanket sleeper over pajamas. However, don't purchase oversized pajamas, regardless of how comfortable you think they might look. If the pajama top rides up on the neck and head or is too loose around the shoulders, the extra space between the material and baby's skin may increase the risk of suffocation.

Some pajamas are made with chemically treated fabric that makes them flame resistant and can help prevent burn injuries in the case of a fire. If you're concerned about these chemicals in your baby's clothes, you can opt instead for snug-fitting pajamas — the kind that taper down from the shoulders to the ends of the sleeves and from the thighs to the hems of pant legs. Tight-fitting sleepwear is less likely to catch fire than the loose-fitting kind. Most importantly, take appropriate fire prevention measures, such as installing smoke detectors in your home, not smoking and not leaving an open flame unattended.

Safe swaddling

Many young babies fall asleep and sleep better when swaddled. If you swaddle your baby, use a breathable 100% cotton blanket or a swaddling sleep sack. A blanket is breathable when you can hold one layer of the blanket up to your mouth and your breath can easily pass through the fabric. This is the best option for a baby because the baby can still breathe if the fabric slips and covers the face. Cotton also allows body heat to escape, which prevents overheating.

When swaddling your baby, make sure to allow room for the hips and legs to move freely. If you wrap your baby too tightly around the hips and legs, it can interfere with proper growth and joint development. Your baby's legs should be able to bend up and out into a frog leg position.

It's time to stop swaddling when your baby first shows signs of rolling over, generally around 4 months. Ideally, babies need to be able to control their arms when rolling. But they can't do that when swaddled.

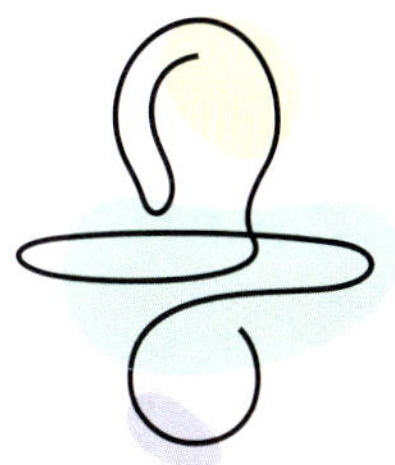

Try a pacifier

Sucking on a pacifier at nap time and bedtime may reduce the risk of SIDS. If you're breastfeeding, you may want to wait to offer a pacifier until you and your baby have settled into a nursing routine. For some babies, this takes 3 to 4 weeks. Some babies have no difficulty breastfeeding despite using a pacifier soon after they are born. If your baby isn't interested in the pacifier, don't force it. Try again another day. If the pacifier falls out of your baby's mouth while baby is sleeping, there's no need to pop it back in.

Smart monitors

Baby monitors have become a nearly standard tool to help parents hear a baby crying and to look in on them while in their crib. Thanks to technology, monitor options now go far beyond audio and video. A growing number of "smart" devices are designed to monitor babies while in the crib. You can find cameras and wearable devices that sense your baby's temperature, as well as mattresses and wearables that track breathing oxygen levels, heart rate, and more.

As a new parent, it's tempting to think that more information about your baby is always better. But you don't need smart monitors to help your baby sleep safely. For healthy full-term infants, the American Academy of Pediatrics (AAP) discourages the use of these smart monitors and other devices marketed for SIDS prevention. They do not prevent SIDS and should not be used in place of safe sleep practices. In addition, they can be overly sensitive or even incorrect, leading to excessive alarms that can further disrupt sleep for parents and babies.

GOOD SLEEP HABITS

A question that new parents often get from friends and family is "Is your baby sleeping through the night yet?" But honestly, no one "sleeps through the night." Everyone experiences nighttime arousals, but most of the time people go right back to sleep after these brief awakenings.

Babies have the same nighttime arousals. In the first few months, a number of biological factors impact these awakenings. For example, new babies need to feed every few hours — including at nighttime. Although their stomachs are tiny, they're growing fast and they need frequent feedings to sustain their growth and development.

MAKE TIME FOR TUMMY TIME

Just because your baby should sleep on the back doesn't mean they should never spend any time on the tummy. Being on the tummy is good for babies. It prepares them for the time when they'll be able to slide on their bellies and crawl by encouraging them to lift their heads and build strong head, neck and shoulder muscles. As babies grow older and stronger, they'll need more time on their tummies to build their strength.

While baby is awake and being supervised, place your baby on the floor on the tummy. Place yourself or a toy on the floor for baby to look at or play with. Another option is to lay your baby tummy-down on your tummy or on your lap.

As babies get older, they're able to take in larger amounts of calories during the day and require fewer feedings at night. At the same time, their biological rhythms are getting used to day and night cycles. By 4 to 6 months, their sleep patterns are becoming more and more like those of adults.

During this process of getting used to the "real world," babies are learning many things based on the repetition of patterns. Examples include making connections between the sound of your voice and loving attention or the smell of breast milk or a fresh bottle and the satisfaction of being fed. Likewise, your baby also is developing associations with falling asleep. Maybe every time you nurse or give a bottle, your baby falls asleep. Or you snuggle together in a chair until your baby falls asleep. Or you rock your baby to sleep.

There's no denying that having your baby fall asleep on your chest can be deeply fulfilling. But if this happens every time your child falls asleep, it can become a condition your child needs to fall asleep. So at 6 months, when your baby wakes at night, they need to be against your chest to feel "right" about falling back to sleep. This is called a sleep association.

You can help create positive sleep associations that allow your baby to fall asleep without your help. This is called self-soothing — a skill that can be especially useful in the middle of the night! Here are steps you can take that have proved to help babies and toddlers get a good night's rest.

Develop a bedtime routine

Bedtime routines, which can start in the early months, become very important to a child by age 1. A winding down of the day's activities signals that it's time for bed. Your routine could include soothing activities such as having a bath, reading or making up stories, and a good-night hug or kiss. Avoid watching TV or using electronic devices with your baby before bed, as these activities can be overly stimulating. Finish the bedtime routine before your child falls asleep. The whole process might last 20 minutes.

Establish a consistent bedtime. The more consistent you can be with when you begin and end your bedtime routine — and all the steps in between — the easier it will be for you and your child. Children thrive on structure, so it's OK to do the same thing every night.

Consider a rule — for yourself and your child — that your child should not leave the crib at night unless it's for a feeding or a diaper change. After age 2, a healthy child doesn't need to leave the bedroom on a typical night except to go to the bathroom.

Allow self-soothing

Drooping eyelids, rubbing the eyes and fussiness are the usual signs that a baby is tired. When you notice these signs, put your baby in the crib while drowsy but still awake. If your baby can fall asleep in bed without assistance when first laid down, it's more likely that baby will fall asleep without help after waking in the middle of the night.

It's common for babies to cry when put down for sleep. But if left alone for a few minutes, most will eventually quiet themselves. If you leave the room for a while, your baby will probably stop crying after a short time. If not, try providing comfort and allowing time for baby to settle again.

During sleep, babies are often active, twitching their arms and legs, smiling, sucking, and generally appearing restless. And while sleeping, infants may cry and move about when entering different sleep cycles. Parents sometimes mistake a baby's stirrings as a sign of waking up, and they begin unnecessary feeding. Instead, wait a few moments to see if your baby settles back to sleep.

Adopt a security object

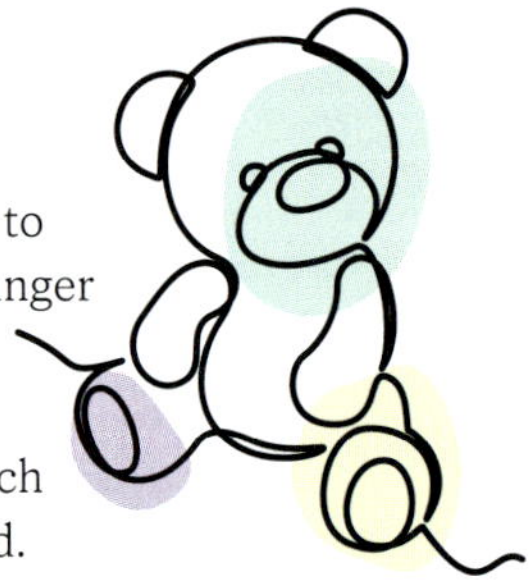

After age 1 or so, your baby has likely developed enough motor skills to have a small blanket or stuffed animal nearby at night without the danger of suffocation. A favorite teddy bear or other safe object can help comfort and soothe your child when you're not present. Offer a simple, breathable blanket. Choose soft toys without decorations, such as buttons or ribbons, that might come off and pose a choking hazard.

Pay attention to naps

Naps are just as important to young children as a good night of sleep. Napping helps your baby get the total amount of sleep needed and prevents exhaustion before bedtime. At nap time, you can use some of the same steps you use for your bedtime routine. For example, read a story, tuck your child in and leave the room. Allow a few minutes for your child to settle and fall asleep.

Some babies sleep for a long time at night but take fewer naps during the day. Other babies take more but shorter naps during the day. If your baby sleeps well at night, it's fine to allow napping for as long as desired. If your baby isn't sleeping at night for as long as you wish, it may help to shorten the nap time. Or if baby takes three naps a day, try to change the habit to two naps a day. Most children between the ages of 12 and 18 months shift to taking one midday or afternoon nap a day. As early as age 3 years, many children drop naps entirely, and most do so by age 5.

Transition to separate bedrooms

As babies grow into toddlers, parents and kids often find that both parties sleep better if they're in separate rooms. If you've had your child sleeping in your bedroom for the first six months to a year, you might be ready to transition your child to a separate bedroom. Here are some suggestions to make this change easier.

Start with naps. Place your child in their bedroom at each nap time. Close the child's bedroom door when you leave the room. This keeps most household noise out of the room so that your child can sleep better. Using a monitor can help you hear or see how your child is doing.

After a week or two of successful napping in the child's own room, begin to put your child to bed at night in the bedroom. If your child is older than a year, make it a grand occasion. Tell the child, "Starting tonight, you get to stay in your own room during the night. You're old enough to do that now!" Kids are usually very happy to "grow up." Let your child choose which blanket or stuffed animal to use on the bed.

Give a small reward if needed when a toddler or older child has stayed in the room overnight. Some examples are reading a new book together, going to the park, or doing a puzzle or game together. Try to avoid using sweets or extra treats as a reward. Tell your child the reason for the reward.

Drop a nap as needed

A nap — or two or three — is a crucial part of your child's day. Frequently, it may be the only thing standing between your child and a full-blown tantrum. And there's evidence to suggest that a nice long nap can improve a child's attention span and ability to learn. But as kids grow, they need less sleep during

TOTAL SLEEP NEEDS: NIGHTTIME + NAPS

The chart below provides general sleep and nap guidance to help you prepare for your child's changing sleep requirements.

Age	Total sleep per 24 hours
Newborns to 4 months	About 16 hours, in the form of sleep periods up to 4 hours, spaced between feedings. Starting a regular nap schedule at this age is difficult because the biological rhythms that control sleep are still maturing.
4 months to 12 months	12 to 16 hours, including at least two naps, usually once in the morning and once in the early afternoon. Some babies take a third nap in the late afternoon, which should be stopped around age 9 months to prepare for an earlier bedtime.
1 to 2 years	11 to 14 hours. Your toddler has probably dropped the morning nap by now, and afternoon naps are typically one to two hours.
3 years	10 to 13 hours. Afternoon naps tend to shorten; some toddlers may stop napping altogether.

the day, and getting too much can affect bedtime. So how many naps are enough?

First things first: Don't panic if your baby or toddler doesn't follow the guidelines exactly for typical nap schedules. Napping, like everything in the first few years, is different from child to child. While one child may go down easily for a nap, another may fight daytime sleeping with every ounce of energy.

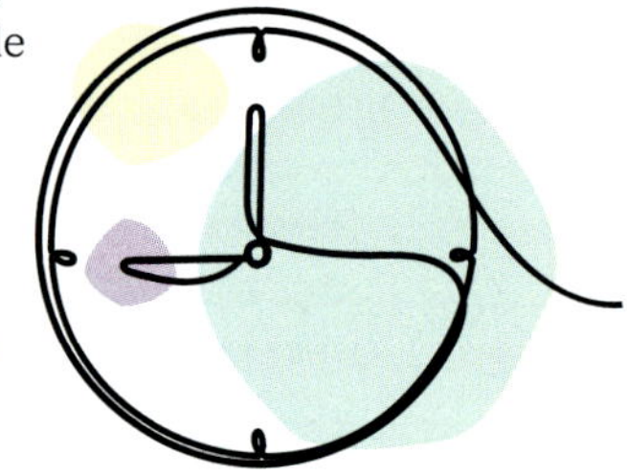

Nap schedules can be influenced by a parent's work schedule, whether the child attends day care and a range of other factors. Sometimes events, such as a family vacation, will temporarily interrupt nap times. Though it may involve some trial and error — and perhaps many tears — children will eventually find the best nap schedule for their needs. A good rule of thumb: A nap should be long enough to be restorative, whatever that may be for your child.

Around age 2, naps start to become less necessary, though the age where naps are phased out varies significantly by child. Eventually children phase out the morning nap, followed by an end to napping entirely. This is OK, provided a child seems rested without the nap and is getting enough sleep at night. Some children go through phases and will try to resist nap time, even though they still need it. In this case, you can try adjusting bedtime earlier or later and see if that helps with naps the next day.

If your toddler is giving up the last remaining daily nap time, you can help ease this transition period by providing a regularly scheduled quiet time to look at picture books or listen to soothing music to help relax. This can be an independent time for your child, as long as they are in a safe space. You can also move bedtime up to help compensate for less daytime sleep. Nighttime sleep will become even more crucial as your child becomes more active and naps less.

Switch from crib to bed

It's time to switch from a crib to a bed when your child learns how to climb out of a crib with the mattress at its lowest setting. This is usually around age 2 or 3. If you keep your child in the crib and the child falls while climbing out, your child could be injured.

Some cribs convert to a toddler bed. Other parents choose to switch to a new, different toddler bed or a bed they think their child can grow into. For example, some toddler beds are designed to adjust in length or width as your child grows. But you also can put a mattress on the floor until you decide on a more permanent arrangement.

TROUBLESHOOTING

Establishing healthy sleeping habits for everyone in the family is often easier said than done. All babies sleep through the night eventually, but each one reaches this milestone at a different time. Try to be patient. In the meantime, expect some trial and error and nights of interrupted sleep because of teething, illness and other disruptions. As your toddler approaches preschool age, they may even experience growing pains — an aching or throbbing feeling in the legs that can wake a child.

There are no hard-and-fast rules for getting your child to sleep consistently through the night, but here are some suggestions that might help.

Phasing out nighttime feedings

It's common for young babies to wake at night to feed. But by about 6 months of age, many babies can sleep five to eight hours or more without a feeding. By this age, babies should be able to get enough calories during the day so that they don't need nighttime feedings.

If your child is 6 months old and cries one or more times a night to be fed, try these suggestions:

- Try to dissociate nursing or bottle-feeding from falling asleep. You might feed your baby an hour or so before bedtime, and do it in a room separate from the bedroom. After feeding your baby, go through your regular bedtime routine, such as reading or singing, at your chosen bedtime. Do this even if it feels a little contrived. Put your baby to bed drowsy but still awake. If your baby needs to suck on something to go to sleep, offer a pacifier.
- Increase the volume of feedings during the day and try to increase the spacing of feedings, too. If your baby consumes small volumes frequently throughout the day, your baby will be used to that feeding pattern. This may lead to your child waking up hungry during the night.

Reducing nighttime waking

If your child is older than about 6 months and repeatedly wakes during the night crying for attention, you can help your child learn to self-soothe. But it does require patience and consistency. If your child is sick or going through a transition, such as attending a new child care center, it may not be a good time to teach self-soothing. When you're ready, here's what to do.

First, be sure your child's basic needs have been met, such as feeding, appropriate clothing, and a dry diaper or a trip to the toilet. Go through your usual bedtime routine.

If your child cries when you leave, wait a few minutes before you decide to go back into the room. Stay out of sight meanwhile.

If your child is still crying after several minutes, go into the room but don't turn on the lights. Comfort your child with a soothing pat or two and a few loving words. But avoid picking up your child. Then say, "It's time to go to sleep now" and leave the room. You should be in the room no more than a minute or two. Don't be surprised if your child cries louder as you leave; this is to be expected.

Wait again, increasing the length of your wait by a few minutes before going back in. Repeat this process, increasing the wait each time. When your child falls asleep, make a note of the last time frame you waited before you entered the room — for example, five minutes.

The next night, if your child cries, repeat the entire process. Start with the last wait from the previous night — five minutes in the preceding example — and go from there. Over the next few days, repeat the process. It may take several nights, but your child will gradually learn to self-soothe.

While it can be difficult to hear your child cry, research has shown that children who learn to self-soothe this way have no more stress or emotional or behavioral problems than others. Their attachment with parents also is just as secure. Learning to self-soothe and fall asleep independently is an important and positive development that will serve your child and your family well in years to come!

If you've tried this method and night waking still isn't improving after about a week, talk with your child's medical professional.

Staying in bed

Toddlers may have a hard time staying in bed even after going through their usual sleep routine. There are just so many interesting and exciting things to do and see! This can be especially true when your child has just learned a new skill or is at a developmental turning point. Some toddlers get upset when it's time to sleep. They may refuse to lie down. Generally, it's best to ignore these protests, as well as any other questions or demands, and leave the room.

Stick to the rule that your child should stay in bed after being tucked in. Once your child starts potty training, you can make an exception for going to the bathroom, of course. If your child leaves the bedroom, calmly tell your child, "You need to go back to your own bed now."

If your child won't do as you directed, walk alongside the child with a hand placed gently on the shoulder. If your child refuses to go to the bedroom, carry the child back to the room without saying anything. Avoid showing frustration or anger. Place your child in the bed and walk away. Close the door to the bedroom.

If your child doesn't know when it's morning and gets up before you do, try using a "good morning light." This is a night-light with a timer. You can set the light to turn on or change colors when you want your child to wake. Explain that your child can get out of bed when the light changes from red to green or when the light turns on.

If you follow these suggestions every time, after just a few days your child will learn that delaying bedtime doesn't lead to more "fun" or extra playtime.

Lastly, being consistent doesn't mean being inflexible. If your child is sick, has had a nightmare or is truly afraid for some reason, spend some time with your child to provide a sense of security.

Sleep terrors

The aptly named sleep terrors can be extremely upsetting to see. One minute, your toddler is sleeping peacefully. The next, your child is sitting up, screaming and sobbing for a solid 10 minutes. No amount of soothing works, either. In fact, your attempts to comfort only seem to increase the crying and yelling. After what seems like an eternity, your little one finally settles down and goes back to sleep.

This scenario is typical of sleep terrors. Sleep terrors occur one to three hours after falling asleep or when the sleep cycle shifts from deeper to lighter sleep. Children may seem fully awake while having a sleep terror, but they're not. And most won't remember the incident the following day.

More than a third of young children experience sleep terrors. They may occur as infrequently as one to two times a month or as regularly as a few times a week. Extreme tiredness, sleep schedule changes and fevers can trigger sleep terrors. Also, if you or anyone else in your family had sleep terrors, your toddler is likelier to have them, too.

If sleep terrors occur once or twice a month, it's worth mentioning to your child's healthcare provider. Infrequent incidents typically don't need treatment, and many children outgrow them in childhood. But it's an excellent opportunity to discuss with the provider how to ensure your child gets the recommended amount of sleep, including naps.

MELATONIN

Melatonin is a natural hormone the brain produces that uses darkness to help the human body regulate sleep-wake timing. Usually the darkness of your toddler's bedroom would trigger melatonin production, signaling to the body it's time to go to sleep. On the other hand, sunlight streaming into your child's bedroom — or light from a screen — suppresses melatonin, telling the body it's time to be awake.

Of course, some children seem to struggle with sleep no matter the conditions, making melatonin supplements a tempting sleep aid to try.

But there are caveats. Although melatonin can help children fall asleep, it won't necessarily help them stay asleep. And if your child is prone to nightmares, melatonin may make these more vivid and lead to poorer-quality sleep.

In addition, the safety and possible long-term effects of using melatonin in young children aren't yet demonstrated by scientific studies. While research has established that melatonin is generally safe for short-term use in adolescents and adults, little research has been conducted on its safety in children. Complicating this is that over-the-counter melatonin is not FDA regulated, and the amount of melatonin in a supplement can vary widely, especially in chewable products. Additionally, some products even contain chemicals that should be consumed only with a medical prescription.

Because of this, experts recommend that you consult with your toddler's healthcare professional to determine if taking melatonin is a good choice. In many cases, focusing on improving sleep habits can work better than a supplement. In certain children, melatonin may be of benefit, including those with autism spectrum disorder or developmental differences.

If you decide to use melatonin, your child's healthcare professional can recommend a product, an appropriate dosage and when to take it.

Depending on your situation, you may also consider scheduled awakenings. Note when your toddler tends to have sleep terrors. Then plan a wake-up for 15 to 20 minutes before this, providing comfort afterward as you usually would to encourage falling back to sleep. This preventive measure can shift the sleep cycle and stop the sleep terrors from occurring.

If your toddler tends to get up during sleep terrors and can get out of bed, you'll need to take steps to ensure a safe home environment. This can include measures such as clearing the bedroom of objects that could be tripped over and securing doors and windows so that your child can't leave the house during an episode.

If your toddler's sleep terrors or other nighttime awakenings occur more frequently or are severe, an evaluation is needed. In addition to possible sleep issues, a health condition such as obstructive sleep apnea, restless legs syndrome or medication can trigger sleep disturbances.

CHAPTER 9

Comforting a crying baby

The dream: Your baby starts sleeping through the night just a few weeks after birth, gurgles happily while you run errands and only fusses when hunger strikes. The reality: Your baby's favorite playtime is after a 2 a.m. feeding, and crankiness peaks whenever you're out and about.

Babies cry. The average newborn cries 1 to 4 hours a day — and for lots of reasons. Babies cry because they're tired, hungry, lonely, too hot or too cold, or simply because it's that time of day. All this crying can be particularly baffling for first-time parents. You might think you should know what your screaming bundle of joy is trying to tell you — and be able to do something, quickly! But it's not always easy to figure out why your baby is crying and what to do about it. It takes time and experience to learn to read your baby's cues.

Don't take the tears personally. If your baby's crying is causing you stress or anxiety, take a deep breath and try to relax. Ask for help if you feel you need it, and remember this stage won't last forever. Crying usually peaks around six weeks or so and then gradually decreases. So hang in there!

WHY BABIES CRY

Babies typically cry to tell you something. Crying is how babies communicate that they are hungry, tired, uncomfortable or overstimulated.

In general, it's best to respond quickly to your child's cries — especially when your child is a newborn. Don't be afraid that you'll spoil your baby by giving too much attention. Just the opposite: Studies show that being responsive to a child's needs might lessen crying overall and reduce aggressive behavior in toddlers.

Here are some of the more common reasons babies cry.

Hunger

Most newborns eat every few hours round the clock and usually wake for feedings during the night. Quiet babies may squirm and root around or fuss gently when they're hungry. More active babies can become almost frantic when hunger strikes. They may get so worked up by the time feeding begins that they gulp air with the milk. This can cause spitting up, trapped gas and more crying. Some babies are intensely bothered by having air in their stomachs, while for others it isn't as much of a problem.

Discomfort

Babies may feel uncomfortable for many reasons. A common cause of baby discomfort is a wet or soiled diaper. Some babies don't mind it. Other babies do, and they'll let you know right away that they're unhappy. Tummy troubles such as gas and indigestion are another common source of discomfort. If your baby fusses after being fed, it could be due to tummy pain. Often the crying will stop after a burp or the passing of gas. Temperature — if baby is too hot or too cold — can be another reason for fussing. So can tight, binding or itchy clothing. Make sure the waistband around baby's stomach isn't too tight, the collar doesn't rub on baby's face, and the legs or sleeves don't pull when baby moves.

Loneliness, boredom or fear

Sometimes babies cry because they're lonely or bored, or because they're frightened. Your baby may calm down simply by seeing or hearing you, feeling your touch, or being cuddled. Babies like to be held. They like to see and hear their parents and listen to the sound of their parents' heartbeats.

Overtiredness or overstimulation

When a baby is overtired or overly stimulated, crying becomes a way to unwind or release tension. (This may be true for adults, too!) Tired babies generally fuss. And you may find that your baby needs more sleep than you think. Newborns often sleep for 16 hours a day. Too much noise, movement or visual stimulation also might drive your baby to tears. In addition, many babies have predictable periods of fussiness. They cry at certain periods of the day and often for no apparent reason.

UNDERSTANDING BABY'S CRIES

Many new parents find that as they get to know their child's developing personality, they understand what different cries mean. You'll likely find the same to be true. In the meantime, here are a few clues that may help if you can't figure out what your little one is trying to tell you.

- A hungry cry might be short and low-pitched.
- A cry of pain might be a sudden, long, high-pitched shriek.
- If your baby is making lip movements or rooting, hunger might be the problem.

- Rubbing the eyes might be a sign that baby is tired.
- If your baby cries after hearing a loud noise, it could be because your baby was startled.

Picking up on patterns can help you better respond to your baby. Getting to know your child's crying triggers also can help you notice unusual distress — when baby is crying about something other than the typical reasons.

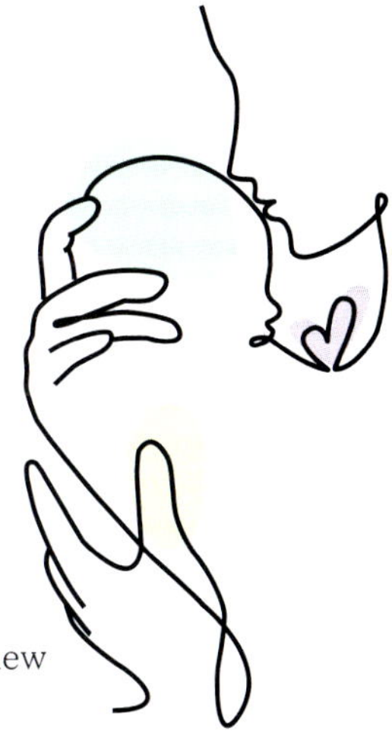

COMFORTING STRATEGIES

When your baby is crying, what do you do? Sometimes the cause is obvious, and you can quickly fix the situation. In other cases, you may have to experiment with calming techniques until you find out what brings comfort to your baby. It's often more art than science. What works for one baby doesn't always work for another (or for the same baby on a different day).

Check baby's diaper

Check your baby's diaper to make sure it's clean and dry. A new diaper may be the answer to the problem.

See if baby is hungry

A hungry baby likely will stop crying when you offer the breast or a bottle, or even a clean finger. Keep in mind, however, that crying is a late sign of hunger that can interfere with feeding. You might need to calm your baby before starting the feeding. To avoid this situation, try to respond to early signs of hunger, such as lip smacking, rooting, disgusted looks or fussing. If your baby begins to gulp during the feeding, take a break. During and after each feeding, burp your baby.

Look for signs of discomfort

Feel your baby's hands and feet. If baby seems too hot or too cold, remove or add a layer of clothing. You also might remove clothing to see if tight elastic or irritating material might be the cause of the tears. If air or gas is the problem, burp baby or gently massage baby's tummy. If your child remains warm, take your baby's temperature to check for a fever.

Caress baby

A gentle massage or light pats on the back can often soothe a crying baby. You might do this while baby lies tummy-down across your lap.

Keep baby moving

Babies generally like movement. Sometimes just that feeling of motion can help soothe your baby. You might rock baby or walk through the house. Keeping safety precautions in mind, try placing baby in an infant swing or vibrating infant seat, or experiment with an infant sling. If the weather permits, head outdoors with the stroller or a baby carrier. You might even buckle baby into the car seat and go for a ride in the car.

Sing or play music

White noise — such as a recording of ocean waves or even the sound of an electric fan or vacuum cleaner in a nearby room — sometimes can help a crying baby relax. Babies often like soothing, muffled sounds similar to the amniotic fluid waves or pulsing sounds they heard in the womb.

Let baby suck

Offer a clean finger or pacifier. Sucking is a natural reflex. For many babies, it's a comforting, soothing activity.

Seek quiet

If your baby is overly tired or has had too much stimulation, provide some quiet time by moving to a calmer environment. You may want to dim the lights or find a darker spot. At times baby just needs a break with less sensory input.

If baby is still crying

Hearing your baby cry and not being able to "fix" it can be really hard. If you've tried everything and your baby is still upset, it doesn't mean you're doing anything wrong. It's OK to let your baby cry while being held.

If you need a break for yourself, put your baby in a safe place, such as the crib. If you've fed, burped and changed your baby and baby appears otherwise OK, letting your baby cry for 10 or 15 minutes in the crib won't do any harm.

COLIC

All babies cry, but some cry more than others. And for a few babies, no matter what you try to do to stop the crying, nothing seems to work. If this description fits your baby, it's possible you're dealing with colic. Colic is the term for periods of intense, inconsolable crying that last for three hours or more, at least three days a week (sometimes every day) and for at least three weeks. The crying episodes typically start a few weeks after birth and generally begin to improve by age 3 months.

Causes

The big question with colic is what causes an otherwise healthy child to cry so much. And the answer is, experts really don't know. There are a variety of theories, and not all medical professionals agree about what may be potential triggers. It's possible the cause may be a combination of factors, and it may differ between infants.

- *Temperament.* Some babies are naturally irritable or sensitive, which might contribute to colicky behavior.

- *Immature nervous system.* An immature nervous system might cause a baby to be unusually sensitive to stimulation. These babies become overloaded by all the sights and sounds, and they aren't able to console themselves. As a result, they cry and they may have difficulty sleeping. Premature babies may exhibit their sensitivity in the form of fussiness rather than crying.
- *Food sensitivities.* Data linking food sensitivities and colic are limited. Talk to your child's medical professional if you have questions or concerns about your diet (if breastfeeding) or formula contributing to colic.

THE 5 S'S

Pediatrician Harvey Karp has combined five techniques for soothing a fussy baby into the "5 S's." Dr. Karp proposes that a baby's first three months are more like a fourth trimester. Creating womb-like conditions — warm, cozy and fairly noisy — can ease a baby's transition to the big, open world. You can find detailed information in Dr. Karp's book *The Happiest Baby on the Block*, but here's a quick rundown. One or two of these steps might do the trick, or you can try several at once.

Swaddle

Wrap your baby snugly in a blanket, with arms tucked in straight at the sides and legs wrapped loosely so they can move and bend.

Side or stomach position

Try holding a fussing baby in a side or stomach position, or over your shoulder. Don't use this position for sleeping, though. Always place your baby on the back to sleep.

Shush

The womb is actually quite a noisy place, with the sound of blood pulsing through nearby blood vessels. Producing a loud shushing noise or white noise near the baby's ear can help soothe fussiness.

Swing

Re-create the motions inside the womb by gently jiggling your baby in fast, tiny motions. Keep your baby's head and neck supported and your motions small. To avoid bodily harm, make sure not to shake your baby too hard.

Suck

Sucking is a relaxing activity for most babies. Offer your baby a pacifier or a clean finger to suck on.

- *Underlying health problem.* Rarely, persistent crying might be a sign that your baby has a health problem, such as a hernia or an infection.

Many other theories about what makes a child more susceptible to colic have been proposed, but none has been proved. Gas was long thought to be a cause because many colicky babies have gas. However, colicky babies may develop gas by swallowing too much air while crying. What medical professionals do know is that birth order doesn't matter — colic doesn't occur more often among firstborns than in later children. Girls and boys experience colic in similar numbers.

And there are no lasting effects or complications from the crying episodes. Babies with colic grow and develop as expected. They also aren't any more likely to cry when they become older infants or toddlers, compared with other children.

Common signs

Some babies are fussy but they don't have colic. Although the behavior can vary, a baby with colic generally displays these signs:

- *Predictable crying episodes.* A baby with colic often cries at about the same time every day, often in the late afternoon or evening. The crying usually begins and ends for no clear reason.
- *Intense or inconsolable crying.* Colic crying is intense and often high-pitched. Your baby's face might flush. Baby might be extremely difficult to comfort.
- *Posture changes.* Babies with colic tend to curl up their legs and clench their fists during crying episodes. You also may notice that the baby has tensed abdominal muscles.

Diagnosis

If you think your baby may have colic, check in with your child's medical professional. This is especially important if your baby is inconsolable or you notice signs of illness, such as a fever, vomiting, changes in eating or sleeping patterns, or other worrisome symptoms. Your baby's medical professional can help you tell the difference between typical tears and something more serious. Explain when and how often the crying episodes occur, how long they last, and

TUMMY HOLD

Some babies find comfort by being held on their tummies, a position sometimes referred to as the colic hold or colic carry. If your baby is fussy, try this position to see if it helps. Place baby facedown along your forearm with your arm firmly between the baby's legs. Baby's cheek should be resting on your palm. Hold your arm close to your body, using it to brace and steady your baby. Just don't let baby sleep in this position.

any observations about your baby's behavior before, during and after the episodes. Your baby's medical professional may ask about your efforts to soothe your baby, as well as your baby's diet and feeding schedule.

Your baby may have a physical exam to identify any possible causes for the distress, but other tests generally aren't necessary. If your baby is otherwise healthy, colic might be identified as the problem.

MANAGING COLIC

Caring for an infant who has colic can be exhausting, confusing and stressful — even for experienced parents. Try to go easy on yourself. Colic isn't a result of parenting skills. Instead, focus on ways to make this difficult stage a little more bearable. Remember, this will pass.

Unfortunately, there are few treatment options for colic. Over-the-counter drugs, such as simethicone (Infants' Mylicon Gas Relief, Little Remedies Gas Relief Drops, others), haven't proved helpful for colic, and other medications can have serious side effects.

Some studies suggest that treatment with probiotics — substances that add "good" bacteria to the digestive tract — might soothe colic. Probiotics can help balance bacteria in the gut to improve digestive health overall. For colic, some research suggests that a bacterium called *Lactobacillus reuteri* may help. But results have been mixed. Most experts agree there's not enough evidence yet to recommend using probiotics to treat colic. However, more research is needed to determine the effects of probiotics on infants.

Some parents want to try alternative therapies, such as herbal teas, herbal remedies such as gripe water, or glucose. Some claim benefits for baby massage, acupuncture and chiropractic treatment. Still, there's not enough evidence for any of these therapies to judge the potential benefits over the risks. For example, regular use of herbal teas or liquid therapies may lead to decreased milk intake or a drop in sodium levels in an infant's blood. Before giving your baby any substance or trying alternative medicine to treat colic, consult your child's medical professional.

While you might not be able to cure colic, there are things you can do to soothe your baby and reduce or lessen the severity of the crying episodes. Consider the following suggestions. (Meanwhile, make sure you're prioritizing self-care during this challenging phase. Ask for help to get the support you need. Take breaks, eat nourishing food and do what helps you feel like you again. See "Keeping your cool" for other tips.)

Feeding

During bottle-feedings, hold your baby as upright as possible. Burp baby often to reduce the chances of swallowing air. Use a curved bottle, designed to minimize the amount of air your baby takes in while feeding. A bottle with a collapsible bag also might help. If bottle-feedings typically take less than 15 to 20 minutes, consider using a nipple with a smaller hole.

If you use formula, you might consider giving your baby a hypoallergenic formula, such as whey hydrolysate formula, for one week. If your baby's symptoms don't improve, continue using the original formula. Avoid frequently switching your baby's formula.

If you breastfeed, try to empty one breast completely before switching to the other breast. This will give your baby more hindmilk, the fattier and potentially more satisfying milk at the end of a feeding.

Your diet

If you breastfeed and you suspect that a food or drink you consume may be making your baby fussier than usual, avoid it for several days to see if it makes a difference. Consider eliminating dairy products or other allergenic foods, which can cause allergic symptoms in breastfed infants. Research suggests that in some special cases avoiding foods such as cow's milk, eggs, peanuts, tree nuts, wheat, soy and fish for a week can reduce infant fussiness. Also, try to eliminate or reduce the amount of caffeine in your diet. Caffeine in your breast milk can keep your baby awake for prolonged periods or cause agitation. Some moms say avoiding spicy foods or foods that cause gas can help — but this hasn't been proved.

Smoke exposure

Research suggests that exposure to cigarette smoke can increase your baby's risk of colic. Living around smoke has many other health risks for you and your baby, too. If you or your partner smoke, ask for help to quit. Keep in mind that smoke from marijuana is smoke, too.

Calming techniques

For most babies with colic, soothing techniques can often help calm the child and lessen the crying — at least for a while. The trick is finding out which

ALWAYS BE GENTLE

When your crying baby can't be calmed, coping with the stress as a parent — and keeping yourself calm — can be incredibly hard. But remember the importance of treating your baby gently. Never yell at, hit or shake your baby.

Newborns have weak neck muscles and head support. Shaking your baby out of sheer frustration can have devastating consequences — including brain damage that leads to seizures, learning disabilities or mental disabilities. And severe shaking can be life-threatening or even fatal.

If you're worried about your ability to cope with a crying baby, contact your medical professional or your baby's medical professional, a local crisis intervention service or a mental health help line for support. If you need to, take your baby to a place where baby will be cared for and safe.

techniques your baby likes. Experiment with the comforting strategies on pages 141 and 142 to see if they help. Also see "The 5 S's" on page 143.

Keep in mind that babies with colic often like motion. Anything you can do to keep baby moving may help. Sit with your baby in a rocking chair, bounce on an exercise ball, carry baby around the house in a baby sling, or take a walk with the stroller. In addition, babies with colic often find certain sounds calming. A steady background of soft noise or shushing sounds may help. Turn on the kitchen or bathroom exhaust fan, run the vacuum in the next room, use a white noise machine, play music, or play environmental sounds such as ocean waves or a gentle rain. Sometimes the ticking of a clock or a metronome does the trick.

KEEPING YOUR COOL

Listening to a baby cry is stressful. When it seems to go on for hours, it's extremely stressful. Even for experienced parents, coping with colic or not being able to figure out what's wrong is tough. And if you're sleep-deprived, that can make it even harder to regulate your own emotions and reactions. That's why it's important to take care of yourself while you're taking care of your baby.

If you're struggling to cope, you're not alone. Parents often need to build on their own ability to manage emotions (self-regulate) while raising babies and toddlers. Improving this skill helps your child learn to self-regulate, too. But it's a process.

When you're feeling overwhelmed by your baby's crying, take steps to calm yourself. Remember that this phase will end. In the meantime, you don't have to do it alone. Ask for and accept extra support to help you through the tough moments, so that you can be the soothing comfort your baby needs.

Take a break

If your baby's cries are getting to you, take deep breaths. Repeat a calming word or phrase, such as "You've got this." Imagine yourself in a calm, relaxing place. Play soothing music in the background. Or take turns with a partner. When you need to, put baby in the crib while you walk into another room and give yourself a break. If baby is with another adult, get away for a while — somewhere out of earshot.

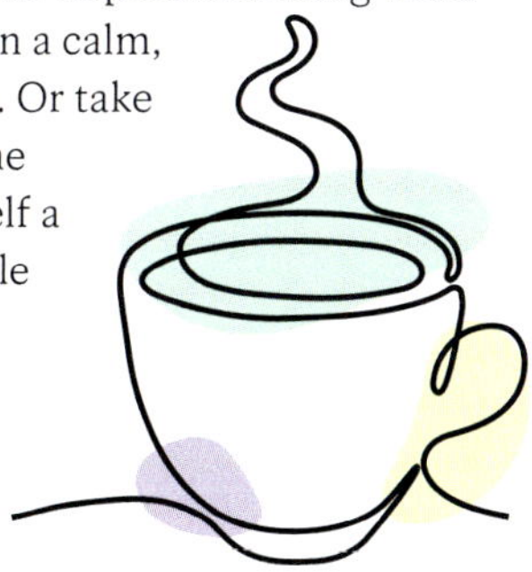

Get out of the house

Put your baby in the stroller or a baby carrier and go for a walk together. The exertion might take your mind off the tears — and the movement or change of scenery might soothe your baby. You might even buckle the baby into the car seat and take a drive.

Ask for help

Take advantage of baby-sitting offers from trusted relatives, friends or neighbors, or make a rescue plan with someone to step in when needed. Use the time to take a nap or do something you enjoy. Even an hour on your own can help renew your coping strength. Expressing yourself can help, too. When you're getting frustrated, speak up. Saying the words out loud can help ease the tension. The more relaxed you are, the more able you'll be to handle baby's crying spells. It's also good for baby. Babies can sense when you're tense and stressed out. A calm presence helps them find calm.

Don't judge yourself

Most of all, don't measure your success as a parent by how much your baby cries. Colic isn't a result of poor parenting, and inconsolable crying isn't a sign of your baby rejecting you. You and your baby will get through this phase. Colic often improves on its own by age 4 months.

CHAPTER 10

Bonding and behavior

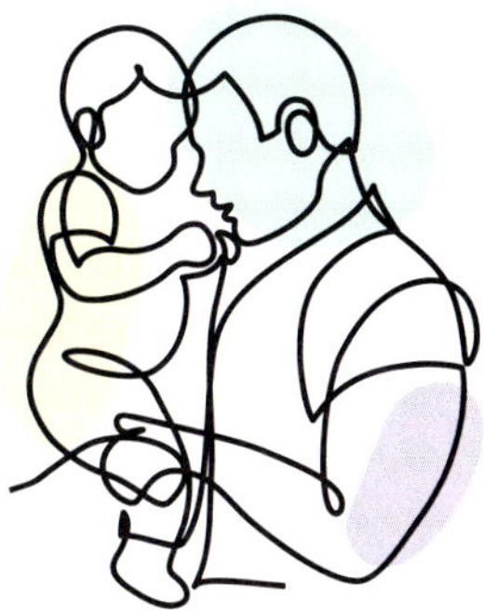

Some days you gaze at your baby and feel a connection deeper than you ever thought possible. Other days you stare at this little person crying inconsolably in your arms and have no idea what's wrong. Then there's the toddler stage. One moment you're enjoying a book with your sweet, cuddly kiddo. The next your child is staging an all-out war because it's time for bed.

When your child was born, you embarked on one of the most rewarding, challenging and complex relationships you'll ever experience. Like any relationship, your connection is a two-way street. Your child's behavior, personality and moods affect you just as much as yours affect your child. There are good days and bad days. After all, no child or parent is perfect.

What matters is not perfection but a commitment to consistently engage with your child and do your best to respond to your child's needs with empathy and sensitivity. Whether that means comforting a crying baby or calming a frustrated toddler, your attention and affection help build the strong, secure and nurturing relationship your child needs to thrive.

NURTURING YOUR BOND

Your baby was born to bond with you. From the start, baby instinctively has sought a connection through each cry, nuzzle or gaze into your eyes. As babies grow and become more interactive, they strengthen the parent-child relationship by smiling, cooing and imitating facial expressions. Even when little ones begin to scoot, crawl or walk, they will continually loop back to you, drawing comfort from the security of your special bond.

Each time you respond to your baby's instinctive connection-seeking behaviors, you build and deepen a stable, nurturing relationship with your child. Experts refer to this healthy child-parent bond as secure attachment.

A securely attached child is easily comforted by a parent and trusts that the parent will respond to those needs.

Benefits of a strong bond

When babies feel secure in their relationship with a parent, they start to feel secure in their relationship with their world. This sense of security helps a child to thrive long after the first year of life. In fact, the positive impact of a baby's connection with a parent can last well into adulthood. That's why you can never spoil a baby with too much attention or affection.

Babies who have a secure, nurturing relationship with a parent in the first year of life may be more likely to:

- Handle brief separations from parents more easily and with less distress
- Explore their surroundings with greater confidence and experimentation
- Adapt to new situations and people more easily
- Tackle challenges with greater pleasure and persistence, leading to the mastering of new skills
- Manage their emotions and stress more successfully in childhood and beyond
- Show greater resilience in the face of obstacles
- Gain a greater capacity to form close, lifelong relationships

Connecting with your baby

Creating a secure attachment with your baby takes a conscious effort. If you strive to be a responsive, dependable and nurturing presence in your baby's life, your bond will grow naturally. Your baby will feel safe, secure and loved knowing that you'll offer comfort or fill a hungry tummy.

It's important to note that bonding with a child comes easier to some parents and is harder for others. It might be particularly difficult for adults who had a difficult childhood or adverse experiences. Certain support groups and therapies can effectively help parents bond with their babies.

Here are some things you can do to keep the connection between you and your baby strong:

- ***Respond to your baby's cries.*** Babies cry to communicate their needs, not to manipulate. There may be times when your baby needs to cry it out, but generally it's best to respond quickly to cries if possible. The reassuring comfort of your smell, touch and voice strengthens your baby's attachment to you.
- ***Spoil away.*** Don't be afraid that you'll be spoiling your baby. Studies show that young babies who are picked up consistently and held in response to their cries tend to cry less by 1 year of age and show less aggressive behavior as toddlers. What's more, soothing babies in this way can teach them to even-

tually soothe themselves. (For tips on how to soothe a crying baby, turn to page 141.)

- *Tune in to your baby's cues.* Being attuned to your baby means paying close attention to the different facial expressions, sounds and movements that communicate their needs. Learning to understand these cues and responding to them with sensitivity helps your baby feel loved and secure.
- *Talk, sing and read frequently to your baby.* Coo or chatter cheerfully to your little one while changing a diaper. When your baby coos back at you, respond in kind. Sing a silly song at bath time. Read a book together. These shared experiences will bring you closer and contribute to your baby's brain development.
- *Make time for playtime.* Playtime offers an opportunity for positive, fun interaction with your baby. Delight your baby with a game of peekaboo or patty-cake. Dangle objects for your baby to observe, touch or grab. Get down on your child's level to stack toys or roll a ball back and forth.

POSTPARTUM DEPRESSION AND ANXIETY

Many people experience some form of "baby blues" in the first few days or weeks after giving birth. This commonly includes mood swings, crying spells, anxiety and difficulty sleeping. But some new parents experience a more severe, long-lasting form of depression known as postpartum depression. Postpartum anxiety is also common.

Postpartum depression or anxiety usually develops during the first few weeks after baby arrives, but it also can appear during pregnancy (called peripartum depression) or anytime during baby's first year. And fathers or partners who didn't give birth can experience it, too. It isn't a character flaw or a weakness, and there's no clear cause. Genetics, hormone changes and emotional issues may all be factors.

Untreated, postpartum depression and anxiety can affect how closely you bond with your baby. The good news is that safe and effective treatment options are available, even if you're breastfeeding or pumping milk.

If you're feeling persistently sad, anxious, irritable or withdrawn, or if you're having severe mood swings in your baby's first year, it's important to talk with your medical professional. Treatment can help you manage your symptoms and continue to build a strong relationship with your baby. Turn to Chapter 37 for more information on caring for your mental health as a parent.

If at any point you have thoughts of harming yourself or your baby, call 911 or your local emergency number to get help. In the United States, you also can call or text 988 at any time to reach the 988 Suicide & Crisis Lifeline. Have your partner or a trusted adult help care for the baby.

- *Give plenty of physical affection.* Whether a newborn or a sturdy 1-year-old, your child benefits from your touch. Hold, cuddle, rock and massage your baby — not only in times of distress but also in peaceful or playful moments.
- *Offer gentle guidance.* Your baby doesn't understand the concepts of right or wrong, good or bad just yet. It's up to you to teach acceptable behavior. If your young baby yanks on a fistful of your hair, gently remove that little hand or distract your baby with an appealing toy. If your baby's old enough to understand language, you can explain, "That hurts."
- *Be a dependable home base.* Once babies are mobile, they want to explore their environment. This newfound freedom is both thrilling and overwhelming. Your baby may periodically seek eye contact with you, call out to you, or return to your side for a quick hug or cuddle. When you're responsive to these ways of reconnecting, you're helping your child feel safe and secure. This allows your little one to continue exploring the world with confidence.
- *Be mindful of screen use.* When interacting with your baby, try as much as possible to set aside your smartphone, turn off the TV and minimize other distractions. If you're making more eye contact with your phone than with your child, both of you will miss out on crucial parent-infant interactions that help your baby thrive.

Setting reasonable expectations

Keep in mind that you won't be able to meet every one of your baby's needs perfectly or immediately, and that shouldn't be your expectation. You aren't

SERVE AND RETURN

Your baby babbles at you. You respond by looking into baby's eyes and imitating the sounds. Your toddler laughs with delight, causing you to giggle. Experts sometimes call this simple back-and-forth interaction serve and return, and it's an important way that parents form close, nurturing relationships with their children.

What's more, serve-and-return interactions provide vital support for the rapidly developing connections in a young child's brain. These interactions can improve the ability to control impulses, regulate emotions and navigate social encounters later in childhood.

Here are some serve-and-return behaviors you can engage in every day:

- Return your child's gaze or smile.
- Mirror your baby's expressions, vocalizations and actions.
- Talk to your child and describe what's happening.
- Play interactive games like peekaboo.
- Participate in imaginative play with your toddler.

causing harm if you can't hold your baby because they're crying in the car seat on the drive to the playground. You won't weaken your bond if it takes you a while to realize that baby is fussing because of a scratchy sweater instead of an empty tummy or a wet diaper.

In addition, keep in mind that your baby needs a happy and rested parent, not a "perfect" parent. Prioritize what needs to be done for baby, and keep your own needs in mind as well. As long as you're generally responsive to your baby's needs, your baby will flourish.

UNDERSTANDING TEMPERAMENT

To read cues and know how to best respond to your child's needs, it helps to gain a deeper understanding of your child. Many factors shape who your child is, including genetics, your home environment and your parenting style. Your child's personality or temperament is another factor.

Your child's temperament includes many traits, including activity level, adaptability, sensitivity, intensity, mood, distractibility and persistence. The predictability of your child's bodily rhythms, such as hunger and tiredness, and how cautious your child typically is, are part of temperament too.

Trait clusters

Researchers have observed that certain temperament traits tend to cluster together to form general temperament styles. For example, some kids are naturally easygoing. They quickly develop regular sleeping and eating schedules, fuss infrequently, smile easily, and adapt well to new situations. Caring for these children is often smooth sailing.

Other kids are naturally slower to warm up. These little ones may be less active and not too intense, approach new things slowly and with caution, and have a harder time transitioning from one activity or person to another. These children tend to be more serious.

Then there are children who keep you on your toes. They display fierce emotion, may have tons of energy, and approach things and people with either avid curiosity or determined caution. They become easily frustrated and have difficulty making changes. Caring for these feisty children is naturally more challenging than caring for more even-tempered ones.

Many children have mixed traits. For example, their overall temperament may be moderate to easygoing, but they may score high on intensity, activity or persistence.

Blending temperaments

As a parent, you might find a particular temperament trait in your child to be pleasing, challenging or somewhere in between. A highly active child might be a blast on an outing but nonetheless a handful for a busy parent juggling multiple responsibilities. By keeping an open mind and staying flexible, you can engage positively with your child in ways that meet both of your needs.

Do you have an extremely focused or persistent child? Consider working together on a fun challenge, like building a colorful block tower or completing an age-appropriate puzzle. For a curious child who's always on the move, visit a place you personally love, such as a scenic park. Play a simple game of hide-and-seek or I Spy. Everyone has different talents and abilities. If your partner or another caregiver naturally fits better with some aspects of your child's temperament, work as a team to help your child develop.

Getting to know your baby's temperament better also can help you adjust your parenting to better fit your child's needs. Is your baby high on the intensity and sensitivity scale? Those long bouts of crying might reflect temperament. Do you have more difficulty redirecting your child's attention than other parents seem to? It might be a sign of a powerful persistence on your baby's part. Learning these ins and outs will help to guide you in your baby's first years of life, and in the years to come.

YOU AND YOUR TODDLER

The foundation of love, security and trust that you've built for your baby takes on new importance as you enter the toddler stage. Parenting children this age is a balancing act. Toddlers crave both a close connection with a parent and greater independence. They're realizing that they are their own person, with their own wants and needs — and they're ready to take charge of their world. Of course, this eagerness to strike out on their own often conflicts with their limitations.

Toddlers can't always move as swiftly and skillfully as they'd like, or clearly express their feelings or needs in words. They also are learning to deal with limits, compromise and disappointment. This can naturally lead to intense emotions, tantrums and difficult behaviors.

Children at this age benefit from a parent who understands and honors their desire for autonomy while also helping them learn how to cope with negative emotions, listen to directions and accept limits. Continue to provide a secure relationship based on love, stability and consistency. This will help your toddler learn to manage the ups and downs of this stage of life.

Little person, big emotions

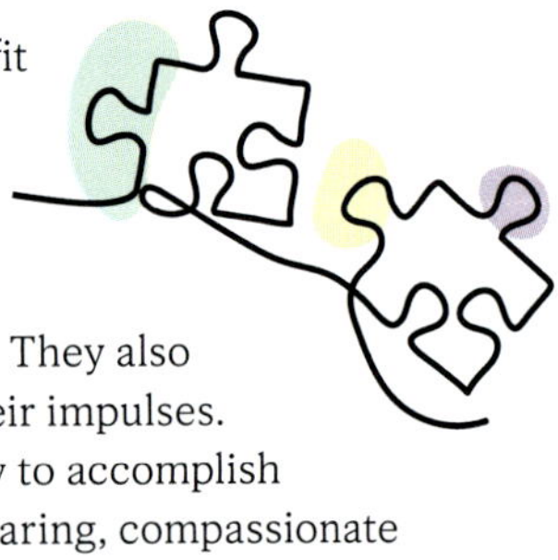

Your toddler is putting together a puzzle but can't seem to fit in the last piece. With each failed attempt to jam it into place, frustration builds.

Toddlers want to do so much — and they want to do it all by themselves, right now. This is what they see you do every day. But they don't yet know how to do it themselves. They also don't know how to handle intense emotions and control their impulses.

That's where you come in. You can teach your child how to accomplish tasks and how to remain calm by word and by example. A caring, compassionate parent can be an anchor in stormy seas. When your child is overcome with strong feelings, your calm presence can help to bring down the intensity level and teach your child how to understand and cope with emotions.

To support and soothe your child in moments of frustration, sadness or disappointment, try these techniques:

- *Get close.* Calmly and slowly move closer to your child. Being nearby reassures your child that you're present and available. You also can say something encouraging, such as "I'm here to help."
- *Validate emotions.* Let your child know that you're listening. You understand those big feelings. Label your toddler's emotions: "You seem frustrated that the puzzle piece won't fit." Remember that downplaying the situation — "Don't get worked up. It's just a puzzle!" — may be confusing for toddlers. They may then escalate their reaction to be believed. Validating your child's feelings helps them start to recover while teaching how to identify strong emotions.
- *Soothe with a calming touch.* Try rubbing your child's back, stroking their head or offering a hug. A parent's touch can be extremely comforting.
- *Offer guidance.* If your child is frustrated with a specific task, gently provide some help. Avoid solving the problem for your child right away. A bit of guidance may be all that's needed for your child to complete the task. Or you can offer to work on the problem together.

When emotions explode into tantrums

Sometimes your child's emotions are just too big to contain. Despite your best efforts to understand and soothe your child, there are times when a tantrum seems unstoppable. What's a parent to do?

First, it's important to understand that temper tantrums are a common way toddlers express frustration with the challenges of the moment. Your toddler might be upset about taking turns at the playground or having to share a toy. Your child could be struggling to transition from playtime to bedtime. Or perhaps the problem is hunger, tiredness or jealousy. These everyday obstacles can be hard for a toddler to deal with, at times sparking a full-blown meltdown.

Experts recommend that parents avoid punishing a toddler's tantrum. Tantrums are developmentally normal — not a sign of misbehaving. In addition, toddlers are still learning cause and effect. Being punished for a strong reaction may only be confusing. Instead, try these strategies to manage a child's meltdown:

- *Keep your cool.* If you react with anger or frustration, you'll likely cause more stress for you and your child. Take some deep breaths to calm yourself. If that doesn't work and you're at home, leave the room for a minute to gather yourself. Let your child know you're taking a moment to calm your body. By staying calm, you're modeling self-control in the face of powerful emotions. In time, your child will learn from your example and gain more emotional control.
- *Try distraction.* You may be able to redirect your child's negative behavior with a positive distraction, especially with young toddlers. Try moving your toddler to another room or a different part of the playground. Offer a book or toy, or ask your child to join you in a different game or activity.

- *Give your child space, with support.* Sometimes a child needs time to self-regulate. If your toddler can't stop crying, screaming or stomping, don't continue to react to the behavior. Sit quietly near your child and say, "I am here when you need me." Wait for your child to calm down a little and then try to redirect.
- *Know when to step in.* If your child starts hitting, kicking or throwing things at others, stop the harmful behavior. Move your toddler away from the situation. Calmly acknowledge the feelings but explain that the behavior is unacceptable: "It's OK to be mad, but it's not OK to hit."
- *Stand firm.* Avoid giving in to your toddler during a temper tantrum. Stick to the limit or rule you have set. If your refusal to buy your child ice cream set off the tantrum, don't appease your child by buying the ice cream. Giving in sends the message that negative behavior works. You'll also make it harder to enforce the rule or limit next time.
- *Reconnect.* Once the flood of emotion has passed, see if your child is willing to accept some comfort. A kind word and some physical affection can help your child move on.

CAN TANTRUMS BE PREVENTED?

There's no foolproof way to prevent tantrums, but there is plenty you can do to encourage good behavior in your toddler.

- *Be consistent.* Establish a daily routine so that your child knows what to expect. Stick to the routine as much as possible, including nap time and bedtime. Set reasonable limits and follow them consistently.
- *Plan ahead.* Run errands when your child isn't likely to be hungry or tired. If you're expecting to wait in line, pack a small toy or snack to occupy your child.
- *Pick your battles.* If you say no to everything, your child is likely to get frustrated. Look for times when it's OK to say yes.
- *Offer choices when possible.* Encourage independence by letting your child pick out a pair of pajamas or a bedtime story. Offer a choice between two options: "Do you want strawberries or blueberries?"
- *Praise good behavior.* Provide extra attention when your child behaves well. Give your child a hug or praise when your child follows directions or does something positive: "Great job coming right away." "I love how you're sharing with others."
- *Avoid situations likely to trigger tantrums.* Don't provide toys that are too advanced for your child. If your child begs for toys or treats when you shop, steer clear of tempting areas. If your toddler acts up in restaurants, pack a picnic or eat at home. Save restaurants for date night, for now.

SETTING LIMITS

Walking, running and climbing toddlers can have a lot of fun exploring their world, but they also can get into a lot of trouble. Just because they can open cabinets, jump on beds and race down sidewalks doesn't mean they know how to stay safe. Your toddler needs clear limits to keep out of danger and learn what behavior is and isn't acceptable.

Now is a good time to establish family rules. Start with two or three core rules related to safety, such as "no hitting" or "no jumping on furniture." Agree on these limits with your partner ahead of time and communicate them to other caregivers. That way you'll be on the same page and can enforce the rules consistently. If you're co-parenting and your child has more than one home, it's helpful to have consistent core rules at both homes.

You'll also need to clearly express these expectations so that your child can successfully understand them. Be prepared to repeat the rules regularly to help your child remember and act on them. As your toddler begins to master a rule, you can add a new one to the list.

Rules that are age-appropriate, consistently enforced, and balanced with warmth and affection will help your child navigate life within your family and beyond the walls of your home.

Encouraging good behavior

Part of a toddler's job is to test the limits, including breaking rules or ignoring directions. But don't assume that your child is being deliberately defiant when disobeying you. Toddlers aren't known for their spectacular listening skills. They're still learning how to understand language, pay attention to what's being said and think about their effect on others.

Positive behavior doesn't happen overnight. It's developed through hundreds of small exchanges with your child. These daily interactions teach your child how to exert emotional self-control, make good choices and behave appropriately, even when you're not around.

Whether you're reinforcing a no-hitting rule or asking your child to put away a toy, rely on these positive techniques to communicate your expectations and encourage good behavior:

- *Get close.* Whenever possible, get down on your child's level and make eye contact. Placing a gentle hand on the back or head can set a positive, caring tone.
- *Speak calmly.* Get your child's attention by using your child's name or a term of affection. Keep your voice neutral when reminding your child of a rule or asking your child to do something.
- *Keep it simple.* Use simple, clear language and short sentences, such as "Please sit down" or "It's time to get your coat." Try to avoid negative statements, such as "Don't get out of your chair."
- *Be patient.* It might take your toddler a moment to focus on you and process what you're saying. Give your child time to figure it out and transition to the new behavior.

CHOICES, LIMITS AND CONSEQUENCES

Toddlers are hardwired to assert their independence and test the limits. When they aren't cooperative, you may be able to appeal to their independence by giving two choices. If that doesn't get results, you'll need to set a limit — also called a boundary — and let your child know the consequence. A natural consequence may be enough. Otherwise, you must be willing to follow through. For example, at dinner you might say:

- "Strawberries are for eating, not throwing. Do you want to eat your strawberries with your fork or with your fingers?"
- "We don't throw food. If you keep throwing the strawberries, you won't have any left to eat."

Or if your child is having trouble sharing a toy with another child who wants to use it, your script might sound like this:

- "We share and take turns with toys. Do you want to play with this for two more minutes, or switch toys now and play with the car instead?"
- "It's time to give someone else a turn. If you don't share the toy, I will take it."
- "It's time to take a turn with another toy." Then calmly remove the toy.

- *Model the behavior.* If your toddler doesn't respond to a request or reminder, try modeling the behavior. Repeat your request: "Time to put away your toys." Then put away one of the toys yourself and say, "Your turn." Another technique is to say, "I'll show you." Then physically guide your child in the task or expected action.
- *Reward with praise.* If your child does as you ask, offer warm praise. Explain how much you appreciate your child's efforts.

PLAYING WITH YOUR TODDLER

Teaching your child how to manage emotions and follow rules is a lot easier when you're doing it in the context of a secure, loving relationship. One way to keep your connection going strong is to spend one-on-one time together. After all, you are your toddler's favorite playmate.

Aim for 5 to 15 minutes of uninterrupted, one-on-one playtime with your toddler each day. You may find it works best to schedule the playtime into your daily routine. But be flexible. Your time together will go better when your child is rested and fed and you have the energy.

Playtime with a parent has many important benefits for children. It serves a vital role in their social, emotional and cognitive development. It also improves their self-control and helps them form close relationships with other children and adults in their lives. Consider these suggestions for making the most out of playtime:

- *Put away devices.* Spend this special time with your child without distractions or interruptions. Silence your phone, turn off the television and set aside any other devices that could compete for your attention.
- *Let your child take the lead.* This is a time when you can focus on what your child wants to do. Let your child set the agenda while gently discouraging activities that are aggressive, competitive, frustrating or destructive. Do things that allow you to be together in a relaxed and happy manner.
- *Show that you're fully engaged.* If your child picks up a doll and says "doll," repeat the word and build on the conversation: "Doll. You're hugging the doll." You also can describe your child's actions out loud during play: "You're stacking red and blue blocks. Now you're knocking them down."
- *Mirror your child.* Another way to connect with your child is to imitate what your child is doing. If your child is moving a train on the tracks and making tooting sounds, grab a train and do the same. If your child gets up to dance to some music, mimic the movements.
- *Describe emotions.* Label the emotions you're observing with phrases like "You look happy." You can label your feelings, too: "I'm excited to play this game." You might also point to a character while reading a picture book or watching a show and ask, "What do you think this person is feeling?" These exchanges can help your toddler learn to identify and express feelings.
- *Enjoy yourself.* Take time to notice and think about how amazing your child is. Show your enjoyment with positive words, an enthusiastic voice and animated facial expressions. Offer an extra hug and a kiss. Savor these special moments together.

CHAPTER 11

Screen time and your child

Sometimes you need just a little uninterrupted time before you can devote your full attention to your toddler again. But try getting your child to understand that! As you attempt to send out important emails for work — or quiet the baby down for a nap — your toddler is begging you to play dinosaurs. That's when you break out the tablet or turn on the TV to keep your little one occupied.

In a perfect world, toddlers wouldn't be so magnetically drawn to electronics, and parents would always have extra support in the moments they need it. But the world, of course, isn't perfect. Sometimes, using a device to keep your toddler occupied buys you time to finish a task — or simply take a deep breath — so you can feel successful at juggling the many demands of parenthood. It's a familiar situation for many parents.

However, it's never too early to think about appropriate media usage in your home. As a parent, you play a crucial role in this. A good place to start is with expert recommendations and how you can make them work for your family.

THE GUIDELINES — AND WHY THEY MATTER

The American Academy of Pediatrics recommends these general screen time limits for digital media:

- Under 18 months, avoid screen time other than video chats.
- From 18 to 24 months, continue to avoid screen time except for video chats. However, if you want to introduce digital media at this age, opt for educational programming, such as content from the Public Broadcasting Service (PBS). Oversee your child's use of the content and avoid leaving your child alone with a device.

BE AWARE OF YOUR OWN SCREEN TIME, TOO

Children aren't the only ones who can go overboard with technology. Research suggests that there are a variety of health risks for adults with more screen time, too. In addition, parents who spend a lot of time on smartphones and other devices limit meaningful interactions with their children, which may affect children's development.

Parents' screen use may be linked with the following outcomes for their families and themselves:

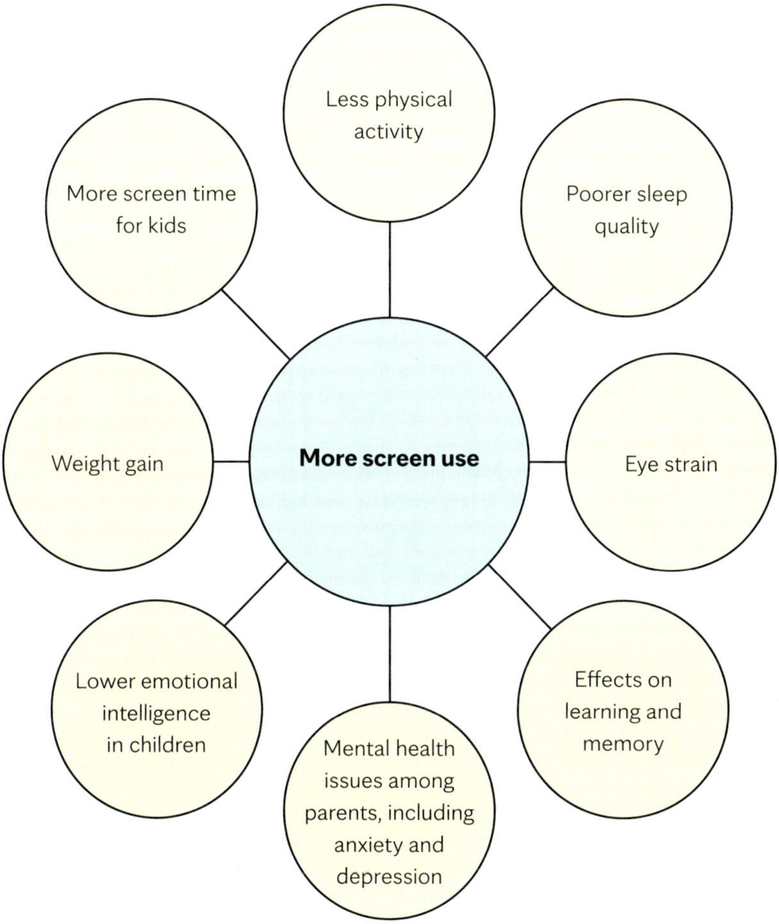

- From 2 to 5 years, limit screen time to one hour a day of educational programming. Ideally, parents should watch or play alongside children, helping them understand what they're watching.

Keep in mind that every child is different. Some may quickly grow bored with a device and need little encouragement to switch activities. Others may cling to their device and have a meltdown if asked to turn it off. Some children may have special needs requiring additional restrictions when using technology. Consider your family and any additional guardrails or support your children may need around screen time.

Though the guidelines seem a little daunting, there is science behind them. Using digital media more than the recommended amounts has been linked to certain risks.

Obesity Researchers have found that the risk of obesity increases with the amount of screen time a child has. It's possible that a child engrossed in watching a show on TV or using a tablet is more likely to eat unhealthy foods or eat mindlessly.

Sleep Studies also have linked screen time with disrupted sleep in children. The blue light from electronic devices can disrupt sleep patterns, cutting sleep time.

Language and development Too much screen time is associated with delays in children's cognition, language, and social and emotional development. Children may choose electronics over engaging in free play or interacting with peers or family, missing out on crucial creative, social and language opportunities.

The timing and type of screen time also matter. Using technology to soothe toddler meltdowns can worsen behavior, as children won't learn how to self-regulate their emotions.

Even when you know the potential pitfalls of screen time, you may still struggle with how (and when) to set limits. Creating a well-structured media plan is an excellent place to start. But also be prepared to concede that even with a carefully crafted media plan, there will be times when you have to loosen the tech reins.

Making screen time count

Not all technology is created equal. There's passive technology, which involves little thought or engagement — think watching a funny YouTube video or scrolling through a social media feed. Then there's active screen time. Active screen time includes interactive games or shows that are designed to build skills such as problem-solving or encourage physical activity. Educational apps tend to fall under this category.

It's ideal to watch or play alongside your child at this stage and create additional learning opportunities. For example, as your child navigates through a vocabulary-building app, you may help them identify words and how they're spelled and used. Some research suggests that using educational content with a parent or caregiver is linked to improved language skills in children.

As your child ages, you can use compare-and-contrast techniques to teach how to evaluate quality programming. Point out advertising that appears on TV and explain how these ads differ from educational content.

But even among apps labeled "educational," careful consideration should be given. Some apps appear educational but might be loaded with ads or encouragement to make in-app purchases. If you're unsure of an app's appropriateness, you can visit a site such as Common Sense Media (commonsensemedia.org), which lists recommended apps for children. Just keep in mind that the app should never take the place of one-on-one time with your child, such as reading and cuddling.

MEDIA MELTDOWNS AND "TECHNO-TANTRUMS"

It's your toddler's nap time, and you make a move to take the tablet away in preparation. Even after a warning that it's almost time, an epic meltdown ensues as your child screams, cries and clings desperately to the device. But why exactly does this happen? It might be the dopamine.

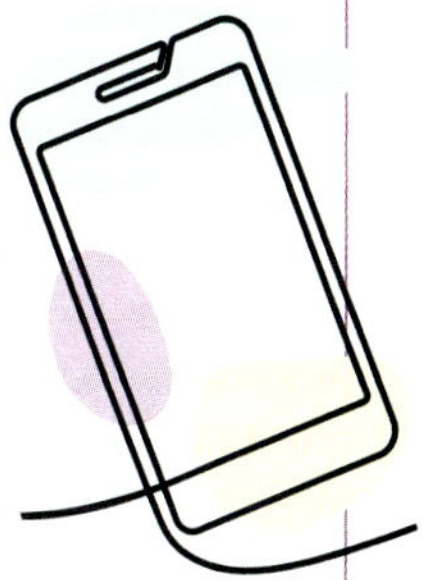

As your child watches an engaging video or plays an exciting game on the tablet, the reward center in the brain releases dopamine — a powerful neurotransmitter that helps maintain interest and attention — in response to these pleasurable or exciting experiences. When the activity ends, dopamine levels drop, and the good feelings associated with the activity disappear.

The brain continues to associate the activity with dopamine. Each time your child experiences that video or game, more dopamine is released, and your child is driven to seek out the same pleasure again and again. It's not an easy cycle to break. Digital media companies often create content that's easily accessible and designed to hold the attention of young children for long periods.

Creating a solid media plan can help curb this, but not always. If your child does act out when screen time ends, stay calm and let the tantrum pass. Don't give back the device; this will only fuel a vicious cycle. When your child calms down, you can allow them to express their feelings while gently reminding them that these are the rules. Then consider moving on to a quiet activity, like looking through a book, coloring or doing a puzzle.

If you're concerned that your child's tech habits are creating constant meltdowns, changes in sleep patterns or eating habits, or your child is finding it increasingly difficult to go without technology for even short periods, contact a healthcare provider to talk through the best ways to handle these issues.

FAMILY MEDIA PLAN

Creating a family media plan is crucial for setting screen limits. You can set daily or weekly time limits and restrictions on when and where screens can be used.

For example, an hour in the afternoon, after nap time, may be a good time to watch an episode of *Sesame Street* on the iPad. But devices might be off-limits for an hour before bedtime. You might also decide not to have TVs, phones or tablets in a child's bedroom.

Children often do best when they know they have a scheduled time to use devices and may be less likely to beg to use them outside these set times. You can also involve your child in creating some of the rules. If your child feels they have some input in drafting a plan for screen time, they may be more likely to follow it.

The American Academy of Pediatrics has created a media plan tool (search for "family media plan" at www.healthychildren.org) in English and Spanish to help you further customize a plan for your family and each child. For example, you can select an activity to complete before kids can use a device. That could be playing outside for at least 30 minutes or looking through picture books for a certain amount of time.

Here are a few tips for success:

- *Stick to the plan.* Being able to use devices only during approved screen times will likely stir up some protest at first. Remind your family that everyone agreed on the plan, which applies to everyone — even the grown-ups.
- *Be a role model.* Being aware of your habits can help you be a better role model. Resist the urge to check email or glance at the screen instead of watching your kids dance around the living room. This includes avoiding using your phone in bed, too.
- *Fill the device gap.* Simply unplugging isn't the point. It's about breaking free of devices to connect with friends and spend time together as a family. Use screen-free time to talk, make pizza from scratch, play games, go for a walk, do puzzles, plan a "someday" trip, rediscover favorite toys, make a scrapbook or volunteer to clean up a local park as a family.

Over time, kids will reap the benefits of having a media plan. Critical thinking skills and executive functions necessary for academic success later on — including regulating and controlling emotions and impulses — are learned through play that's not on a computer, tablet or phone. They're learned through one-on-one interactions with you and the world around them.

PART 2

Health and safety

CHAPTER 12

Finding the right medical care

During your baby's first year, you and your baby will likely spend a lot of time with your baby's medical professional. Beyond the recommended checkups every couple of months, it's likely that your baby will get an illness at some point this year. In addition, you may have questions about newborn care or your baby's health and development.

In the second and third years, you'll see your baby's medical professional less often than in the first year. But between scheduled vaccinations, well-child checkups, and the ever-present colds and other viruses children so often get, there still will be plenty of visits.

While finding a medical professional for your baby might sound simple, it's worth the effort to find an individual who can best meet your baby's and family's needs. Determining what you're looking for can help you find a pediatric medical professional whom you feel comfortable with and with whom you can build a good relationship as your child grows and matures.

GETTING STARTED

If you haven't already chosen a medical professional for your baby, now is the time to do so. If you don't have a specific medical professional in mind, start by asking for recommendations from trusted family members, friends or co-workers who have children. Your own medical professional might be a good referral source, too. You also may be able to find information about pediatric medical professionals by calling a nearby hospital or other community health resources. Note that some clinics and healthcare systems will assign you a medical professional, depending on availability.

Keep in mind that your health insurance company may require you to choose from its approved network of medical professionals. Check to see if the company provides information about who is in the network to help you make your decision.

Whatever you do, don't put off finding a medical professional for your baby. Even if you're about to move or change insurance providers, do your best to find a medical professional as soon as possible. Waiting until your baby becomes sick can be stressful for you and might delay your baby's care. Establishing a relationship with a medical professional for your baby also will make it easier for you to schedule regular visits and keep your child's vaccinations up to date.

MEDICAL PROFESSIONAL OPTIONS

When it comes to choosing a medical professional for your baby, you have options. Many types of medical personnel treat babies and children.

Pediatricians

Many parents choose a pediatrician to be the medical professional for their children. Pediatricians specialize in the care of children from infancy through adolescence. After medical school, pediatricians go through a three-year residency program. Some pediatricians receive further training in subspecialties such as the care of sick and premature newborns (neonatology), children's heart conditions (pediatric cardiology), children's skin issues (pediatric dermatology) and others. If your baby ever needs to be treated by a subspecialist, the regular medical professional can provide a referral.

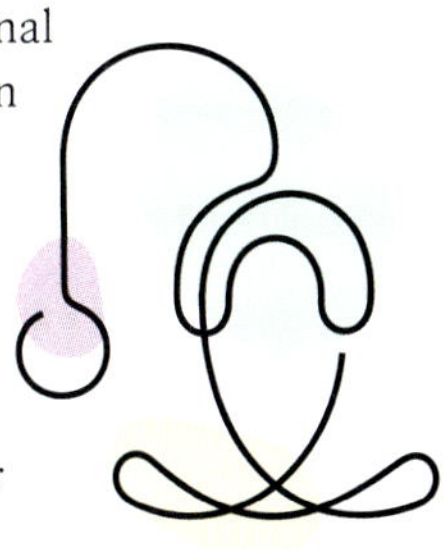

Family physicians

Family physicians are trained in adult and pediatric medicine. They provide healthcare to people of all ages. After medical school, they complete three years of family medicine residency. A family physician can see your child from infancy all the way through adulthood. Family physicians take care of most medical problems. In addition, a family physician who treats everyone in your family will gain an overall health perspective on you and your loved ones. If you already have a family physician you trust, ask if infant healthcare is available.

Midlevel professionals

Midlevel professionals include nurse practitioners and physician assistants.

Nurse practitioners are registered nurses who have completed additional training in an area of practice, such as pediatrics or family health. After nursing school, a nurse practitioner must go through a formal education program in a specialty field. A pediatric nurse practitioner focuses on caring for infants, children and teens. Family nurse practitioners often see all family members, including children.

Physician assistants are medical professionals who are trained and licensed to diagnose illness, develop and manage treatment plans, and prescribe medications. Physician assistants work in all areas of medicine, including pediatrics and family medicine.

Nurse practitioners and physician assistants often work with or under the supervision of a physician. But they may practice independently, depending on state guidelines, and may serve as your primary medical professional.

FACTORS TO CONSIDER

Before you choose a medical professional for your child, think about what you're looking for.

Your needs and preferences

Would you prefer your child to see the same medical professional who takes care of the rest of your family's health or someone who specializes in pediatrics? Would you like a medical professional who is older and may have more experience, or an individual who is younger and also may have young children at home? For parents who have children with complex care needs, a medical professional with the relevant experience and training may be the best fit.

Cost

Do you need to choose someone from among your insurance company's list of approved medical professionals?

Location, accessibility and hours

Is the medical professional's office in a convenient location for you? Would you prefer an office that has extended hours? Is it important for you to be able to contact the medical professional at night or on the weekends or by an online patient portal message? Would you like your child's medical professional to have privileges at a particular hospital? Would you prefer an office that has separate waiting rooms for children who are well and those who are sick?

EVALUATING YOUR OPTIONS

Once you've thought about what you're looking for and compiled the names of some possible medical professionals, do some research to confirm that they are accepting new patients and that they work with your insurance company. This information may be available on each office's website, or you may need to call each office.

Next, call to schedule an appointment with the medical professional. Try to schedule the visit at a time when you and your partner can attend, so you can both ask questions. If you're given a recommendation by friends or family, you may be able to get some basic information from them before talking to the medical professional. For example, you might ask about:

- *Bedside manner.* Does the medical professional interact well with both adults and children? Does the child of your friend or relative like the medical professional?
- *Office atmosphere.* Is the office staff helpful? How do staff members manage phone calls, particularly when it comes to emergencies? Is it difficult to make an appointment when a child is sick? Is there generally a long office wait before being seen?

Issues to consider

Before your visit with a new medical professional, think about what questions you have. Check out the clinic's website, which might provide some answers. You also can ask office staff general questions about the clinic. During your visit, don't feel embarrassed about asking questions that might help you get to know the medical professional and make the right decision for your family.

Training and style How long has the individual been treating children? At what hospitals does the medical professional have privileges? Does the medical professional have any particular area of expertise or interest? Does the medical professional listen to your questions, answer them thoughtfully and appear interested in your concerns?

Knowledge Does the medical professional seem to know about medical advances, and offer helpful advice?

Accessibility and referrals How does the medical professional handle emergencies, including those that occur after hours? Does the office have guidelines for what kind of questions can be resolved with a phone call or email and what requires a visit? Is the medical professional part of a group practice? If so, will you be able to request an appointment with a specific medical professional? If you choose someone who is part of a group practice, make sure you feel comfortable with other members of the practice who might treat your baby.

KEEP MEDICAL INFORMATION HANDY

Write down key information about your child's medical professional, such as contact information, the office's hours and location, and any policies for making appointments. Keep this information in a place that will be easy to access for you and anyone caring for your child. Also, create a file or notebook or an electronic record for your child's medical information. Include information such as the vaccination record, measurements, and any prescriptions or lab test results.

Ask the medical professional about the referral process for specialists. Some medical professionals may be limited to referring your child to someone who is practicing in the same healthcare network or at certain medical institutions.

Making your decision

After your appointment, consider the medical professional's overall approach to healthcare and your interactions with the staff. Most important, would you trust this person to treat your child? Trust your instincts. If you don't feel comfortable, consider another medical professional.

Once you've selected your child's medical professional, you may want to discuss topics such as breastfeeding, circumcision or child care. If you feel it would be helpful, schedule an appointment to discuss these issues.

A TEAM APPROACH

If you're ever unhappy with the care your child receives, talk to the medical professional about your concerns. Chances are, once the issue is discussed, you can agree on a solution.

If you can't resolve the problem, you might consider finding another medical professional for your child. In the coming months, your child's medical professional will help you make healthy choices for your baby, as well as determine what to do about any health problems. While you may have certain viewpoints, don't forget that your child's medical professional is trained in infant care and likely has considerable experience. It's important that you work together as a team to stay on top of your child's health.

CHAPTER 13

Checkups

Frequent checkups with a medical professional are an important part of your baby's first few years. These checkups — often called well-child visits — are a way for you and your child's medical professional to keep tabs on your child's health and development, as well as spot any potential problems. Well-child visits also give you a chance to discuss any questions or concerns you might have and get advice from a trusted source on how to provide the best possible care for your child.

At first, well-child visits aren't always easy on you or your baby. Your baby may not like getting undressed and measured — and then there are immunizations.

TIPS FOR SCHEDULING APPOINTMENTS

When scheduling appointments, consider avoiding the medical professional's busiest times. You might have the best chance of getting in and out of the office quickly if you ask for the first appointment of the day or choose a time right after lunch. On the other hand, if you'd like to have extra time to speak with your child's medical professional, you might ask for an appointment at the end of the day. Also, consider avoiding appointments on Mondays and Fridays, as well as on holidays when the office is open. These days tend to be busier than others. The end of summer vacation also tends to be a busy time for medical professionals, since many children are required to have physicals before the start of the new school year.

These visits may be stressful initially, but visiting the medical professional will soon become part of the routine for you and your child. The visits will become more enjoyable as your baby becomes familiar with the office, and you will likely look forward to finding out just how big your baby is getting. You'll also find the guidance invaluable in the months and years ahead.

CHECKUP SCHEDULE

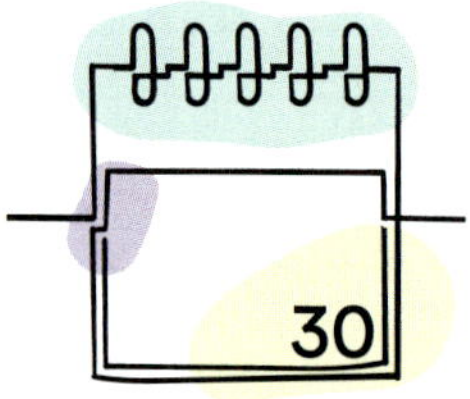

Most newborns have their first checkups within 48 to 72 hours of being sent home from the hospital, or at 3 to 5 days old. This timeline is important to have their feeding, weight gain and skin color — in case of jaundice — evaluated. After that, your child should see a medical professional at the following ages:

- Within 1 month
- 2 months
- 4 months
- 6 months
- 9 months
- 12 months
- 15 months
- 18 months
- 24 months
- 30 months
- 36 months

After age 3, most children move to a yearly exam schedule. Some children need more frequent visits. Plus, you can make an appointment for your child to see a medical professional anytime your child is sick or you're concerned about your child's health and development.

If possible, both parents should try to attend baby's first few checkups together. This will give both parents a chance to get to know the medical professional and ask basic questions. If it's just you, ask a family member or friend to help you navigate these early visits. Remembering your questions and listening to the medical professional's advice can be difficult when you're trying to undress or calm a fussy baby. An extra set of hands also may prove useful during your first few outings.

WHAT TO EXPECT AT A WELL-CHILD VISIT

Early on, the medical professional likely will pay extra attention to measuring height, weight and head circumference and doing a thorough physical exam. Over time, as the medical professional gets to know you and your child, things will likely go faster and exams may become more routine. The benefit of seeing your child's medical professional regularly is that each visit adds critical information to your child's health history. Over time, you and the medical professional will get a good idea of your child's overall health and development.

In general, the medical professional will be more attentive to your child's pattern of growth over time, rather than to specific one-time measurements. Typically, what you'll see is a smooth curve that arcs upward as the months and years go by. Regularly reviewing your child's growth chart also can alert you and the medical professional to unexpected delays in growth or changes in weight that may suggest the need for additional monitoring. You can see examples of growth charts on pages 578 and 579.

Each medical professional does things a bit differently, but here's what's generally on the agenda during a well-child exam.

Growth

Checkups usually begin with growth measurements. During first-year visits, a nurse or your baby's medical professional will measure and record your baby's length, head circumference and weight. Once your child is upright and walking, height measurements generally replace length measurements.

Starting after age 2, head circumference measurements are no longer routine, but your child's medical professional may start measuring your child's body mass index (BMI). This is a screening tool based on population averages. It uses weight in relation to height to estimate whether body size falls into categories of underweight, overweight or obese. BMI for children is expressed in percentiles, which is different from the BMI measurements we are used to seeing in adults.

Your child's measurements will be plotted on a growth chart. This will help you and the medical professional see how your child's size compares with that of other children the same age. However, try not to fixate on the percentages too much. All kids grow and develop at different rates. In addition, babies who take breast milk gain weight at a different rate than do babies who are formula-fed.

Keep in mind that a child who's in the 95th percentile for height and weight isn't necessarily healthier than a child who's in the 5th percentile. What's most

PREMATURE BABIES

If your baby was born prematurely, growth and development will be measured using corrected age — your baby's age in weeks minus the number of weeks your baby was born premature. For example, if your baby was born eight weeks early, then at age 6 months, or about 24 weeks, your baby's corrected age is 4 months, or 16 weeks. This adjustment will be necessary until your baby reaches 2 years of age or so. Immunizations, however, will be given to your baby according to chronological age, which is the number of weeks since they were born.

important is steady growth from one visit to the next. If you have questions or concerns about your child's growth rate, discuss them with your child's medical professional.

Physical exam

Your child's medical professional will give your child a thorough physical exam. Be sure to mention any concerns you have or specific areas you want checked out. The more information you can provide about your child's health, the better. Here are the basics of what medical professionals commonly check for during an exam.

Head In the beginning, your child's medical professional likely will check the soft spots (fontanels) on your baby's head. These gaps between the skull bones give your baby's brain plenty of room to grow in the coming months. They're safe to touch and typically disappear within two years, when the skull bones fuse together.

The medical professional also may check baby's head for flat spots. A baby's skull is soft and made up of several movable bones. If the head is left in the same position for long periods of time, the skull bones might move in a way that creates a flat spot. If flat spots are a concern, continue to place your baby on the back to sleep. However, your baby's medical professional may recommend alternating the direction your baby's head faces in the crib, giving your baby more tummy time while awake, and limiting the amount of time your baby spends in a car seat outside of the car. If these types of changes are made, the flattening typically improves in three to four months. Occasionally, babies need to wear a positioning helmet to improve head shape.

Ears Using an instrument called an otoscope, the medical professional can see in your child's ears to check for fluid or infection in the ears. The medical professional may observe your child's response to various sounds, including your voice. Be sure to share any concerns about your child's ability to hear or if there's a history of childhood deafness in your family. Unless there's cause for concern, a formal hearing evaluation isn't usually needed at a well-child exam.

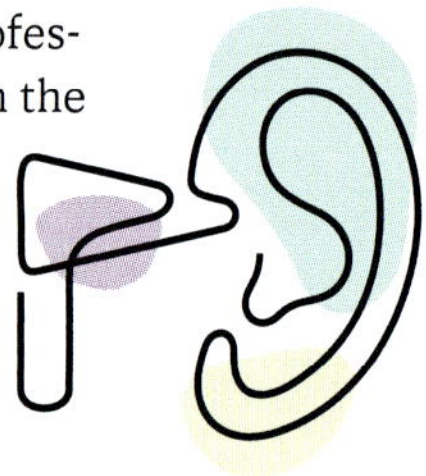

Eyes Your child's medical professional may use a flashlight to catch your child's attention and then track eye movements. The medical professional also may check for blocked tear ducts and eye discharge and look at your child's eyes with a lighted instrument called an ophthalmoscope. Share if you've noticed that your child is having any unusual eye movements, especially if they continue beyond the first few months of life.

Mouth A look inside your baby's mouth may reveal signs of oral thrush, a common and easily treated yeast infection. The medical professional also might check your baby's mouth for signs of tongue-tie (ankyloglossia). This is a condition that affects the tongue's range of motion and can interfere with a baby's oral development as well as the ability to feed.

As your baby gets older, the medical professional may ask whether your child has started to drool more than usual, become fussy or irritable, or lose appetite.

These are often the first signs of teething. Your child will be checked for emerging teeth. After teeth erupt, the medical professional likely will discuss with you the importance of regularly cleaning your baby's new teeth with a small amount of fluoride toothpaste to strengthen the teeth and prevent decay. Your child's medical professional also may recommend making an appointment for your baby with a pediatric or family dentist.

Skin Various skin conditions may be identified during the exam, including birthmarks, rashes and jaundice, a yellowish discoloration of the skin and eyes. Mild jaundice that develops soon after birth often disappears on its own within a week or two. Cases that are more severe may need treatment (see page 36).

Heart and lungs Using a stethoscope, your child's medical professional can listen to your child's heart and lungs to check for irregular heart sounds or rhythms and for breathing difficulties.

Abdomen, hips and legs By gently pressing a child's abdomen, a medical professional can detect tenderness, enlarged organs, or an umbilical hernia, which occurs when a bit of intestine or fatty tissue near the bellybutton breaks through the muscular wall of the abdomen. Most umbilical hernias go away on their own by the toddler years. The medical professional also will move your infant's legs to check for dislocation or other problems with the hip joints, such as hip dysplasia.

Genitalia Your child's medical professional likely will inspect your child's genitalia for tenderness, lumps or other signs of infection. Your baby may be checked for an inguinal hernia, which results from a weakness in the abdominal wall. For girls, the medical professional may ask about vaginal discharge. For boys, the medical professional will make sure a circumcised penis is healing well during early visits. The medical professional also may check to see that both testes have descended into the scrotum and that there's no fluid-filled sac around the testes, a condition called hydrocele.

"FAILURE TO THRIVE"

Failure to thrive is a term — not a disease — that's used to describe a baby or toddler who isn't growing or developing at an appropriate rate. It's an older term without a specific definition, but it's usually used to mean that a child's weight or height appears below the 5th percentile on a growth chart or that a child's growth rate is lower than expected. The term *weight faltering* has been proposed as an alternative.

Multiple issues may play a role, such as an underlying health problem or environmental problems. If your child's medical professional is concerned about growth and development, you may be asked about your pregnancy and delivery, your child's medical and dietary history, and your family history. With early intervention, many children respond well and catch up in their growth.

Nutrition

Your child's medical professional likely will ask you about your child's eating habits. If you're breastfeeding, you may be asked how often you're feeding your baby during the day and night and whether you're having any problems. If you're pumping, the medical professional may offer suggestions for managing pumping frequency and storing breast milk. If you're formula-feeding, the medical professional likely will want to know how often you feed and how many ounces of formula your baby takes at each feeding. In addition, you may discuss your baby's need for vitamin D and iron supplements.

Although breast milk or formula will be the main part of your baby's diet throughout the first year, eventually you'll want to discuss introducing your baby to solid foods. A medical professional can offer advice on the best foods to start with, the importance of making healthy choices and how to feed your baby. Once your baby starts eating solid foods, the medical professional may check to see if you're having any problems feeding your child or if your child has had any allergic reactions.

As your child gets older, discussion topics may include drinking from a cup, weaning your baby from the bottle by age 1, and when and how to start giving your baby whole milk. You also may want to mention any concerns about picky eating in your toddler (see Chapters 3 and 4).

Bowel and bladder function

In the first few visits, your child's medical professional likely will ask how many wet and dirty diapers your baby makes on a daily basis. This information offers clues as to whether your baby is getting enough to eat.

As your child gets older and you move closer to toilet training, usually between ages 2 and 3 years, your child's medical professional can offer advice on when to start. The medical professional also may have some tips to help you and your child transition successfully to using the toilet (see Chapter 6). A well-child visit also is an opportunity to discuss any concerns you might have about your child's bowel functions and any irregularities, such as frequent loose stools or constipation.

Sleep

Your child's medical professional may ask you questions about your child's sleep habits, such as your regular bedtime routine and how many hours your child is sleeping during the day and night. Don't hesitate to discuss any concerns you may have about your child's sleep, such as when it's OK for your baby to sleep through the night, when to stop napping, switching your toddler from a crib to a bed or getting your child to stay in bed (see Chapter 8). Your child's medical professional also may help you figure out how to find rest for yourself, especially in the early baby months.

Development

The progress of your child's development is important. Your medical professional will monitor your child's development in the following five main areas. (For a list of developmental milestones by age, see chapters in Part 3 of this book.)

Gross motor skills These skills, such as sitting, walking and climbing, involve the movement of large muscles. Your child's medical professional may ask you how well your baby can control the head. Is your baby attempting to roll over? Is your baby trying to sit without help? Is your child starting to walk or throw a ball? Can your toddler walk up and down steps?

Fine motor skills These skills involve the use of small muscles in the hand. Does your baby reach for objects and bring them to the mouth? Is your baby using individual fingers to pick up small objects? Does your child use a cup? Can your toddler draw a straight line?

Personal and social skills These skills enable a child to interact and respond to surroundings. Your child's medical professional may ask if your baby is smiling. Does your baby relate to you with joy and enthusiasm? Does baby play peekaboo? Is your toddler starting to explore without help or show signs of independence?

Language skills These skills include hearing, understanding and using language. The medical professional may ask if your baby turns toward voices or other sounds. Does your baby laugh? Is baby responding when called by name? Is your toddler starting to say "No" or point to named objects in a book?

Cognitive skills These skills allow a child to think, reason, solve problems and understand surroundings. Your child's medical professional might ask if your baby can bang together two cubes or search for a toy after seeing you hide it. Can your child point to a body part or follow simple one-step instructions?

Behavior

Your child's medical professional may ask you questions about your child's behavior or whether your child has started throwing tantrums or misbehaving.

DEVELOPMENTAL DELAYS

Before an appointment, you may be asked to complete a questionnaire about your child's developmental skills. This can help the medical professional track your child's milestones. If your child doesn't reach a specific milestone by an expected age, there may be a developmental delay.

Delays can occur in one or several areas of development. Your child's medical professional might recommend certain tests to check for underlying problems. You also may meet with a specialist, such as a developmental pediatrician. If your baby or toddler has a developmental delay, the medical professional can recommend a type of developmental therapy that may help your child make progress. Most children are eligible to receive a wide range of therapies in their homes, often at no cost. Early identification of a developmental delay is important because it will enable you to get your child help as soon as possible. For more information on developmental delays, see Chapter 45.

Explain what you've noticed so far and anything that seems out of the ordinary to you or is causing you concern. Your child's medical professional can help reassure you about what's OK and how to handle your child's budding sense of autonomy.

As your baby gets older and begins exploring everything in sight, you may find yourself setting greater limits. Your toddler also might get frustrated as a growing desire for independence conflicts with a limited vocabulary and physical abilities. Your child's medical professional might discuss the importance of creating a safe home environment and predictable routine, as well as how to handle your toddler's meltdowns without having one yourself (see Chapter 10).

Immunizations

Your baby will need a number of immunizations during the first years. The medical professional or a nurse will explain how to hold your baby as each shot is given. Be prepared for possible tears. Keep in mind, however, that the pain caused by a shot is typically short-lived but the benefits are long-lasting. Keeping up with immunizations and vaccines, including flu shots every year, is important throughout your child's life. Chapter 14 provides more detailed information on the immunizations given during the first 36 months.

Safety

Your child's medical professional may talk to you about safety issues, such as the importance of placing your baby to sleep on the back and using a rear-facing infant car seat as long as possible. As your child becomes more mobile, you may be given tips for babyproofing your home. The medical professional also may explain how to prevent falls, the importance of water safety and how to prevent infections by washing hands.

KEEP A RECORD

Some medical offices have the option for parents to review their child's medical records electronically on a secure online account. If not, consider starting a file, notebook or electronic record for your child's medical information, such as the immunization record, measurements, and any prescriptions or lab test results.

Taking time to organize your child's health history will give you a chance to review any information the medical professional gives you. It's also a good habit to start early because when your child enters preschool or kindergarten, you'll likely need to provide certain medical details. Plus, your notes about your baby's growth make for a cherished keepsake.

QUESTIONS AND CONCERNS

During checkups, it's likely that you'll have questions, too. Ask away! Nothing is too trivial when it comes to caring for your baby or toddler. Write down questions as they arise between appointments so that you'll be less likely to forget them when you're at your child's checkup. Feel free to ask your child's medical professional for advice on topics that aren't medically related, too. For example, if you're looking for child care, ask the medical professional for advice.

Also, don't forget your own health. If you're feeling depressed, stressed out, run-down or overwhelmed, describe what's happening. Your child's medical professional is there to help you, too.

Before you leave the office, make sure you know when to schedule your child's next appointment. If possible, set the next appointment before you leave the office. If you don't already know, ask how to reach your child's medical professional in between appointments. You also might ask if the medical professional has a 24-hour nurse information service. Knowing that help is available when you need it can offer peace of mind.

CHAPTER 14

Immunizations and vaccines

Before childbirth, did you think about your baby's health? Of course you did. Think back to your pregnancy — the things you did to keep yourself healthy and to prevent problems from occurring, so that the baby inside you could grow and develop. This most likely included receiving one or more immunizations to help protect you and your baby.

Prevention is crucial to good health. It's far better to prevent a disease than to treat it. And one of the best ways to protect your family from many diseases is to get immunized. Immunization is the best line of defense against diseases such as tetanus, hepatitis, influenza and many other infections.

Thanks to immunizations and vaccines, many infectious diseases that were once common in the United States are now rare or nonexistent. As a parent, you no longer have to fear that your child will die of or become disabled by smallpox or tetanus. And you no longer have to keep your children away from swimming pools to avoid getting polio.

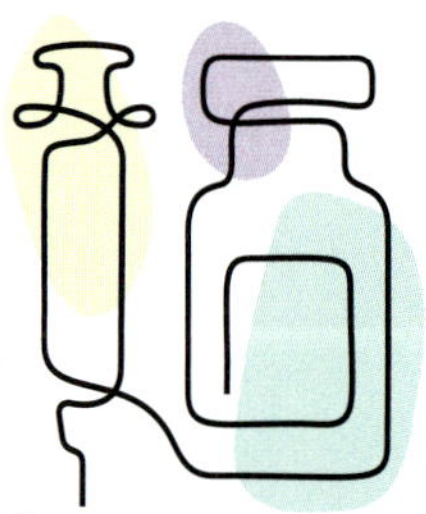

Truth be told, immunizations aren't exactly fun — for children or parents. It's hard to see your little one cry after getting a series of shots. But as much as you want to shield your child from tears, keep in mind that the discomfort is temporary and minor compared with the potential harm of a serious illness.

Immunizations prevent millions of deaths worldwide each year. However, despite the availability of vaccines, many people remain underimmunized. One reason is that some people have concerns about the safety and risks of immunizations. In addition, some people feel it's dangerous to give more than one vaccine at a time, and others feel certain vaccines are no longer needed. These concerns are the result of incorrect information.

HOW IMMUNIZATIONS AND VACCINES WORK

Every day, the human body is exposed to bacteria, viruses and other germs. When a disease-causing microorganism enters your (or your child's) body, your immune system mounts a defense, producing proteins called antibodies to fight off the harmful germ. The goal of your immune system is to neutralize or destroy the germ, making it harmless and preventing you from getting sick.

One way the body's immune system fights off harmful germs is through what's called post-exposure immunity. After you've been infected with a certain organism, your immune system puts into play a complex array of defenses to prevent you from getting sick again from that type of virus or bacterium.

Another way to get the immune system to fight bad germs is through vaccines. With this method, a person becomes immune without getting sick. A vaccine contains just enough of a killed or weakened form or derivative of the infectious germ to trigger your immune system's infection-fighting ability. But it's triggered without the harmful effects of an actual infection. The vaccine makes your body think that it's being invaded by a specific organism. Your immune system begins building defenses against that organism. In this way, vaccination is one way to provide immunization.

Another form of providing these defenses — immunization — is to provide the defenses ready-made. This is also called passive immunity. One example of this is the RSV immunization, nirsevimab (see page 187). Providing vaccination to a pregnant person is another way to provide defenses to an infant. The pregnant person's immune system creates the defenses and then passes them to the developing infant, where the defenses are active for several months after birth.

If you're exposed to a disease for which you've been immunized, the invading germs are met by antibodies and other defenses prepared to defeat them. And immunizations can be given without the risk of the serious effects of disease.

Sometimes it takes several doses of a vaccine for a full immune response — this is the case for many childhood vaccines. Some people fail to build immunity to the first doses of a vaccine, but they often respond to later doses. In addition, the immunity provided by some vaccines, such as tetanus and pertussis, isn't lifelong. Because the immune response may decrease over time, you may need another dose of a vaccine (booster) to restore or increase your immunity. And for some diseases, the organism evolves, and a new vaccine is needed against the new form. This is the case with the annual flu (influenza) shot.

WHY GET IMMUNIZED?

Because many vaccine-preventable diseases are now uncommon in the United States, some people feel less urgency about getting themselves or their children immunized. If you wonder if it's necessary to immunize your family and to keep everyone up to date with immunizations, the answer is yes. Many infectious diseases that have virtually disappeared in the United States can reappear quickly. The germs that cause the diseases still exist and can be

WELL-CHILD IMMUNIZATION SCHEDULE

The following chart lists the recommended routine childhood immunizations. Immunization guidelines for children change fairly often as new immunizations are developed, recommendations on timing and dosages are revised, and combination vaccines are created. Check with your child's medical professional to make sure that your child is up to date on immunizations.

Recommended immunization schedule for children 0-3 years*

	Ages			
Immunization	**Birth**	**1 mo.**	**2 mos.**	**4 mos.**
RSV	1 dose if mother did not receive dose of RSV vaccine (Abrysvo) at 32-36 weeks gestation and at least 14 days before birth			
Hepatitis B	HepB (1st dose)	HepB (2nd dose)		
Rotavirus (2-dose or 3-dose series)			RV (1st dose)	RV (2nd dose)
Diphtheria, tetanus and pertussis			DTaP (1st dose)	DTaP (2nd dose)
Haemophilus influenzae type b (3-dose or 4-dose series)			Hib (1st dose)	Hib (2nd dose)
Pneumococcal conjugate			PCV (1st dose)	PCV (2nd dose)
Inactivated poliovirus			IPV (1st dose)	IPV (2nd dose)
Flu (influenza)				
COVID-19 (2-dose or 3-dose series depending on the brand)				
Measles, mumps and rubella				
Varicella				
Hepatitis A				

*Based on 2024 recommendations.

Source: Centers for Disease Control and Prevention

You also can view current immunization schedules on the CDC's website. Health insurance usually covers most of the cost of immunizations. A federal program called Vaccines for Children provides free immunizations to children who lack health insurance coverage and to other specific groups of children. Ask your medical professional about it.

Recommended immunization schedule for children 0-3 years*

Age					
6 mos.	**12 mos.**	**15 mos.**	**18 mos.**	**19-23 mos.**	**2-3 yrs.**
HepB (3rd dose)					
RV (3rd dose if 3-dose series)					
DTaP (3rd dose)		DTaP (4th dose)			
Hib (3rd dose if 4-dose series)	Hib (Final dose)				
PCV (3rd dose)	PCV (4th dose)				
IPV (3rd dose)					
Flu (annually, 2 doses for the first season 28 days apart beginning in September and at 6 months of age or older; subsequent years only 1 dose needed)					
Begin 2-dose or 3-dose series depending on the brand					
	MMR (1st dose)				
	VAR (1st dose)				
	HepA (2 doses at least 6 mos. apart)				

acquired and spread by people who aren't protected by immunization.

As travelers unknowingly carry disease from one country to another, a new outbreak may be only a plane trip away. From a single entry point, an infectious disease can spread quickly among unprotected individuals. Outbreaks of mumps and measles have repeatedly occurred in just this way in the United States in the past few years.

IMMUNIZATION SAFETY

As a new parent, you might have some misgivings about giving your child immunizations. You don't want to do anything to harm your child, and it's even difficult to do things that can cause discomfort or distress for your baby. And while you know that immunizations are important, perhaps you've also heard that they could be harmful, too — possibly causing side effects. You may worry after hearing or seeing reports about a severe "reaction" that occurs shortly after a child's immunization visit that's said to be a side effect or complication of a vaccine. Theories and stories such as these frequently circulate on the internet.

The fact is, immunizations are extremely safe. Before they can be used, they must meet strict safety standards set by the Food and Drug Administration (FDA). Meeting these standards typically requires a lengthy development process lasting 10 to 14 years, from exploratory work in laboratories through

ALTERNATIVE IMMUNIZATION SCHEDULES

Some people tout what they call alternative immunization schedules. These typically delay immunizations by spacing them further apart than they need to be and skipping some altogether. For parents who may be skittish about giving their children so many immunizations due at once, such schedules may seem reasonable.

But health experts, including those at Mayo Clinic, point out that these approaches leave the children unprotected for too long and put the children through more pain and anxiety because they receive more shots at older ages. Furthermore, none of these alternative schedules has undergone scientific study. They are dangerous because of the increased risks they pose. Delaying and skipping immunizations dramatically increases the child's risk of illness.

If you're concerned, talk with your child's medical professional to make sure that you're getting the correct information. In the end it must be your decision, but you must have your questions answered with the best information we have.

years of testing in humans, all before the immunization can be licensed. These studies, unlike drug studies, involve tens of thousands of individuals. The FDA licenses immunizations that meet these requirements. Then the Advisory Committee on Immunization Practices (ACIP, part of the Centers for Disease Control and Prevention, CDC) examines the current rates of risk of a specific infection for individuals and determines whether or not to recommend immunizations based on that risk.

Once immunizations are licensed and made available to the general public, the FDA and the CDC continue to monitor their safety. Furthermore, immunizations are subject to ongoing research, review, and refinement by doctors, scientists and public health officials. Those who provide immunizations, such as medical professionals, must report any side effects they observe to the FDA and the CDC.

The bottom line is, your child's chances of being harmed by an infectious illness are far greater than the chances of being harmed by an immunization used to prevent that disease.

Additives

In addition to the killed or weakened microorganisms that make up vaccines, small amounts of other substances may be added to an immunization to

COMFORTING BABY DURING AND AFTER IMMUNIZATION

It can be difficult to see your baby cry or be uncomfortable as a result of immunization. Try to keep in mind that protecting your baby against serious disease is worth the short-term discomfort. Studies have shown that giving all the immunizations due at once actually reduces a baby's pain and anxiety rather than giving them at separate visits. Studies also show parents do not successfully make all the visits as planned when they space out the immunizations.

During each injection, hold your baby close. Offer a pacifier, blanket or other comfort object. Your calm presence can help your baby feel secure.

Your baby may experience mild side effects from the immunization, such as redness, pain or swelling at the injection site. Ask the medical professional what to expect. If your baby develops discomfort from fever or soreness at the injection site, you may give your baby acetaminophen (Tylenol, others) beginning at 2 months of age. If your child is 6 months or older, you can use ibuprofen (Advil, Motrin, others). Follow the label instructions for the correct dose (see dosage charts on pages 580 and 581). Years ago parents were encouraged to give such medicines before the immunizations were given and before any discomfort appeared. Experts no longer recommend this, as the medications decrease the baby's immune response to the immunization. Use the medications only when needed.

enhance the immune response, prevent contamination, and stabilize the immunization against temperature variations and other conditions. Immunizations may also contain small amounts of materials used in the manufacturing process, such as gelatin.

One additive that received much attention is a preservative called thimerosal, which is a derivative of mercury. Thimerosal has been used in medical products since the 1930s and in small amounts in some vaccines to prevent bacterial contamination. Several very large studies have shown clearly that children have not been harmed by its use in vaccines. Nonetheless, childhood immunizations are now made without thimerosal or with only trace amounts.

Vaccines and autism

Many parents have heard claims that vaccines cause autism. The most common and specific claims are that autism stems from the measles, mumps and rubella (MMR) vaccine or from vaccines that contain the preservative thimerosal. An ex-physician who lost his license invented this claim, which has since been exposed as a fraud. Studies conducted around the world have shown without a doubt that the MMR vaccine doesn't cause autism. In the meantime, researchers have learned a great deal about autism itself. For example, it's now known that the signs of autism often appear well before the first dose of the MMR vaccine is given. And several causes of autism have been identified — some are genetic in nature, while others act early in pregnancy. Unfortunately, the claims about autism and the MMR vaccine persist, and they've led some parents to refuse to immunize their children.

Some people also worry that receiving too many vaccines early in life can overwhelm a baby's immune system and that this might somehow harm the baby. Such reasoning doesn't fit with what we know about the remarkable capacity of the immune system. From the day a child is born, the immune system begins battling microorganisms in the form of bacteria, viruses and fungi. A system that effectively copes with exposure to countless everyday bacteria can easily withstand exposure to the antigens in vaccines.

MISSING AN IMMUNIZATION

If your baby falls behind on immunizations, catch-up schedules can address the problem in most cases. Make an appointment with your child's medical professional to determine the immunizations your baby needs and when to get them.

An interruption in the schedule doesn't require a child to start a series over or redo any doses. But until the entire vaccine series is given, your child won't have the maximum possible protection against diseases.

CHILDHOOD IMMUNIZATIONS

Fortunately, many of the most problematic diseases of childhood —including influenza, RSV, COVID-19, whooping cough, tetanus, chickenpox, measles and mumps — can be prevented through immunization (see recommended schedule on pages 182-183).

Respiratory syncytial virus (RSV)

RSV causes infections of the lungs and respiratory tract. It's so common that most children have been infected with the virus by age 2. In adults and older, healthy children, RSV typically causes mild, cold-like symptoms. However, it can cause severe infection in some people, including babies 12 months and younger, especially premature infants, older adults, people with heart and lung disease, or anyone with a weak immune system. Severe RSV symptoms can lead to dangerous difficulty breathing, pneumonia and other complications.

Recommendation An RSV vaccine is available for pregnant people to help protect their baby from birth through 6 months of age. If that was not given during pregnancy, an antibody product called nirsevimab (Beyfortus) is recommended for babies younger than 8 months born during or entering their first RSV season. This single-dose immunization is given in the month before or during RSV season. Nirsevimab also can be given to children 8 months through 19 months old who are at higher risk of severe RSV disease through their second RSV season.

Hepatitis B

The hepatitis B virus can cause a short-term (acute) illness marked by loss of appetite, fatigue, diarrhea, vomiting, jaundice, and pain in muscles, joints and the abdomen. More rarely it can lead to long-term (chronic) liver damage (cirrhosis) or liver cancer.

The virus is spread through contact with the blood or other body fluids of an infected person. This can happen by sharing personal items, such as toothbrushes or razors, or having unprotected sex. It also can happen during birth, when the virus passes from an infected mother to her baby. Twenty percent of people in the United States with hepatitis B contract it from exposures other than birth, sex or known blood exposure. The infection can be silent for decades before the liver shows signs of the infection.

Recommendation The hepatitis B vaccine is given to children in three doses — at birth, at least one month later (1 to 2 months of age) and then at 6 to 18 months. Most people who are vaccinated with hepatitis B vaccine are immune for life.

Diphtheria

Diphtheria is a bacterial infection that spreads from person to person through airborne droplets. It causes a thick covering (membrane) to develop in the back of the throat and can lead to severe breathing problems, paralysis, heart failure and death. It used to be the most common cause of school-age death from infection. Due to vaccination, the disease is now rare in the United States.

Recommendation The diphtheria vaccine typically is given in combination with the tetanus and pertussis vaccines (a DTaP shot). Vaccination should begin when a child reaches 2 months of age. A child should receive five shots in the first six years of life, a booster shot of tetanus, diphtheria and pertussis (Tdap) at age 11 or 12, and then a tetanus and diphtheria (Td) booster every 10 years after.

Hib disease

Haemophilus influenzae type b (Hib) disease is primarily a childhood illness, but it also can affect some adults. It's caused by bacteria that spread from person to person through the air. This infection can cause serious and potentially fatal problems, including meningitis, sepsis, severe swelling in the throat, and infections of the blood, joints, bones and membranes around the heart (pericarditis).

Recommendation The Hib vaccine is given to children at ages 2 months, 4 months, and 12 to 15 months. Some brands of vaccine also need a dose given at 6 months.

Pneumococcal disease

Pneumococcal disease is the leading cause of bacterial meningitis and ear infections among children younger than 5 years. It also can cause blood infections and pneumonia. Children below the age of 2 are at greatest risk of the most serious complications of this disease.

WHY SO MANY SO SOON?

Newborns need multiple immunizations because infectious diseases can cause more serious problems in infants than in older children.

While a mother's antibodies help protect newborns from many diseases, this immunity may begin to disappear as quickly as one month after birth. In addition, children don't receive maternal immunity from certain diseases, such as whooping cough. If a child isn't immunized quickly and is exposed to a disease, the child may become sick and spread the illness.

Research shows that it's safe for infants and young children to receive multiple immunizations at the same time, as recommended by the Centers for Disease Control and Prevention. In addition, giving several immunizations at once means fewer office visits. This saves time and money for parents and may be less traumatic for the child.

Remember, newborns and young children can be exposed to diseases from family members, child care providers and other close contacts, as well as during routine outings — such as trips to the grocery store. Immunizations can often be given even if your child has a mild illness, such as a cold, earache or mild fever. It's important to keep your child's immunization status up to date.

Pneumococcal disease is caused by *Streptococcus pneumoniae* bacteria. The bacteria spread from person to person through physical contact or by inhaling droplets released into the air when a person with the infection coughs or sneezes. Because many strains of the bacterium have become resistant to antibiotics, the disease can be difficult to treat.

Recommendation Pneumococcal conjugate vaccine (PCV) can help prevent serious pneumococcal disease. It also reduces the child's risk for ear infections and the resulting need to have tubes placed surgically in the eardrums. The vaccine is given in four doses between ages 2 months and 15 months.

Polio

Polio is caused by a virus (poliovirus) that enters the body through the mouth. Polio affects the brain and spinal cord and can result in paralysis or death. Polio vaccination began in the United States in 1955. Rare polio cases have been reported in this country recently, as the disease still occurs in some parts of the world. Because the virus can be brought to the United States through travelers, getting vaccinated against polio continues to be critical. The vaccine, called inactivated poliovirus vaccine (IPV), contains the chemically killed virus. IPV is given by multiple injections.

Recommendation IPV is given in four doses, at ages 2 months, 4 months, 6 to 18 months, and 4 to 6 years. The last vaccination is a booster dose. Contrary to the fears of some people, the shots can't cause polio.

Rotavirus

Rotavirus is a common cause of severe diarrhea among infants and children. Almost all children are infected with rotavirus before their fifth birthday. The infection is often accompanied by vomiting and fever. It can cause severe dehydration, especially in infants and toddlers.

Recommendation Rotavirus vaccine is a swallowed (oral) vaccine medication, not a shot. The vaccine is very good at preventing diarrhea and vomiting caused by rotavirus. Since the vaccine was introduced, it has significantly decreased the number of rotavirus infections in young children. It won't prevent diarrhea or vomiting caused by other germs, however.

There are two brands of rotavirus vaccine. A baby should get either two or three doses, depending on which brand is used. The first dose is given at 2 months, the second at 4 months and the third dose, if needed, at 6 months.

Tetanus

Tetanus causes painful tightening of the muscles, usually all over the body. It can be difficult to open your mouth (lockjaw) or swallow. Tetanus isn't contagious. The tetanus bacteria enter the body through deep or dirty cuts or wounds.

Recommendation The tetanus vaccine typically is given in combination with those for diphtheria and pertussis (DTaP vaccine). Immunization is acquired through a series of five shots beginning when the infant is 2 months old and continuing to between ages 4 and 6. Starting at age 11, people should boost their immunization every 10 years with the adult form of the vaccine.

Whooping cough

Whooping cough (pertussis) is a disease that causes severe coughing spells, making it hard for infants and toddlers to eat, drink or even breathe. The word *pertussis* is from the Latin word for "cough." These coughing spells can last for weeks and can lead to pneumonia, seizures, brain damage and death. Severe whooping cough primarily occurs in children younger than 2 years and is contracted by inhaling infected droplets, often coughed into the air from an adult with a mild case of the disease.

Recommendation The DTaP vaccine combines vaccines for diphtheria, tetanus and pertussis. It's given as a series of five shots beginning when the infant is 2 months old and continuing to between ages 4 and 6. The DTaP vaccine is a better-tolerated version of an older vaccine called DTP. The "a" in DTaP stands for "acellular," meaning that only specific parts of the pertussis bacteria are used in the vaccine. This has reduced the reactions to this vaccine, including fever and irritability.

An adolescent-and-adult form of the vaccine, called Tdap, is recommended starting at age 11 years. It is also recommended in pregnancy to protect the infant in the first seven months of life. Infants are not fully protected until they have had all three doses at 2, 4, and 6 months of life.

IMMUNIZATIONS FOR PRETERM BABIES

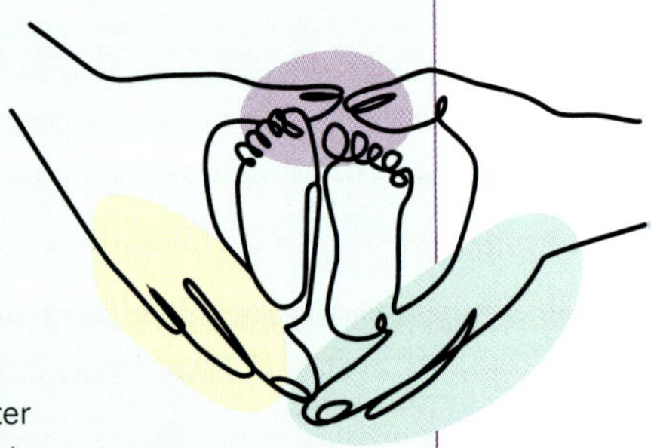

If your baby was born early or with a low birth weight, you might be concerned about having your baby immunized on the standard schedule. However, it's recommended that even premature babies should be given the routinely recommended immunizations based on their chronological age without delay. They respond well and the immunizations are safe for them to receive.

Keep in mind that premature babies have a greater chance of having disease-related problems, putting them at particular risk if they acquire a preventable infection. All the vaccines and immunizations that are currently available are safe for premature babies and those with low birth weight and pose the same minimal risk of side effects as in full-term babies and babies with normal birth weight.

There is only one exception to this: the hepatitis B vaccine that is given soon after birth. For an infant who weighs less than 2.2 pounds at birth, your medical professional may need to give your baby a fourth dose in the first six months. Or, depending on your prenatal testing, the medical professional may delay the first dose for one month or until hospital discharge.

COVID-19

COVID-19 is an illness caused by the virus known as severe acute respiratory syndrome coronavirus 2, or more commonly, SARS-CoV-2. The virus spreads most commonly through the air in tiny droplets of fluid between people in close contact. Many people with COVID-19 have no symptoms or mild illness. But for older adults and people with certain medical conditions, COVID-19 can lead to the need for care in the hospital or death.

Recommendation The Centers for Disease Control and Prevention (CDC) recommends a COVID-19 vaccine for everyone age 6 months and older. While rare, some children can become seriously ill with COVID-19. Staying up to date on your COVID-19 vaccination helps prevent infection and especially protects against serious illness and the need for hospital care due to severe COVID-19.

Flu (influenza)

Influenza is a viral infection that sickens millions of people each year and can cause serious complications, especially in children and older adults. Flu vaccines are designed to protect against strains of flu virus expected to be in circulation during the fall and winter of that year. Flu season varies across the United States. For most of us, it's best to get vaccinated in September or October, so that you and your child receive protection before the start of the flu season.

Recommendation The influenza vaccine is recommended yearly for infants and children, beginning at age 6 months. Children require two doses of the flu vaccine the first time they receive it. That's because they don't develop an adequate antibody level the first time they get the vaccine. Antibodies help fight the virus if it enters your child's system.

Chickenpox

Chickenpox (varicella) is a once common childhood disease that in years past every child got. Mayo Clinic studies in the 1970s showed how harmful chickenpox could be to healthy children. Chickenpox often resulted in impetigo, ear infections and pneumonia. A significant proportion needed medical care and hospitalization. It also can affect adults who aren't immune, and the disease is even harder on adults. Furthermore, chickenpox can lead to recurrences of viral inflammation later in life called shingles (herpes zoster).

The chickenpox virus is spread by breathing in infected droplets from the air or by direct contact with fluid from the rash, which is the best-known sign of the disease. The rash begins as superficial spots on the face, chest, back and other areas of the body. The spots quickly fill with a clear fluid, rupture and turn crusty.

Recommendation Children should receive one dose of the chickenpox (varicella) vaccine between 12 and 15 months of age and a second dose between 4 and 6 years of age.

German measles

German measles (rubella) is a contagious disease that spreads through the air from people sick with the infection. It's typically a mild infection that causes a rash and slight fever. However, women who develop rubella during pregnancy may have miscarriages or give birth to children with severe, irreversible birth defects. By vaccinating all children, including boys, young women who are raising children, caring for them, living next door to them, or teaching them are protected from this infection. In this way this vaccine prevents congenital rubella syndrome.

Recommendation Two doses of the combination measles, mumps and rubella (MMR) vaccine are given, the first at ages 12 to 15 months and the second at 4 to 6 years.

Hepatitis A

Hepatitis A is a highly contagious liver disease caused by the hepatitis A virus. The virus is found in an infected person's stool. It's usually spread by eating or drinking contaminated food or water or by close personal contact.

Children do not get sick when they contract hepatitis A, but diaper-wearing children easily spread it. Adults caring for them can get very sick from hepatitis A, with jaundice, fever and malaise lasting weeks to months.

Recommendation The two-dose series of the hepatitis A vaccine is recommended for all children in the United States. The first dose is generally given at 12 to 23 months and the second dose 6 to 18 months later.

Measles

Measles (rubeola) is primarily a childhood illness, although adults also are susceptible. It's the most contagious human virus known. The measles virus is transmitted through the air in droplets, such as from a sneeze. The virus can remain suspended for hours in the air of a room where an infected person was.

Symptoms include rash, fever, cough, sneezing, runny nose, eye irritation and a sore throat. Measles can lead to an ear infection, pneumonia, seizures, brain damage and even death.

Recommendation Typically, two doses of a combined measles, mumps and rubella (MMR) vaccine are given, beginning at ages 12 to 15 months and then again at 4 to 6 years.

SIGNS OF A SEVERE REACTION

After immunization, watch for any unusual conditions, such as a serious allergic reaction (anaphylaxis). Symptoms of a serious allergic reaction include difficulty breathing, hoarseness or wheezing, hives, paleness, weakness, a fast heartbeat, dizziness, and swelling of the throat. Severe reactions are rare and usually occur in the first 15 minutes after the immunization is given. But if you think that your baby may be experiencing one, call your child's medical professional or go to an emergency department immediately.

Mumps

Mumps is a childhood disease that also can occur in adults. Mumps is caused by a virus that spreads through inhaled droplets. The disease causes fever, headache, fatigue and swollen, painful salivary glands. It can lead to deafness, meningitis, and inflammation of the testicles or ovaries, with the possibility of sterility.

Recommendation Two doses of a combined measles, mumps and rubella (MMR) vaccine are given, usually beginning at ages 12 to 15 months and then again at 4 to 6 years. Use of this vaccine has markedly decreased the incidence of mumps in the United States.

SIDE EFFECTS OF IMMUNIZATIONS

Although immunizations are considered very safe, like all medications they aren't completely free of side effects. Most side effects are minor and temporary. Your child might experience soreness or swelling at the injection site or a mild fever. Serious reactions, such as a seizure or high fever, are very rare.

According to the CDC, serious side effects occur on the order of 1 per 1,000 doses to 1 per 1 million doses. The risk of death from an immunization is so slight that it can't be accurately determined. When any serious reactions are reported, they undergo careful review by the Food and Drug Administration and the CDC.

Some vaccines are blamed for chronic illnesses, such as autism or diabetes. (See page 186 for more on autism and vaccines.) However, decades of vaccine use in the United States show no credible evidence that immunizations cause these illnesses. Researchers have, on occasion, reported a link between vaccine use and chronic illness. But when other researchers have tried to duplicate those results — a test of good scientific research — they haven't been able to produce the same findings.

When to avoid immunizations

In a few circumstances, immunizations should be postponed or avoided. Talk to your child's medical professional if you question whether your baby should be immunized.

Immunization may be inappropriate if a child has:

- Had a serious or life-threatening allergic reaction (anaphylaxis) to a previous dose of that immunization
- A severe allergy (anaphylaxis) to an immunization component, such as gelatin
- A medical condition or treatment that has compromised the child's immune system and could allow a live-virus vaccine (MMR, chickenpox, or rotavirus) to cause severe illness

Immunization may need to be delayed if a child has:

- A moderate to severe acute illness with or without fever
- Received a transfusion of blood or plasma or been given blood products within the past year that might prevent a live-virus vaccine (MMR, chickenpox, or rotavirus) from working

THE IMPACT OF VACCINATIONS

Thanks to the use of immunizations, many childhood illnesses are no longer common concerns. This graph shows the number of U.S. cases of certain childhood illnesses before vaccines were available, compared with recent numbers.

However, high rates of immunization are needed to keep case case numbers low. For example, in areas with lower vaccination rates, measles can spread more easily, leading to local outbreaks.

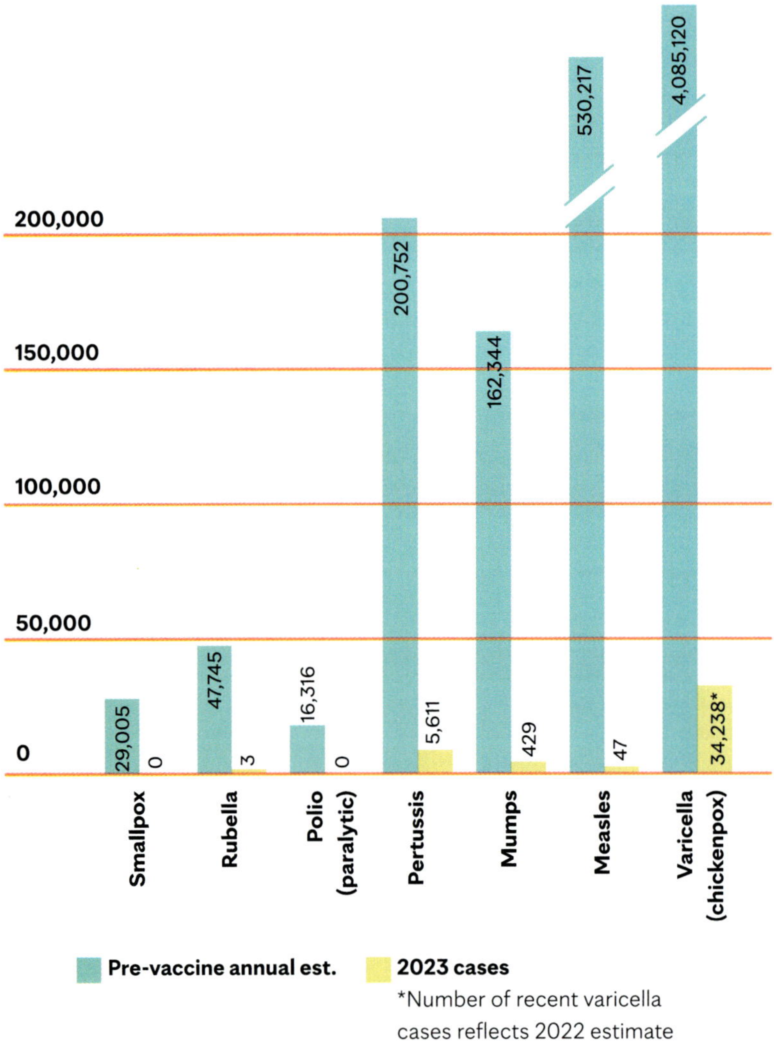

Source: Vaccine-Preventable Disease Morbidity in the United States. Centers for Disease Control and Prevention, 2024.

Immunization shouldn't be delayed because your baby has a minor illness, such as a common cold, an ear infection or mild diarrhea. The immunization will still be effective, and it won't make your child sicker.

WEIGHING THE RISKS AND BENEFITS

The consequences of getting a disease that can be prevented by immunization are far greater than the extremely rare risk of a serious side effect resulting from an immunization. For example, if your child gets mumps, the risk of developing encephalitis is 1 in 300. For measles, the risk is 1 in 2,000. Encephalitis is a brain inflammation that can cause permanent, serious brain damage. In contrast, the risk of contracting encephalitis from the mumps and measles vaccines is virtually nonexistent.

If a child gets serious Hib disease, the chances of death are 1 in 20. The vaccine for Hib disease, meanwhile, hasn't been associated with any serious adverse reactions and is highly effective.

Most childhood immunizations are effective in 85% to 99% or more of children who receive them. For example, a full series of measles vaccine protects 99 out of 100 children from measles, and a polio vaccine series protects 99 out of 100 children from polio. The graph on page 194 shows how effectively these and other vaccines have prevented childhood diseases since the vaccines were introduced in the 20th century.

CHAPTER 15

Child care

When you first get home from the hospital, it might be hard to imagine trusting anyone else to take care of your baby. You might have a difficult time feeling comfortable taking your baby with you as you run errands, let alone picturing yourself dropping your baby off at a child care center. But for many families, child care is a necessity at some point — whether in the form of the occasional babysitter, full-time nanny, child care center or other option. So how do you find child care that will promote your baby's health, safety and development but won't completely empty your bank account?

To begin, determine how much you can afford to spend on child care, and identify your needs and expectations — what's important to your family when it comes to child care. Then begin looking around at the available options in your area, usually the sooner the better. To make the most of your visits, make sure you know how to identify quality child care providers.

GETTING STARTED

Whether you need full-time child care after your baby is born or just need some help a few days a week, it's never too early to start thinking about child care arrangements. Even if you're not sure about your plans, begin exploring and researching your options early.

Start by asking your friends, your co-workers or your child's medical professional for recommendations. Your local child care resource and referral agency can be a great source of information, too. It can provide resources about licensing requirements, and also assess whether your family may qualify for financial assistance. See the additional resources on page 575.

You might want to visit multiple child care centers to find the right one for your child — and many child care centers have long waiting lists. If you're looking for in-home care, you might need time to find a child care agency, interview caregivers, and set up health insurance or workers' compensation for your child's caregiver.

Before you return to work, you might want to have your child spend time at a child care center or with a child care provider. This will allow you to see how your child handles the situation and whether the arrangement works for your family.

CHILD CARE OPTIONS

There are a variety of child care options. Generally, they tend to include the following arrangements.

In-home care

Under this arrangement, a caregiver comes to your home to provide child care. The person might live with you or come to your home each day, depending on the agreement you work out. Some examples of in-home caregivers include babysitters, nannies and au pairs. Au pairs are typically people who come to the United States on a student visa and provide child care in exchange for room and board and a small salary.

Pros One of the big advantages of this type of arrangement is that your baby can stay at home. You don't have to bundle up your baby early in the morning to drop off baby on your way to work. In addition, you set your own standards, and you might have more flexibility with your work hours.

Other advantages of an in-home arrangement are that your child will get individual attention and won't be exposed to other children's illnesses or poor behaviors. Plus, you likely won't need backup care if your baby becomes ill. You won't need to worry about transportation for your baby unless you want your child care provider to take your baby somewhere. An in-home caregiver also might be able to help with light housework or preparing meals during your baby's naps.

If you use an agency to find a child care provider, you may have the comfort of knowing that someone has already checked the backgrounds and references of potential candidates. If you have more than one child, in-home care might not be significantly more expensive than other care options.

Cons This type of care isn't well regulated and typically is more expensive than other options. If you use an agency to find a child care provider, you'll likely have to pay a hefty fee. Your caregiver might have minimal training in child development, first aid or CPR. As an employer of a child care provider, you also might have certain legal and financial obligations, such as meeting minimum wage and tax-reporting requirements or providing health insurance. Some people also feel uncomfortable having a caregiver spending time in or living in their homes.

There might not be as much opportunity for your baby to socialize with other children, which becomes increasingly important as your baby develops into a toddler. You may need to provide your child's caregiver with an allowance for gas and arrange daily activities you'd like your child to be involved in. And when your child care provider becomes sick or goes on vacation, you'll need to find backup care.

Family child care

Many people provide child care in their homes for small groups of children, sometimes in addition to caring for their own children. Typically, family child care centers provide care for children of mixed ages. Small programs provide care for up to 6 children at one time, while large programs are for 7 to 12 children.

Pros One of the main attractions of family child care is that it allows your baby to be in a home-like setting with other children. In addition, family child care is often less expensive than care provided by an in-home caregiver or a child care center. Homes that offer child care usually have to meet state or local

CARE FOR CHILDREN WITH SPECIAL NEEDS

If your child has a developmental disability or chronic illness, finding quality child care may require additional considerations. The best programs encourage regular activities and also meet each child's special needs. To find a child care program, ask your child's medical professional or your state's department of health or education. Your child's medical professional also can help you determine what kind of care will best address your child's needs. Look for a program that meets the basic requirements you'd want in a child care program. Here are several other things to look for.

Specialized staffing and equipment

Has the program's staff been trained to meet your child's specific needs and recognize when your child might need medical attention? Does the program have a medical consultant who is involved in the program's development? What kind of specialized equipment does the program provide, and is it in working condition? Has the staff been trained to use it? Does the program tailor emergency plans to the needs of its children?

Confidence-building activities

What kinds of activities will your child be able to participate in? Does the program include children who don't have special needs? Programs that care for children who have different levels of ability can help encourage social confidence and sensitivity.

safety and cleanliness standards. Some places might be able to cater to your baby's and family's specific needs, providing extended hours or offering care for children with special needs.

Cons The quality can vary widely. While many family child care providers undergo background checks and participate in ongoing training, not all may be required to do so. Family homes may not have the same facility resources as larger child care centers. You may have to drop off and pick up your baby at the home at specified times.

Child care centers

Child care centers — also called day care centers, child development centers, or sometimes preschool or pre-kindergarten programs — are organized facilities with staff members who are trained to care for groups of children. In these settings, care typically is provided in a building — rather than a home — with separate classrooms for children of different ages. Programs can be large or small, based on their maximum capacity. A child care center can be part of a chain or independent, for-profit or nonprofit, state-funded or part of a federal program such as Head Start. Some child care programs also have religious affiliations or income eligibility requirements.

Pros Child care centers offer many advantages. They're generally required to meet state or local standards. Many have structured programs designed to meet the needs of children at different age levels. Child care centers often have high education requirements for staff. And because most centers have several caregivers, you likely won't need backup care if a child care provider becomes sick. In addition, child care centers provide opportunities for socialization with other children. Some centers might provide extended hours or allow you to enroll your baby for less than a full week if you work part-time. Some child care centers also allow you to check in on your baby during the day via secure online video systems.

Cons A drawback of larger facilities is that they might have long waiting lists for admission. Also, spending time with other children can increase your baby's risk of getting sick. Because of this, some child care centers might not let you bring a mildly ill child to the center. Child care centers can be expensive, depending on the services offered. Regulations vary, too. If the program is large or the ratio of care providers to children is low, your child might not receive a lot of individual attention. You may have to drop off and pick up your baby at the child care center at specified times. Some centers charge fees if you don't pick up your baby on time.

Relative or friend

Many people rely on relatives or friends to provide part-time or full-time care for their children. While having someone you know and trust take care of your child is comforting, there are advantages and disadvantages to this type of arrangement, too.

Pros Chances are your baby will receive plenty of individual attention. You might even be able to have your relative or friend care for your baby in your own home, so you don't need to worry about transportation. Your baby won't be exposed to other children's illnesses or misbehaviors, and you may not need backup care if your baby becomes ill. This type of arrangement might give you some flexibility with your work hours, too. It's also possible, depending on the agreement you work out, that you might not need to pay your friend or relative for child care services, or you can pay a discounted rate.

Cons Your friend or relative might not have any training in CPR or other emergency care. If you pay your friend or relative and they provide care in your home, you'll want to check out your local employment laws to make sure you meet requirements for matters such as tax withholding, health insurance and workers' compensation.

Sometimes the main drawback of having a family member or a friend provide care is that it can cause tension. You might not feel comfortable talking to your relative or friend if you have differing opinions about how to care for your child. Your relative or friend also might offer unwanted parenting advice.

FACTORS TO CONSIDER

Before you look at facilities or interview care providers, think about what kind of child care might work best for your family. Knowing your priorities will help you in the process.

Expectations

Think about your family's needs and what's most important to you in a child care provider. Here are some questions to ask yourself: How many days and hours a week do you expect your child to need care? How do you want your child care provider to approach misbehavior in your child? If you're considering hiring a nanny, do you want the nanny to be able to drive and do light housework? If you're considering out-of-home care, how far away from your home or place of

SICK CARE

When your child becomes ill and you need backup care, you might have options beyond staying home to provide care. Some child care centers or family child care programs offer care for sick children in a separate area. Your community might have child care centers or family child care programs that specialize in providing care only for sick children. Some employers also provide sick care for their employees' children. Investigate your options before your child becomes ill. When looking for this type of care, ask about how much individual care your child will receive, how the facility and equipment are cleaned, and whether the facility has a medical professional on call.

work would you like your child to be? How will you handle transportation to and from the child care center or access to transportation your caregiver and child might need during the day? What kind of backup arrangements can you make if your child or care provider becomes sick? Do you want your child to be exposed to a specific language? How much free playtime will your child have? How much time outdoors?

Budget

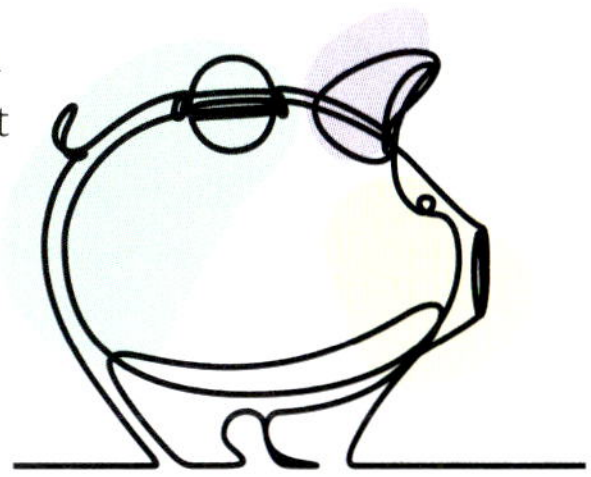

Think about how much money you can afford to spend on child care and how different types of child care will affect your budget. Are you eligible for any state subsidies or assistance from your employer, such as employee discounts or dependent care spending accounts? If you're considering in-home care, are you prepared to pay any necessary state taxes and the cost of backup care during your child care provider's vacation and sick days? If you're concerned about the expense of child care, could you or your partner adjust work hours or schedules to reduce your need for child care?

EVALUATING YOUR OPTIONS

Once you've thought about what kind of child care will work best for your family, compile a list of potential caregivers or facilities in your area. Next, call, interview or visit the caregivers or facilities. During your visit, pay special attention to the way staff members treat the children. After a tour, be prepared with a list of questions. If you're evaluating several different settings or child care providers, consider taking notes.

In-home care

When looking for someone to come into your home to care for your baby, checking references is crucial — especially if vetting by an agency hasn't already occurred. Talk to several of the child care provider's previous employers and ask questions about the person's strengths and weaknesses, as well as any problems or concerns the employer might have had. Do a background check. Search for information about the person online via a search engine or social networking sites. Ask about the care provider's approach to child care. What will the care provider do if your baby won't stop crying? How will the care provider manage tantrums? What kind of hours can the provider work? What kind of salary does the child care provider expect? Does the provider need health insurance? Does the provider have CPR and first-aid training?

Family child care

Look for a facility that's certified and licensed and provides a safe environment for children. Ask about how many child care providers are on staff and if they have undergone background checks. Request references. Ask about the provider's training, how many children are enrolled and the facility's hours. Discuss the facility's approach to child rearing. How many child care providers are currently certified in CPR and have first-aid training? Who lives in and visits the home? What are their backgrounds, and how might they interact with your child? How does the staff plan to deal with emergencies? What safety measures are in place? Are there daily activities for the children? Find out what happens if the care provider becomes ill or goes on vacation. How much does the program cost?

Child care center

When evaluating child care centers, find out about each program's practices. Many child care centers provide pamphlets or have websites to answer your questions. You can also speak to the program's director. Consider asking about the following topics.

Credentials and staff qualifications Make sure the program is licensed and has a recent inspection certificate. Programs that are accredited have met voluntary standards for child care that go beyond most state licensing requirements. The National Association for the Education of Young Children and the National Association for Family Child Care are the two largest organizations that accredit child care programs. Staff should have training in early child development, CPR and first aid. References should be available upon request. Ask if there are frequent staff changes, since high staff turnover might be a sign of a problem and changing care providers can be hard on a child. If possible, talk to at least one parent whose child was in the program in the past year.

Adult-to-child ratios Ask about the ratio of adults to children. The fewer the children for each adult, the better the child care experience may be for your child. For infants, look for an adult-to-child ratio of 1 to 3 or 1 to 4. Also, look for a group size that's no larger than 6 to 8 infants or 6 to 12 young toddlers. Keep in mind that infants and young toddlers do better in smaller groups.

Health and sanitation practices Ask whether the program requires children and staff to have standard vaccinations and regular checkups. Is the staff prohibited from smoking inside and outside the building? What happens if your baby becomes ill during the day? Are parents notified when a child or staff member gets a communicable disease, such as chickenpox? When should you keep your sick child home? How are medications and first aid administered? How often are a baby's diapers changed? Are diapering areas and toys cleaned and sanitized on a regular basis? Do staff members regularly wash their hands? How are babies put to sleep? How regularly is bedding cleaned?

Safety and security Ask what kind of security system the facility has to ensure that strangers don't enter the building. What happens if a child becomes injured or lost? Are outdoor play areas secured? Do outdoor play areas have sturdy structures and safe surfaces? What kind of security measures are taken during field trips? How are children transported? What is the program's emergency evacuation plan? How are other emergencies handled?

Daily activities Ask what your child's daily routine would be like. Is there a mix of group play and individual attention? Is there a balance between physical activity and quiet time? Is there time for free play? Are there activities appropriate for different age levels? Do care providers read to the children? Are meals and snacks provided? If so, what kinds? What are the program's overall goals? Is parental involvement expected or encouraged?

Additional details What is the program's admissions policy? What kind of information will you need to provide? If the program has a waiting list, how long is it and how does it work? What are the program's hours of operation and cost? Can you pay in installments? Will you need to pay if your child is absent for a vacation? What is the policy for withdrawing a child from the program? How are parents notified of weather cancellations? Do parents need to provide any supplies? Can you drop in and visit your child during the day?

Preschool

Some preschools begin enrollment at 2 years, while others require children to be at least 3. Think about whether this is something that might be a good fit for your child. This will depend on your child's personality and needs, as well as the resources in your community. At this age, preschool curriculums are almost entirely play-based. But ideally, preschool teachers encourage expanded thinking and language skills through frequent conversation with your child, reading and use of new words to expand vocabulary.

CONTACT INFORMATION

Whenever you leave your child with a child care provider or a sitter, make sure you provide a list of important contact information, including your phone number and how to reach you at all times. Also, provide the phone numbers of any other close family members or friends who can be contacted in the event of a problem. Explain what you want your child's care provider to do in the case of an emergency.

If you're leaving your child with a care provider in your home, show the care provider the locations of all exits, the smoke detector, the fire extinguisher and the poison control hotline number. Make sure that anyone who provides care for your baby understands the importance of putting your baby to sleep on the back. Make sure the care provider knows how to use a car seat properly, if necessary.

It's also a good idea to write down your address and your child's full name and birth date in the event of an accident. The stress of an emergency may make it difficult for a child care provider or sitter to remember those details.

WORKING TOGETHER

In the coming weeks, monitor the performance of the child care provider you hire or the child care providers at the center your child attends. Pay close attention to your child's adjustment and interaction with the care provider or providers. Establishing a good relationship with your child's care provider benefits everyone involved. You may worry that your child will come to love a care provider as much as or more than your child loves you. Remember, no one can replace you in your child's heart.

Showing your child's care provider warmth and courtesy will make the provider, as well as your child, comfortable. This also will make it easier for you and your child's care provider to communicate. Try to set aside a few extra minutes to discuss any relevant issues when you leave your child with the care provider and when you return. If your child didn't sleep much the previous night, is teething or has another issue that might affect behavior that day, let your child's care provider know. If your child is taking any medications, explain what the medication is for and provide written instructions detailing how it needs to be stored and administered and what side effects might occur. If there are certain activities you'd like your child's care provider to do with your child, or not do — such as watch TV — talk with the care provider.

When you return, you'll want to find out what happened with your child that day. How much did your child drink and eat and at what times? How many diapers did your child wet and soil? What activities did your child do? How many naps did your child have, and how

HANDLING THE SEPARATION

Babies up to age 6 months often adjust well to being taken care of by a new child care provider. Older babies and toddlers, however, might have a harder time with the transition. Between ages 7 and 12 months, babies begin to develop stranger anxiety. They might need extra time and help getting used to a new child care provider and setting. If possible, arrange for an in-home care provider to spend time with your child while you're at home. Or take your child to visit the family child care or child care center before regularly attending it. Stay nearby while your child plays, and steadily increase the length of your visits. When you begin dropping your child off at the program, create a goodbye ritual. You also might let your child bring a reminder of home, such as a stuffed animal or a picture of you, to the program. Always say goodbye to your child before leaving. If your child shows persistent fear about being left alone with a caregiver, talk to your child's care provider.

Separation is sometimes harder for the parents than the child. Checking in regularly with your child care provider to see how your child is doing might help reassure you. The care provider may be able to send you pictures, videos and updates throughout the day. Ask your child care provider about the best way to check in, as visiting in person may cause repeat separations for your child or may be disruptive. Talk to friends and family who've been through it before.

long were they? Did your child achieve any new milestones or display any behavior that's of concern? Are any necessary baby supplies running low? Going over these topics regularly will help ensure consistency in your child's care and might help eliminate some confusion.

For instance, if you're unaware that your child skipped an afternoon snack, you might be bewildered when your child has a total meltdown due to hunger just before dinner. Some child care centers provide daily logs with this information. You also can ask your child's care provider to write down basic information in a daily log for you.

Beyond going over your child's daily activities, make time occasionally to have longer talks about your child's changing needs and how to meet them. This also will give you and your child's care provider a chance to discuss any other issues or concerns. Be sure to listen to your child care provider's thoughts on each topic and, if possible, work together to come up with solutions. If you're happy with your child's care, don't forget to mention that, too. Showing appreciation for your child's caregiver can help strengthen your relationship.

Finding good child care can be a stressful process. By considering your family's needs at the outset and thoroughly researching your options, you'll save time and energy. Carefully reviewing each candidate's background and evaluating different child care settings will help you feel more comfortable with your decision and ease your concerns about spending time apart from your child.

CHAPTER 16

Traveling

Whether you're bringing your baby home from the hospital, taking your child for a stroll around the block or going on your first family flight together, you and your child are likely to do some traveling in the months and years ahead.

Traveling anywhere with a child takes some planning. Your child may never have a leaky diaper, spit up all over or stray from mealtime when you're at home, but it always seems to happen when you're out and about. Then you reach toilet training days, and — well, you're bound to need supplies on the go.

It's a good idea to prepare for anything when you're traveling with your child. In addition to knowing what to bring with you to meet your child's needs while you're away from home, you'll have to figure out which modes of transportation work best and how to use them safely. You probably have more options than you might realize.

Before you hit the road, find out what you need to know about traveling with a baby or a toddler. Then have fun!

HEADING OUT

Both you and your baby are likely to benefit from getting out of your home. While you may feel nervous at first about leaving the comfort of your home as you learn to care for your baby, a change of scenery may be good for you. Taking small trips to uncrowded places with a young baby also will help you gain confidence and help you prepare for bigger adventures later on.

At the same time, if you've been up all night with your baby, your baby is having a fussy day or you can't face figuring out how to work the stroller yet, that outing you planned can always wait until tomorrow. There's no gold medal for the new parent who gets out of the house first. Take your time and head out with your baby when you feel ready. Consider the following tips to help things go smoothly.

Limit contact

When you first take your newborn out, consider avoiding places where baby will come into close contact with a lot of people and, as a result, germs. Or head to a destination when it's least likely to be crowded.

Dress for the weather

Young babies have trouble regulating their body temperatures when exposed to extreme heat or cold. As a rule, dress your baby in one more layer than you're wearing. Infants should wear hats when it's cold because they can lose a large amount of heat from their exposed heads.

If you're unsure about your baby's temperature, check the hands, feet and skin on the chest while you're out. Your baby's chest should feel warm, while the hands and feet should feel slightly cooler than the body. If your baby feels cold, remove the outer clothing layer and hold baby close to your body. Feeding your baby something warm also might help. Dressing your baby in layers and bringing extra layers will help you adapt if the weather changes.

Provide sun protection

Babies have sensitive skin. Before age 6 months, avoid exposing baby to direct sun for long periods of time. At any age, protect your child from sun exposure by dressing baby in lightweight, light-colored protective clothing and a hat with a brim. Apply sunscreen on exposed areas of your child's skin, remembering to reapply as needed. For more information on young children and sunscreen, see page 457.

SHOPPING CART SAFETY

Grocery shopping with a baby or toddler can be an adventure, to say the least. While your baby is young, it may be less stressful to shop online. But a quick errand run on the way home is bound to happen sometime. Be sure to take proper precautions with shopping carts. They can easily tip over when a child is in the shopping cart seat. A child who isn't properly buckled in also could fall out of the shopping cart seat. If possible, look for an alternative to placing your child in the shopping cart. Avoid placing an infant carrier on top of the cart. Consider using a front pack carrier instead. If you must place your child in the cart, use the seat buckle. Look for carts that have kid seats closer to the ground, such as the model car carts. Don't allow your child to ride in the basket or ride on the outside of the cart.

Keep child equipment cool

Avoid letting your child's car seat or stroller sit uncovered in the sun for long periods of time before using it. Plastic and metal parts may become hot enough to burn you or your child.

Be prepared

Take along diaper supplies, a change of clothes for your child (and maybe even yourself) and food for your baby — just in case. Bring a water bottle for yourself and for a child old enough to drink water, especially in warm weather. If you're nervous, ask a family member or a friend to go with you on your first few outings. As your child gets older, a snack and a favorite toy or book in the diaper bag often come in handy.

BABY CARRIERS

One of the most convenient and intimate ways to carry your baby around is in a baby carrier. These carriers can be used around the house, on a hike, and most anywhere that you're mainly standing or walking. If you're considering purchasing a baby carrier, you've got options, including:

- *Backpack or front pack.* This device allows you to carry your baby in an upright position on your back or against your chest.
- *Wrap carrier.* A wrap is a long strip of fabric that's designed to wrap around your shoulders and torso to hold baby against your body.
- *Baby sling.* This is a baby carrier made of soft fabric that you wrap around your body, often over one shoulder and around your torso. The sling cradles your baby at an angle.

Choosing a baby carrier

Not all carriers are the same. Some carriers aren't appropriate for young babies. Others are quickly outgrown. When looking for a carrier:

- *Find the appropriate size for your baby.* A newborn's head and neck should be supported. The carrier's leg holes should be small enough so that your baby can't fall through them. Some carriers may need an insert for a young baby but can be adjusted to fit as your child gets older.
- *Check the weight minimum and maximum.* Different models have different weight limits. Keep in mind that some models aren't appropriate for newborns. Also, consider how long you'd like to use it.
- *Look at the construction.* Will the carrier provide adequate support for your baby's head and neck? Is the material sturdy? Is it breathable? If you're looking for a hiking backpack, does it transfer the child's weight to your hips comfortably? Is it adjustable enough to be comfortable for more than one parent to use it?
- *Try it out.* Is the carrier comfortable for you and your baby? If you plan to use the carrier for a while, consider how the straps will feel as your baby grows, gains weight and becomes more restless.

Baby carrier risks

When used incorrectly, a baby wrap or sling can pose a suffocation hazard to an infant younger than 4 months. Babies have weak neck muscles and can't control their heads during the first few months after birth. If the fabric of the baby carrier presses against a baby's nose and mouth, baby may not be able to breathe. This can quickly lead to suffocation. In addition, a baby wrap or sling can keep a baby in a curled position, bending the chin to the chest. This position can restrict the baby's airway and limit the oxygen supply. In turn, this can prevent a baby from being able to cry for help. If your baby was born prematurely or has respiratory problems, don't use any carrier that keeps your baby in an upright position until you talk to your baby's medical professional.

Safety tips

When using any baby carrier, take the following precautions:

- *Be careful when bending.* Bend at the knees, rather than at the waist, when picking up something. This will help keep your baby settled securely in the carrier and protect your back.
- *Keep up with maintenance.* Keep an eye out for wear and tear. Repair any rips or tears in the carrier's seams and fasteners. Also, check the Consumer Product Safety Commission's website to make sure the carrier hasn't been recalled (see page 576).
- *Keep your baby's airway clear.* If you use a baby wrap or sling, make sure your baby's face isn't covered by the fabric or pressed into your chest, and is visible to you at all times. Check your baby's position frequently. If you breastfeed your baby in a baby carrier, change your baby's position afterward so that the head is facing up and is clear of the fabric and your body.

STROLLERS

You'll likely want to get at least one stroller for your child. But the options can be overwhelming. What's the best stroller for your baby, family and lifestyle? Here are questions to keep in mind as you're looking.

Where and how will you use it?

If you live in or near a city, you'll need to be able to maneuver your stroller along crowded sidewalks and down narrow store aisles. You also might need to be able to collapse your stroller in a pinch to get on a bus or down stairs to the subway. Parents in suburban and rural areas, on the other hand, might want to look for a stroller that fits into their car trunks.

If you have twins or an older child, you might consider getting a double stroller or a stroller with an attachment that allows your older child to stand or sit in the rear.

Frequent travelers also might want a collapsible tri-fold stroller or an umbrella stroller — either in addition to or as the primary stroller. Plan to take your baby along on your runs? You might look for a jogging stroller, too.

Is it appropriate for a newborn?

If you plan to use a stroller while your baby is a newborn, make sure that the stroller offers enough of a recline — since newborns can't sit up or hold up their heads. Some strollers fully recline or come with bassinet attachments. Strollers that can be used in combination with an infant-only car seat also are a good choice. However, most umbrella strollers typically don't provide adequate head and back support for young babies. In addition, most jogging strollers aren't appropriate for a baby until age 5 to 6 months.

Do you need a travel system?

Some car seats and strollers come in matching sets, to be used together. Others require separate attachments that allow the strollers to be used with certain car seats. Once you strap your baby into the car seat, these strollers will allow you to move your baby (and car seat) easily between the stroller and the car. This type of stroller also can be helpful in an airport if you plan to take your baby's car seat on the plane or check it at the gate.

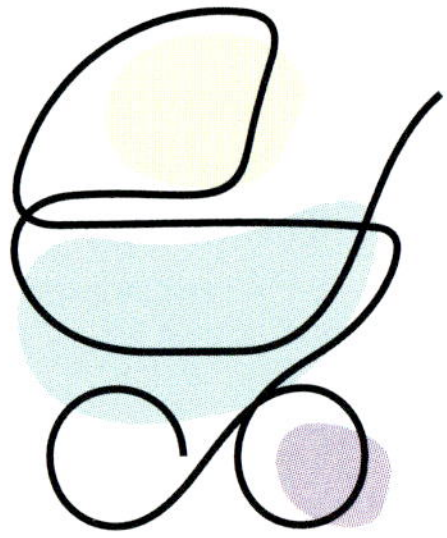

What kinds of accessories are available?

You might consider whether you'll want features or accessories for your stroller, such as a large cargo basket, a rain cover, a stroller blanket, stroller gloves, a sunshade or a cup holder. Some strollers can have a second seat or a stroller board attached to use as your family grows.

Other features

Strollers with wide bases are less likely to tip over. Look for a stroller with practical brakes that you can lock easily when the stroller is stopped. Avoid strollers with hinges or latches that might readily pinch or damage a child's fingers. Always read the stroller manufacturer's weight guidelines, especially when looking for a stroller with an area for an older child to sit or stand.

Safety tips

Once you find the right stroller, remember never to leave your child unattended in the stroller and follow these safety tips:

- *Take caution when unfolding.* Always make sure the stroller is locked open before you put your child in it.
- *Buckle up.* Always buckle the safety harness when taking your child for a stroller ride. Make sure your child can't unfasten the safety harness or slide out from underneath it. Most stroller-related injuries occur when a child falls out of the stroller.
- *Be careful with toys.* If you hang toys from a stroller bumper bar to keep your baby entertained, make sure that the toys are securely fastened.
- *Properly store belongings.* Don't hang a bag from the stroller's handlebar, which can make a stroller tip over. Place items in the stroller's cargo basket.

CAR SEATS

Whenever you travel by car with your child, a car seat is a must. Not only are car seats required by law in every state, but they're essential for your child's safety. Traveling with your baby in your lap could put baby at risk of serious injury in case of an accident.

The best time to get a car seat is before baby is born. This will allow you to install the car seat in your car — which might be a more complicated process than you realize — and have it ready for your baby's trip home from the hospital.

A good fit

When choosing a car seat, you'll have lots of options. Don't assume that the pricier models are best. Instead, look for a car seat that will keep your baby safe and best serve your family's needs. Keep these important points in mind:

- *Find the right fit.* Make sure the car seat fits your child's current height, weight and age. Also, make sure the car seat fits your vehicle, behind the front seat and alongside any car seats for other children. You'll want the car seat installed and used correctly every time.
- *Follow height and weight limits.* Carefully adhere to your car seat manufacturer's guidelines on height and weight limits. Follow your vehicle's owner manual on installing the car seat using the seat belt or lower anchors and a tether, if available.
- *Maximize safety.* The American Academy of Pediatrics (AAP) and the National Highway Traffic Safety Administration (NHTSA) recommend that all infants and toddlers ride in a rear-facing car seat as long as possible, until they've reached the maximum height or weight limit allowed by the specific car seat model. Some state laws require rear-facing car seats up to at least age 2. Many children should remain rear-facing to maximize safety even longer — sometimes up to age 4 or more, depending on their height and weight as well as the car seat limits. In a car crash, a rear-facing seat helps cradle and protect your child's delicate neck and spinal cord. Once your child outgrows the rear-facing limits, switch to a forward-facing car seat with a harness for as long as possible, up to the manufacturer's allowed height and weight limits.

IS YOUR CAR SEAT TOO OLD?

Yes, car seats do expire — typically after six years. The expiration date is usually stamped in the plastic on the bottom of the seat. With time, pieces of the car seat may become worn, jeopardizing the seat's ability to keep your baby safe in a crash. As technology improves, safety recommendations change, so check the expiration date of your specific car seat. It really does matter.

Types of car seats

Several types of car seats can accommodate the needs of babies and toddlers.

Infant car seat An infant car seat, sometimes called a bucket seat, is made specifically for newborns and small babies. It comes with a five-point harness and can be used only in the rear-facing position. It typically has a handle and can be installed using the seatbelt or snapped in and out of a base in your car. This allows you to carry the car seat with you wherever you go; just lock the car seat in place when in the car. Some models also snap into a stroller base. When your baby reaches the maximum weight or height allowed for an infant car seat, you'll need to move your child to a rear-facing convertible or all-in-one car seat.

Convertible car seat A convertible seat can be used rear-facing or forward-facing and typically has a higher rear-facing weight and height limit than an infant-only seat. This type of car seat also has a five-point harness.

When your child reaches the rear-facing weight or height limit recommended by the car seat manufacturer, you can turn the seat to face forward.

All-in-one car seat This seat can be used rear-facing, forward-facing or as a booster seat, so you can use it through preschool and beyond. Just be sure not to switch positions too early, before your child has reached the maximum height and weight limits. The booster seat, which secures the child with the car's seat belt, should not be used until a child is 4 years or older and has exceeded the height and weight limit for a convertible seat.

Other considerations

If you have two cars, you may want to buy two car seats or, for an infant car seat, two bases. Otherwise, for each car trip you'll need to move the car seat to the

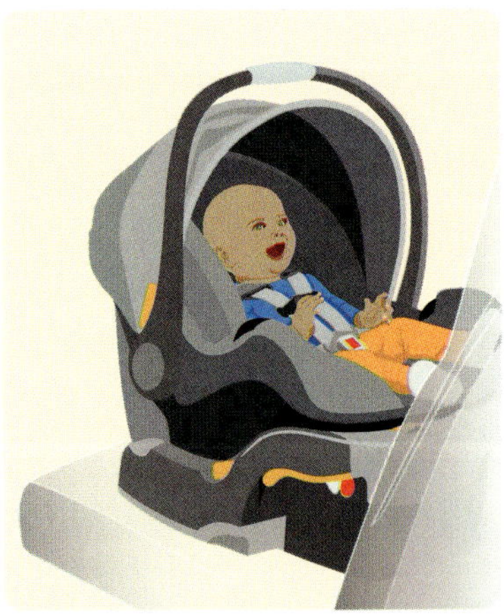

Infant-only seat

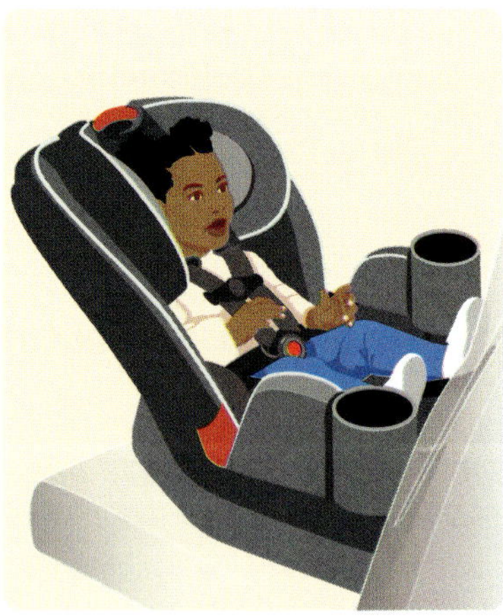

Convertible seat

car in which your child will be traveling. Also, look for a model with a cover that's easy to wash — in case your child spits up, vomits or spills food in the car seat at some point. No matter what kind of car seat you choose, make sure the label says that it meets all federal safety standards. Register your car seat online or by filling out the manufacturer's product registration card so that you can be notified of any recalls.

Used car seats

If you're considering borrowing or buying a used car seat, take extra precautions to make sure the car seat is safe. If you don't know the car seat's history, don't use it. Look for a car seat that:

- Comes with instructions and a label showing the manufacture date and model number
- Hasn't been recalled
- Isn't expired or more than six years old (the expiration date is usually stamped in the plastic on the bottom of the seat)
- Has no visible damage or missing parts
- Has never been in a moderate or severe crash

If the car seat has been recalled, find and follow instructions for how to fix it or get the necessary new parts.

SAFE CAR SEAT USE

Choosing the correct car seat is important. But it's equally important to install and use car seats appropriately. Here are some tips for getting it right.

Back seat is best

The safest place for your child's car seat is the back seat, away from active airbags. If the car seat is in the front seat and an airbag inflates, it could hit the back of a rear-facing car seat — right where your child's head is — and cause a serious or fatal injury. A child who rides in a forward-facing car seat also could be harmed by an airbag.

If it's necessary for a child to travel in a vehicle with only one row of seats, deactivate the front airbags or have a power switch installed to prevent airbag deployment during a crash. Otherwise, airbag power switches should be used only if your child has certain health problems and a medical professional recommends it.

If you're placing only one car seat in the back seat, the safest spot to install it is in the center seat — if possible — rather than next to a door. This minimizes the risk of injury in case of a crash.

Installing and buckling

Properly installing a car seat and correctly buckling your child into it before the start of every car ride are crucial. Before you install the car seat, read the manufacturer's instructions and the section on car seats in your vehicle's owner manual. Find out if your vehicle has the Lower Anchors and Tethers for Children (LATCH) system. Make sure the seat is tightly secured — facing the correct direction and allowing no more than 1 inch of movement from side to side or front to back when grasped at the bottom near the attachment points. It should be this tight whether installed with the LATCH system or the seat belt.

Rear-facing If you're using an infant seat or a convertible seat in the rear-facing position, keep these tips in mind:

- Install the car seat in the back seat according to the manufacturer's instructions, using either the seat belt or the LATCH system.
- Recline the car seat based on the manufacturer's instructions so that your child's head doesn't flop forward. Babies must ride semi-reclined to keep their airway open. Most seats include angle indicators or adjusters to guide you. Keep in mind that as your child grows, you might need to adjust the angle.
- Use the harness slots as described in the car seat's instruction manual, usually the slots at or below the child's shoulders. Place the harness straps over your child's shoulders.
- Buckle the harness straps and chest clip, with the chest clip even with your child's armpits. Make sure the straps and clip lie flat against your child's chest and over the hips with no slack. Most infant car seats include head positioning accessories to prevent slouching.

Forward-facing Resist the urge to place your child's car seat in the forward-facing position just so that you can see your child's face in your rearview mirror. Although it's natural to want to interact with your child during a trip, remember that your child's safety is of ultimate importance. Riding rear-facing is recommended until a child reaches the highest weight or height allowed by the car seat manufacturer.

When your child in a convertible seat reaches the weight or height limit, you can face the seat forward. When you make the switch:

- Install the car seat in the back seat according to the manufacturer's instructions, using either the seat belt or the LATCH system.
- Use the tether strap — a strap that hooks to the top of the seat and attaches to an anchor in the vehicle — for extra stability.
- Adjust the harness straps so that they're at or above your child's shoulders and fit snugly.

After you install the car seat, consider having a certified child passenger safety technician check your handiwork at a local car seat clinic or inspection event. Before each trip you take, check that the car seat is installed tightly.

The NHTSA's website is an excellent resource for help choosing

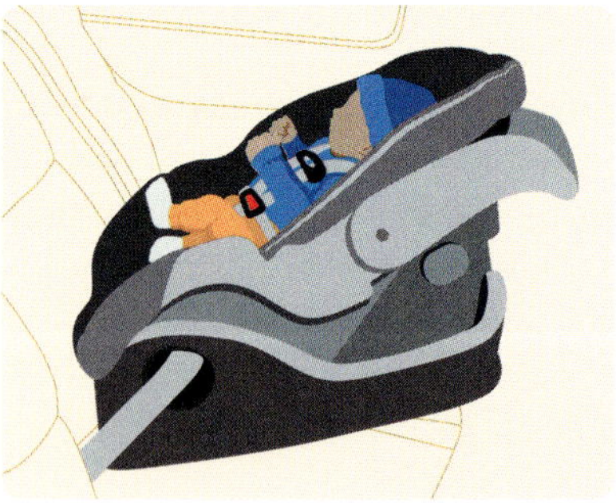

Correct installation of rear-facing infant seat with a base

an appropriate car seat. It also offers information on finding a car seat inspection station and other car seat safety information, including video demonstrations.

Remove heavy outerwear

Bulky coats and blankets prevent harness straps from snugly securing your child. Buckle the harness, then place a coat or blanket over the harness to keep your child warm.

Stay together

Remember, never leave a child alone in a car. Children can quickly become overheated, cold or frightened. Even though it might be hard to imagine forgetting your child in the back of the car, it can happen. To remind yourself of your precious cargo, place your cellphone or bag in the back whenever your child rides in the car with you so that you'll have an extra reason to check the back seat before leaving the car.

Be a force of nature

At some point, your child may protest riding in a car seat. Don't be afraid to draw the line when it comes to your child's safety. Help your child understand that riding in a car seat is non-negotiable and that even grown-ups must wear seat belts to stay safe.

To keep your child entertained during travel, bring a favorite toy or book. You also can talk, play music or sing songs together.

PREEMIES AND SMALL BABIES

A baby born prematurely or at a low birth weight might need to be monitored while sitting in a car seat before being discharged from the hospital. This is because sitting semi-reclined in a car seat can increase the risk of breathing problems or a slow heartbeat. To make sure your baby is safe in a car seat, you'll need to bring your baby's car seat to the hospital prior to discharge. If this test is recommended, your baby will be placed in the seat and have the vital signs recorded for a certain period of time.

If your baby has a health problem that requires lying flat, a vehicle bed may be recommended. Look for a

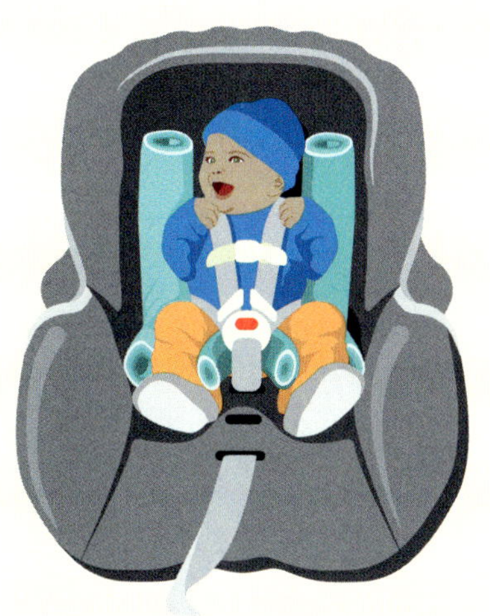

If allowed by the car seat manufacturer, tightly rolled receiving blankets can be placed alongside baby for added support.

vehicle bed that's been crash-tested. Position the bed lengthwise in the back seat so that your baby's head will be in the center of the car. Always use the buckle and harness to secure your baby in the bed.

When you have the OK to use a car seat, you may need an infant car seat — not a convertible seat — to accommodate your small baby. Use it only during travel, and don't let your child sleep in it outside of the car.

If your baby needs to travel with devices such as an oxygen tank, secure them in the vehicle so that they don't become flying objects in case of a sudden stop or accident.

AIR TRAVEL

Your first flight with your child will likely be a lot different from your previous flights. Instead of worrying about whether you have enough reading material, you may now be worried about entertaining your baby or toddler. While there's no telling how your baby will react to the first time on an airplane, careful planning can go a long way toward calming you and your child's nerves.

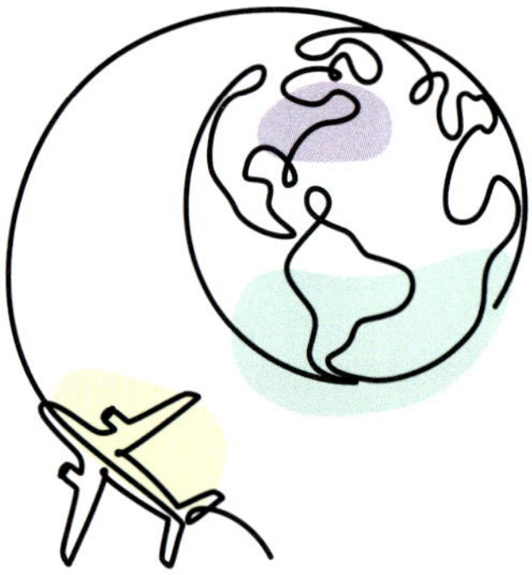

Identification

For domestic travel, consider bringing a copy of your child's birth certificate with you. If leaving the country, your child will need a passport. If you know you'll be traveling outside the country with your child in the future, consider applying as soon as possible. The application process typically can be expedited for a fee.

IS IT SAFE FOR YOUR BABY TO FLY?

Generally, age doesn't affect an infant's ability to handle air travel. While it's always a good idea to avoid enclosed, crowded spaces when you have a newborn, most healthy full-term babies are OK to fly at age 1 week to 2 weeks. If your baby was born prematurely or has a history of lung disease, however, talk to your baby's medical professional before flying with your baby. If your baby has an underlying respiratory condition, a medical professional might recommend supplemental oxygen.

Ear infections and ear tubes aren't thought to pose problems during air travel. However, if your baby is ill, you might want to consider postponing the trip.

Where you are traveling from, and to, does matter. If you live at lower elevation, talk to your child's medical professional before traveling with a young infant to high elevations.

Seat safety

Although airlines typically allow children younger than 2 years old to ride on a caregiver's lap during flight (called infant in arms), the Federal Aviation Administration (FAA) recommends that infants ride in properly secured safety seats. Most infant car seats are certified for air travel. In order for your little one to travel in a car seat, your child will need a separate seat on the plane. Though airlines typically will let you use an empty seat if available, the only way to guarantee a spot for your child is to buy a ticket. After your child turns 2, you'll always need to buy a separate seat.

When booking flights with a baby, call to check if there are any discounts for infant children. Keep in mind that car seats must be secured in a window seat so other passengers will be able to exit the row. Car seats need to be secured in the seat using the plane's seat lap belt.

If you don't bring a car seat for your child on the plane, ask a flight attendant for instructions on how to hold your child during takeoff and landing. If you sit in an aisle seat with your child, protect your child's head, hands and feet from getting bumped by service carts or other passengers. Most airlines do not allow infants to be worn in a baby carrier during takeoff and landing.

Many traveling families seek out the bulkhead of the plane, which offers extra space. Others prefer the back of the plane, which is typically noisy enough to drown out crying and may even lull a baby to sleep.

Many airlines offer bassinets called sky cots for use during flights. These are secured to a vertical wall, such as the bulkhead wall, in front of a seat. However, bassinets are not available on all airlines or all routes, and many airlines do not allow them to be reserved in advance. The FAA states that an approved child seat, secured in the child's own plane seat, is safest.

Getting through the airport

If you plan to bring a car seat on the plane or check it at the gate, a stroller that allows you to attach the car seat to it is a smart investment. You'll be able to wheel your child in the car seat until you board the plane. Then you can collapse the stroller base and check it at the gate. You will, however, have to take your child out of a car seat and carry your child through security while the stroller is screened.

While the Transportation Security Administration limits the amount of fluids you can bring on a plane, exceptions are made for baby-related items, such as medications, formula, baby food and breast milk. Toddler snacks are often not included in these exceptions, but if they are medically necessary, be sure to carry appropriate documentation. Notify security officials about what you're carrying and expect it to be inspected. Also, let security officials know if your child is using or has any special medical devices.

Boarding

Many airlines offer families priority boarding. However, some families prefer to board last to minimize the amount of time spent on the plane. Consider what seems best for your family.

Keeping baby happy

Some airlines don't count a diaper bag as one of your carry-on items on the plane, so make sure to check ahead of time. Dress your child in comfortable, easy-to-remove layers. This will help you keep baby warm or cool enough and make diaper and clothing changes easy. Nursing or sucking on a pacifier or bottle might ease discomfort during takeoff and landing. This is because babies and young children can't intentionally "pop" their ears by swallowing or yawning to relieve ear pain caused by air pressure changes. A sippy cup of water can help a toddler with the same issue.

If your child is restless, take an occasional break to walk up and down the aisle — as long as the crew approves moving throughout the cabin. Although you might hear parents joke about giving a child a sedating over-the-counter medication to induce sleep during the flight, this isn't recommended. In some cases, the medication could end up producing the opposite effect and make your child agitated.

If your child does cry during the flight, do your best to figure out what's wrong — just as you would at home — and try to stay calm. Chances are that many passengers on the plane have been in your situation before and likely sympathize.

PLAN FOR SUCCESS

Taking your child on a trip — particularly those involving flights, overnight stays and different time zones — requires some planning ahead. When you schedule your trip, think about your child's usual routine and what you can do during your travels to accommodate those daily needs.

Minding your child's internal clock

If your child is an early riser, consider booking an early morning flight and scheduling morning activities during your trip. Think about what times your child typically naps and eats and how you'll be able to keep this schedule intact while away. Keep in mind that if you cross time zones during your trip, it might take your child a few days to adjust to new sleeping and eating schedules.

Gathering essentials

If your child is still in diapers, start by packing your diaper bag because you'll need it with you at all times. Fill it with diapers, wipes, diaper ointment and a changing pad. If you feed your baby with a bottle, make sure you have bottles, nipples and formula or properly stored breast milk. Bring enough to cover your travel time and well beyond, just in case you encounter delays. If you're breast-feeding, a blanket or nursing cover might come in handy. If your baby uses a pacifier, bring more than one. (And if baby uses it to go to sleep, bring at least two.) Bring all medications onboard with you.

For older toddlers, bring easy snacks and a sippy cup that you can fill with water. Small toys, books, crayons and paper, or a tablet loaded with a few select games or videos that are accessible offline can help you entertain your child while at the airport and onboard.

It's always smart to pack an extra change of clothes — or two — for your child and yourself in your carry-on, just in case. Don't forget hand sanitizer and disposable bags for dirty clothes.

For your stay

When packing your child's clothes for the trip, think about the weather you're likely to encounter, how many outfit changes your child typically needs in a day, and whether you'll have access to a washer and dryer. You might bring along a few familiar items, such as small toys, books or a white noise machine, to help your child feel comfortable in the new environment. If you'll be staying at a hotel, call ahead and see if you can reserve a crib for your room. Otherwise, bring a collapsible crib with you or arrange to rent or borrow one during your stay. In addition to the bottle supplies you bring with you on the plane, consider what kind of sterilizing or pumping equipment you might need to bring for the rest of your trip. Some families prefer to purchase disposable items, like diapers, at their destination, or have them delivered to their lodging.

Traveling with a little one takes some thought and — often — a lot of luggage. Think about what your child might need, and do your best to prepare for the worst. And don't forget to enjoy your trip!

CHAPTER 17

Home and outdoor safety

As your baby becomes more mobile, exploration will become the name of the game. Rocking, rolling and sitting will give way to crawling, climbing and cruising along the furniture. And then come walking and running.

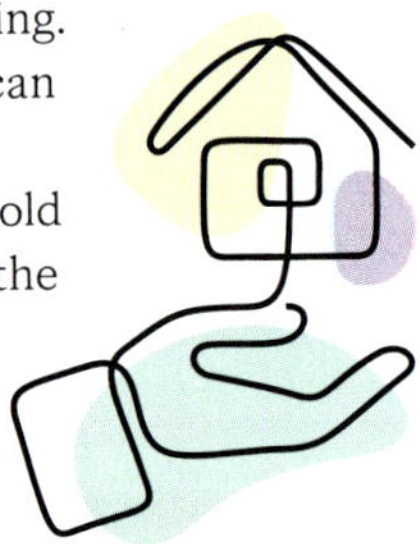

Your child's budding curiosity and inexperience, however, can prove to be a dangerous mix. Power cords, dresser drawers, kitchen cabinets, dish soap and the toilet are just a few household items that your child might touch, grab or try to climb onto in the coming months. Small toys, hot drinks, slippery surfaces and furniture with sharp edges also can pose hazards for your little explorer. To help prevent injuries, you can take lots of steps to safeguard your home and keep your child safe outdoors.

To get started childproofing your home, consider your family's lifestyle and the layout of your home. Think about which rooms your child will spend time in and what dangers each room poses. Sit on the floor in each room to get an idea of what might catch your child's attention or be within your child's reach. If you don't childproof every room in your home, you'll need to be extra vigilant about keeping your child away from un-childproofed areas. As your child gets older, reassess each room and your childproofing measures to make sure they still meet your needs.

NURSERY SAFETY

Your child will spend a lot of time in the nursery. To help keep your child safe while in that room, here are some helpful tips.

Secure furniture

Bookshelves, open dresser drawers and other furniture can look like ladders and stairs to kids, who are eager to reach the top. Climbing may cause the furniture to tip, even if it is heavy or sturdy. Always use furniture anchors to secure furniture taller than 27 inches high to the walls. The U.S. Consumer Product Safety Commission's website Anchor It! (www.anchorit.gov) provides additional information.

SAFE TOYS

Playing with toys helps little ones learn and grow, but you want to make sure the toys around them don't pose any hazards.

Choose toys carefully

Don't let your child play with balloons, marbles, coins, toys that contain small parts or other small items. Balloons, in particular, pose a major choking hazard when uninflated or broken. Avoid projectile toys, extremely loud toys, and toys with cords, long strings and small magnets. Remove plastic wrapping and stickers from new toys, and make sure any decorations or small parts — such as eyes, wheels or buttons — are tightly fastened to the toy. Regularly check your child's toys for small parts that could come loose, sharp edges, and mechanical parts that could trap a child's finger, hair or clothes.

Safely store toys with small pieces

If you have an older child, you likely have toys in your home with small pieces that your younger child could easily choke on or swallow. Gather up games and toys that have small parts, and do your best to keep them out of your baby's reach. Make sure your older child plays with these toys in a designated area and picks up all of the pieces afterward.

Take care with electronic toys

Don't allow small children to play with toys that need to be plugged into electrical outlets. Make sure battery covers are securely fastened with screws. If the toy contains a button battery, make sure your child cannot access the battery. If you suspect your child swallowed a battery, seek care immediately.

Avoid baby walkers

A young child may fall down the stairs, reach dangerous objects, or access bathtubs or pools while using a walker. The American Academy of Pediatrics has called for a ban on the manufacture and sale of baby walkers with wheels. In addition, walkers don't help children learn to walk. Choose a stationary activity center or playpen instead.

Take crib precautions

It's important to keep your baby's crib free of loose items, especially during the first year or at least until your baby can move easily around the crib. This helps avoid a risk of suffocation. Put your baby to sleep on the back on a firm mattress, without a soft comforter or pillow. Don't allow your baby to sleep with loose blankets or toys. For more on crib safety, see page 128.

Stay with your child during changes

Never leave a child alone on the changing table. Even at young ages babies can move suddenly and flip over the edge of a high surface. Keep diapering supplies within your reach but beyond your child's reach. If you need to retrieve an item that requires you to step away, never leave your child unattended, even if there's a strap or guardrail.

Safely store disposable diapers

If you use disposable diapers, keep them out of your child's reach. Swallowing plastics or absorbent materials can pose significant risks.

Avoid powders

Powders, such as talcum powder or cornstarch, contain fine particles that can cause lung irritation.

Window safety

In the nursery and throughout the house, avoid window coverings such as blinds that have long cords. These can present a strangling risk when little hands can reach them.

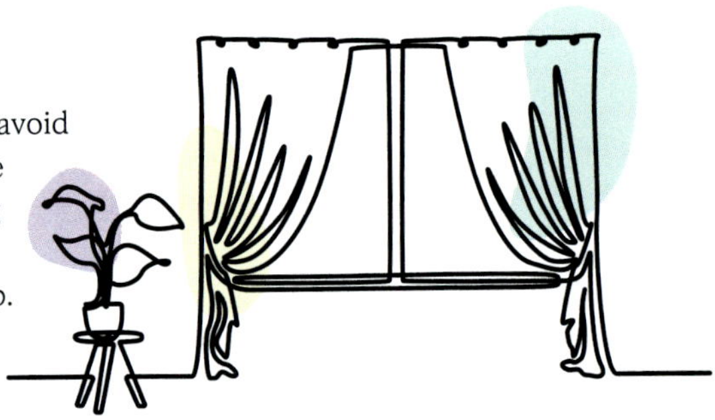

If possible, open windows from the top. If windows open only from the bottom, consider installing a window guard that prevents opening beyond 4 inches. Screens are not sturdy enough to prevent falls.

Watch toy box lids

If you use a toy box, look for one with no top, a lightweight lid, or sliding doors or panels. If you have a toy box with a hinged lid, make sure the hinge allows the lid to stay open at any angle. In addition, look for a toy box with ventilation holes, in case your child gets trapped inside it. Don't block ventilation holes by storing the toy box against the wall. Rounded edges are also a plus.

Check or install smoke and carbon monoxide detectors

You should have smoke detectors on each floor of your home, outside each sleeping area, and in each bedroom. Carbon monoxide alarms should be installed outside each sleeping area and on every level of the home. Refer to your local laws and codes to determine if either of these is needed in additional locations. Check these devices regularly to ensure proper functioning.

KITCHEN SAFETY

The kitchen is often the center of the home. Most parents spend a good amount of time there, and it can be a fun place to do activities with your child. But the kitchen also poses a number of hazards. Take these steps to prevent accidents.

Find a safe spot for your child

When you need to spend time in the kitchen, consider placing your baby in a high chair with a few toys on the tray. For a toddler, fill a low kitchen cabinet with safe items to play with — such as plastic bowls and cups, wooden spoons, spatulas, and other items without sharp edges or small pieces. Or set up a play yard for your child that's in your line of vision.

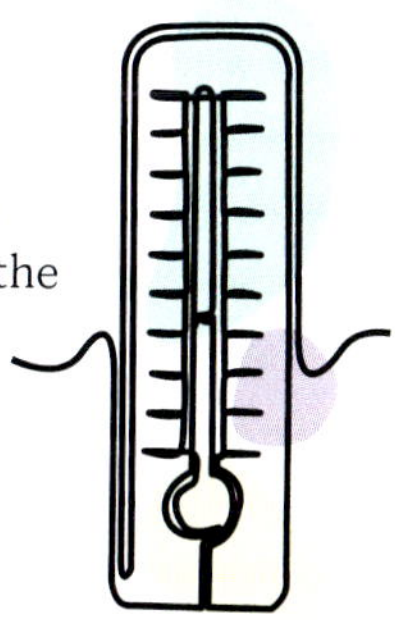

Reduce water temperature

Set the thermostat on your water heater to less than 120 F. If you bathe your baby in the kitchen sink, never run the dishwasher at the same time — in case hot water from the dishwasher backs up into the sink. Don't run the faucet while your baby is in the sink.

Safely store hazardous items

Keep sharp instruments in a drawer with a latch or a locked cabinet. Make sure appliances are unplugged and out of your child's reach. Don't allow electrical cords to dangle where your child could tug on them. Keep hazardous substances out of sight, out of reach and — whenever possible — in a high cabinet that locks automatically every time you close it. Hazardous substances in the kitchen might include dishwasher soap, cleaning products, medications and vitamins, alcohol, liquid nicotine or other products for vaping, and marijuana (especially edible products).

Avoid hot spills

Don't cook, drink or carry hot beverages or soup while holding a child. When you're walking with a hot liquid, use extra caution around your child. Keep hot foods and liquids away from table and counter edges. Don't use tablecloths, place mats or runners, which young children can pull down. When you're using the stove, use the back burners and turn the handles of your pots and pans inward. Don't leave food cooking on the stove unattended.

Safeguard your oven

Try to block access to the oven. You might use oven latches made to secure the oven door closed or a gate to block the whole area. As your baby gets older, place tape on the floor around the oven and call it a "no-kid" zone. Never leave the oven door open. If you have a gas stove, turn each dial to the off position and — if possible — remove the dials when you're not cooking. Otherwise, use childproof knob covers.

Look around

Watch out for other situations that could be hazardous:

- Put away small refrigerator magnets. A young child could choke on or swallow them.
- Address slippery or uneven surfaces and clean spills quickly.
- Keep a fire extinguisher handy.

FEEDING SAFETY

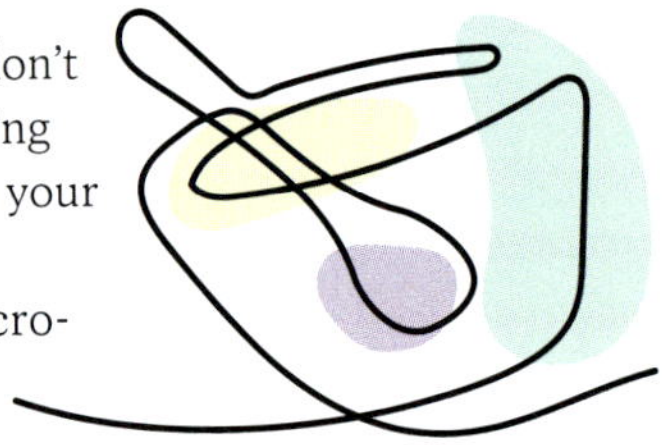

Feeding your child is often a messy experience, but you don't want it to be a dangerous one. If you use a high chair during feedings, always use the chair's safety straps to buckle in your child. And before you feed your child, always check the temperature of the food. Food or liquids warmed in a microwave may heat unevenly, so never use the microwave to warm milk or formula.

For more information about feeding your child, see Chapters 3 and 4.

Choking prevention

Choking is a common cause of injury and death among young children, primarily because their small airways are easily obstructed. It takes time to master the ability to chew and swallow food. Babies and even toddlers may not be able to cough forcefully enough to dislodge an airway obstruction.

Sometimes health conditions increase the risk of choking as well. Children who have swallowing disorders, neuromuscular disorders, developmental delays or a traumatic brain injury, for example, have a higher risk of choking than do other children. To prevent choking:

- *Introduce the right foods at the right time.* Giving solid foods before your baby has the motor skills to swallow them may lead to infant choking. Wait until your baby is at least 4 to 6 months old and shows signs of readiness to introduce pureed solid foods. Soft solids and harder solids can be introduced as feeding skills mature.
- *Stay away from high-risk foods.* Don't give babies or young children small, slippery foods, such as whole grapes and hot dogs, which can block the airway and be difficult to dislodge; dry foods or foods that are hard to chew, such as popcorn and raw carrots; or sticky or tough foods, such as peanut butter, marshmallows and chunks of steak.
- *Supervise mealtime.* Secure your child in a high chair or on an adult's lap when eating. Avoid eating when in the car, or if your child is playing, walking, running or lying down.

For more information about feeding safely, see page 78.

In addition, keep in mind that young children often put small toys and other objects into their mouths as they explore their environments. That can easily lead to choking. For guidance on how to respond if your child chokes, turn to page 236.

BATHROOM SAFETY

The easiest way to avoid bathroom injuries is to make sure your child can't access bathrooms in your home without an adult. Consider these precautions around the bathroom.

Keep the bathroom door closed

Bathrooms can be dangerous for many reasons. The best way to avoid accidents is to keep out young children. Install a safety latch or doorknob cover on the outside of the door. Keep the toilet seat down after use. Also consider installing childproof locks on toilet lids.

Reduce water temperature

If possible, make sure the thermostat on your water heater is set below 120 F. Don't run the faucet while your child is in the tub. Instead, fill the tub and test the water temperature with your wrist or elbow before placing your child in the water. Consider installing anti-scald devices on bathtub faucets and shower heads.

Supervise bath time

Never leave a child alone or in the care of another child in the bathtub — even for a short time. If you need to turn away, remove the child from the bath. A child can drown in just an inch of water. Drain water from the tub immediately after use. Remember, infant bath seats or supporting rings aren't a substitute for adult supervision.

Safely store hazardous objects and substances

Make sure electrical appliances, such as hair dryers, are unplugged and out of your child's reach. Don't allow electrical cords to dangle where your child could tug on them. Keep hazardous substances in a cabinet that locks automatically every time you close it. Hazardous substances in the bathroom might include nail polish remover, mouthwash, medications and bathroom cleaners. Dispose of unused, unneeded or expired medicines.

Address slippery surfaces

Use a rubber pad or slip-resistant stickers in the bathtub to help prevent slipping. Place a bathmat with a nonskid bottom on the bathroom floor. Clean splashes and spills quickly.

GARAGE AND BASEMENT SAFETY

Accidents and injuries also can happen in areas where kids don't spend a lot of time. Don't forget to childproof areas of the house such as the garage and basement. Once your child can move around, securing these areas to block access is strongly recommended.

AVOIDING LEAD POISONING

Lead is a metal that's found in many places — including old homes, drinking water and some children's products (usually older ones) — and it can be hard to detect. Children are at especially high risk of lead exposure because they tend to put their hands and objects in their mouths, and their growing bodies readily absorb lead. If you suspect that your home contains lead hazards, you can take simple measures to minimize your child's risk of exposure.

If you think your child has been exposed to lead, even if they seem healthy, ask your child's medical professional about a blood test to check for lead.

Check your home

Homes built before 1978 are most likely to contain lead. Professional cleaning, proper paint stabilization techniques and repairs done by a certified contractor can reduce lead exposure. Before you buy a home, have it inspected for lead.

Keep out of potentially contaminated areas

Don't allow your child near old windows, old porches or areas with chipping or peeling paint. If your home contains chipping or peeling paint, clean up chips immediately. Cover peeling patches with duct tape or contact paper until the paint can be removed.

Test and filter your water

Plumbing systems installed before 1986 may contain lead parts, and even newer "lead-free" pipes may contain small amounts of lead. Ion exchange filters, reverse osmosis filters and distillation can effectively remove lead from water. If you live in an older home and don't use a filter, run cold tap water for at least a minute before using it. Use cold, flushed tap water for cooking, drinking or making baby formula. Accredited laboratories can test your water for lead; sample kits can be purchased directly from laboratories. Your state department of health is a good resource for finding a qualified testing lab.

Avoid certain products and toys

Lead may be found in some children's toys — especially antique toys, some imported toys or toy jewelry. Lead testing of infant and children's products was required as of 2008. However, lead can still be used in plastics. A child can absorb lead found in these products by mouthing or chewing on them or can inhale lead if the product is burned, damaged or deteriorating. Avoid buying old toys or unbranded toys from discount shops or private vendors, unless you can be sure that the toys have been produced without lead or other harmful substances. Don't give costume jewelry to young children; in addition to containing lead, it can pose a choking risk.

Safely store hazardous objects and substances

Keep them in a cabinet that locks automatically every time you close it. Hazardous substances in the garage or basement might include cleaning products, windshield washer fluid, paint and paint thinner, and garden or lawn care products. Always unplug and store tools after using them. Store sharp and pointy objects high and out of reach.

If you have a chest freezer, or an unused refrigerator or freezer, secure the doors with a childproofing device or remove the door so that a child can't become trapped inside.

Don't allow your child to play near the garage

It might be difficult for a driver to see a small child. Automatic garage doors can pose a danger for children. Always keep the garage door opener out of reach.

Carefully store ladders

Put ladders away after each use, as well as anything else that a young child could climb on. Always store a ladder on its side.

FRONT YARD AND BACKYARD SAFETY

To protect children from outdoor hazards in a yard:

- *Set boundaries.* If your backyard doesn't have a fence, make sure you keep your child within a safe area. Your child should always be closely supervised when outdoors.
- *Check for dangerous plants.* If you're not sure about the plants in your yard, contact your regional poison control center or the National Capital Poison Center (www.poison.org/articles/plant) for advice and lists of potentially hazardous plants. If you have poisonous plants in your yard, remove them.
- *Be cautious with pesticides and herbicides.* Wait at least 48 hours before allowing your child to play in an area that's been treated.
- *Keep children away from power mowers.* Mowers may throw yard debris with enough force to injure a child. Keep your child away when mowing. Also, don't allow your child to ride on a riding mower.
- *Safeguard grills and fire pits.* Don't allow children to play near these potential hazards. If you have a grill, screen it so your child can't touch it. Make sure charcoal is cold before you dump it.

GENERAL SAFETY TIPS

To reduce the risk of injury in other areas in and outside your home, consider the following suggestions. Keep in mind that curious babies and toddlers can often still find trouble in a babyproofed area. Especially as toddlers grow, adequate supervision is needed even with safety barriers in place.

Use furniture bumpers

Cover sharp furniture and fireplace corners with corner or edge bumpers, just in case your child falls. Consider removing items with sharp edges from high-traffic areas while your child is learning to walk.

Secure furniture

Pieces of furniture around the house, as well as in the nursery, should be secured due to the risk of tipping. See page 230 for resources. Consider moving floor lamps behind larger furniture items or putting them into storage for a while.

Use doorknob covers, locks and stops

Doorknob covers and door locks can help prevent your child from entering a room with hazards. Look for a doorknob cover that's sturdy but can be used easily by adults, in case of an emergency. Make sure any locks you use on a door can be unlocked from the outside. Consider temporarily removing swinging doors and folding doors or keep your child away from them.

Keep hazardous objects out of reach

Common household items that may pose a choking hazard include safety pins, coins, pen or marker caps, buttons, small batteries, baby powder, and bottle tops. Always safely store all potentially poisonous substances in a high, locked cabinet. Always keep products in the original containers, which might contain important safety information. Don't allow your child to play with plastic bags or to play around recycling bins. Consider placing your trash can in a locked cabinet or getting a childproof lock for it.

Address outlets and electrical cords

Insert plastic plugs — which are designed not to be a choking hazard — into electrical outlets, or cover the outlets with plates. Keep electrical cords, including cellphone chargers and other electronic cables, out of the way so that children don't chew on them or grab them.

Keep cords out of reach

Keep electronic device, lamp and window blind cords secured and inaccessible — especially near your baby's crib. Safety tassels and inner cord stops for window blinds and draperies can help prevent strangulation. When buying new window coverings, be sure to check on safety features.

Watch out for liquid containers

Keep your child away from fish tanks and coolers. Empty buckets, small pools and other containers immediately after use. Don't leave them outside, where they may accumulate water and create a drowning hazard.

Avoid certain houseplants

Some plants — poinsettias, English ivy and peace lilies, for example — can be hazardous to children (as well as pets). So can fertilizers and some soils. Consider removing plants or placing them well out of reach. See page 227 for additional resources and advice.

Safely store firearms

The risk of gun injury is lowest in homes where there are no firearms. If you do keep firearms in your home, it is best to keep the unloaded gun(s) and ammunition in separate locked cabinets. Trigger locks also help reduce the risk of accidental injury. Remember to ask about firearms in other settings where your child plays or is cared for, too.

PREVENTING BURNS

Children get burned because they don't know certain objects may be hot. To prevent burns, follow these burn-safety tips:

- *Establish "no" zones.* Block access to the fireplace, fire pit or grill so a child can't get near it.

SAFETY AROUND PETS?

To prevent your child from being bitten or injured, follow some basic animal precautions:

- *Never leave your child alone with a pet.* Even if you know your pet and its temperament well, your child might inadvertently provoke an animal to bite through roughhousing, teasing, mistreatment or just curiosity.
- *Teach appropriate behavior.* Don't allow your child to tease pets. Never let your child pull an animal's tail or take away its toys or food. Don't let your child's face get close to a pet.
- *Get your pets vaccinated.* Make sure your pets are fully immunized according to their veterinarian's recommendations, including against rabies.
- *Be cautious around new animals.* Don't allow your child to approach unfamiliar animals without permission and guidance from the pet owner. Stay close to your child in case you need to move them away quickly.
- *Show your child how to greet animals.* For example, demonstrate how to let a dog sniff you and then slowly extend a hand to pet the dog.
- *Think twice about petting zoos.* Young children are at higher risk of contracting an infection through contact with cattle, sheep, goats, and other domestic and wild animals. If you choose to take your child to a petting zoo or other venue where animals might be present, be sure to wash your child's hands after leaving the animals' area, and even sooner if their hands are dirty.

WHICH CHILD SAFETY PRODUCTS SHOULD YOU BUY?

Your child needs your close attention to stay safe, no matter where you are. But certain products can help reduce the chance of accidents and injuries at home or other places where your child spends significant time.

The types of safety products that are most useful will be different for everyone, depending on your lifestyle and the features of your home. Here are some of the most commonly needed items.

Furniture anchors

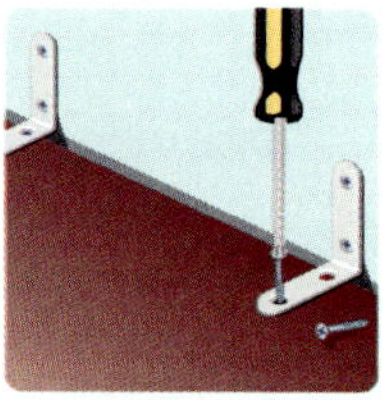

If a dresser, bookshelf or other piece of furniture comes with anchors, use them to attach the top of the furniture to the wall. A variety of anchors are sold separately, too. They're sometimes called anti-tip kits or furniture straps. Installing anchors is key in child-proofing your home. In the United States, thousands of children each year go to the emergency department after tip-over accidents.

Outlet covers

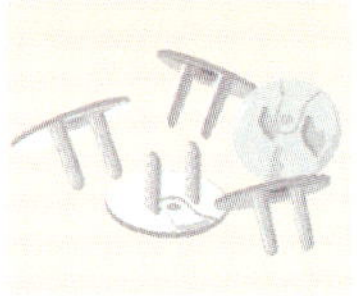

Basic plastic plugs are all you may need. For outlets that are frequently in use, other options include sliding cap covers and outlet cover boxes.

Safety gates

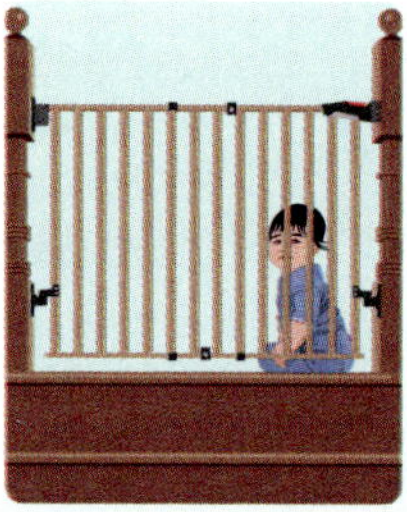

A wide range of gate designs are available at different price points, so it's worth doing some research to figure out what will fit your home and family best. Options beyond standard gates include extra-wide gates, retractable mesh gates and panels that connect to form a freestanding play yard.

Child-safe locks for drawers and cabinet doors

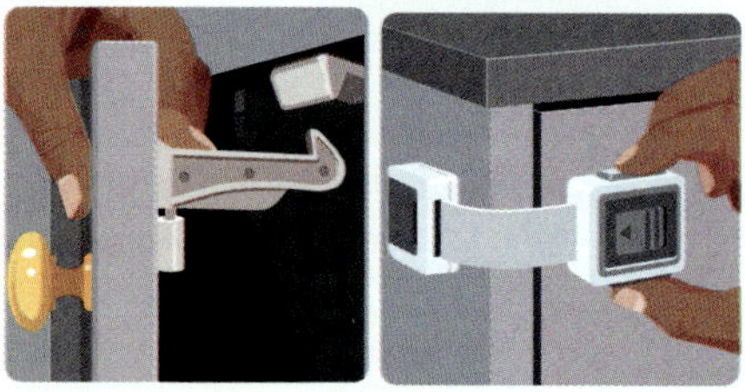

Many varieties of drawer and cabinet locks are available. Install them in the kitchen, bathroom and anywhere else your child might be exploring. Leave one drawer or cabinet unlocked and full of child-friendly items. Pro tip: As your child's awareness grows, you may want to be discreet while opening locks.

Corner bumpers and edge protectors

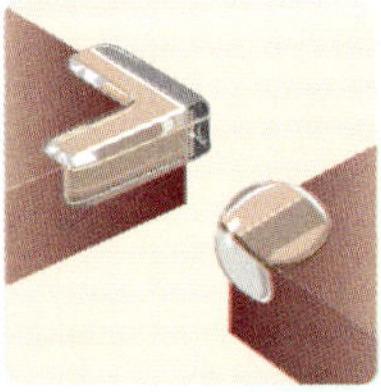

Tables, counters, and other furniture with hard corners and edges can cause surprising injuries as your child grows and becomes more curious and capable. Bumpers can help prevent cuts and more serious accidents.

- *Use space heaters with care.* Make sure a child can't get near a space heater. Also keep the heater at least 3 feet away from bedding, drapes, furniture and other flammable materials. Never leave a space heater on when you go to sleep or place a space heater near someone who's sleeping.
- *Watch where you park.* If you park in direct sunlight, cover the car seat with a towel or blanket. Before putting your child in the car seat, check the temperature of the seat and buckles.
- *Lock up matches and lighters.* Store matches, lighters and flammable liquids in a locked cabinet or drawer.
- *Choose a cool mist humidifier.* Steam vaporizers can burn a child.
- *Unplug irons.* Store items designed to get hot, such as clothing irons, blow dryers and hair irons, unplugged and out of reach.
- *Practice fire safety.* Install smoke alarms on every level of your home, and regularly maintain all alarms in your home. Keep extinguishers near places where a fire might start.

PREVENTING FALLS

There's plenty you can do to help prevent dangerous falls. Follow these simple tips to reduce your child's risk.

Beware of heights

Never leave a small child alone on a piece of furniture. Always use the safety strap on strollers and other infant seats. Don't allow a young child to play alone on a high porch, deck or balcony. Keep curious children away from bunk bed ladders. As your baby grows, provide safe places to climb. Stairways are of particular interest to young kids. Under your close supervision, teach your child how to go up and come back down the steps safely.

Install safety gates

Unless you can constantly supervise your child, or you can secure an area without access to stairways or other dangers, consider installing safety gates. Install gates at the top and at the bottom of each flight of stairs, if possible. Look for a safety gate that a child can't easily dislodge but which adults will be able to open and close easily. If you're putting a safety gate at the top of a staircase, attach it to the wall.

Lock windows and secure screens

A young child may squeeze through a window opened as little as 5 inches. Limit window openings to 4 inches or less. Although all windows that open should have guards or screens, screens often aren't strong enough to keep a child inside. Discourage young children from playing near windows and patio doors. Consider moving things a child could climb on, such as couches or tables, away from windows. When opening windows for ventilation, open them from the top if possible.

Use night-lights

Consider using night-lights in your child's bedroom, the bathroom and hallways to prevent falls at night. Night-lights can be especially helpful for toddlers who are learning to use the toilet or dealing with nighttime fears.

PREVENTING DROWNING

Swimming pools, hot tubs, ponds and other bodies of water are very dangerous to young children. Buckets of water, toilets and fish tanks also can be hazardous if kids climb in headfirst and are unable to get back out. Close supervision of a child around water is imperative. Multiple layers of protection can help ensure water safety and prevent drowning.

If you have a pool or hot tub, consider these general safety tips.

Fence it in

Completely surround your pool or hot tub — whether it's aboveground or in-ground — with a fence that's at least 4 feet tall. Make sure slatted fences and openings under fences have no gaps wider than 4 inches, so kids can't squeeze through. Install self-closing and self-latching gates with latches that are beyond a child's reach. Make sure the gate opens away from the pool or spa. Check the gate frequently to make sure it's in working order.

Install alarms

If your house serves as part of your pool or hot tub enclosure, outfit any doors leading to the pool or hot tub area with an alarm. Consider adding an underwater alarm that sounds when something hits the water. Make sure you can hear the alarm inside the house.

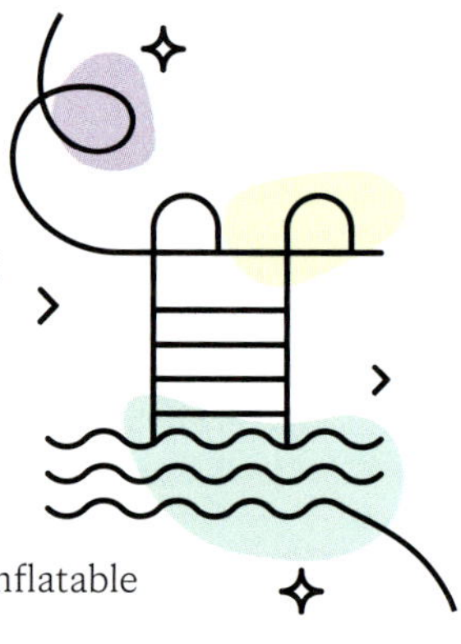

Block pool and hot tub access

If your house serves as part of your pool enclosure, use a power safety cover to block access when the pool isn't in use. Always secure a cover on a hot tub when it isn't in use. Sliding glass doors that need to be locked after each use aren't effective pool or hot tub barriers. Install self-closing, self-latching devices on all house doors that provide access to the pool area.

Remove aboveground pool steps or ladders or lock them behind a fence when the pool isn't in use. In addition, empty inflatable pools after each use.

Use life preservers

Young children should always wear life preservers when in a watercraft. Don't use inflatable toys to keep your child afloat, since they can deflate suddenly or your child might slip out of them. Even if your child is wearing a life preserver, always keep a hand on your child while in the water.

KEEP YOUR HOME (FULLY) SMOKE-FREE

The risks of secondhand smoke for babies and young children are well known. Exposure to smoke from cigarettes and other tobacco products can cause sudden infant death syndrome (SIDS), asthma, respiratory infections, ear infections and other problems.

In recent years, vaping and marijuana use have been on the rise, and these are often touted as safer options than cigarettes. There hasn't yet been as much research on the health effects of secondhand vape or marijuana smoke. But the evidence we do have is clear: the smoke particles and aerosols are still dangerous for young children's lungs. These particles pose some of the same risks as tobacco smoke and contain other potentially harmful chemicals. Data shows that even thirdhand exposure — from particles left behind on surfaces such as walls and floors — is dangerous, especially for infants and toddlers.

Beware of drains

Don't allow children to play near or sit on a pool or hot tub drain. Body parts and hair may become entrapped by the strong suction. Use drain covers, and consider installing multiple drains to reduce the suction.

Keep your eyes peeled

Never leave children unsupervised in or around a pool, pond or other body of water. An adult — preferably one who knows cardiopulmonary resuscitation (CPR) — should always provide supervision. Child supervision near water is a full-time job. Stay off your phone and other devices, and don't multitask.

Keep emergency equipment handy

Keep pool safety equipment beside the pool. Always keep a phone in the pool area in case of an emergency.

BE CAUTIOUS, NOT PANICKED

It might seem as if everything in your home and outdoors poses a potential threat to your baby. But don't panic. You can do plenty to childproof your home in a single afternoon or evening. As your baby gets older, stay on the lookout for new hazards. Go through your home from top to bottom every few months to make sure you're doing everything you can to keep your child safe. Be alert when visiting new places and friends' or family members' homes. If your child is going to spend a lot of time at grandparents' homes, you might consider asking them to do some childproofing, too. The most important safeguard, though, is adult supervision.

CHAPTER 18

Emergency care

Every parent wants to keep their child healthy and safe, but occasional accidents or injuries can happen. Even parents who have plenty of experience with children can have a tough time telling routine illnesses from more serious problems.

You can prepare for emergencies by asking your child's medical professional during a scheduled checkup what to do and where to go if your child needs emergency care. It's also important to learn basic first aid, including CPR, and to keep emergency phone numbers handy.

WHEN TO SEEK EMERGENCY CARE

Seek immediate care for:

- Bleeding that can't be stopped
- Poisoning
- New seizures
- Trouble breathing
- Severe head injury
- Unresponsiveness
- A sudden lack of energy or an inability to move
- Large cuts or burns
- Neck stiffness with fever, persistent crying or a lack of energy (called lethargy)
- Persistent blood in the urine
- Bloody diarrhea or persistent diarrhea
- Skin or lips that look blue or gray

In case of an emergency, call 911 or your local emergency care number immediately. If it's not possible to call for emergency assistance, take your child to the nearest emergency facility. In case of possible poisoning, if your child doesn't require emergency care, call the Poison Help hotline at 800-222-1222 in the United States. Have this number stored in your cellphone and written down in an obvious place in your home. You also can use the online tool at www.poisonhelp.org.

BLEEDING

You generally can judge the seriousness of bleeding by the rate of blood loss. Rapid blood loss from injured arteries is serious. Slower bleeding — a steady trickle of dark red blood — generally comes from injuries to veins or the body's smaller blood vessels (capillaries). Bleeding that stops with applied pressure within a few minutes is less likely to be serious. Bleeding can be the result of a cut, puncture or abrasion.

How serious is it?

The rate of blood loss is a good indicator of how severe the injury is. Remember, because babies have a much smaller volume of blood, they can't afford to lose as much blood as an older child or adult. Serious injuries that result in bleeding from the arteries can cause death in minutes if untreated.

What you can do

If the bleeding is serious and it doesn't stop on its own or if the cut or puncture is large or deep or has rough edges, apply pressure directly to the injury with a sterile gauze pad or clean cloth. Keep pressure on the wound until the bleeding stops. In most cases, you can stop bleeding with direct, firm pressure to the wound. Follow these steps:

1. Remain calm. This can be difficult, but it's important.
2. Immediately apply steady, firm pressure to the wound with a sterile gauze pad, a clean cloth or your hand until the bleeding stops. Don't clean the wound first or remove any embedded objects.
3. When the bleeding stops, keep a bandage or cloth in place over the wound by taping, tying or wrapping it securely. If blood seeps through the dressing, place more absorbent material over the first dressing.
4. If possible, elevate the wounded area.
5. If the bleeding continues, call 911 or your local emergency number. If this isn't possible, take your child immediately to the nearest emergency department. In the meantime, keep pressure on the wound and apply pressure to the nearest major artery above the wound, if you can identify it.

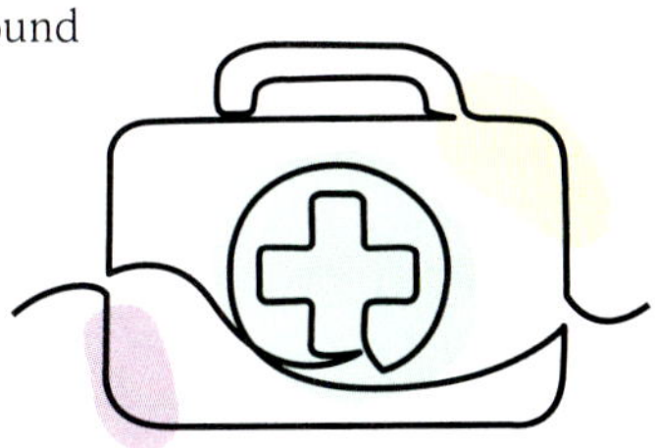

CHOKING

Most of the time when something blocks your child's throat, your child will instinctively cough, gasp or gag until the object clears the windpipe. Usually children will breathe on their own, and you don't need to interfere. But if your child cannot make sounds, stops breathing or turns blue or grayish, you must act immediately.

Babies and toddlers most commonly choke on small objects or foods that "go down the wrong way." Keep from a young child's reach anything that the child can choke on. This includes nuts, whole grapes, hot dogs and any small toy parts or objects that can obstruct a child's airway.

How serious is it?

When your child's airway is blocked and your child cannot clear it, the situation is life-threatening. The longer your child is deprived of oxygen, the greater the risk of permanent brain damage or death. If you cannot clear the airway, call 911 or emergency medical help, or ask someone else to call.

What you can do

Let your child continue coughing until the windpipe is clear. If your child can't make sounds, stops breathing or turns blue or grayish, act immediately. Look into your child's mouth. If you can see something that's blocking the throat, carefully pinch and grab the object to remove the blockage. If nothing is visible, don't stick your fingers into your child's throat. You don't want to push the object farther back and have it become more deeply lodged in your child's airway.

For infants To clear the airway of a choking infant:

1. Sit down. Hold the infant facedown on your forearm, which you'll rest on your thigh. Support the infant's head and neck with your hand, and place the head lower than the trunk.
2. Thump the infant gently but firmly five times on the middle of the back using the heel of your hand. The combination of gravity and thumps to the back should release the blocking object. Keep your fingers pointed up to avoid hitting the infant in the back of the head.
3. If the previous steps don't work, hold the infant face-up on your forearm, with the head tilted downward. Using two fingers placed at the center of the infant's breastbone, give five quick chest compressions. Press down 1½ inches, and let the chest rise in between each compression.
4. If breathing doesn't resume, repeat the back blows and chest thrusts and call 911 or emergency medical help.
5. Begin CPR (see page 237) if these techniques open the airway but the infant doesn't resume breathing. Call 911 or emergency medical help.

For toddlers To help a child over age 1 who's choking:

1. Stand or kneel behind your child. Place one arm across your child's chest for support. Bend your child over at the waist so that the upper body is parallel with the ground. Deliver five back blows between the child's shoulder blades with the heel of your hand.

2. Do five abdominal thrusts (Heimlich maneuver). Make a fist with one hand and position it slightly above your child's navel. Grasp your fist with your other hand and press hard into your child's abdomen with a quick upward thrust — as if trying to lift the child up.
3. Do this until the blockage is dislodged.

If your baby or toddler becomes unconscious, lay your child down on the back and begin CPR or call 911 or emergency medical help. If you're alone, attempt CPR for two minutes, and then call 911. If someone is with you, have that person call for help while you continue to do CPR. Continue doing CPR until your child starts coughing, crying or speaking. If your child resumes breathing within a minute or two, the child will most likely not experience any long-term effects.

After your child is breathing again, look for continued coughing or choking. This may mean that something is still preventing proper breathing. If you are worried your child may have choked on or swallowed a button battery, seek emergency care. Call 911 or local emergency services.

CARDIOPULMONARY RESUSCITATION (CPR)

Cardiopulmonary resuscitation (CPR) is most effective when delivered by a person who's trained in CPR. It's a good idea for all parents, and for anyone who provides child care, to take a certified course in CPR. You can contact your local

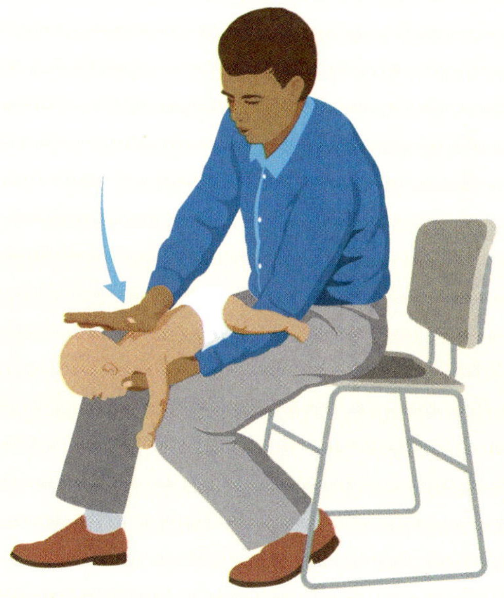

A firm, gentle thump on the back can help clear the airway of a choking infant.

American Red Cross or American Heart Association chapter to sign up for a course.

You may need to give CPR if a child:

- Has no pulse or heartbeat
- Has blue lips or skin
- Has difficulty breathing or stops breathing entirely
- Is unresponsive

The sooner you start CPR, the greater the chances of saving your child's life or avoiding permanent injury.

What you can do

The procedure for giving CPR to a child is similar to the one used for adults. Loudly call out the child's name and stroke or gently tap the child's shoulder. Don't shake the child.

If you're alone and you didn't see the child collapse and you can't find a pulse, provide CPR for two minutes — about five cycles — before calling 911 or your local emergency number. If you see the child collapse and CPR is needed, call 911 immediately and then begin CPR as quickly as possible. If another person is available, have that person call for help immediately while you attend to the child.

Circulation: Restore blood circulation

1. Place the child on the back on a firm, flat surface, such as a table. The floor or ground also will do.
2. Imagine a horizontal line drawn between the child's nipples. For an infant, place your hands around the sides with your thumbs in the center of the chest, just below this line. If the child is over a year old, place the heel of your hand in the center of the chest.

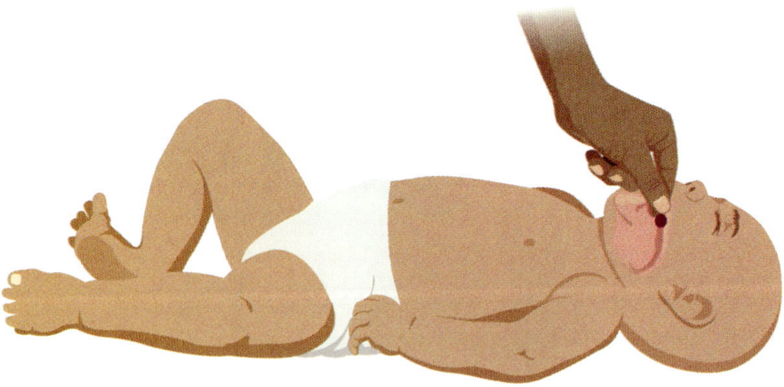

Before giving CPR to an infant, tilt the child's head back to open the airway. If you see an object in the infant's mouth, try to pinch it out without pushing the object farther back in the airway.

3. Gently compress the chest about 1½ inches or one-third the depth of the chest.
4. Count aloud as you perform 30 compressions, pumping at a rate of about 100 to 120 compressions a minute.

Airway: Clear the airway

1. After 30 chest compressions, gently tip your child's head back (head-tilt maneuver) by lifting the chin with one hand and pushing down on the forehead with the other hand.

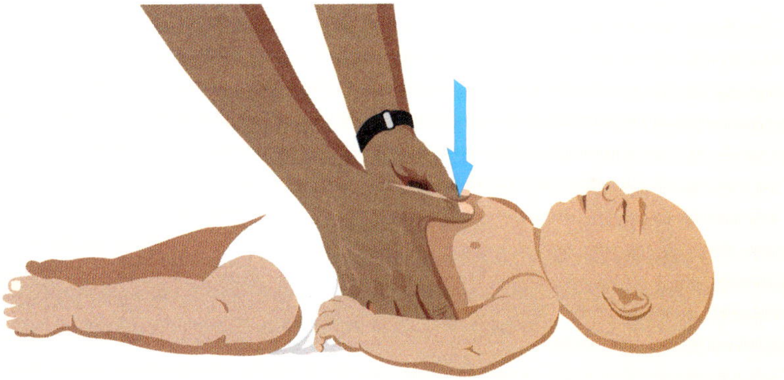

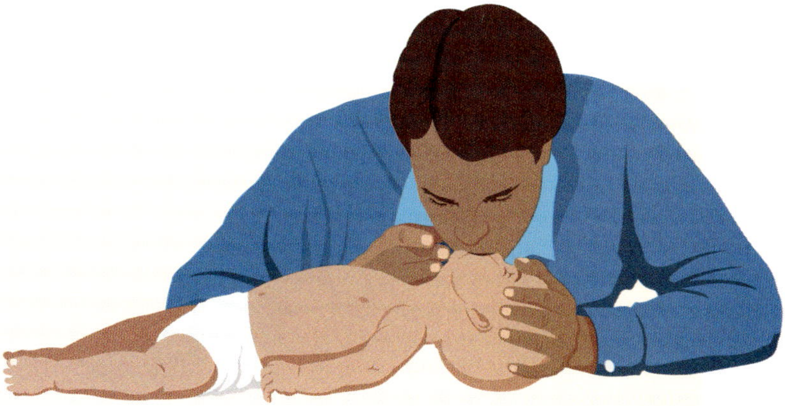

During infant CPR, alternate compression of the infant's chest with gentle breaths from your mouth. When breathing for the infant, cover the infant's mouth and nose with your mouth.

Breathing: Provide ventilation

1. Cover the child's mouth and nose with your mouth.
2. Prepare to give the child two rescue breaths. Use the strength of your cheeks to deliver gentle puffs of air (instead of deep breaths from your lungs) to slowly breathe into the child's mouth one time, taking one second for the breath. Give a deep enough breath to cause the child's chest to rise gently. If it does, give a second rescue breath. If the chest does not rise, repeat the head-tilt maneuver and then give the second breath.
3. If the child's chest still doesn't rise, resume chest compressions. After another 30 compressions, examine the mouth to make sure no foreign material is inside. If an object is seen, pinch it out with your finger and then give two breaths. If the airway seems blocked, do first aid for a choking baby or toddler (see page 236).
4. Give two breaths after every 30 chest compressions.
5. Do CPR for about two minutes (about five cycles) before calling for help, unless someone else can make the call while you attend to the child.
6. Continue CPR until you see signs of life or until medical personnel arrive.
7. If you're unable or unwilling to do the rescue breathing portion of CPR, continue chest compressions until there are signs of movement or until medical personnel take over.
8. If you have someone who can help you do CPR, have one person do chest compressions while the other does rescue breaths. For two-person CPR, do 15 compressions followed by two breaths. Repeat this cycle for two minutes (10 times) before switching roles.

BURNS

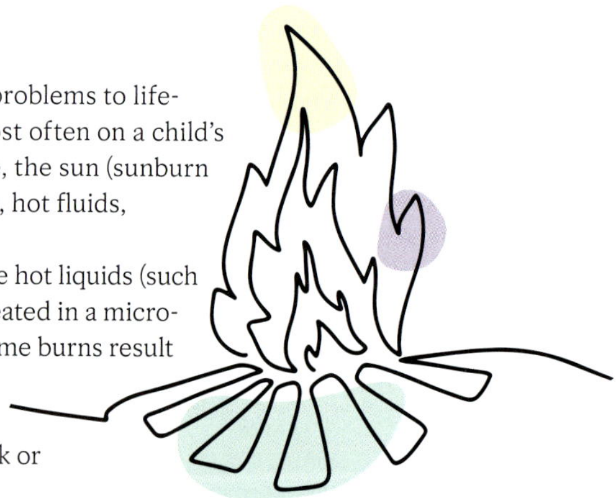

Burns can range in severity from minor problems to life-threatening emergencies. They occur most often on a child's hands or face. Burns may result from fire, the sun (sunburn is discussed on page 456), heated objects, hot fluids, electricity or chemicals.

Common causes of burns in infants are hot liquids (such as coffee or tea), bottles that have been heated in a microwave, stoves, fireplaces and cigarettes. Some burns result from water heater temperatures that are too high (above 120 F). Be cautious about a child's clothing catching fire from a spark or ashes.

How serious is it?

Burns can range from mild to serious and are classified in three categories, according to their severity.

Superficial burns They cause redness and slight swelling of the skin. These are the mildest types of burns, affecting only the outer layer of skin.

Superficial partial-thickness and deep partial-thickness burns They generally cause blistering, intense reddening, and moderate to severe swelling and pain. The top layer of skin has been burned through, and the second layer also is damaged.

Full-thickness burns Full-thickness burns appear white or charred and involve all the layers of skin. There may be little pain with these burns because of substantial nerve damage.

What you can do

Minor burns often can be taken care of at home. Major burns require emergency treatment.

Minor burns For minor burns, take the following steps:

- Remove any constricting items. Since burned areas can swell, take off any jewelry, belts and similar items. Try to do this quickly and with care.
- Hold the burned area under cool (not cold) running water for 10 to 15 minutes or until the pain eases. If this isn't possible, cover the burn in cool water or use cool compresses. Cooling the burn reduces swelling by pulling heat away from the skin. Don't put ice on the burn.
- After cooling the burn for comfort and cleaning, cover the burn with antibiotic ointment. This will prevent bandages or dressings from sticking to the burn.
- Cover the burn with a sterile nonstick gauze bandage. This provides comfort by keeping air off the injury, and it reduces the risk of infection. Don't use fluffy cotton or other material that may get lint in the wound. Wrap the gauze loosely to avoid putting pressure on burned skin.
- To ease pain, you can give your child an appropriate dose of acetaminophen or ibuprofen. Refer to dosage instructions on the bottle (see pages 580-581). Talk to your child's medical professional if you have questions or concerns.

Minor burns usually heal without further treatment, but watch for signs of infection, such as increased pain, redness, fever, swelling or oozing. If infection develops, seek medical help.

Major burns For full-thickness burns or superficial partial-thickness and deep partial-thickness burns that involve a large area of skin, call 911 or your local emergency number. Until an emergency unit arrives, follow these steps:

- Don't immerse large severe burns in cold water. This could cause a drop in body temperature (hypothermia) and deterioration of blood pressure and circulation (shock).
- Check for signs of circulation (breathing, coughing or movement). If there is no breathing or other sign of circulation, begin CPR.
- Cover the area of the burn. Use a cool, moist, sterile bandage; a clean, moist cloth; or moist towels.
- Elevate the burned body part or parts above heart level, if possible.
- Remove jewelry, belts or other items that can become too tight if a burned area rapidly swells.

ELECTRICAL SHOCK

The most common ways that infants and young children receive electrical shocks are by biting into electrical cords and by poking metal objects or their fingers into unprotected outlets. Some holiday decorations provide another source of possible injury, when electrical cords and lightbulbs may be within a child's reach.

Electrical shock often results in injury only at the point of contact, similar to a burn. For example, a less severe shock may burn a child's mouth or skin. However, a stronger electrical shock may cause your child to stop breathing and may stop the heart's beating. Internal organ damage is possible but may not be obvious.

How serious is it?

Depending on the voltage and the length of the contact with electrical current, an electrical shock may range from being mildly uncomfortable to causing serious injury or death.

What you can do

If you see that your child is in contact with electricity, attempt first to disconnect the source. If you cannot disconnect the source, use an insulating material such as rubber, plastic or wood to attempt to move your child away from the electricity. Don't attempt to handle a live wire — or a child in contact with electricity — with your bare hands. Use something made of insulating material that won't conduct electricity.

As soon as your child is away from the source of electricity, check your child's breathing and heart rate. If either is stopped or erratic, or if your child is unconscious, begin CPR (see page 237) and call or have someone else call for emergency help. If your child is conscious, look for evidence of burns and notify your child's medical professional.

You can prevent accidental electrical shocks by childproofing your home and using safety plugs in all electrical outlets. In addition, avoid stringing long extension cords or electric lights where your child can reach them.

ANIMAL OR HUMAN BITES

If your child is bitten, try to discover the source of the bite as quickly as you can. Household pets are the cause of most animal bites. Although pet dogs are more likely to bite than cats, cat bites are more likely to become infected. Bites from some wild animals are dangerous because of the possibility of rabies. Most human bites that children get are only bruises and not dangerous. However, human bites can lead to infection if they break the skin.

How serious is it?

An animal bite can cause serious wounds — especially to the face — as well as emotional trauma. Consider any animal or human bite that breaks the skin to be a serious injury. Fortunately, cases of rabies are uncommon today; still, any animal bite caused by a dog, cat, skunk, raccoon, fox or bat should be evaluated for rabies risk. Bites by rabbits, gerbils and hamsters generally are harmless and require only typical wound care.

What you can do

If your child is bitten, follow these guidelines.

For minor wounds If the bite barely breaks the skin and there's no danger of rabies, treat it as a minor wound. Wash the wound thoroughly with soap and water. Apply an antibiotic cream or ointment to prevent infection and cover the bite with a clean bandage. Contact your child's medical professional to see if your child should receive a medical evaluation and treatment with antibiotics.

For deep wounds If the bite creates a deep puncture of the skin or the skin is badly torn and bleeding, apply pressure with a clean, dry cloth to stop the bleeding. See your child's medical professional or go to your local emergency department. If you're concerned about the possibility of rabies, tell your child's medical professional. Your child may need a series of shots to prevent rabies infection.

Also seek medical assistance if you see any signs of infection: pus draining from the wound, increased redness and swelling several days after the bite, or red streaks extending from the wound.

DROWNING

Infants and toddlers can drown in very shallow water. Never leave your child alone in the bathtub, even briefly. If a phone call, doorbell or something else interrupts your child's bath, either ignore the interruption or bring the child with you, wrapped in a towel. Keep the toilet lid and bathroom door closed. Fence swimming pools with automatic latching gates, and constantly supervise your infant when near lakes, pools or rivers. Toddlers have even drowned after falling into buckets used for cleaning.

What you can do

If your child has been submerged in water and isn't breathing or has breathing difficulty, has bluish skin or lips, is unconscious, or has a decreased level of consciousness, call for emergency help or have someone call for you. If your child has no pulse or isn't breathing, begin CPR immediately (see page 237). Continue CPR until medical help arrives.

INJURY FROM A FALL

Infants and toddlers can fall for many reasons. Falls tend to occur when a baby is able to roll or to tip an infant seat — often more easily than a person realizes! — or in the early days of crawling or walking.

How serious is it?

If your child cries immediately after a fall that involves the head and remains alert, chances are the fall didn't cause serious injury. Falls can be serious, but babies' and toddlers' soft bones don't fracture as easily as those of older children. Important factors that can affect the seriousness of a fall are the force and distance of the fall.

What you can do

Use ice to control swelling, but be careful not to freeze your child's skin. In case of a head injury, observe your child carefully for 24 hours for any behavior changes. If the injured body part looks different than usual, or if your child cannot move it, seek immediate care. Also seek immediate care if you notice any of the following signs:

- An inability to crawl or walk, if the child was able to do so before the injury
- Persistent irritability, possibly indicating a severe headache
- Blood or new watery fluid discharge from the ears or nose
- Persistent vomiting

Call 911 or emergency help if your child experiences:

- Irregular breathing
- A lack of energy (lethargy) or excessive sleepiness
- A seizure
- Loss of consciousness

If your child stops breathing or if you can't detect a heart rate, begin CPR immediately (see page 237) and call 911.

SWALLOWED POISON

While toxicity varies, almost any nonfood substance is poisonous if taken in large doses. Babies and toddlers are at risk of being poisoned because they explore by putting things in their mouths. Thankfully, with immediate treatment most children aren't permanently harmed from poisons they swallow.

In the United States, keep the Poison Help hotline number (800-222-1222) nearby. Tell anyone who takes care of your child about the number. Also keep the hotline number in your cellphone.

Some common items you may keep around your house can be quite dangerous to an infant or toddler. These include plants, medications (including pain relievers and aspirin), alcohol, mouthwashes that contain alcohol, detergents and detergent pods, pesticides, antifreeze and cleaning substances. Button batteries — the round type used in watches and many small devices — also are extremely dangerous if swallowed.

Suspect poisoning if you find your child with an open or empty container of a toxic substance. Look for behavior differences; burns or redness of the lips, mouth or hands; unexplained vomiting; breath that smells like chemicals; breathing difficulties; or convulsions.

How serious is it?

Substances vary widely in the seriousness of their effects and the amount needed to do harm. Remember, though, that a small amount of some products or medications can be much more damaging to an infant or toddler than it would be to an adult. If you have any questions about whether a substance may be toxic, call the Poison Help hotline for advice.

What you can do

If your child is in obvious distress (unconscious, convulsing, experiencing breathing difficulties), call 911 or your local emergency number immediately. If possible, have the container in front of you when you call so that you can tell emergency personnel what substance caused the problem. If you need to go to the emergency department, bring the product or container with you or take a picture of it, including a close-up of the label.

If your child does not appear to be in immediate danger, remove your child from the source of the poison and immediately call Poison Help at 800-222-1222 in the United States. Be prepared to share as many details as possible. The operator may ask you to read the labels on the container and to describe the substance and amount ingested and when and how your child came into contact with it. Describe any physical changes you detect in your child.

Don't give your child anything by mouth until you've talked to someone at the Poison Help hotline. Inducing vomiting in your child isn't recommended, as it can cause more damage in some instances.

If your child is vomiting, turn the head to the side — or forward if your child is upright — to prevent choking.

Prevention

Any medication and many products in your house can be harmful to your child. If you don't need the medication or product, remove it to avoid accidental ingestion. Store medications, chemicals and batteries in a locked cabinet out of reach of children. Be especially cautious when visiting grandparents or non-childproofed homes. Be sure that all substances are in their proper, child-resistant containers and clearly labeled. Check the label on medicine bottles each time you give a medication, especially in the middle of the night, to confirm that you're giving the proper medicine and dose.

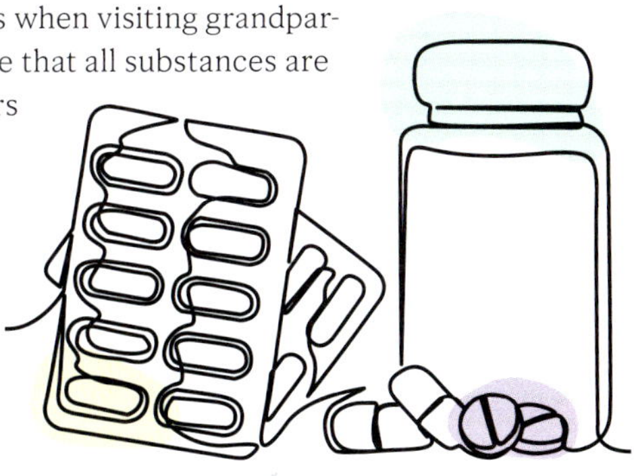

INHALED POISON

Inhaling poisonous substances can cause various reactions, including nausea and vomiting, loss of or decreased consciousness, headache, breathing difficulties, coughing, or lack of energy. A child's reaction will vary, depending on the amount of exposure and the substance inhaled.

Numerous substances are toxic when inhaled. They include carbon monoxide, smoke and fumes from fires, propellants, gasoline, kerosene, turpentine, furniture polish, charcoal, lighter fluid, glue, paint remover, and lamp oil.

It can be dangerous for your child to inhale toxic substances. Act quickly when you suspect that your child has inhaled a dangerous substance.

What you can do

Avoid using aerosol products near your child, because young children can react more severely to a small amount of inhaled poison. Never run your car in a closed garage, and maintain coal, wood or kerosene stoves regularly. Make sure you have a working carbon monoxide detector on each floor of your home.

If you smell a strong natural gas odor or if you hear a carbon monoxide alarm, turn off any gas burner or oven, leave your house immediately and call the gas company. Avoid breathing the fumes yourself, and get your child to a well-ventilated area. Check your child's breathing and pulse; if needed, begin CPR.

Call 911 or your local emergency number immediately if your child is having difficulty breathing or showing a lack of energy or a decreased level of consciousness, is without a heartbeat, or is convulsing.

POISON ON THE SKIN

If you suspect that your child's skin has come into contact with a poison, look near your child for evidence of the poison. Spilled household cleaners probably would leave a young child's skin looking irritated. The chemicals in many household cleaning substances, especially oven and drain cleaners, can easily damage your child's skin.

What you can do

Keep all cleaning solutions in a childproof cabinet out of reach. If your child comes into contact with a poison, check with the Poison Help hotline at 800-222-1222 in the United States for treatment advice.

If your child is experiencing obvious distress — unconsciousness, lack of energy, hallucinations, convulsions, or breathing difficulties — call 911 or local emergency services immediately.

POISON IN THE EYE

Poison can get in a child's eye when a liquid splashes into it. Many substances can damage your child's eyes, but your infant or toddler may not be able to tell you about the problem. Be alert to possible situations in which this can happen. Acting quickly could make the difference between a temporary problem and a long-term disability.

What you can do

Use a large glass or pitcher filled with cool tap water to flood your child's eye for 10 to 20 minutes. Try to get your child to blink frequently as you flood the area. Keep the child's hands out of the eyes. You may need to wrap your child in a bedsheet or large towel to keep the hands out of the affected eye. Get another adult to help you, if possible.

Call the Poison Help hotline at 800-222-1222 in the United States if you're unsure whether the liquid that splashed in your child's eye is poisonous or if you're unsure whether to seek emergency help.

PART 3

Growth and development

CHAPTER 19

Month 1

The first month of your baby's life can feel like a whirlwind — coming home from the hospital, getting your baby settled in your home, learning the rhythms of parenting, recuperating from childbirth, and so much more. There's a lot going on!

At the same time, being with a newborn can make you feel like time has slowed down to a crawl. After all, newborns spend most of their time sleeping and eating, with a diaper change and a crying spell here and there. The most exciting times may be when your child's eyes are open for a few minutes and you can interact. Even then, you may wonder: Should baby be moving more? Is baby getting enough to eat?

But that's what the first month is all about — slowing down enough to rest, recover and get to know each other. By the end of the first month, you'll be surprised at the changes that have occurred in your little one and the jump in your self-confidence as a parent.

DID YOU KNOW?

Babies usually have a couple of growth spurts within the first month or two, generally around 7 to 10 days and at 3 to 6 weeks of age. During a growth spurt, your baby may want to eat more often, so don't be surprised if your baby seems to have gone on a feeding frenzy. Hang in there. The frequency of feedings will soon even out again.

GROWTH AND APPEARANCE

During the first few days of life, your newborn loses the excess body fluid present at birth. As a result, by the time you go home your baby will weigh slightly less than at birth. Most babies will regain this weight quickly. In about 10 days to 2 weeks, your baby likely will be at birth weight once again. And growth certainly won't stop there. Most babies grow rapidly in their first few weeks. By the end of the first month, your baby is likely to weigh around 10 pounds. Your baby's length will increase by 1½ to 2 inches.

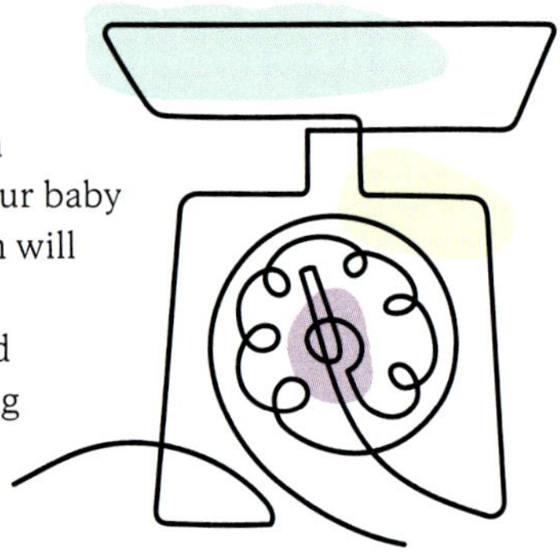

Many people envision newborns as cute, round and smooth-skinned, but that's not always the case. Passing through the birth canal isn't an easy journey, and it takes a while for baby's skin to adjust to the outside world. Most newborn appearance issues pass quickly.

To help you know what to expect, here are some brief descriptions of how a typical newborn is likely to appear.

Head

Forging headfirst through the birth canal can put a lot of pressure on a baby! Literally, pressure from the tight birth canal can cause the bones in your baby's skull to shift and overlap. This can leave your newborn's head looking slightly elongated or cone-shaped at birth. Don't worry, though. Your baby's head should round out in a few days. Babies born buttocks or feet first or by C-section are more likely to have round heads at birth. Pressure on your baby's face may leave your newborn's eyelids puffy or swollen.

The size of your baby's head is important because the growth rate of your baby's head reflects the growth of the brain. Both the brain and the skull grow incredibly fast in the first few months. In the beginning, the average newborn's head measures about 13¾ inches around and grows to about 15 inches by the end of the first month. At birth, baby's brain accounts for about 20% of body weight. By adulthood, this decreases to about 2 percent.

At the top and back of your baby's head, you'll notice two soft areas where the skull bones haven't yet grown together (see page 28). These soft spots, called fontanels, allow a baby's relatively large head to move down the narrow birth canal. They also accommodate a baby's rapidly growing brain. You may notice slight bulging from these spots when your baby cries or strains.

Skin

A newborn's skin can cause considerable distress to new parents. It's just more blotchy, flaky, pimply and wrinkled than they expected. But most of the time, this is completely typical. For example, switching from the moist environment of the womb to the relatively dry air outside it can cause the top layer of your baby's skin to flake off shortly after birth. You may notice plenty of dry, peeling skin for the first few weeks.

Your newborn's skin also may look slightly mottled, with some patches looking paler or darker than others, especially near the hands and feet. Your baby's hands and feet may also be colder than the rest of the body, and may appear a little blue or purple. But if you reposition your baby or move your baby's arms and legs a little, they should regain typical color.

In some cases, your baby's complexion may remind you more of an adolescent's than a newborn's, due to the appearance of tiny white bumps. These harmless bumps are called milia. Later, your baby may develop newborn acne, which causes small pimples on the face. A common, harmless rash called erythema toxicum often appears in the first few days of life as well. For more on common infant skin conditions, see page 119.

Many newborns have birthmarks (see page 29). You may notice reddish or pink patches above the hairline at the back of the neck, on the eyelids or between your newborn's eyes. These marks — nicknamed salmon patches or stork bites — are caused by collections of blood vessels close to the skin. Sometimes babies are born with a large flat brown or bluish-gray mark on the buttocks or lower back. This type of birthmark is called a slate gray nevus.

Umbilical cord

The stump of a newborn's umbilical cord is usually yellowish-green at birth. As the stump dries out and eventually falls off — usually within two to three weeks after birth — it'll change in color from yellowish green to brown to black. In the meantime, keep the stump clean and dry. Make sure it is not covered by the diaper. It's OK to get the cord wet in the bath. Just make sure to pat it dry completely afterward. When the cord falls off, there may be a few drops of blood, similar to a healing scab, but this should stop quickly. The cord may also be quite smelly as it is drying up — this is typical! Don't pull on the cord to help it separate faster.

INFANT JAUNDICE

It's not uncommon for a healthy newborn to develop a yellow tint to the skin and eyes in the first few days of life (jaundice). This occurs when the baby's blood contains too much of a yellow-colored substance formed during the breakdown of red blood cells (bilirubin). Jaundice typically develops because a baby's liver isn't mature enough to properly get rid of bilirubin in the bloodstream. Your baby's care team will check for jaundice in the first days and at baby's checkup during the first week. Mild infant jaundice is harmless and usually resolves on its own within a few weeks. If your baby's jaundice doesn't go away after a couple of weeks or gets worse, contact your baby's medical professional promptly. See page 36.

Breasts and genitalia

Before birth, the birthing person's hormones pass through the baby's system. This may lead to swollen breasts at birth for both boys and girls. Newborn girls may have a swollen vulva and light mucus-like or bloody vaginal discharge. The swelling typically disappears within two to four weeks. Vaginal discharge may last several days. For some newborn boys, fluid can accumulate around a testicle. This swelling, known as a hydrocele, usually disappears within a few months. Frequent erections are common, too. For information on circumcision care, see page 40.

Legs and feet

A newborn's legs and feet often look bowed or bent, thanks to the cramped quarters of the womb. As long as your newborn's legs and feet are flexible and can easily be moved about, there's no need for concern. These curves typically straighten on their own as your baby becomes more mobile. When a child is born, part of a newborn checkup includes an evaluation of a baby's hips, legs and feet.

Hair

Don't be alarmed if that great head of hair your baby was born with falls out within the first few weeks. Almost all newborns lose at least some of their baby hair. It will grow back in a few months. Plenty of babies also develop temporary bald spots on the back of the head from regular contact with the crib mattress or other sleep surface. Once your child starts rolling over and moving around, this won't be a problem anymore.

Some newborns are covered by fine, downy hair at birth — known as lanugo — especially on the back, shoulders, forehead and temples. Tiny hairs may also appear on your newborn's ears or in other spots. Lanugo is most common in premature babies. It typically wears off from friction within several weeks.

MOVEMENT

In this first month, your baby doesn't have a whole lot of control over movements, which are likely to be jerky and quivering. Your baby also may startle easily and even cry at sudden movements or loud noises. Swaddling or holding your baby close will help bring comfort.

Because your newborn's brain and nervous system are still immature, movements are largely involuntary or reactive. In order for your baby to move purposefully, the brain must send messages via nerve cells to muscles with specific instructions for movement. In the first few weeks of life, brain and nerve cells are rapidly developing, but they haven't achieved fluid communication yet.

Over time, the maturation of your child's nervous system will allow your baby to gain control over different parts of the body. This follows an orderly sequence from head to toe, so your baby's first major milestone is gaining head control, followed later by sitting, crawling and walking. By the end of the first month,

SPOT CHECK: WHAT'S GOING ON THIS MONTH

Here's a snapshot of what your baby's basic care looks like in the first month.

Eating

Baby will need breast milk or formula generally every two to three hours, although the frequency at first can be pretty variable. The goal is a minimum of 8 to 12 feedings a day to make sure your newborn is getting enough to eat. (Chapter 3 discusses nutrition in more detail.)

Sleeping

Expect your newborn to sleep about 16 hours a day, in one- to three-hour spurts, fairly evenly distributed throughout the day and night. Place your baby on the back to sleep to decrease the risk of sudden infant death syndrome (SIDS).

Sample newborn sleep schedule

In the first few weeks of life, there is no set schedule. Follow your baby's cues as you get to know each other. Here's just one example of what your newborn's sleep and awake time might look like over a full day.

7:30 a.m.	Feeding & awake time
8:15 a.m.	Sleep
10:45 a.m.	Feeding & awake time
11:45 a.m.	Sleep
1:30 p.m.	Feeding & awake time
2:20 p.m.	Sleep
5:20 p.m.	Feeding & awake time
6:15 p.m.	Sleep
7:15 p.m.	Feeding & awake time
8:00 p.m.	Sleep
9:05 p.m.	Feeding
9:20 p.m.	Sleep
10:15 p.m.	Feeding
10:45 p.m.	Sleep
1:05 a.m.	Feeding & awake time
1:55 a.m.	Sleep
4:15 a.m.	Feeding & awake time
5:30 a.m.	Sleep
8:30 a.m.	Awake

your baby's neck muscles will have developed considerably. When lying face-down, your baby may lift up the head and turn it from side to side.

In the first few weeks, your baby's hands are apt to be curled up into tight little fists much of the time. By the end of the first month, you may catch your baby trying to bring those fists toward the face for closer inspection. Over time, the hands will relax and spread wide, allowing your baby to use them more deliberately.

Baby reflexes

From birth, your baby comes hard-wired with a number of automatic responses (reflexes). Some of these reflexes help your baby survive entry into the big, new world.

Rooting reflex If you stroke your baby's cheek or the corner of the mouth, your baby will turn toward your hand and move the tongue in that direction. This helps your baby find the nipple of the breast or bottle and initiate feeding. This reflex usually disappears around 4 months of age.

Sucking reflex This reflex is present even before birth, and you may have even seen your baby sucking a thumb during an ultrasound examination. After

SOOTHING BY SUCKING

Most babies have a strong sucking reflex. Beyond nutrition, sucking often has a soothing, calming effect. That's where a pacifier can come in handy.

Some babies are interested in pacifiers; others aren't. If your baby isn't enthralled at first, you can try invoking your baby's natural sucking reflex. Gently stroke the side of your baby's mouth while holding the pacifier in the mouth until the sucking gets going.

If a pacifier seems to help your baby, feel free to use it. The American Academy of Pediatrics gives pacifiers the go-ahead for soothing between feedings and helping baby fall asleep. Pacifiers used during sleep may even help reduce the risk of sudden infant death syndrome (SIDS). The downside is that you may be woken up more often during the night to retrieve a lost pacifier.

In the beginning, be sure that pacifier use doesn't interfere with your breastfeeding routine, especially while you and your baby are still learning the ins and outs of nursing. Choose a pacifier that's made as one piece to avoid any choking hazards and that's dishwasher safe for easy cleaning. It helps to have several identical pacifiers handy so that you're not searching for the lone favorite in a desperate time of need. Also replace pacifiers that have worn or cracked nipples, as the nipples can tear off and pose a choking hazard. You may wish to stop using pacifiers by 18 months, but most kids do this on their own between ages 2 and 4.

your baby is born, placing a nipple in the mouth will cause your baby to automatically begin sucking. At first baby squeezes the area around the nipple between the tongue and palate to force out the milk. Next, your baby moves the tongue toward the end of the nipple to move the milk into the mouth.

The American Academy of Pediatrics reminds parents that even though this rhythmic sucking is a reflexive action, it generally takes a bit of practice for your baby to turn the reflex into an effective voluntary skill. So don't get discouraged if you and your baby don't seem to nail breast-feeding at first pass. Give yourselves a little time to practice and adjust.

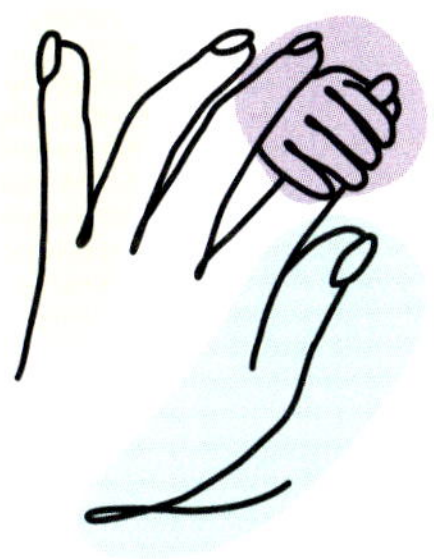

Grasp reflex Placing your finger in your newborn's palm causes your baby to grasp your finger. You'll find that if you try to remove your finger, baby will grasp it even tighter. A similar reaction occurs in the toes and foot if you press your thumb on the sole of baby's foot, just behind the toes. These reflexes generally disappear by 6 months and 12 months of age, respectively.

Startle reflex Upon hearing a loud noise, your baby will react by throwing out the arms and legs and then drawing in the arms. This reaction is also known as the Moro reflex. Another time it occurs is if your baby's head suddenly falls back. Doctors may check this reflex to make sure your baby's development is healthy. The startle reflex usually disappears by about 2 to 4 months of age.

Tonic neck reflex This reflex occurs when your baby turns the head to the side. Simultaneously, the arm and leg on the same side will extend out, while the opposing arm and leg flex, giving your baby the look of a fencer. It's a fairly subtle reflex, though, so don't worry if you don't notice it every time. The tonic neck reflex disappears around 4 to 7 months.

Stepping reflex If you hold your newborn upright and let the feet touch a flat surface, your baby will pick up one foot and then the other, as if walking. Of course, your baby's not ready to walk yet, and this reflex will disappear around 2 months. It will become a controlled skill when your baby starts walking, usually around a year or so of age.

SENSORY DEVELOPMENT

From the first moments, your baby may use all five senses to learn about the surrounding environment. Baby also uses them to form emotional attachments with you and others. By identifying your face, your smell and the sound of your voice, your baby establishes a connection with you.

In addition, your baby rapidly begins using multiple sensory skills to explore and interact with you. For example, your baby will quickly connect the sight of the breast or bottle with a particular scent, all of which equals food!

In the first month, your baby is likely to perceive the world in the following specific ways.

Vision

At birth, your baby is fairly nearsighted, with the ability to focus on objects that are roughly 8 to 12 inches away. Coincidentally, this is just about the distance between your baby's eyes and your face when you're nursing or holding baby. Thus, from early on, your baby is able to gaze at your face and quickly learns to recognize it. In fact, at this stage, your baby prefers the human face to any other patterns. This is an early opportunity for bonding with your baby. Make eye contact while feeding your baby or changing diapers.

Right after birth, your baby is very sensitive to bright light and is likely to close the eyes tightly to keep the light out. Over the next few weeks, though, vision will develop enough so that your baby can see a widening range of lights and darks. The higher the contrast in a pattern, the more likely it is to catch your child's attention during this first month.

Hearing

Your baby's hearing is fully mature at birth, but it takes a little while for your baby to learn how to recognize and react to different sounds. As with your baby's visual preference for the human face, your baby favors the sound of human voices, reacting especially to high-pitched voices. It's possible that your baby may even recognize your voice from having heard it during pregnancy and will turn toward the sound of your voice from the beginning. Talk and sing to your baby.

Some babies are more sensitive to noise than others. Too much noise, for example, and your baby may start to cry. In general, low, rhythmic tones are most likely to soothe your baby.

Smell

Your baby already has a keen sense of smell and quickly becomes able to discern their parent's breast milk from others' breast milk. Other smells new babies seem to like include sweet or fruity smells, such as vanilla and banana.

Taste

As a newborn, your baby has more taste buds than does an adult. Therefore, your little one can be fairly picky about different taste sensations, including the temperature of breast milk or formula. Most babies also prefer sweet tastes to sour ones.

Touch

New babies have a fully developed sense of touch as well. For example, they prefer soft, smooth surfaces to coarse or scratchy ones. And they can feel pain at the prick of a needle.

Most importantly, they respond to the way they're touched. In essence, this is the first form of communication between you and your baby. Gentle handling, snuggling and holding are not only soothing to your baby but a sign of your love and affection as well.

COGNITIVE DEVELOPMENT

Your baby's brain has been on a development fast track — generating new brain cells (neurons) at a rate of 250,000 a minute — ever since the early days of your pregnancy. By birth, your baby has virtually all the brain cells that will be used in a lifetime.

But having all these brain cells is just the beginning. As your baby is exposed

TOYS AND GAMES

During the first month, your baby doesn't need a lot of toys to be entertained — there are so many other things to take in. Still, you can provide different things for your baby to look at and listen to, which will help the brain cells develop more and better connections.

Chitchat

Since your face is one of your baby's favorite things to look at, why not make it available? Position yourself to be face-to-face and have a conversation. Talk to your baby about your day and what you're planning for dinner. Make faces, smile and sing. Eye contact is important, so try to minimize distractions such as TV or phones.

Listen to music

Play soft music while your baby lies in a crib or swing and you fold laundry or take care of some other chore.

Provide a view

During the first few weeks to months, your baby's neck muscles are still developing. But your baby can look from side to side. Hang a picture with bold graphic lines near the changing table at baby's eye level.

Read a book

Although your baby isn't ready to interact with a book yet, it's never too early to start reading together. Your baby will enjoy the rhythmic sound of your voice as you read, whether it's Dr. Seuss' *Hop on Pop* or your usual news source.

Get some tummy time

Place your baby on the tummy for a short time while awake. This will encourage your baby to hold the head up and strengthen those neck muscles. Some babies cry at first with tummy time. Stick with it! Try lying next to your baby or placing a mirror or toys on either side of your baby's head.

to a whole new world, brain cells rapidly start making connections called synapses. These connections create pathways between brain cells that, when reiterated through day-to-day experiences and activities, form the basis for knowledge and thought and for skills such as remembering, analyzing and problem-solving. These connections also set the foundation for communication and the interpersonal skills your child will use when relating to others.

Remember, it's never too early to set the foundation for essential skills such as language. It will still be a number of months yet before your newborn will be talking, but baby is already forming necessary connections for language development. You can encourage such development by talking and reading to your child. Provide plenty of face-to-face time when your baby is awake and alert.

STATES OF CONSCIOUSNESS

Scientists have observed, and you will too, that new babies fluctuate between different states of consciousness throughout the day. Some of these states are during sleep, and some occur while your baby is awake. There's no need to memorize them, but understanding the different states of consciousness may help you better understand your baby's moods.

- *Deep sleep.* During the deep sleep state, your baby sleeps quietly and does not move.
- *Active or light sleep.* In this state, your baby moves while sleeping, and may be startled or wakened by loud noises.
- *Drowsiness.* Drowsiness may occur before or after a sleep state. You'll notice your baby's eyes become a little droopy, and baby may yawn or stretch. Keep this one in mind for when you want to put your baby down to sleep.
- *Quiet alert.* In this state, your baby looks bright-eyed and bushy-tailed, but the body is quiet.
- *Active alert.* During active alert, your baby is wide-eyed and moving actively. Baby may be busy with self-entertainment.
- *Crying.* This state of consciousness is not hard to recognize because of the wails coming from your baby's mouth. During crying, baby also tends to flail or thrash about.

The best time to talk and play with your baby usually is during the quiet alert state. In this state, baby is most likely to be receptive to play and outside stimulation. Be warned, though, that new babies tend to cycle through states of consciousness fairly quickly. So don't be surprised if a toy elicits attention for a short while and then quickly becomes a source of irritation, and soon your baby starts crying. Just move on to what your child wants next, which is probably comforting or napping.

Your baby's environment has a tremendous impact on how the brain develops. While your baby's genetic makeup and physical development provide the essential "nature" ingredients, you provide the "nurture" components. You'll read more in the following chapters on how you can create the best environment for your child's mental growth and development. But the one thing that is essential to know, especially now in the first month, is that all children thrive in an environment of consistent warmth and positive attention, no matter how old they are.

Communication

Of course you knew your baby wouldn't be able to talk for quite some time. But who knew it would be such an adjustment to stare at your newborn and realize you were temporarily going to have to rely on something other than words to communicate?

You'll quickly discover, however, that your baby has a few different ways of communicating during this first month.

Crying This is the only way your baby can verbalize needs and feelings. All babies can and should cry, because this helps them receive the care they need. Adults, in turn, have a strong drive to respond when a baby cries, making this form of communication between you and your baby fairly natural. Responding warmly to your baby's cries helps your baby feel safe and secure in the new environment, as well as develop a secure attachment to you.

Lots of crying can be hard to take, of course. If you've run through your mental checklist and your baby is dry, full, comfortable and snug, then maybe baby just needs comforting. Or your baby may need some downtime without any stimulation, even if crying goes on for a few minutes. Sometimes you may not know why your baby is crying, and that's OK, too. Keep in mind that young babies don't cry to manipulate their parents or make them do things. They

1ST MONTH MILESTONES

In this first month, new babies are usually working on the following skills:

- Turning head from side to side
- Lifting head for a second while lying on belly
- Bringing fists in toward face
- Checking out human faces and maybe high-contrast patterns
- Visually tracking moving objects that are in close range (eyes may cross at this age, as eye muscles are still developing)
- Perhaps turning head toward familiar voices and sounds

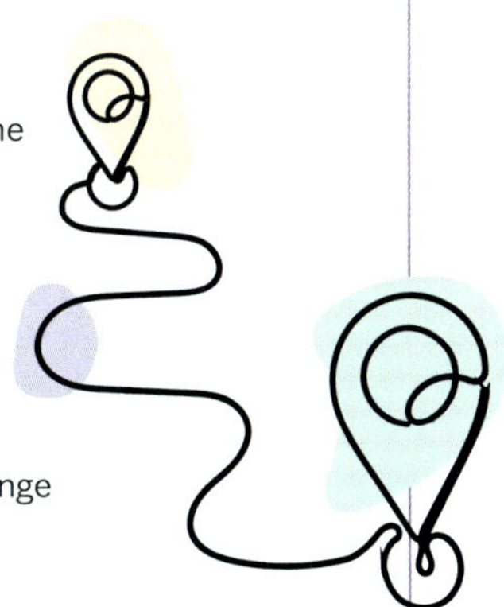

generally cry to communicate their needs, whether they're hungry, uncomfortable or overstimulated.

If your baby cries a lot, it's OK for you to take a break. Let your partner take over for a while, or lay your baby in a safe place for a few minutes of alone time. Your baby may need a bit of downtime. Crying usually increases over the first few weeks, peaking at about three hours a day at 6 weeks of age. Then crying gradually decreases to about an hour a day at 3 months old (see Chapter 9).

Body language During these first few weeks, your baby also communicates through body language. For example, when awake and alert, your baby may make eye contact with you and carefully scan your face. Or if your baby thinks there's simply too much going on at the moment, your baby may react by turning away from the source of stimulus, closing the eyes or becoming irritable.

Although new babies aren't capable of responding in many vocal ways yet, they're able to receive information and interpret nonverbal signals. Your baby can "read" signals you send, such as the expression on your face and the way you hold baby.

SOCIAL DEVELOPMENT

The main social event on your baby's calendar this first month is getting to know you. While you're occupied trying to figure out your baby, your baby is busy using the senses to become acquainted with you — how you smell, sound, look and feel.

Becoming attached

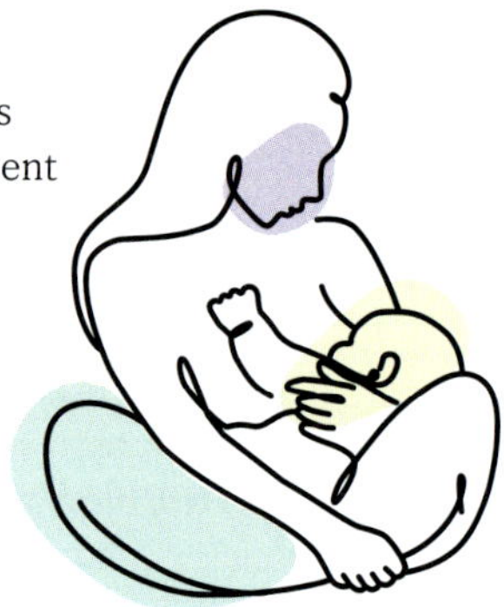

Babies' bodies are pretty amazing self-functioning packages when they arrive, but babies still depend on their environment for survival. Every time you feed your baby, change your baby's diaper, respond to your baby's cries or simply hold your baby close, you're establishing a pattern of consistent availability to your baby's needs. This creates a bond of trust and confidence between the two of you. This bond is the primary building block for your child's early social and emotional development. It's also your baby's template for future relationships. As a primary caregiver, you become your child's "home base," to which your child will repeatedly return over the years for comfort, help and support.

Breastfeeding can be a natural way of bonding with a newborn because it covers many of the baby's needs at once — food, warmth, comfort and security all rolled into one. But breastfeeding is only one way to bond. You also can connect with your baby when you're feeding your baby a bottle or doing any of the other activities involved in baby care. It's your general approach of love and gentle care that communicates safety to your child.

For some people, bonding comes more easily than for others. If you don't feel immediate attachment to your baby on day one, don't worry too much. After all, this is a new person in your life. As you spend time together and get to know each other's traits and characteristics, you'll develop a unique relationship that will be strengthened in the months and years ahead.

In addition, many people who have recently given birth have a mild case of the blues, not to mention fatigue and soreness. If you don't start feeling better and more involved in your parenting role after a few weeks, talk to your medical professional about treatment options. (See Chapter 37 for more information about caring for your mental health.)

Building up to smiles

Smiles actually take a while to develop. But you may notice over the course of this first month that your baby sometimes smiles during sleep or after a feeding. Around 4 weeks or so, your baby's smile may evolve a little further, involving the eyes more, and come several seconds after hearing your voice or feeling your touch. Next month, you can look forward to full-blown happy smiles involving the whole face that come in response to your own smiles.

CHAPTER 20

Month 2

By the beginning of your baby's second month, you're probably starting to get a handle on having a new baby in your home. You're better at basic caregiving activities, such as changing diapers or fixing bottles, and you've almost gotten your swaddle technique down. If you're breastfeeding, you've probably started ironing out some of the kinks, and you and your baby are feeling a lot more confident.

During month two, you'll still be perfecting a lot of these activities, but you'll also see your baby's personality begin to emerge. Your diligent efforts are more apt to be noticed by your little tyke, and you'll likely be rewarded with the beginnings of true interactive smiles. What's nice about month two is that the cogs of family life are slowly sliding into place and yet the excitement of it all is still bright.

GROWTH AND APPEARANCE

During the second month of life, your baby keeps growing at about the same rate as during the first few weeks, gaining about 5 to 7 ounces a week and growing about ½ inch a month. Your baby is starting to fill out — cheeks are getting chubbier and arms and legs fuller!

The head and brain are still growing rapidly, so head circumference increases by about ½ inch a month. It's typical for your baby's head to be proportionally larger than the rest of the body — it's still growing faster than anything else. The soft spot on the back of your baby's head is still open, but toward the end of this month and into the third month, it should begin to close.

Keep in mind that healthy infants come in a range of sizes. Although it's easy to cite averages, it's hard to predict your baby's exact growth. Your medical professional will monitor your baby's growth at each well-child visit. Where your child's numbers fall on the growth chart or how they compare with other babies' numbers isn't as important as whether your baby is maintaining a steady growth curve.

Baby skin issues will start looking a little better. Any jaundice should be gone by the second month. If not, contact your child's medical professional. Other newborn skin conditions, such as the little white pimples known as milia, are largely disappearing, although newborn acne may stick around for another month or two. If your baby has acne, gently cleanse your baby's face with baby soap several times a week, and avoid using lotions and oils.

Growth spurts

Just when your baby is finally sleeping for several nighttime hours at a stretch, baby may go back to waking up every two hours again. What's going on? Nothing out of the ordinary, probably. Infant growth and development occur in spurts. Usually a pause in learning happens before a new leap forward. For example, your baby may be subtly working out how to roll over. But until the technique is mastered, your baby may not fall or stay asleep like before.

SPOT CHECK: WHAT'S GOING ON THIS MONTH

Here's a snapshot of what your baby's basic care looks like in the second month.

Eating

Feed your child with breast milk or formula exclusively. Breastfed babies likely still want to eat every two to three hours. As the second month progresses, however, your baby's stomach capacity grows, and baby may take in more milk at each feeding. This may lead to a dropped nighttime feeding and hopefully more sleep! Formula takes longer to pass through the stomach, so formula-fed babies are more likely to eat every three to four hours. Within a month or two, though, the difference in nighttime feedings between breastfed and formula-fed babies tends to even out.

Sleeping

Your child may sleep between 15 and 16 hours a day. As your baby's nervous system matures and stomach capacity increases, more of these sleep hours will become part of nighttime sleep. At 2 months, your baby may be sleeping for five to six hours at a stretch during the night. Always place your baby on the back to sleep in a crib with no blankets, pillows or toys to decrease the risk of sudden infant death syndrome (SIDS).

TOYS AND GAMES

During the second month, your baby will gradually be awake for longer periods of time and have more quiet alert times. You can take advantage of these times by interacting in ways that encourage your child's development.

But let your baby guide playtime. Watch for clues that baby is tired or overstimulated, such as turning away, closing the eyes or becoming irritable. Also, keep in mind your baby's physical limitations. During physical play, be gentle, and be careful not to shake your baby or toss baby in the air. These activities can cause severe injury to your baby's eyes, neck and brain.

Here are a few suggestions for playtime with your 1- to 2-month-old.

Keep up tummy time

Regularly placing your baby on the belly for a short time while awake helps develop neck muscles and increase head control. You can share in tummy-time fun by lying on the floor facing your baby and talking to baby. Your baby will work neck and arm muscles to lift up and be face-to-face with you. You also can encourage your child to work those muscles by putting toys just within reach.

Set up a mobile

Your baby can better hold the head steady enough to look straight up while lying on the back. Mobiles can become particularly fascinating. When choosing a mobile, look at it from your baby's perspective. Keep in mind a child's preference for simple shapes, high contrast and bright objects. Some models will even twirl around to music, engaging your baby's eyes and ears. Be sure all items are secured completely and placed out of baby's reach.

Introduce color

As vision improves, baby will become more interested in bold, vivid colors in addition to high-contrast patterns. Visit your local library to borrow books containing brightly colored art or photographs. Or arrange a still life with brightly colored fruits and vegetables — say, oranges, apples and asparagus — for your baby to check out.

Encourage familiarity

Try reading the same story several nights in a row to your baby, and see if baby starts to show signs of recognition. Or play a favorite song several times during the week and see how your baby reacts after hearing it multiple times.

OUT OF SIGHT, OUT OF MIND

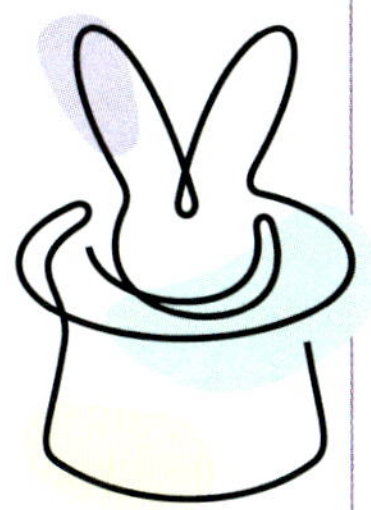

At this age, your baby's mind has yet to grasp the concept that things continue to exist even if they're out of sight (object permanence). For example, if a dog wanders into your 2-month-old's field of vision and then out again, your baby may stare for a few seconds at the spot where the dog was. Baby won't understand that the dog still exists once it can no longer be seen.

In other words, once something is out of sight, it's also out of your baby's mind. It isn't until later during the first year — around 8 months or so — that your baby will understand that even if you hide your face behind a blanket, you are still there. Up until that point, peekaboo games can feel pretty magical!

MOVEMENT

Most of your baby's movements are still jerky and involuntary (reflexive) at this point. But as the month progresses, these newborn reflexes will give way to more purposeful movements. Your baby may seem less active for a short period until major muscle coordination becomes natural. You'll see your baby practice new positions by stretching, moving and watching.

Your baby's neck muscles are getting stronger, too. When pulling your baby gently to a sitting position, you'll notice that the head still lags behind a bit. But when upright, your baby can probably hold the head steady for a few seconds, although not much longer. Continue to support your baby's head when holding or carrying your baby. When lying belly down, your baby may raise the head to look straight ahead for a few moments, rather than just side to side. Lying on the back, your baby can keep the head centered and look straight up — a handy skill for watching mobiles and looking up at you!

At this age, most babies aren't ready to roll from front to back or side to back yet — that generally happens around 3 to 4 months of age. But you cannot be certain that your baby will stay in one place, either. Babies this young can use their feet to push off surfaces and scoot around. And even though they're just learning controlled maneuvers, they can unexpectedly flip themselves over by sudden, startled movements. Don't leave your baby unattended in a car seat, on a changing table or other elevated surface, and take proper precautions to securely strap your baby in while on a changing table.

Toward the end of the second month, your baby also may become aware of their own hands and fingers and try to bring them together to play with them.

SENSORY DEVELOPMENT

During the second month, your baby's eyes are getting better at moving and focusing on objects at the same time. This makes it easier for your child to visually track moving objects. Your baby's brain isn't mature enough to process visual information speedily, but baby can track a toy if it's moving very slowly. Although your baby is still likely to prefer the sight of human faces, baby also will enjoy patterns that are more complex and colorful than simple black-and-white checkerboard images.

When you talk to your baby, you'll find that baby is actively listening and watching the movements of your lips with interest as you speak. In return, your baby may move arms and legs excitedly or try to make sounds.

COGNITIVE DEVELOPMENT

So far, your baby has been taking in a lot of information. But baby may be ready for some outward expression as well. Child psychologists refer to incoming

BIG SIBLINGS

Having a new baby in the house brings a special excitement for families that already have kids. Although caring for other children as well as a newborn can be challenging, you'll also have the rich experience of watching your children's sibling relationships grow.

Generally, children are quite excited at the prospect of having a real live baby in the house. But what they may not realize is that they'll need to share you, their parent, with another person. Sometimes this can lead to older children acting out to get more attention, or even lashing out at the baby. With time, though, most children learn to adjust to the household reorganization and find their own special place. You can help them with this in several ways.

Postpone major changes

During the weeks following your baby's arrival, avoid any drastic changes in older children's routines. This may mean waiting a while to potty train, switch from a crib to a bed or move to another home.

Let each child set the pace

Despite being raised in the same family, each child can react differently to a new baby. Responses may vary from excited giggles to hyperactivity to lack of interest. Sometimes a child's reaction is delayed for weeks. Allow your children to become accustomed to the baby in their own time.

language as "receptive" and outgoing speech as "expressive" language. Receptive language, where your baby listens and absorbs speech and sounds, almost always happens first. Then baby begins to use expressive language by vocalizing thoughts. This is why it's so important for you to talk to your baby even before baby can talk. In general, children understand language much earlier than they can clearly use it themselves.

Cooing and gurgling

One of the most gratifying developments for parents this month — generally around 6 to 8 weeks of age — is their babies' first attempts at expressive language. These are typically soft, single-vowel sounds that sound like oohs and aahs, or like cooing.

As opposed to crying and grunting, which come from the chest, cooing and gurgling sounds come from your baby's voice box (larynx). Cooing also involves using different mouth muscles than crying does. Eventually your baby will begin to use the tongue and then lips to make more precise sounds. This pattern of language development — starting from the center and moving outward — mirrors baby's motor development (fine-tuning movement from arms to hands to fingers).

Set clear expectations

Let your older children know what behavior is appropriate around the baby. For example, let your child know it's never OK to pick up the baby without permission, but that it is OK to sit next to the baby and talk nicely.

Offer sincere praise

When you find your older child behaving well, acknowledge it. Praise your child for speaking gently to the baby or playing nicely. This kind of positive reinforcement shows that you still value your child's presence and that you appreciate your child's contributions to the family.

Make time for older kids

Siblings of babies need lots of personal attention, too. Make plans to leave the baby with your partner or a reliable sitter, and spend some undivided time with your older children.

Be patient and positive

Some children go back to old behaviors after a new baby arrives, such as sucking a thumb or using baby talk. This is called regression, and it's common. Be patient during this period of change. Treat regression in a matter-of-fact way. For example: "I see you wet your bed this morning. Let's change the sheets together." These simple sentences state the problem and offer a ready solution.

2ND MONTH MILESTONES

During the second month, your baby is busy:

- Working on lifting up shoulders while lying on belly
- Holding head steady while sitting
- Becoming aware of own fingers
- Straightening out legs and strengthening kicks
- Focusing on objects moving across field of vision
- Cooing and making sounds
- Recognizing parents' faces, being reassured by parents' touch
- Learning to smile in response to parents' smiles
- Learning to smile spontaneously to express happiness or contentment

Cooing is a way for your baby to express happiness and contentment. Your baby may coo and gurgle for self-entertainment, but also to attract your attention. If your baby coos at you and you talk back, your baby quickly discovers that this is a two-way game. By talking back, you reinforce the notion that communication is important and often a source of great delight.

Crying at its peak

Your baby still relies heavily on crying to communicate needs and moods. In fact — brace yourself — crying tends to reach a peak of about three hours a day right around 6 to 8 weeks of age. This is typical. A lot of babies develop a period of fussiness and prolonged crying at the end of the day, perhaps as a way of releasing pent-up stress (not unlike adults, if you think about it).

If you've already accounted for all of your baby's needs, listening to your baby cry can be hard. You may feel frustrated with your parenting skills. But it's not always possible to calm a crying baby, especially if your baby is just letting off steam. Remember that your baby's crying is not a rejection of your efforts, nor does it mean you're a failure at parenting. Babies cry; that's what they do. Eventually your baby will fall asleep or change moods. By the time your baby is 3 or 4 months old, time spent crying will decrease greatly.

If your baby's crying is accompanied by other symptoms, or if you feel the length or intensity of your baby's crying is unusual, trust your intuition. Call your child's medical professional. For more on crying, see Chapter 9.

SOCIAL DEVELOPMENT

During the second month, your baby still spends a lot of time sleeping, and your interactions with each other are fairly limited. But at the same time, your baby is making definite strides in social graces. By the age of 1 month, your baby is learning to recognize you, perhaps reacting with a jerky arm wave or a few bobs of the head at the sight of you. By 6 weeks, many babies start to smile in response to a parent's smile. After weeks revolving around feeding, changing diapers and trying to catch some sleep, seeing your baby smile at you can be very rewarding.

When you react to your baby's smiles with a show of delight, your baby learns that actions have an impact, and that baby has a certain amount of control over what's happening. This initial awareness is the beginning of your baby's ability to distinguish between the self and others.

Baby smiles also can be spontaneous expressions of happiness or contentment even at this stage. For example, your baby is starting to recognize certain objects by sight, such as a bottle or bathtub. Baby may smile or coo excitedly in anticipation of what's to come.

Spoil away

Don't worry about spoiling your baby during the early months of life. Addressing your child's physical needs and desire for attention helps establish a pattern of consistent and predictable loving care in your baby's mind. This allows your baby to establish an emotional comfort level. In other words, your baby is learning to feel safe and secure. Baby also is learning to trust you and to have self-trust. In addition, when you soothe your baby during a crying spell, you're teaching your child how to regulate emotions even in times of intense emotion or stress.

So pick your baby up as often as you like, and hold your baby as much as you want. It's good for both of you!

CHAPTER 21

Month 3

While a solid block of sleep may still seem out of reach by the third month, your baby's range of motor control, mental engagement and social interaction is widening dramatically. A number of factors are affecting your baby's growth and development, including a more mature nervous system, development of the senses, reinforcement of the memory pathways in the brain and expansion of the range of emotions. They all contribute to your baby's growing interest in your family and the world.

GROWTH AND APPEARANCE

In the third month, the rate at which your baby gains weight and grows in length should roughly match last month's rate. Most babies gain between 1 and 1¾ pounds and lengthen by about ½ inch a month during the first six months of life. Head circumference increases by about ½ inch a month during this time as well.

If you're worried that your baby seems too thin or too chubby, be careful not to judge by appearance alone. Since infants tend to carry different amounts of weight at different stages of development, making judgments about baby fat on the basis of appearance alone isn't reliable or effective. Instead, talk to your baby's medical professional about your concerns. The medical professional will plot your baby's growth on charts that show measurements for height, weight and head circumference (see pages 578 and 579). You can use the charts to compare your baby's growth with that of other infants of the same sex and age. What really matters, however, is the trend revealed on growth charts — not any particular percentile. Your baby's medical professional will look mainly for predictable changes in weight over time.

If you're following your baby's hunger cues for feeding and baby's growth is progressing steadily, there's generally no reason to worry about your baby's size.

Baby fat

Babies need a diet high in fat to support growth during infancy. In addition, a diet high in fat helps to build a thick casing (myelin sheath) around nerve fibers in the brain and spinal cord. This sheath offers "insulation" for nerve fibers and helps ensure that nerve impulses are sent efficiently.

It's true that many medical professionals and medical researchers are concerned about the rise in childhood obesity. Some evidence suggests that this problem may arise earlier than previously believed. For example, some studies have linked rapid weight gain in the first year of life to obesity later on in life. Excess baby fat also may have more immediate consequences, such as delaying the development of crawling and walking.

Yet the first year of life is no time to put your baby on a diet or limit calories, unless your baby's medical professional has given you specific feeding instructions. Your baby needs adequate nutrition to develop properly. Steps that may help reduce the risk of later obesity include:

- *Breastfeed for as long as possible.* Several studies have shown a connection between breastfeeding and reduced childhood obesity. The cause for this link isn't clear, but it may have to do with the ability of breastfed babies to self-regulate their intake of milk. In other words, baby decides when to stop eating. If you're bottle-feeding, try to follow your baby's cues about fullness. Don't make your baby finish a bottle just because the milk is there.

SPOT CHECK: WHAT'S GOING ON THIS MONTH

Here's a snapshot of what your baby's basic care looks like in the third month.

Eating

Breast milk or formula exclusively. Longer stretches of sleep at night may mean more frequent feedings during the day. But through this month and the next, you can expect your baby to gradually take in more milk at a single feeding, perhaps resulting in fewer feedings throughout the day. Between 2 and 4 months of age, the average baby eats around 2 ounces per pound of body weight every 24 hours.

Sleeping

About 15 hours a day. By about 3 months old, many babies sleep for a solid six to eight hours during the night. Still, this doesn't always happen when you're sleeping. Expect to be up once or twice during the night, especially if your baby has a growth spurt and needs more frequent feedings.

- ***Avoid juice.*** Don't serve juice until your baby is older than 6 months (and even then, you don't have to). Offering juice before this age may lead to juice taking the place of regular breast milk or formula feeding, which can deprive your baby of necessary nutrients. If you choose to offer juice after your baby is 6 months old, serve it in a cup rather than a bottle, and limit it to no more than 4 ounces a day.
- ***Don't use food as a pacifier.*** If your baby still seems fussy after a feeding, don't automatically try to calm baby with another feeding. Try other methods of distraction first.

MOVEMENT

By the third month, added muscle strength gives your baby new viewpoints from which to peer at the world. As your baby develops more purposeful movements, you'll notice those newborn reflexes fading.

Head and neck

Lying belly down, babies this age can usually lift their heads and shoulders. Some infants may even extend their arms and rest on their elbows. This gives them even more support for looking around. In turn, looking upward and sideways while on their tummies further increases neck strength and head control.

Increased head control means that your baby's head lags less when you pull baby into a sitting position. Also, when you support your baby seated on your lap, your baby can hold up the head for longer periods of time instead of just a few seconds. In the third month, you'll notice your baby's back still rounds forward. But as your child's movement (motor) skills develop, the muscles in the upper and then lower back will strengthen as well. Strong back muscles act as a balance and body brace so baby can eventually sit straight unsupported, crawl, stand and then walk.

Hands and arms

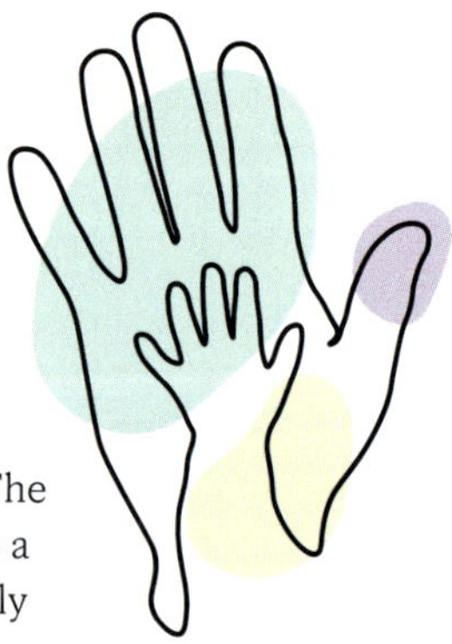

This month your baby is likely to enjoy watching their own hands, bringing them together at eye level and trying to bring them to their mouth.

You may notice that your child's hands begin to uncurl from their previous clenched-fist position. At this age, babies begin to experiment with opening and shutting their hands and spreading their fingers wide to test and inspect them. Your baby also may start to grip objects intentionally rather than reflexively, but then have a hard time letting go. The next step will be to gain enough finger dexterity to hold on to a toy, and then transfer it from one hand to the other. Eventually your baby will be able to pick a toy up and set it down again, firming up basic fine motor skills.

At the same time, your child may start reaching for objects by swiping or batting at them with broad arm movements and clenched fists. As the hands become more open, your child will have better luck hitting the intended target.

Legs

Your baby's legs are becoming impressively strong, and baby is likely to experiment with flexing the legs and knees at will. Some babies, especially when they're excited, may even kick hard enough to flip themselves over. In preparation for purposely rolling over, your baby may start rocking back and forth. In fact, by 3 months of age, many babies start to roll from their backs onto their sides and then onto their backs again. Always take proper precautions to prevent baby from wriggling off a changing table or flipping out of a car seat. Strap your baby in and stay nearby to avoid any accidents.

SENSORY DEVELOPMENT

Although the development of your baby's senses isn't as easy to observe as the development of motor skills and coordination, one is essential for the other. Playing with and watching your baby will help you know how well your child sees and hears.

Vision

Your baby's sight is maturing rapidly. In the next few months, baby will begin to view the world in much the same way you do. By 2 or 3 months old, your

HOLD OFF ON THE PUREES AND SOLIDS

For the first six months, breast milk or formula is generally the only food your baby needs. Its liquid form perfectly matches your baby's eating skills, habits and digestive abilities.

Before age 4 to 6 months, your baby isn't developmentally ready for purees and solid foods. At this stage, your baby still manages milk or formula by moving it from the front to the back of the mouth by sucking, then swallowing. This sucking reflex is aided by the tongue-protrusion reflex, in which the tongue pushes forward to help the baby suck. This reflex is still strong during this month and next, which means that it's difficult for a baby to manage more solid textures. Babies at this age tend to push out cereals or solid foods rather than swallow them, which can make spoon-feeding a frustrating experience for you and baby.

Signs that your baby may be ready for solid foods include good head and neck control, being able to sit supported, and opening the mouth when a spoon approaches. These skills usually come a bit later (see Chapter 4).

baby is steadily developing the ability to simultaneously turn both eyes inward to focus on a close object (convergence). Convergence allows your baby to focus on and play with the hands. At the same time, your baby is learning to focus on distant objects by simultaneously turning both eyes outward (divergence).

As the vision matures, your baby will be able to notice details of a pattern and to tell whether there is more than one object in a picture. As distance vision improves, you may catch your baby studying you across the room or gazing intently at a ceiling fan. Your baby also is getting better at distinguishing between colors, and may especially enjoy primary colors.

Around this time, your baby also learns a skill that encompasses both sensory and social development. Your baby will look at your eyes and then turn to discover what it is that you see. This is called shared attention.

During the third month, if you still see your baby's eyes crossing or if you notice there seems to be a lag in one eye, let your baby's medical professional know. If it happens consistently, you may be referred to an eye specialist, who can take any steps needed to correct the vision problem.

TOYS AND GAMES

As your baby becomes more interactive, it becomes even more fun to play together. This may be especially true in the next month or so when your baby discovers the ability to laugh.

Around this time, your baby also may become more interested in objects or toys that can be touched or held. Choose toys that are lightweight, easy to grasp, drool-resistant, too big to swallow and without sharp edges. Some examples include board books, soft blocks, wooden and plastic spoons, measuring cups, empty containers, rattles, balls, and squeeze toys. As long as the toys are safe, let your creativity flow. (Avoid shiny plastic wrap or plastic bags, though, which can easily cover your baby's mouth and nose and cause suffocation.)

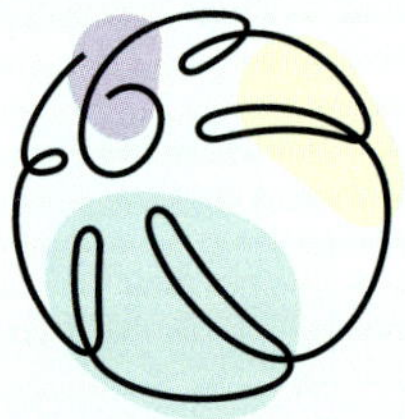

Here are some other ideas for fun and games in the third month.

Get rolling

To help your baby practice rolling skills, lie side by side and encourage baby to roll toward you. Your baby will try to do this with the whole body, which essentially means rolling over. In the beginning, babies usually find it easier to roll from back to side and then back again. Give praise when baby manages a roll. There's no need to push or pull, though. This skill will be perfected when baby is ready.

Hearing

Your baby's hearing contributes to a growing sense of familiarity and comfort with the world. Around the third month, your baby may quiet when hearing your voice or get excited when hearing siblings or a favorite song. You may even notice baby turning toward the sound of your voice or other interesting sounds. Your familiar voice may get a smile out of baby, too.

Taste and smell

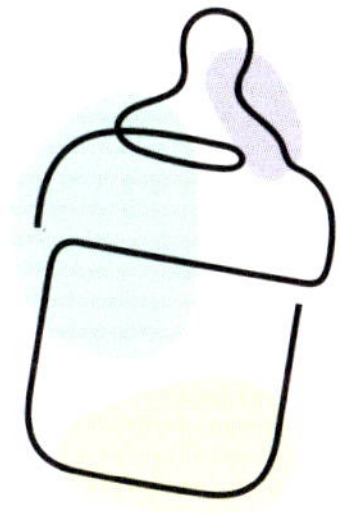

Toward the end of this month, your baby is starting to distinguish between different tastes, such as breast milk versus formula or the usual kind of formula and a new brand. Your baby also is likely to favor certain smells or be turned off by other smells.

These factors can sometimes affect feeding preferences, depending on your baby's temperament. For example, if your baby is very sensitive to odors and finds a smell unpleasant, baby may not want to eat while the smell is present.

Touch and feel

As your baby's hands gradually open up, try placing different textures in the palm — soft, smooth, fuzzy, bumpy. See what textures your baby likes most.

Get a grip

Place a toy or object in your baby's hand. Let baby hold it, feel it and move it. Also, try this with objects that rattle, squeak or make noise. Share in the surprise when baby succeeds in producing sound.

Set up batting practice

Place your baby on an infant floor gym or play mat — the kind that usually has brightly colored, different-shaped objects dangling from it. Your baby can practice reaching and batting at the toys, as well as discover different shapes and textures. Another way to encourage reaching and grasping is to place your baby in an infant seat and offer items that are in front, just above or below, or just to the side of your baby's eye level. These games also help your baby develop depth perception and hand-eye coordination.

Get giggling

Almost all little kids love gentle tickling, especially if you deliver it with laughter and exaggerated facial expressions. Or try blowing a raspberry on your baby's belly. Your baby may be surprised at first, but eventually these activities will likely have your baby laughing.

VIEW TIMETABLES WITH CAUTION

Don't worry if your baby doesn't follow the exact timetable of development milestones outlined in these chapters. In some cases, your baby's development may be well into the next chapter; in other cases the previous chapter may be more appropriate. All babies go through the same progression of milestones, but each baby reaches them at a unique pace (including babies with developmental disabilities). The timing of social development is likely to be even more variable than other aspects of development.

COGNITIVE DEVELOPMENT

As the nerve cells in your baby's brain mature, connect with other brain cells and become insulated with fatty myelin, your baby's brain gains more control over the rest of the body. You can see this when you observe your baby making purposeful movements, such as bringing a hand up for inspection or reaching for a toy.

These intentional motor skills require subtle complexities in thinking, reasoning and planning skills:

- ***Interest.*** What is that thing dangling in front of me?
- ***Speculation.*** What happens if I try to touch it?
- ***Trial and error.*** Moving my arm this way seems to work better than moving it that way.

If your baby succeeds in making the toy rattle or make noise, for example, further information processing and analysis is required: What was that noise? How did it happen? Can I make it happen again?

Laying down tracks

Repetition of experience is how memories are created in an infant's brain. Over time, your consistent response to your baby's needs — feeding, cuddling, bathing, soothing, carrying — lays down pathways among your baby's brain cells. Those pathways become reinforced and streamlined every time you respond in a similar manner.

By the third month, these memory pathways are becoming more clearly defined, and your baby is starting to have a better understanding of the connection between behavior and your reactions. For example, your baby has figured out that crying can get your attention fairly quickly, or that smiling will likely get a smile in response.

Expanding communication

At the same time, your baby is building an increasing number of sounds and gestures as means of communication — squealing, growling, blowing raspberries and experimenting with consonant sounds.

As your baby approaches 3 and 4 months of age, baby may start "conversations" with you by smiling, cooing or squealing. Acknowledging your baby's overtures is sure to delight. Repeat baby's sounds so that baby knows you're listening. Also, talk back to your baby in "parentese" — use real words pronounced correctly and clearly but at a high pitch and with exaggerated tones. This helps your baby learn the sounds of your language. Most parents naturally

RETURNING TO WORK

In the United States many working parents prepare to end family leave and return to work around this time, if they haven't already. It's certainly not easy to leave a new little one in the care of someone else, even if temporarily, and especially after spending so much time together. In the meantime, though, nothing can change the fact that you are now a parent and you have a baby who thinks the world of you. To make the transition back to work a little smoother, try some of these suggestions:

- *Let go of the guilt.* Returning to work after having a baby often leaves many new parents feeling particularly torn. But working outside the home doesn't make you a bad parent — and it's OK to look forward to the challenges and interactions of your job.
- *Talk to your boss.* If you're interested, you might ask about flexible hours, working remotely or working part-time.
- *Plan for feeding changes.* If you're breastfeeding and plan to continue doing so after returning to work, ask your employer about a clean, private room for breast pumping. About two weeks before returning to work, change your nursing schedule at home so you're pumping during the day for at least one to two feedings and nursing before and after your upcoming work hours. Have someone else feed your baby a bottle of stored breast milk to help your baby adapt.
- *Start short.* If you can, go back to work late in the week. That'll make your first week back to work more manageable.
- *Get organized.* Sketch out a daily to-do list. Identify what you need to do, what can wait — and what you can skip entirely.
- *Stay connected.* Keep in touch with your baby's caregiver to see how your baby is doing. Some caregivers may be willing to send photos or videos of your baby during the day.
- *Make backup plans.* Know what you'll do if your baby is sick or your baby's caregiver is unavailable. Options might include you or your partner taking the day off or calling a friend or loved one to care for your baby.
- *Maintain a positive attitude.* Show how excited you are to see your baby at the end of the day. Baby may not understand your words but will pick up on your emotions.

use parentese when they talk to babies. So don't be embarrassed; go ahead! Your baby will love it.

Once you've said your piece, pause to allow your baby to respond with a look, wriggle or sound. This will help baby learn the rhythm and timing of effective communication.

SOCIAL DEVELOPMENT

It doesn't take long for parents and family to become the most important people in an infant's life. Your baby's world is centered entirely around you and your family. Baby is involved in your everyday lives, watching, listening and picking up clues on how humans interact. And your family will be the first people with whom your baby interacts.

3RD MONTH MILESTONES

During the third month, your baby is busy:

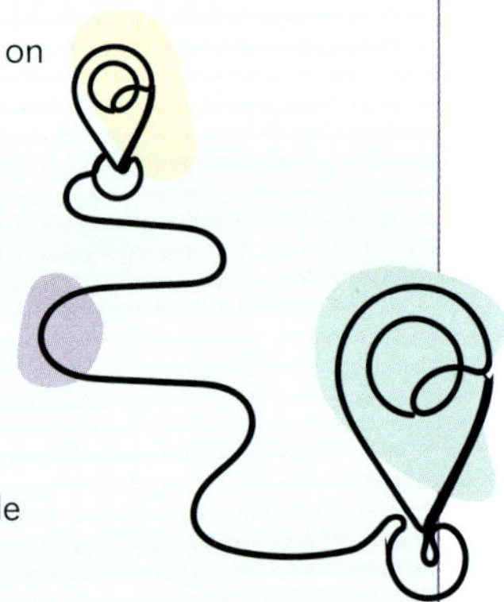

- Raising head and chest to look around while lying on belly
- Working on supporting upper body with arms while lying on belly
- Holding head steady for longer periods while sitting
- Playing with hands at eye level
- Trying to bring hands to mouth
- Swiping at dangling objects
- Opening and closing hands, stretching fingers wide
- Holding toys briefly
- Stretching and kicking legs
- Developing distance vision
- Recognizing familiar people and objects from a distance
- Using eyes and hands in coordination
- Distinguishing between different colors, tastes and smells
- Increasing repertoire of sounds to include squealing, growling, consonant sounds and maybe even giggling
- Turning head toward sound
- Making eye contact
- Enjoying family and familiar faces, maybe even new people
- Using expanding communication skills to express emerging emotions
- Imitating some sounds, movements and facial expressions
- Learning to self-entertain

A real charmer

Around this time, your baby not only is pleased with your attention but also is starting to discover personal powers of attraction. With a smile or a squeal of excitement, your baby can draw you out to respond in kind. Your baby is able to make and maintain eye contact, and interact more vigorously with others. Make your attention available when your baby seeks it. Try to carve out time away from distractions such as phones, TV and other devices.

Some babies even start to giggle or laugh in response to facial and vocal expressions or in response to touch. In general, laughter usually comes about a month after social smiling and is a great addition to your relationship!

At this stage, your baby has yet to develop anxiety about meeting strangers and may even be fairly outgoing and happy to meet other people. This may be a good time to introduce your baby to the concept of staying with grandparents or a babysitter for a few hours and to allow baby to develop a bond with these trusted adults. In a few months, your baby may not want to be separated from you. But if baby is used to the idea that although you may go away for a short while, you always come back, it may make it a little easier when you need to temporarily leave your child in the care of another.

Wanting attention

During this month, you also may notice that your child cries not just to express a need or feeling but also in order to get your attention. In the coming weeks, crying in general will decrease (thankfully), but it's likely to become more purposeful and directed at bringing you back to your baby's side.

Continue to respond quickly (or as quickly as possible) and warmly, even if just by calling out to your child. This will help reassure your baby that you're still there. This continued responsiveness helps to cement the trust and sense of security your baby feels in you.

CHAPTER 22

Month 4

Before you begin month 4, pat yourself on the back. You've made it through the first few months of parenthood, quite possibly one of the biggest transitions of your adult life. At this age, most babies have begun to adjust to life in this brave new world. They've also become much more secure in their relationship with their parents and their own abilities to adapt and react to their environment.

New families often find the next few months to be a joyous time. You've probably settled into a familiar routine, and eating and sleeping schedules are becoming more regular. The amount of time your baby spends fussing is probably on the decline. The brain and nervous system have matured enough that baby is ready to become much more interactive with family and friends, while continuing to explore new sights and sounds. Newborn reflexes are fading and your little one is starting to move and do things by design now. In addition, your infant is getting much better at conveying emotions and desires, and you're getting much better at understanding your child. In other words, the bond between the two of you is truly blossoming!

Take advantage of this time to enjoy each other's company and revel in the little things — a giggle and a smile, a splash in the tub or a bug on a window. Who knew life could be so exciting?

GROWTH AND APPEARANCE

Between 3 and 4 months old, your baby's growth is likely to slow a little. But you can still expect your baby to gain between ¾ and 1½ pounds over the course of the month and grow about ½ inch in length. Some babies may double their birth weight by the end of the fourth month. Head circumference increases by about

½ inch. All babies grow differently. Your baby's 4-month well-child exam is a great time to check in on your baby's growth.

Skin rashes

You're getting ready to change your baby's diaper, and there under your baby's shirt is a rash. Alarm bells go off and you rush to call your baby's medical professional. This happens to just about every parent. And while you should always call your baby's medical professional if you notice something unusual or are concerned about your baby's health, you also should know that most skin rashes in infants are common and usually not serious. If the rash occurs along with a fever, call your baby's medical professional promptly.

Rashes in babies often result from skin irritants, such as soap or scratchy fabric, or an underlying viral infection, such as a parvovirus infection or roseola. Because rashes are so visible, they're a common cause of concern for new parents. Most of the time, though, rashes aren't a sign of a serious problem and

SPOT CHECK: WHAT'S GOING ON THIS MONTH

Here's a snapshot of what your baby's basic care looks like in the fourth month.

Eating

Feed breast milk or formula exclusively. During this month, the number of daytime feedings generally decreases to about four or five, but a midmonth growth spurt may lead to more frequent feedings for a few days. Although it may be tempting to get your baby started on cereal or other solid foods during this month, hold off a little bit longer until your baby shows clear signs of being physically ready for solids (see Chapter 4). Your baby also does not need plain water at this age. They should be getting enough fluid intake from breast milk or formula to keep them hydrated.

Sleeping

Expect your child to sleep about 15 hours a day, including more predictable nighttime hours of sleep — generally six to eight hours, although every baby is different. Around this age, babies become more active sleepers, making noise, scooting around and often waking their parents. It's OK to give your baby a few minutes to settle back down without your help. This allows your baby to learn to self-soothe upon waking at night. Although your baby is moving around more — maybe even starting to roll — it's still important to put your baby on the back to sleep. By this time, your baby also may have settled into two to three daytime naps, lasting an hour or two each. See Chapter 8 for more on sleep.

may not even need treatment beyond proper skin care and perhaps a mild cortisone cream, as indicated by your child's medical professional.

Some general rules of thumb for baby skin include avoiding long, hot baths and staying away from any substances or fabrics that seem to cause a reaction. Using gentle moisturizers daily can help soothe and protect the skin. You can read more about common skin rashes in Chapter 7.

Bedtime routine

It's probably a safe bet that almost all new parents are hoping to find somewhere — in the pages of a book, in advice from a friend or on a website — the secret to getting their kids to sleep. Alas, there is no simple solution. Your child's sleeping habits depend on a number of factors, including age, how long baby can go without a feeding, and personality. Some babies settle down without a peep and wake briefly for feedings. Others cry every time you put them in the crib and have a hard time lulling themselves to sleep.

During the first few months of your baby's life, it's important to respond to your baby's cries and provide enough soothing to optimize sleep. But around the

KEEPING PLAYTIME SAFE

Your baby might not be crawling yet, but it's around this time that babies start putting whatever they can in their mouths. Take advantage of this limited period of immobility to make sure the spaces where you play with baby are free of any potential hazards. Get into the habit of doing a baby-level safety check each time you put your baby down on the floor to play. Get down on your hands and knees, at your baby's level, and look for these items:

- Small objects your baby could accidentally swallow, such as coins, button batteries, magnets, paper clips, or small pieces of food or candy
- Toys with small parts
- Balloons
- Uncovered electrical outlets
- Pulls for window blinds, in which your baby could get entangled
- Electrical cords to irons, lamps or other appliances that could fall if baby tugs on the cord
- Plastic bags or wrappings that could suffocate your baby
- Newspapers and magazines
- A pet's toys or treats
- Houseplants

These safety searches can become fun and helpful activities for older siblings to get involved in. Help them understand the things that can be harmful to a baby. This will increase their awareness about the hazards of leaving toys and objects around the play area.

third and fourth months, you can start taking steps to help your child fall asleep independently, an important skill that every child must eventually learn.

Parents at this stage often worry about letting their babies "cry it out." There is plenty of advice out there on the "best" way to get your baby to sleep. Different methods involve various ways to offer comfort, and at different intervals. See what method works best for you. In the meantime, there are a couple of things to keep in mind. One, a little bit of crying won't harm your baby, and it won't affect baby's attachment to you. Your overall approach of loving care is what bonds the two of you together. Two, if your baby isn't keen on self-soothing at first, hang in there. It can be tough initially, but one thing is for sure: This phase won't last forever. If you establish consistent bedtime practices, your child eventually will be "sleeping like a baby." (Oh, the irony.)

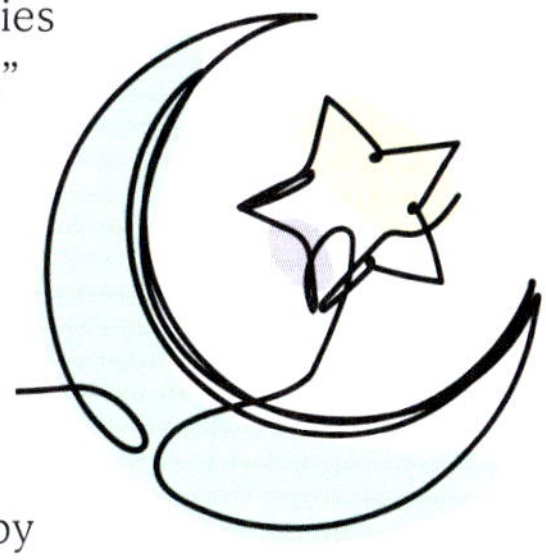

For tips on how to help your little one sleep well, see Chapter 8.

MOVEMENT

Around the fourth or fifth month, the newborn reflex that makes your child look like a baby fencer, called the tonic neck reflex, begins to fade. This clears the way for further development of your baby's gross motor skills — skills that involve the large muscles. At this stage, babies often seem fidgety, but they're really exploring purposeful coordination of their large muscle groups to move around.

At 4 months old, most babies are exercising their arm muscles by pushing up with their elbows or hands when on their tummies. These mini push-ups give your baby a new vantage point and help strengthen muscles necessary for rolling. Some babies may even use this newfound arm power to scoot around in a circle or move around a few inches.

Your baby's fine motor skills — skills that generally involve the hands and fingers, such as the grasp — also are improving.

Head and back control

As the 4-month birthday approaches, baby is achieving good control of the head and neck. Full head control is an important milestone that's essential for other motor skills, including sitting, crawling and walking.

While lying down, your baby is apt to lift the head and shoulders to look straight ahead while resting on the hands and arms (a favorite pose of portrait photographers, and who can blame them? It's downright cute).

When pulled up to a sitting position, about half of 4-month-old babies can keep their heads in line with their bodies. In fact, your baby may even lift the head to try to sit up. By the middle of this month, most babies can keep their heads steady when held in a sitting position.

While sitting, your baby's back muscles are working on keeping the spine straight, reducing the hunched appearance.

Rolling over

On average, this is the month that babies really get rolling. Some may have started rolling even earlier. But don't worry if your baby isn't there yet by age 4 months. You'll probably notice some rolling attempts in the near future. A few babies even skip this milestone altogether.

Rolling from front to back, which requires only a shift in the center of gravity, is generally easier than rolling from back to front. This is why many babies roll from front to back first. Give your baby a little floor space and plenty of tummy time during waking hours to allow for practice.

Rolling from back to front, which tends to occur a little later, requires more complex maneuvering, such as rocking, arching the back, and twisting the legs to flip over. Each baby is different, though. Some roll one way; others roll another. Whether your baby is rolling or not, and which way, isn't as important

LAUGHTER AS A LIFE SKILL

Encouraging laughter and humor in your household can have benefits for both you and your family. The following are some of the science-backed functions of laughter.

Bonding agent

When people laugh together, they bond together over the shared experience and emotion. Laughing with your baby helps you become closer.

Stress reliever

When the house is a mess, your clothes smell like spit-up and dinner is mediocre at best, balancing it all with a good laugh can lessen the stress you might be feeling and unconsciously passing on to your children. Even babies sense when their caregivers are stressed and tend to reflect these emotions. So instead of rushing to load the dishwasher or check your work email, take a few minutes to giggle and laugh with your baby after a long day. It'll make you and your child feel better.

Immune system booster

Evidence suggests that a good belly laugh can increase immune system cells that fight viral illnesses and various cancers.

Resilience maker

If you regularly show your children that you can still laugh despite life's curveballs and momentary imperfections, you're ultimately teaching them about resilience and the ability to withstand distress. This is a skill that will serve them well throughout life.

as whether baby shows interest in moving from one spot to another.

Don't wait until baby has rolled off the couch, bed or changing table to discover your baby's ability to roll. Take precautions not to leave your baby unprotected on elevated surfaces.

Standing

By the end of the fourth month, most babies can, with a little help, bear their own weight on their legs. If held upright, baby likely will push down with the feet. In fact, you may start to feel as if your lap is an infant trampoline as your baby learns to bounce vigorously. Standing and bouncing while well supported won't hurt your baby's legs or hips; in fact, it will give them (and you) a good workout. Just make sure you're not holding a hot cup of coffee or tea at the same time.

If your baby doesn't push off with the feet right away at age 4 months, don't worry. If your child still doesn't do this at 6 months old, you might mention it to your child's medical professional to see if further investigation is necessary.

Reaching and grasping

During this month, your baby likely will be busy waving the arms about, batting at nearby objects and trying to reach them. If you present a rattle or similar toy, baby is likely to grasp it, shake it and maybe even bring it to the mouth.

You may notice that sometimes your baby intentionally looks at and reaches for an object. Other times your baby's hand may touch something and instinctively grab it, and your baby may seem surprised or intrigued by what has unexpectedly appeared in hand. This change from grasping as a reflex to reaching for things voluntarily is gradual.

SENSORY DEVELOPMENT

Throughout these months and until your baby's sixth month, your child will do a lot of exploring by touching, feeling and mouthing whatever comes into grasp. Combined with hearing and seeing, these sensory skills promote the development of your child's motor, mental and social skills. Seeing an object encourages your baby to reach for it. Grasping and touching the object helps your infant become familiar with it. Shaking it and hearing it make noise helps your child learn about cause and effect. Listening to you respond to accomplishments aids in baby's language development and social interaction. You can see how various aspects of development form a complex interplay that contributes to your child's overall growth as a person.

Mouthing

At this stage, your baby's mouth is more sensitive than the fingers to an object's characteristics. Your baby also lacks the dexterity to use the hands to investigate an object, but tongue and lips are perfect! And if your baby can't bring the object of interest to the mouth, baby likely will bring mouth to object by bending down to suck on it.

You can spend a lot of time discouraging your baby from putting things in the mouth. Or you can stockpile a variety of safe toys with interesting textures that will further excite your child's curiosity and encourage oral exploration.

If your baby reaches for something dangerous, your best bet is to quickly remove it from sight and distract your baby with a more appropriate toy. At this age, your baby doesn't understand that something may be harmful and is only interested in its appearance. This is why it's especially important to safeguard your baby's play area and remove any potential hazards.

Hearing

Listening is another way of exploring an environment. By the fourth month, your baby may continue to quiet at the sound of your voice and turn the head toward you as well. Baby also may turn the eyes toward a specific sound, such as a shaking rattle, to find out where the sound is coming from.

Vision

By 4 months old, many babies have improved visual tracking abilities and can watch a brightly colored object as it moves in a slow arc overhead. You also might notice your baby focusing on very small objects, such as a piece of yarn or a crumb, and watching things in the distance with great interest, such as a tree outside the window. Improving hand-eye coordination — being able to both see and reach for an object — further encourages those exploration instincts.

COGNITIVE DEVELOPMENT

Brain activity during these early months is at one of the highest peaks in a person's lifetime. And as your baby becomes more mobile, you can really see curiosity begin to emerge. Everything is an object of interest. Your baby looks, touches, smells and chews to discover and explore whatever's nearby, including the hands, cheeks, legs and other body parts.

Language skills

Since birth, your baby has been building language skills by listening to others and by picking up communication clues from the inflection and tone of their voices. Although words are still a jumble by age 4 months, your baby is familiar with many of the sounds you make and may begin to experiment with making some of these sounds. Warmly encourage these baby "conversations." Talk about your surroundings and what you're doing. Imitate your baby's sounds. These exchanges between you and your baby are key to developing the nerve cell networks that form the foundation of your baby's brain architecture.

Laughter

During this month, your baby probably laughs out loud frequently. Laughter evolves out of cooing and gurgling and usually comes about a month after your baby's first real smile. At first the laugh tends to come in response to something

TOYS AND GAMES

Promote your baby's motor development, excite curiosity, and encourage exploration of the world with some of these activities and toys.

Practice sitting

Once your baby can hold up the head fairly well, try sitting up your infant in a baby seat or against cushions for support. This will improve your baby's sense of balance and help strengthen back muscles. Sit face-to-face and play singing and clapping games together. You can also set up baby against the curve of your own body while you lie on the floor. Don't expect the sitting to last too long at this point, though. After your baby topples over a few times or tires of sitting, switch to a different activity, such as tummy time or reading a book together.

Choose toys that stimulate the senses

Keeping in mind your baby's love for mouthing at this age, choose toys that won't be harmed by a little dampness or chewing. Soft books with textured corners and squeaky pages are both fun and practical. Other ideas include a bumpy teething ring, a ring of big plastic keys, measuring cups or soft blocks. Also, look for toys or everyday objects that your baby can practice holding on to, shaking and manipulating. Make sure the toys you choose have no small parts that can come off and pose a choking hazard to your baby.

Play mimicking games

Starting around this age, your baby studies the sounds you make and tries to copy them. Take the time to listen to your baby's vocalizations, then try to imitate those sounds. Talk back to your baby, speaking slowly and clearly, and allow baby time to try to make the same sounds. If you speak a second language, use it with your child. Mimic facial expressions and laughter, too. This encourages your baby's language skills and social interactions.

Enjoy bath time

As it becomes easier for babies to sit when supported, parents often turn bath time into playtime. The feeling of being weightless in the warm water and the freedom from restrictive diapers and clothing all make for a great sensory experience. However, remember that bubble bath and soap can be irritating to a baby's eyes, skin and genitals. And keep a close eye and good grip on your baby. The water makes your wriggly, active baby extra slippery. Never leave your baby alone in a tub.

— a laugh from you, a funny face from an older sibling. Your baby may also laugh to get your attention or just for the experience of making noise. In the coming months, though, you'll notice the beginnings of a sense of humor. For example, something out of the ordinary may strike your baby's funny bone.

SOCIAL DEVELOPMENT

During the fourth month, your baby likely is starting to show clear signs of recognizing you and other members of your family. If you have other children, they may be your baby's favorite playtime friends. Children can easily make a baby smile and laugh.

For siblings, this is a "honeymoon" time. The baby is old enough to thrill an older brother or sister with smiles and giggles but still too young to be "trouble," getting into toys and interrupting play.

At this age, your baby has yet to develop stranger anxiety and is likely to enjoy meeting new people, smiling, wriggling and laughing with anyone who will respond. This is a comfortable time for most parents. The baby is big enough that you're not overly concerned about safe handling, and you know the baby is comfortable with someone else. At this age, it's easy to share the fun of your baby with others.

4TH MONTH MILESTONES

During the fourth month, your baby is busy:

- Pushing up on elbows and hands to look around when lying on belly
- Sitting supported with head steady
- Practicing moves that enable rolling over
- Bearing weight on legs, bouncing with arms supported
- Grasping and shaking toys, practicing letting go
- Bringing hands to mouth, exploring items with mouth
- Studying small items
- Gazing at things in the distance
- Looking for the source of a sound
- Becoming more communicative with body language and vocalizations
- Laughing
- Imitating language sounds
- Engaging in back-and-forth "conversations" with you
- Enjoying playing with others, capturing attention

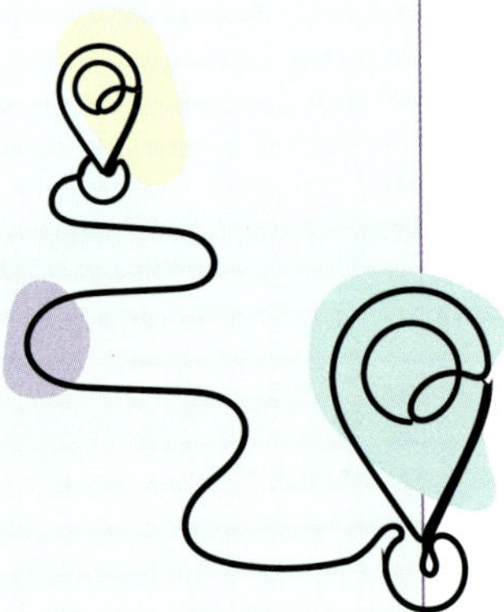

Distractions

As your baby nears 4 months old, feeding times become less frequent, and baby's attention is drawn to other people and activities during feeding. Your baby may move around or stop feeding to play or "talk" to you. This distraction isn't a sign that your baby is rejecting breastfeeding or is bored with formula. As baby discovers and explores the world, distraction is typical. Your baby may discover that feeding time can be more than a time to eat; it's also a time to socialize, experiment and assert some independence. As much as you want your child to learn through exploration and interaction, it can be frustrating to feed a distracted baby. You might try a quiet, uninterrupted feeding place. Early morning feedings — when your baby is still sleepy and the room is dark — may be the best feeding of the day.

CHAPTER 23

Month 5

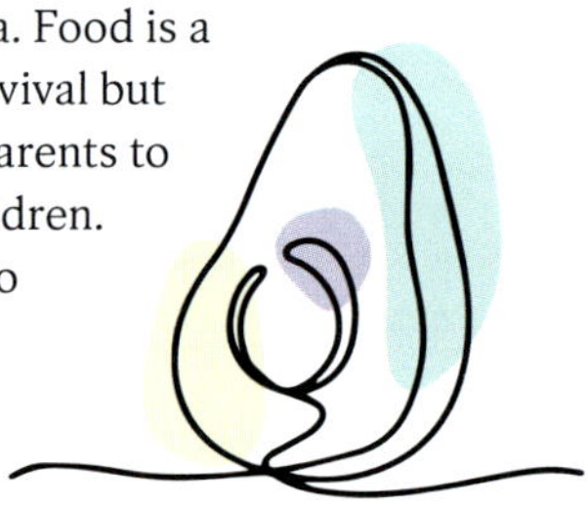

Many parents eagerly look forward to this month because they can finally start introducing baby to foods other than breast milk or formula. Food is a big part of human culture, and it plays a role not only in survival but also in societal traditions and pastimes. So it's natural for parents to want to share the joy of eating favorite foods with their children. When baby gets to join the others at the dining table it's also another step toward becoming part of the family.

As much as you may be excited to embark on culinary adventures with your baby, keep in mind your baby's stage of growth and development. In this chapter you'll read about signs that show that your baby is ready for solid foods, as well as tips on a successful introduction. In Chapter 4 you'll find a more in-depth discussion of infant nutrition and when to introduce solid foods.

During the fifth month, your baby gains increasing control over the body, enthusiastically exploring each newfound function. Baby also is continuing to discover new emotions, ranging from happy to grumpy, and solidly establishing a place in the family.

GROWTH AND APPEARANCE

Between 4 and 5 months old, your baby's growth rate is likely to match last month's. This rate is a little slower than the first three months, but not by much. Most babies gain anywhere from just shy of 1 pound to 1½ pounds or more. Length and head circumference both increase by about ½ inch during this month.

Introducing solid foods

Between this month and next, your baby will begin to develop the coordination to move solid food from the front of the mouth to the back for swallowing. At the same time, your baby's head control will improve, and baby will learn to sit with support — essential skills for eating solid foods.

Breast milk or formula is enough to meet your little tyke's needs in the first four to six months. But eventually additional nutrition is needed for your baby to continue to thrive. After 6 months of age, for example, breast milk alone generally isn't enough to give your baby the necessary energy, protein, iron, zinc and other nutrients.

Is your baby ready?

Sometime between ages 4 and 6 months, most babies are ready to begin eating solid foods as a complement to breastfeeding or formula-feeding. But age should not be the only determining factor. You want to make sure your child is both physically and socially ready. And you shouldn't feel pressured to begin solids. The American Academy of Pediatrics recommends that parents wait until a child is 6 months old to introduce solids, if possible. If you're not sure whether your baby is ready for solids, ask yourself these questions:

- Can your baby hold their head in a steady upright position?
- Can your baby sit well with support?
- Is your baby interested in what you're eating, perhaps eyeing your breakfast toast or opening the mouth if you offer a spoon?

If you answer yes to these questions and you have the OK from your child's medical professional or dietitian, you can begin supplementing your baby's liquid diet. Read more about what to serve when and which foods to avoid in Chapter 4.

Tips for a successful meal

Once your baby starts eating foods besides breast milk or formula, feedings are likely to become a lot more interactive and, most probably, messier! But that's OK. It's all part of the process of exploring new things. Here are some suggestions for when your little one is ready to try solids.

Pick a happy time For your first try, choose a time when your baby is most likely to be open to adventure, such as when baby is alert, dry, comfortable and not starving. If your baby's very hungry, you might want to start off with a little breast milk or formula first and then switch to solids.

Set your expectations Remind yourself that the goal of these first solids is to introduce your baby to the experience of food, rather than to meet your child's nutritional needs. In fact, it will likely be several weeks before the amount of food that actually gets into your baby's belly is contributing to overall nutritional requirements. For a while, baby will still need the same amount of formula or breast milk as the primary source of energy.

Sit up Try feeding your baby propped up in your lap or in a high chair.

Try a spoon The American Academy of Pediatrics recommends encouraging your baby to use a spoon or fingers to self-feed. A small espresso spoon or a silicone-coated baby spoon usually works well. Eating off a spoon helps your baby learn to swallow without sucking, and allows your baby to learn the process of eating in the same way the rest of the family eats. Avoid giving your child cereal in a bottle, which may encourage excessive calorie intake.

Start small For your baby's first meal, start out with just a couple of spoonfuls of food, such as pureed meat or vegetables or infant cereal, in a bowl. Thin the food with breast milk or formula until it's the consistency of heavy cream, to help ease the transition from bottle to spoon. Over the next few meals, you can gradually make the consistency thicker as your baby gets used to swallowing solid foods.

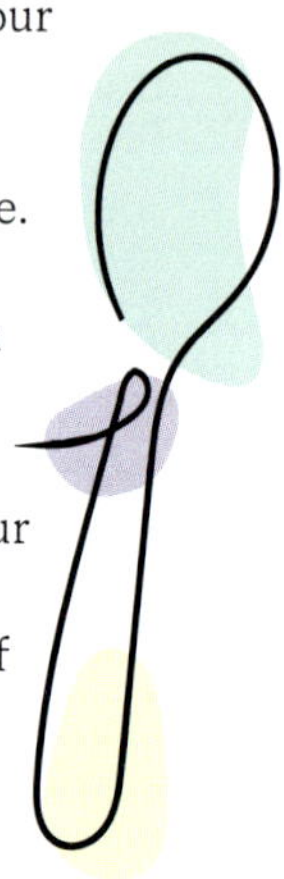

Be patient Although some babies seem thrilled with their first bowl of "big-kid" food, others may not be convinced of its joys the first time around. If your baby flat-out refuses the first feeding, don't give up hope. Clear the food away and try again a few days later. Focus on enjoying mealtime rather than getting your baby to eat solid foods by a certain date.

The scoop on poop

Once you start feeding your baby solid foods, you'll likely notice a difference in the texture, color and smell of your baby's stools. Solid foods make for more solid stools. Foods such as peas, blueberries and beets can make noticeable differences in the color of stool as well. Last but not least, get ready for stinky stools. The added sugars and fats in solid foods can lead to a stronger odor. If you start to notice that your baby's stools become hard or difficult to pass, consider adding more fruits like prunes or pears to your baby's diet.

MOVEMENT

Between 4 and 5 months old, most babies achieve the first big milestone — good head control. By the end of this month, your baby is likely to be able to hold up the head steadily while sitting. Baby also will learn to turn the head from side to side, making it easier to track moving objects and identify different sounds and voices.

Once your baby has full head control, baby has the skills necessary to move on to sitting. And just in time, too. As the months go by, baby may become less satisfied with lying face-up or facedown and will probably want to spend more time upright. During this month and next, your baby is working toward sitting up without help. Tummy time on the floor and lifting the head and chest to see toys are good exercises to help your baby strengthen neck muscles and develop the head control necessary for sitting up.

Rolling over

At this point, most babies are making progress in their attempts to roll over, too. By the end of this month, some babies can even roll both ways without help. Once babies learn to roll from front to back and back to front again, they may start out sleeping on their backs, just as you laid them down, but then flip over in the middle of the night. If this happens, don't feel compelled to flip baby back again. The risk of SIDS begins to decrease once your baby gains head and neck control and is able to roll over.

Reaching and grasping

During the fifth month, you may notice your baby start working for a toy or other object. At first, this may mean reaching for a toy without being able to grasp it on the first try. At 4 months of age, your baby still manipulates objects by batting at them. But eventually baby may try to pick up a larger object by pressing it with the palm of the hand and curling the fingers around the object. When your baby does get hold of a toy, baby may grasp it with both hands and have fun shaking it around. Dangling toys are still a source of entertainment at this age and help your child further develop hand-eye coordination.

Bouncing

Your 4-month-old most likely gets great joy out of being upright and "standing" on your lap, and perhaps bouncing. All the bouncing your baby does is a part of typical development and isn't harmful to your baby's hips, legs or feet. By about 5 months, you will notice that your baby can probably bear full body weight on the legs. Standing alone and walking are still a long way off, but you can see how the small stages of development are preparing your baby for greater mobility.

Encouraging physical activity

Take a look around your local baby supply store and you'll see an amazing range of infant equipment — swings, playpens, infant seats, stationary activity centers,

SPOT CHECK: WHAT'S GOING ON THIS MONTH

Here's a snapshot of what your baby's basic care looks like in the fifth month.

Eating

Breast milk or formula still plays the central role in your little one's nutrition, although some parents begin to introduce solid foods during this month. Be sure your baby is developmentally ready for solid foods before starting them, such as being able to swallow, hold the head steady, and sit with support.

Sleeping

Your baby is more likely to sleep six to eight hours at night with no interruption. Some babies still wake up once or twice during the night for a feeding. Total sleep may add up to between 14 and 15 hours in a 24-hour period, including a couple of daytime naps, usually one in the morning and one in the afternoon. Some babies may need a third nap late in the afternoon.

walkers, baby gyms, bouncy chairs. And with your baby learning so many new skills, it's tempting to try to physically help baby along with the latest gadget. Quite a lot of infant equipment is marketed with the idea of helping your baby reach a new milestone, such as sitting or walking.

Truth? What infants need more than anything to develop their motor skills is freedom of movement in a safe space. They need to explore their surroundings and to practice their budding skills under the watchful eye of a nearby caregiver. Warm interaction with a supportive caregiver during playtime also is important.

Does that mean you have to be constantly down on the floor with baby? Not always. Certain pieces of baby gear can definitely come in handy, such as a stationary activity center where your baby can sit and bounce or play with attached toys, or a molded seat that helps your baby sit up. Swings and playpens also can be essential at times. But keep in mind that these items are mostly for your convenience, allowing time for you to move about unrestricted — to do some chores, say, or eat breakfast. Try to limit the amount of time your child spends in these devices, as extended movement restriction in turn may limit

GETTING KIDS TO LIKE FRUITS AND VEGETABLES

A common battle parents face as their kids grow is getting them to eat their fruits and vegetables. Research indicates that starting early is key.

Since a number of food flavors are transmitted via amniotic fluid or breast milk to a baby, what the birthing person eats affects the baby's early experiences with flavor. Some evidence suggests that the more often a baby experiences a particular flavor — such as carrots, for example — during pregnancy or breastfeeding, the more accepting the baby is likely to be of that taste when starting solid foods. And because breastfeeding offers a child a greater variety of flavor experiences due to a birthing person's varying diet, breastfed infants seem less picky and more willing to try new foods.

Another finding suggests that flavor learning after the introduction of solid foods is based on repeated exposure to new foods. One study, for example, found that with repeated offerings of green beans, expressions of surprise or distaste were fewer, and willingness to eat the vegetables was greater. This is especially true if the green beans were followed by a sweet-tasting fruit.

This type of research is ongoing, but in the meantime, it doesn't hurt to eat well yourself and keep setting the good stuff out there. Chances are good that eventually your kids will enjoy it for themselves. Starting early does actually help — infants are more likely to accept fruits and veggies when they are included with first foods. Those same foods may then get rejected in the toddler years. But kids are more likely to come back later to foods they ate as infants. For example, your broccoli-loving baby is more likely to eat broccoli as an older child, compared with kids who didn't eat it as infants.

your child. Be sure to supervise older siblings around these devices, too, as they may become overenthusiastic in "helping" the baby use them, potentially causing harm (think "Look how fast Sammy can go in the swing!").

The American Academy of Pediatrics (AAP) advises specifically against using mobile walkers. These devices generally have a cloth seat set in a frame with wheels that allow the baby to move around the room even though baby might not be able to crawl or walk yet. A number of studies have shown that these devices can make a baby more prone to injury, such as falling down steps or reaching for dangerous objects. Even under supervision, the AAP contends, walkers are simply too fast for a parent to reach before an accident happens. Other experts have cautioned against the use of door jumpers — seats that hang from a door frame — as well. If you need a place for your baby to safely play for a few minutes, consider a stationary activity center or playpen instead. You also can use a high chair, once your baby is able to sit in it safely.

Keep in mind that if your baby has a developmental disability, a medical professional may recommend certain pieces of equipment to help baby sit with support or move with help.

SENSORY DEVELOPMENT

During this month, mouthing becomes an even more important avenue of exploration for your young child. Keep offering safe toys and everyday objects to practice the art of picking things up and bringing them to the mouth. This helps your baby develop sensory and motor skills. At the same time, keep a sharp eye out for anything that might be a choking or poison hazard for your baby.

Vision

Earlier, your baby was learning to distinguish between bold colors. Improved visual awareness during this month and the next helps your baby discern more subtle shades of color, such as soft pastels, although bold colors may still be favorites. Improved visual tracking and coordination also help your baby become better at reaching and grabbing larger objects and toys. Baby definitely is noticing small objects, but doesn't yet have the dexterity to grab them.

Babies at this age are also starting to discriminate between the different emotions they see in others — such as joy, fear or sadness — and to make similar responses.

Hearing

Between 4 and 5 months, about half of all babies turn their heads toward a voice. Most babies at this age will turn toward a rattling sound to investigate its source. At this age, babies also learn to distinguish emotions by tone of voice.

If by this month your baby doesn't respond to sounds, talk to a medical professional. Although newborns are generally checked right after birth for hearing loss, your observations at home are key to identifying the need for further testing.

COGNITIVE DEVELOPMENT

As the brain develops, and more and more connections are made between brain nerve cells, your baby's memory of faces, sounds, places and event patterns increases. Although your baby has been absorbing information about the surrounding world since birth, baby has had only limited ability to respond. But as motor skills increase, you can watch your infant apply this knowledge.

This is evident in the way your baby reacts to seeing you or to certain daily routines, such as a feeding or a bath. If you sit in your favorite chair for breastfeeding or a bottle, you may notice that your baby quickly settles in with you and may make noises or kick in anticipation of what's coming. And if for some reason what's expected isn't forthcoming, you may hear a squawk or two of displeasure.

Learning how things work

At the same time, your baby's curiosity and attention span are increasing. This allows baby to spend more time examining things and observing how things work. This natural curiosity also drives your baby to start to work for objects that are out of reach. Even if baby can't quite get to a toy yet, you can see the focus and concentration in your child's eyes.

During this month, your baby also is learning more about cause and effect. When baby cries, you come. When baby bangs a toy on the table, it makes noise. When baby giggles, siblings giggle, too.

Like a scientist, your baby may test different actions over and over to see if they always get the same effect. And, like a successful scientist, your baby will be proud every time the response is the one expected. You'll appreciate your baby's smiles and squeals of accomplishment and self-confidence.

Language skills

Your 5-month-old may have already started imitating some of the speech sounds you make, even though it will be a few more months before baby understands how these sounds work together to communicate. During this month and the next, your baby is likely to pick up on a single sound — such as "ah" or "oh"— and repeat it over and over. Then, a few days later, baby will discover a new sound and practice it repeatedly. Babies seem to enjoy playing with a new sound as much as they delight in playing with a favorite toy. Pretty soon your baby will be babbling away at you, excited to create sounds.

Continue talking to your baby every chance you get. Regular face-to-face interaction with your baby is a key building block for mental, emotional and social development. When you respond positively to your baby's bids for interaction, you're showing how relationships work and solidifying the secure attachment your baby has to you.

SOCIAL DEVELOPMENT

At this age, your baby is quickly figuring out how to express a variety of emotions through facial expression, vocalizations and body language. For example, baby now uses laughter to express happiness and excitement. At the same time, your baby may start to show dislikes, making a face or turning away from things. You may notice this latter type of reaction more as you introduce new foods to your child or start to set limits on your child's actions for safety's sake.

TOYS AND GAMES

At this young age, babies are interested in very simple objects and toys. They also don't need a heap of toys to stay busy. In fact, too many toys or too much activity can overwhelm your baby and lead to tears. Limit toys to just a few at a time. That way your baby can take the time to study each one and see what it can do. Following are some of the toys and games your baby may enjoy during this month.

Toys that make noise

By now, your baby is starting to play purposefully with rattles and toys that squeak or make noise. Offer toys that make noise to enhance the discovery of cause and effect as baby bangs and rattles about. Infants also seem to get great joy from pressing buttons that make things happen, such as on a pop-up toy or a baby phone.

Music to bounce, sway or swing to

Music can help express emotions and thoughts when the words aren't quite there yet. Most babies love music and will move along to a rhythm they find catchy. Make a playlist of your favorite kid-friendly (but not necessarily kiddy) songs, and play them for your baby. Better yet, pick your baby up and sing and dance around the room together in accompaniment to the music.

The company of a mirror

Place an unbreakable mirror in front of your baby and watch as your baby and "the other baby" get acquainted. At this age, your baby probably won't know that it's a reflection but may have fun watching.

Stuff to reach for

While your baby is lying prone on the floor or sitting upright, place a couple of bright toys or objects just out of reach. This will encourage your child to practice reaching skills and improve hand-eye coordination.

Growing attachment

By the fifth month, your baby is establishing a solid place in the family structure and clearly knows who loved ones are. Your baby feels comfortable with the family routine and indeed expects it. Spending time with you is still baby's favorite activity. In fact, this closer sense of attachment to you and other family members may lead your baby to feel upset and display unhappiness when you stop playing a game or leave the room. Baby may even need a little extra reassurance that you're still available — perhaps by talking or singing a song — and will return as soon as possible.

This narrowing focus of attachment goes hand in hand with a gradual realization that some people are strangers. Your baby likely still has an accepting, welcoming response to unfamiliar people. But in the months ahead, you'll notice that your baby is becoming increasingly picky about company.

Emerging personality

As your baby matures, personality traits will rapidly become more apparent. Is your baby bouncy and full of energy? Or perhaps more quiet and cautious? Is your baby easily frustrated when a goal can't be obtained? Or is your infant persistent to the point where you might call it stubbornness? Does your baby adjust easily to new environments, or take a while to warm up?

Everyone is born with certain behavioral characteristics that form a basic temperament. Depending on the situation, a temperamental trait can be

5TH MONTH MILESTONES

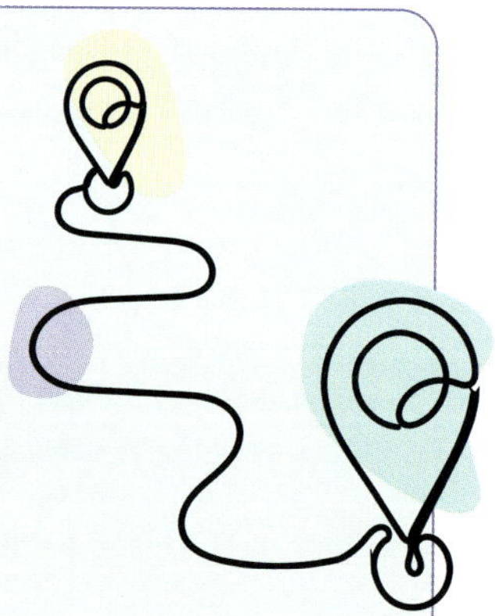

During the fifth month, your baby is busy:

- Perfecting mini push-ups while lying on belly
- Learning to sit, balanced by hands on floor in front (tripod style)
- Bearing weight on legs
- Rolling over from front to back, maybe even back to front
- Working to get to a toy
- Grasping with both hands
- Exploring with mouth
- Studying small objects
- Locating sounds and voices by turning head
- Imitating speech sounds
- Repeating single sounds
- Laughing, squealing
- Expressing dislikes, making faces
- Enjoying playing with others, crying when playing stops

pleasing or frustrating to you as a parent. For example, the same high energy that makes your baby so fun to play with can also make for difficult diaper changes or wriggly feedings!

Generally, your baby's natural traits can't be changed — it would be like trying to change your baby's personality. But by knowing your baby's usual behaviors and baby's temperament, you can better appreciate your infant and adjust your parenting style to bring out baby's best. How you interact with your baby now can set the stage for your relationship throughout childhood, adolescence and even adulthood. You can read more about temperament in Chapter 10.

CHAPTER 24

Month 6

As you approach your baby's half-year mark, think about how far you've both come. By now, that little person in the nursery is no longer a baby but a world-class explorer. And you have become an ever more confident parent, familiar with the rhythms of baby care and more secure in your ability to meet upcoming challenges.

During this month, your baby is becoming more adept with the hands and may even start to sit unsupported by the end of the month. Each aspect of your baby's motor and sensory development gives your baby new tools to explore the world and expand mental and social development. This is a fun time as your baby babbles and laughs, excited to be part of the family.

GROWTH AND APPEARANCE

By the time the sixth month rolls around, many babies have doubled their birth weight. Your baby's growth rate this month is likely to be similar to last month's — weight gain of 1 to 1½ pounds or more and an increase in length and head circumference of about ½ inch. But don't be surprised if the growth rate starts to slow down in a few weeks. Most babies grow a little more slowly during months 7 through 12 than they did in the first six months.

Teeth!

Drooling, crankiness and tears — could it be baby teeth coming in? Although timing varies widely, many babies begin teething by about age 6 months. The two bottom front teeth (lower central incisors) are usually the first to appear, followed by the two top front teeth (upper central incisors). Teething can occur at a wide variety of ages, however. Some babies do not get teeth until after they are a year old.

Classic symptoms of teething often include:

- Drooling, which may begin about two months before the first tooth appears
- Irritability or crankiness
- Swollen gums
- Chewing on solid objects

Many parents suspect that teething causes fever and diarrhea, but researchers say this isn't true. Teething may cause symptoms in the mouth and gums, but it doesn't cause problems elsewhere in the body. If your baby develops a fever or has other symptoms of illness, contact your child's medical professional. Otherwise, teething can usually be handled at home.

If your teething baby seems uncomfortable, consider these simple tips.

Rub your baby's gums Use a clean finger, moistened gauze pad or damp washcloth to massage your baby's gums. The pressure can ease baby's discomfort.

Offer a teething ring Try one made of firm rubber. The liquid-filled variety may break under the pressure of your baby's chewing.

Keep it cool A cold washcloth or chilled teething ring can be soothing. Don't give your baby a frozen teething ring, however. Contact with extreme cold may hurt, doing your baby more harm than good. If your baby's eating solid foods, offer cold items such as applesauce or yogurt.

Dry the drool Excessive drooling is part of the teething process. Saliva is used in the digestion of food. So it makes sense for the body to produce more saliva at the time when infants typically begin to eat solid foods. To prevent skin irritation, keep a clean cloth handy to dry your baby's chin.

SPOT CHECK: WHAT'S GOING ON THIS MONTH

Here's a snapshot of what your baby's basic care looks like in the sixth month.

Eating

Breast milk or formula still plays the central role in baby's nutrition, although most parents will begin to introduce solid foods by the end of this month. Feed your baby in a seated position, and avoid hard, chewy or round pieces of food that could potentially block your baby's airway.

Sleeping

Your baby is more likely to sleep six to eight hours at night without interruption. Some babies still wake up once or twice during the night for a feeding. Total sleep may add up to between 14 and 15 hours in a 24-hour period, including a couple of daytime naps, usually one in the morning and one in the afternoon. Some babies may need a third nap late in the afternoon.

Try an over-the-counter remedy If teething is making your baby especially cranky, acetaminophen (Tylenol, others) may help. Ibuprofen (Advil, Motrin, others) also can help but should not be used until your child is 6 months or older. Don't give your baby products that contain aspirin, however, and be cautious about teething medications that can be rubbed directly on a baby's gums. The medication may be washed away by your baby's saliva before it has the chance to do any good — and using too much of the medication may numb your baby's throat. This may interfere with baby's gag reflex.

Caring for new teeth

Now is a great time to start running a clean, damp washcloth over your baby's gums every day. The washcloth can keep bacteria from building up in your baby's mouth. When your baby's first teeth appear, switch to a small soft-bristled toothbrush. Use a small smear of toothpaste, about the size of a grain of rice. If you have well water or if you use bottled water in your home, your baby may not be getting the fluoride needed for healthy tooth development. Discuss this issue with your child's medical professional.

It's also time to think about regular dental checkups. The American Dental Association and the American Academy of Pediatric Dentistry recommend visiting the dentist after the first tooth erupts. All children should start regular dentist visits by age 3. Your baby's teeth and gums also will be examined at well-baby checkups. Regular childhood dental care helps set the stage for a lifetime of healthy teeth and gums.

MOVEMENT

By 5 or 6 months old, most babies have achieved pretty good head control and are rolling over both ways. By now they may be ready to learn to sit without help. By 7 months or so, most babies have learned to sit independently, but some may wait until 9 months to do so. This is within the typical range.

At the same time, baby's hand control skills are rapidly improving, allowing your child even more flexibility in exploring surroundings, and even other parts of the body.

Tripod sitting

Your baby's first attempts at sitting will probably be very entertaining. At first, baby will sit hunched over, balancing on arms extended to the front. Experts sometimes call this the "tripod sitting" stage. Almost anything will topple a baby in this position — leaning a little to one side, a distraction that makes the baby look in another direction or any attempt to shift weight.

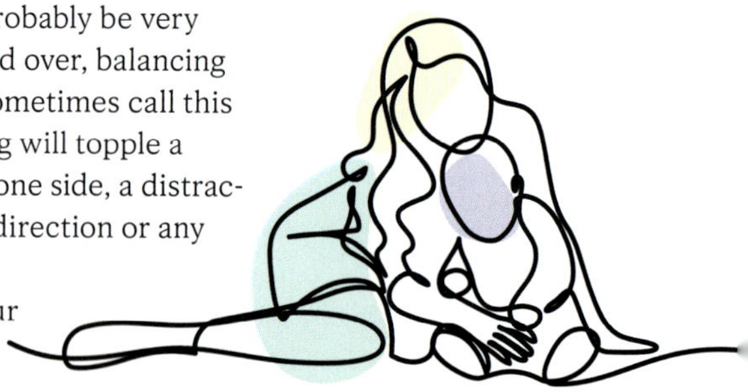

This hunched-over sitting takes all your baby's energy. Baby probably can't do much else but hold up their head without falling over. In a few weeks, though, your baby's strength and balance will improve with practice, and baby will be able to sit upright.

Toes, toes, toes!

If it hasn't happened yet, baby likely will discover the toes this month. When fingers don't seem so novel anymore, baby may catch sight of those wiggly things at the end of the feet and bring them up for investigation.

Picking up and letting go

By age 5 or 6 months, your baby can reach for a desired object using a rake-like motion and grasp it. After learning to grab a toy, your baby will practice moving things from hand to mouth, using both touching and tasting to explore the toy. You may even see your baby repeat the hand to mouth to hand movement, taking the object out of the mouth with alternating hands. By 6 months, your baby may learn to move something directly from one hand to the other.

Your baby will soon discover that letting go of something is as much fun as picking it up. At first, letting go is almost accidental. As soon as your baby learns to hold something, baby will also drop it. But over the next few months, your baby will begin to let go more purposefully. By the end of year one, your baby will develop other ways of getting rid of unwanted objects, such as throwing them or pressing them down on a surface.

At this age, babies still use their whole hands to pick things up. When babies are relaxed, their hands are open; by now, they've outgrown the closed-fist pose of younger babies. You can see the slow progression from that tight-fisted infant to a more mobile and coordinated baby. Right now your baby is just beginning to use hands for small tasks. And it's hard work! Watching your baby, you can probably see the amount of effort that goes into this kind of "play." When your

A LEFTY OR A RIGHTY?

At this age, it's too early to tell whether your baby is left-handed or right-handed. For now, babies may seem to favor one hand for a while, then switch and use the other hand more often. A 1-year-old may use both hands equally. By 18 months to 2 years, toddlers start to show a preference for which hand they use. Still, true handedness isn't usually determined until a child is about 3 years old.

Handedness develops naturally, although scientists still aren't sure what role genes play in it. Children with left-handed parents have an increased chance of being left-handed, but the inheritance pattern isn't clear-cut.

If you do notice during infancy that your child favors one hand over the other, let your medical professional know. Sometimes further investigation is necessary to make sure that both hands do, in fact, work equally well.

baby reaches for an object, the other hand may mirror the movement of the reaching hand. Both hands may close as one hand reaches for and grasps a toy.

SENSORY DEVELOPMENT

Although your baby's senses will continue to mature throughout early childhood, they're now almost as fully developed as those of an adult. Your baby sees and hears the world almost as clearly as you do, and this ability allows the two of you to understand and share many of the same experiences.

Vision

By 6 months of age, your baby has more clearly focused vision and can probably track the course of a falling toy or other object quite smoothly. Ongoing development of your baby's visual system allows for greater depth perception. And now, with the ability to sit upright, your baby can gaze across at you and at other things, rather than just look up. Both of these skills — increased depth perception and the ability to look across — come in handy, such as when baby is learning to eat solid foods and you're aiming a spoon full of cereal at the mouth.

TOYS AND GAMES

Now that sitting upright is more comfortable, your baby has a whole new position from which to watch, play and interact with the world. And as the sensory and motor skills continue to develop, baby will become much more interested in anything that provides opportunities for adventure and discovery.

Colorful books and magazines

Your baby can now focus on an entire pattern and distinguish a range of colors. Reading colorful board books together becomes especially fun at this age. Simple texts allow you to repeat sounds that your baby can try to repeat. Don't be offended if baby decides to take over, though, turning the pages or flipping back to the cover every time you try to read the next page. At this age, the main idea isn't to understand the story line but to make sounds, look at pictures and chew on the covers. Old magazines that you don't mind being torn up can also be fun to look at; just make sure baby doesn't eat the pages.

Short trips

Once your baby is able to sit up in a stroller, walks around the neighborhood or the park take on a whole new dimension. Now your baby can see most of the things you see and will enjoy the sight of a passing dog or a squirrel hopping to the

During this month, your baby also is able to take in more complex visual images and study them. You might notice this increased visual curiosity when your baby picks up a toy and examines it, although eventually it's likely to end up in the mouth for a truly thorough examination. Looking at picture books together is great fun at this age. Sturdy board books can provide visual interest as well as something for your baby to practice manipulating with the hands.

Hearing

By the end of this month, most babies respond readily to sound and turn their heads quickly toward the direction of a voice or other noise. With improving memory and increasing exposure, they may even be able to distinguish between voices.

Touch

In addition to exploring the environment, your baby's body is a new source of discovery. By touching the cheeks, nose, toes and genitals, your baby is becoming familiar with the contours and shapes of the body. Baby also continues to explore textures and shapes. Offer new surfaces and objects for your baby to touch, such as a branch or a smooth rock. Be aware that most objects will quickly go to your baby's mouth, so be sure to supervise baby's tactile exploration.

nearest tree. With a turn of the head, your baby can locate different sounds, too, such as the honk of a goose or the sounds of children playing. If it's nice out, place your baby on a patch of grass and let baby feel the different textures. Trips to the zoo or your local library also become more entertaining at this age, but don't expect them to last too long. It's probably best to keep them to under an hour or two to match your baby's limited energy and short attention span.

Bouncy lap games

Good head control also allows for slightly more physical games. Almost all babies seem to love bouncing around on a grown-up's lap. Have your baby sit on your lap facing you, hold the hands, and bounce baby gently on your knees while singing a song. If you don't know any kid songs, ask your parents or grandparents. They'll probably remember some, and it will be fun to hear what they sang to you at one point. Or try looking up nursery songs and rhymes.

Reach!

Once baby can raise the body up on straight arms while lying belly down on the floor, you can start encouraging baby to reach out with one arm for a toy just ahead. Eventually, your baby will lean on one arm and reach for toys with the other. This act of reaching forward is generally the first step toward crawling. Rolling balls or other toys also provide an incentive for chasing.

PLAYING WITH SIBLINGS

An older sibling can get a lot of enjoyment out of a 5- to 6-month-old baby. By 6 months, the baby has moved beyond face-to-face interaction and may even play with toys offered by an older child. Your baby probably can get a sibling to pick up dropped toys or play passing games.

At this age, it's important that your baby have personal toys separate from an older sibling's toys. Illnesses can be easily spread from one child to another through shared toys. Keep the baby's toys clean. Plastic toys should be washed often, and fuzzy toys that aren't as easily washed should be reserved just for the baby's play.

Babies love older kids mostly because they're fun to watch. Although babies will play some turn-taking games, they delight in being an audience and responding to what older children do. For safety reasons, always supervise playtime between your baby and an older child.

COGNITIVE DEVELOPMENT

Between 5 and 6 months, your baby is working out some of the first inklings of an identity — what it feels like to be a separate person with individual powers of action and reaction. In parallel with these discoveries, your baby is uncovering the possibilities that exist for interaction with others.

As the memory expands, your baby can roughly start to catalog experiences — the kitchen floor is hard, a beard is prickly, this toy is fun to gum, the music comes from there, and so forth.

Me, myself and I

Combining sensory, motor and mental skills, your baby begins to realize that moving certain muscles always produces physical sensations that correspond with specific visual results. For example, baby's effort to kick the legs is always accompanied by the sight of these legs moving.

Sensations associated with self are easier to make with regularity than sensations associated with others. Every time your baby kicks, the legs move. But every time your baby cries, you may or may not appear immediately.

Playing becomes serious business

At the same time, playing rises to a new level. Toys that stimulate the senses and simple games, such as peekaboo or mimicking games, become the tools and experiments of your small adventurer. Even the process of getting your attention requires a certain amount of strategy and can become a game for baby.

Again, you don't need expensive toys to stimulate your child's mind and senses. Common household items with different shapes and textures — such as cardboard boxes, egg cartons, lids, paper towel rolls, spoons, tea towels and nesting bowls — offer plenty of opportunities for sensory exploration and discovery. Homemade noisemakers (think tightly capped containers filled with rice) are fun to shake and prod, and a plastic lid filled with water placed on the high chair tray is sure to intrigue.

Peekaboo is still fairly magical because your 5- to 6-month-old hasn't quite grasped the concept that you're still there behind the blanket even though you can't be seen. This memory of things not immediately visible is called object permanence. Your little one may, however, look for a dropped toy but give up quickly if it's not in sight.

Mimicking games become more important as your baby strives to match your facial expressions and imitate the sounds and cadences of your voice.

Babbling

Babbling usually begins with babies trying out vowel sounds, something you may have already noticed your baby doing. A few weeks later, baby may start to add in consonant sounds. By 6 months, about half of all babies babble by repeating one syllable over and over, such as "mah" or "bah." Some babies may even have started adding more than one syllable to their babbling. You may hear your baby cheerfully practice one kind of sound, then move on to something else and not repeat the first sound for several days.

6TH MONTH MILESTONES

During the sixth month, your baby is busy:

- Maintaining good head control
- Rolling both ways
- Working toward sitting independently
- Raking small objects toward self
- Picking up toys with both hands
- Bringing toys to mouth
- Exploring with the mouth
- Learning to self-feed
- Perhaps transferring an object from one hand to the other
- Repeating single syllables, maybe even combining sounds
- Giggling, laughing
- Exploring their own body
- Differentiating between self and others
- Enjoying simple games
- Looking briefly for dropped toy
- Mimicking and sharing your emotions

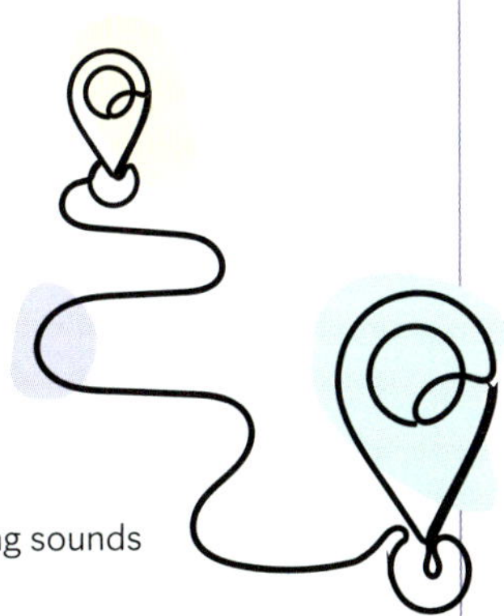

Much of your baby's "talking" may seem more like sound effects than babbling. Squeals, sliding pitches and bubbling sounds are all common for babies at this age. Giggles and laughter are favorite sounds for both babies and parents.

SOCIAL DEVELOPMENT

This is a fun age for socializing and playing with your baby. Adults have the remarkable ability to show almost any emotion through facial expressions, and babies love to watch and try to imitate these expressions. Sharing emotional states with someone else is vital for social development and is one of the basic foundations for communication.

Don't be discouraged if playing with your baby seems uncomfortable at first. Remember, it's been a few years since you spent your evenings on the floor with rattles and a box of blocks. Watch the "expert," observing which toys your baby is drawn to and what baby does with them. Then join in. Soon you'll know what games and toys make playtime fun for your baby. Your baby will give you the kind of immediate response — giggles, turn-taking, smiles — that make playtime rewarding for both of you.

Your baby will let you know if playtime is too intense or has gone on too long. Watch for clues that baby is overstimulated, such as turning away or becoming grouchy or tense.

Don't be surprised if you feel your baby needs even more attention now than in the newborn days. Your baby wants and needs stimulation, especially from you. Left alone in a playpen, crib or infant seat, your baby likely will become bored. But life doesn't have to be all games and playtime. You can meet many of those social needs by including baby in your daily tasks or just by positioning baby to watch you at work.

CHAPTER 25

Month 7

The next few months are a time of growing independence for your little one. This can be both exhilarating and frightening for an infant. You may find your baby boldly venturing into new things but afraid to be too far away from the security of what's known — you. By sharing in your child's curiosity while still providing lots of affection and comfort, you can help your baby become more confident and competent in these evolving skills.

From month seven on, mobility starts to take off. Day by day, your baby will build on existing motor skills, such as reaching, rolling over and sitting. Your baby also will move on to new ones, such as crawling and standing (some faster than others).

Since you can't predict when your baby will make the first move across the floor, now is a good time to review your home safety. (See Chapter 17 for more information on childproofing your home.) Keep an eye out for dangling cords and unsteady furniture. As mobility progresses, your baby will latch on to nearby items to move along faster or even up. Removing treasured or breakable items and creating a safe environment will give your baby the freedom and confidence to explore and learn. At this age, it's generally easier to change the environment than to teach a child not to touch.

GROWTH AND APPEARANCE

During these past months, your baby's growth rate was on fast-forward. Once your baby reaches 6 months, though, you'll find that growth tends to slow a bit. Previously, your baby was likely to gain over a pound a month. Now, the weight increase is more likely to be just under 1 pound each month, and the increase in length around $^{3}/_{8}$ inch or less. You can expect the growth of your baby's head to begin to slow, too.

From here on out, your child will continue to grow steadily, with additional growth spurts here and there. But your baby will never again grow quite as fast as in those first six months.

MOVEMENT

When your baby was younger, signs of developing motor skills were subtle, with some so basic as to go almost unnoticed. Fidgeting, for example, is a typical phase of growth and development, but it isn't nearly as exciting as the motor skills that are now blossoming. Between now and baby's first birthday, noticeable changes take place that transform your child from a dependent infant to a toddler who's becoming more independent.

Around 7 months of age, your baby may be sitting alone with no support, even working to put arms to the side to avoid toppling over. By 9 months, your baby may be steady and strong enough to play for longer periods while seated on the floor, even pivoting and reaching to get to different toys.

By the seventh month, babies are refining their hand and finger coordination, moving beyond the basic mitten grasp (clumsy hand movements and picking up objects by pressing all their fingers against their thumbs). They begin to develop a more sophisticated pincer grasp between now and the ninth month, using their thumb and index finger to pick up small objects.

The transition from a mitten grasp to a pincer grasp is gradual. First, you may notice your child using a cross between the two, picking up objects with the thumb, index and middle fingers. You also may see baby resting the arm and hand on a surface to steady the hand and pick up a small object.

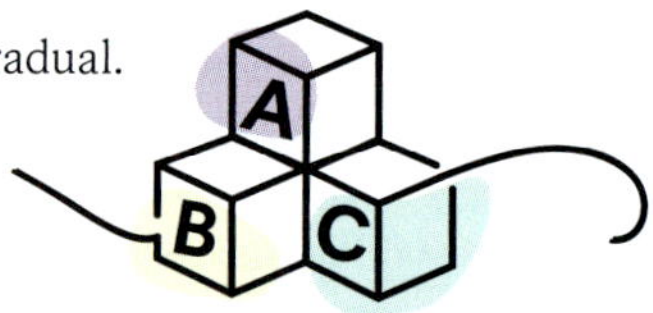

At the same time, your baby is also getting better at transferring an object from one hand to the other, turning it around and upside down, holding it this way and that, and getting to know how it feels. About half of babies this age begin to hold an object in each hand. Eventually they'll delight in banging objects against each other. But for now your baby may simply enjoy banging things against their leg or a table.

SENSORY DEVELOPMENT

By 7 months of age, your baby's eyesight is nearly mature. Distance vision continues to improve, and faraway people and objects appear clearer and more distinct. Your baby's eyes also can track faster movements and closely follow moving objects. In fact, if you roll a ball, your baby can monitor its path and probably put a hand out to it as it gets near.

By age 6 or 7 months, your baby's hearing is almost fully developed. Baby also is becoming more selective about reacting to sounds. For example, your baby at this age can quickly and accurately locate you when you speak. Baby also may stop to listen to quieter sounds.

Watch to see if your baby turns toward a sound, even if the sound comes from beyond the line of vision. If you notice that baby doesn't respond to surrounding sounds, talk to your baby's medical professional. If there's a problem with your baby's hearing, it's better to identify it sooner rather than later. Untreated, hearing loss can interfere with other aspects of development, such as language and social development.

COGNITIVE DEVELOPMENT

During month seven, your baby continues to pick up on language skills from listening to you and others speak. Before, your baby may have focused on imitating specific sounds, such as "mmm" or "bbbb." In these next few weeks, you may notice baby start to combine different sounds, such as consonants and

SPOT CHECK: WHAT'S GOING ON THIS MONTH

Here's a snapshot of what your baby's basic care looks like in the seventh month.

Eating

Breast milk or formula is still the primary part of your baby's diet, but by this time you should be introducing additional foods. Around 7 months, most babies who have not already begun eating solid foods can start to transition to soft foods or foods with tiny lumps without gagging. Your baby's airway is still very small, so avoid foods that could pose a choking hazard, such as those that are small, round, hard, chewy, slippery or crunchy. See Chapter 4 for more on introducing new foods.

Sleeping

Baby is more likely to sleep six to eight hours at night with no interruption. Some babies still wake up once or twice during the night for a feeding, although they're unlikely to need middle-of-the-night feedings by this age. Total sleep may add up to between 14 and 15 hours in a 24-hour period, including a couple of daytime naps, usually one in the morning and one in the afternoon. Some babies may need a third nap late in the afternoon. As your baby becomes more curious and mobile, it may be harder for baby to settle down to sleep at night. Establish and maintain a consistent, relaxing bedtime routine. Give baby a bath, read books together or sing a quiet song. This can be a great help in getting your child used to the idea of going to sleep at night.

vowels. By 6 or 7 months, your baby should make more complex sounds such as "dadada" and "mamama." As tempting as it may be to think your baby is referring to you when saying these sounds, it will likely be several more weeks before baby is able to attach names to people.

The art of conversation

In addition to imitating sounds and even combinations of sounds, your baby also may begin to follow your pattern of speech. For example, your baby may pause between "sentences" or end a string of sounds with an upward inflection, as if posing a question. You can encourage the art of conversation by talking to your baby and acknowledging baby's efforts with your own warm responses.

An infant's understanding of words is far ahead of the ability to use them. At this age, your baby understands the meaning of what you say by listening to your tone of voice. Even the word no (which you may find yourself using more often as your baby starts to push against the limits you've established) is understood by your inflection and tone and not necessarily by the word itself.

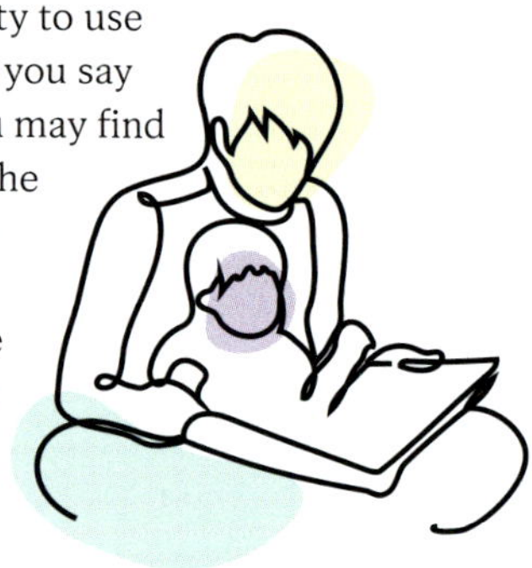

The more you talk to your baby — whether it's while you're driving, doing chores around your home, or during a changing or feeding — the more your little one learns about all aspects of communication. This includes sounds, inflections and tone of voice, as well as facial expression and body language.

The science of experimentation

As your baby's understanding of the power to make things happen grows, you can see how baby begins to test the limits of what's possible. How far can I push this train over the edge of my tray before it falls out of sight? Will my parent bring it back intact every time? How much can I kick during a diaper change before I receive a frown?

Amid all this experimentation, you will find that your baby is likely to waver between feeling confident and exuberant at times, and needy and cautious at other times. By helping baby feel secure — creating a safe environment to explore and practice, offering warm praise and support, setting firm yet practical limits — you can encourage experimentation and promote competence. In this type of setting, your baby learns to tackle challenges with enthusiasm, adding skill upon skill.

Finding the energy to repeat the same game or story over and over again can be challenging. But keep in mind that the process of repetition is essential to your baby's learning and mastering key skills.

SOCIAL DEVELOPMENT

Between 6 and 7 months, your baby is becoming quite the expert at nonverbal communication, expressing emotions in a variety of ways — laughing, crying, shrieking, squealing and cooing.

Stranger anxiety

Even as your infant becomes more expressive around you, baby may start to become quiet around strangers. Your child has come to associate you with comfort and happiness and is increasingly reluctant to let you go. Baby also is becoming keenly aware of who is familiar and who isn't. By 8 or 9 months, your baby may openly reject strangers, clinging to you and even crying if unknown people come too close.

This is a typical phase of development and is a sign of the strong bond your baby has developed with you. Shyness toward strangers can last months and even years, depending on your child's personality. Some children are shyer than others.

Discipline in infancy?

Discipline is something every parent thinks about at some point, perhaps even before a baby is born. You may have definite ideas about guiding your child's behavior, or you may not. It can be a fuzzy topic, especially if you have little previous experience. During the first six months, distracting your baby from unwanted behavior is usually enough to stop it. But by the time your baby reaches the seventh month, you may need to start setting some additional limits.

Keep in mind that true discipline — throughout the childhood years — is positive in its approach, with the ultimate goal of teaching rather than simply punishing. Your goal as a parent is to help your baby become a secure, independent and well-adjusted adult who is able to successfully navigate almost any social environment. You can start this process early on by establishing a trusting relationship between you and your child and setting simple, consistent limits.

Create a foundation of trust During your baby's first year, you can set the foundation for a pattern of parent-child interaction that will serve you well in later, potentially more trying times. This is done in the way you nurture and react to your infant, including simple things such as following a consistent schedule, attending to your baby's needs promptly and spending time bonding as a family.

As your baby gets a little older and more independent, baby will likely start testing the boundaries you've carefully created. This is not "misbehaving" — it's how a baby explores the world. If you manage that exploration safely, you can prepare the way for your child to become a happy, competent and confident member of your family and, ultimately, of society at large.

Be gentle yet firm By this time, your child's needs and wants have already started to separate. For example, your baby still might like to have a nighttime feeding, but probably doesn't need a midnight snack. If you haven't yet done so, start phasing out nighttime feeding (see page 135). Establish a consistent bedtime routine that helps your baby learn to self-soothe rather than rely on you to fall asleep (see page 131). This is a first step toward independence and will make bedtime much easier in the future. In addition, it's likely that your baby will get better rest this way, and so will you.

Likewise, at this age your baby's sense of curiosity and touch have kicked into a higher gear. As your baby discovers the use of the hands, those hands will

TOYS AND GAMES

As your baby becomes more interested in interacting with the outside world, provide new opportunities to do so.

Introduce the high chair

By this month, your baby is likely to sit well while supported. Putting your baby in a high chair can be a great way to include baby in family mealtimes. It can also be an interesting new place for your baby to sit and watch daily household activities and play with small toys on the high chair tray (baby can start working on thumb-finger coordination). Choose a high chair that has a comfortable seat and straps to keep your baby safely positioned. A detachable tray that you can take to the sink to wash is convenient. Experienced parents may recommend removable washable parts in general, as high chairs often become a backdrop for bits of cereal, splattered applesauce and mashed-up yams. Hosing off the entire apparatus in the backyard or shower isn't unheard of.

Provide warm-up time

If baby is shy or cautious, offer plenty of time to warm up to a new activity. Allow your child to observe on the sidelines for a while and assess the situation. This will give your child time to approach the activity in a way that's comfortable. Once secure, your baby will become more involved in what's going on.

Make new friends

If you haven't already done so, now might be a good time to introduce your baby to other children. Although they likely won't play together for some time yet, at this age babies will play side by side. Also, they're intrigued by others who are similar in size and behavior. Exposure to other children can help expand your baby's social horizon. But watch for when your baby has had enough "socializing."

Check out activities at your local library

Many libraries have special activities for infants, such as story time. Often a staff member will read a book aloud and include activities, such as singing silly songs and interacting with puppet shows. Libraries also may have play areas designed especially for younger children. This may be a good place to meet other parents and children. Plus, having all those books to look at can't hurt, right?

grab keys, hair, earrings, a nose — anything within reach. Baby will judge what's OK by your reaction. Use your tone of voice and facial expressions to express disapproval. If baby pinches your nose and it hurts, make a funny face or set your baby down and say "No" or "Ouch." Your baby can't control the impulse to touch and grab, so provide gentle guidance to what is acceptable.

Being consistent and firm in your limits will make it easier for your child to remember what's OK and what's not. Establishing your authority now — showing that you have the final say — will make life easier as your baby grows up.

Be proactive Once your baby is crawling — then walking — your baby thinks everything in the home is there to be touched, pulled, mouthed, opened and, in general, spread around the room. This is typical and expected behavior. Take a proactive approach and prevent problems before they happen. Set up boundaries by childproofing your house. Gates, cabinet locks and outlet covers can help you establish a positive learning environment for your baby and you won't have to constantly say no.

What to avoid Day-to-day management of an active, curious child can be frustrating at times. If you lose your patience with your infant, give the baby to your partner or set the baby in the crib and take a break to cool off. Never shake your baby. If you're struggling with your child's behavior or how to handle your frustrations, talk to your child's medical professional. If your child has a physical or developmental disability, managing behavior can be even more challenging. You may need more intensive strategies, so don't be afraid to ask for help.

7TH MONTH MILESTONES

During the seventh month, your baby is busy:

- Learning to sit unsupported
- Sitting and looking around
- Perhaps getting into a crawling position, while reaching out with one hand
- Using hands to rake up small objects
- Getting better use of thumb and fingers
- Transferring objects from one hand to the other
- Visually tracking rapid movements
- Readily responding to sounds
- Looking for sounds outside field of vision
- Starting to look for dropped toys
- Combining different sounds
- Imitating patterns of speech
- Distinguishing strangers from loved ones
- Starting to test limits and boundaries

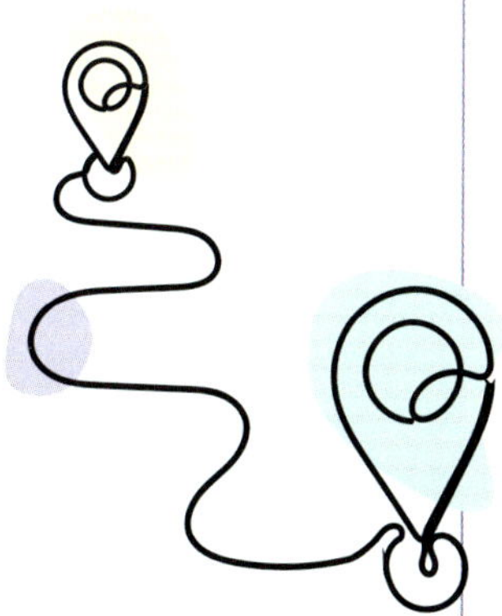

CHAPTER 26

Month 8

By month eight, most of your baby's newborn reflexes have faded away and are now replaced by intentional, purposeful movements. This is a result of your baby's maturing nervous system. As more and more nerve endings become encased in protective coverings (myelin sheaths), the nerves become efficient at carrying messages from the brain to muscles. This makes your baby's movements increasingly "smarter" and more refined.

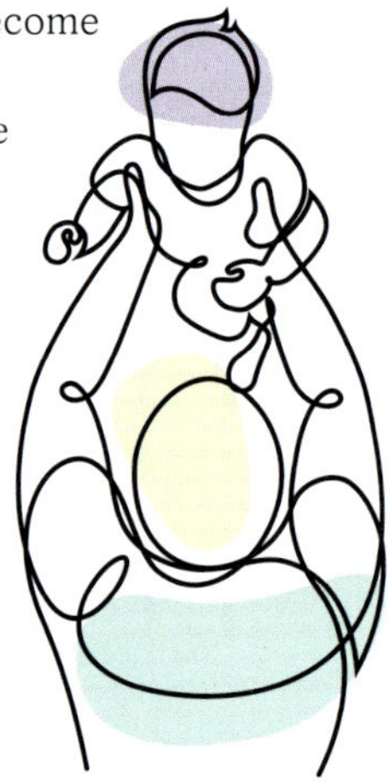

At the same time, your 7- to 8-month-old's brain is developing the ability to attach meaning to different sounds and gestures. For example, your baby might become quiet upon hearing their own name. Similarly, if you have a pet at home and frequently say its name when it appears, your baby may start associating the pet with its name.

Your baby's thinking processes are becoming ever more complex. You can see this by the way your baby begins to show likes and dislikes and to be fairly clear about them. This may be especially apparent in your infant's social preferences, as baby becomes increasingly aware of the difference between familiar and unfamiliar people.

Your baby is also developing an understanding of objects. Your baby is starting to realize that although people and things may temporarily disappear from the line of vision, that doesn't mean they're gone forever. This realization tends to coincide with less tolerance for being separated from you (separation anxiety), making transitions to child care and babysitters a little more challenging for a while.

GROWTH AND APPEARANCE

During this time, your baby is growing steadily but probably at a slightly slower rate than in previous months. The average baby at this age tends to gain just under 1 pound over the course of the month and grow about $^3/_8$ inch in length. Your baby's head circumference is still increasing, but only slightly compared with early months.

SPOT CHECK: WHAT'S GOING ON THIS MONTH

Here's a snapshot of what your baby's basic care looks like in the eighth month.

Eating

As you continue introducing solid foods into your baby's diet, you may wonder whether breast milk or formula still plays an important role in your baby's diet. Even though solid foods are beginning to supplement some of your baby's feedings, they can't completely replace the balance of nutrients that breast milk or formula provides. Breast milk is designed to be an excellent source of nutrients for your baby through the baby's first year and beyond.

Many parents wonder whether their babies can drink whole milk at this age. It's best for your baby to have breast milk or formula for the first year. Avoid cow's milk until your baby is 1 year old. Your baby's delicate digestive system isn't able to adequately handle the type and concentration of some nutrients found in cow's milk. And cow's milk is lower in iron and vitamins C and E than breast milk or formula.

Sleeping

Most babies are able to sleep well through the night — between 10 and 12 hours — around age 8 months, to the relief of their weary parents. Total sleep for baby may add up to about 14 hours in a 24-hour period, including a couple of daytime naps, usually one in the morning and one in the afternoon.

But beware: New skills such as pulling up to stand and cruising are near if not already learned, and your baby may wake during the night and want to practice. If your baby can't quite return to a sleeping position independently, your help may be needed.

In addition, if your baby gets anxious when separated from you during the day, that anxiety likely will be worse at bedtime and in the middle of the night. You're caught in the dilemma of wanting to reassure your baby and also wanting your baby to learn good sleep habits. For more information about helping your child develop good sleep habits, see Chapter 8.

As long as your baby is following a steady growth curve based on measurements by your baby's medical professional, there's no need to be overly concerned about specific numbers. At this stage, there is more variety in what your baby eats. But keep in mind that your baby still needs a proper balance of fats, carbohydrates and protein.

Establishing good eating habits

As you introduce new foods to your child, take the opportunity to establish good eating habits right away. Here are some tips to help your baby develop healthy eating patterns. (You can find much more guidance in Chapter 4.)

Offer a wide variety of foods You still want to introduce new foods one at a time, but that doesn't mean you have to stick to a single food for weeks on end. By this age, you can experiment with a variety of foods. If your baby does well with pureed yams, try some ground chicken after a few days. Or after a successful course of mashed peas, provide a dessert of mashed bananas.

Include a good balance of foods Prioritize fruits, vegetables, meats and healthy carbohydrates over processed foods and baked goods. Instead of a cut-up hot dog, for example, offer bits of turkey. Or instead of a soft cookie, offer pureed peaches. Minimize salt and offer sweet foods in moderation. Examples of not-so-obvious salt-rich foods include processed cheese, cold cuts, pizza, canned vegetables, canned beans and canned soups.

Avoid overfeeding Watch for cues that your baby is full. While you control what and when your baby eats, let your baby determine whether to eat each food you offer and how much.

Enjoy food for its nutrition But avoid using food as a reward or as a comfort item. Instead, reward and comfort your baby with hugs, kisses and attention.

Introducing a cup

You can provide a cup as soon as your baby starts eating solid foods. A two-handled sippy cup is usually easy for baby to use. This will help your child become familiar with the idea of using a cup. But at this age, your baby will probably bang, drop and dump the cup more than drink from it. It will probably be another few months before baby uses it properly.

Even if your baby uses a cup at mealtimes, you may decide to continue breastfeeding or using a bottle for supplemental feedings, simply because baby can't get much out of the cup just yet. Feeding your baby breast milk or formula from a cup at mealtime may help pave the way for weaning when you're ready.

MOVEMENT

Your baby's rapid development during these months can be astonishing. In just a few weeks, your baby may go from barely sitting up without your help to bustling around the room by scooting, crawling and cruising.

TOYS AND GAMES

Around this age, most babies enjoy toys they can bang, poke, twist, squeeze, drop, shake, open, close, empty and fill. Toys should be lightweight with no sharp edges. Remember that all toys will end up in your baby's mouth, so don't give your baby toys with small parts.

For the most part, your child's playtime will center around playing on the floor, working on crawling, sitting and standing. You can encourage these skills by putting a toy just beyond your baby's reach and encouraging baby to move toward it. Here are some other playtime ideas.

Peekaboo

Games of peekaboo take on a new dimension around the time your baby develops a sense of object permanence. Your baby will enjoy games in which objects and people "disappear" and your baby finds them again. Use a small blanket to cover toys, and let your baby uncover and discover them. Your baby may even cover them up again only to rediscover them.

Mirror games

Your little one is starting to learn the concept of three-dimensional space. Contrast two-dimensional images with three-dimensional ones by playing games in the mirror. If your baby is looking in a mirror and you suddenly appear in the mirror, too, baby is likely to turn around and look for you instead of believing you're in the mirror itself.

Buckets of stuff

Your baby is also learning how objects relate to one another. Infants at this age start to understand that smaller objects fit inside bigger ones. Stacking toys appeal at this age. Games in which toys can be put into a container and dumped back out again are popular as well. For a quick and easy version, fill a plastic mixing bowl with odds and ends from the kitchen — measuring spoons, plastic lids, small containers and empty baby bottles. Let your baby sort through them, dump them out and put them all back in again.

Book of animals

As your baby begins to understand that things have names and labels attached to them, introduce baby to a book with simple pictures of various animals and their names. You can read it together. As you point to the picture and name the animal, your baby will eventually start to associate the name with the animal. In time you can introduce animal sounds, too. For a more lyrical version, read *Brown Bear, Brown Bear, What Do You See?* by Bill Martin Jr. and Eric Carle, which contains rhythmic prose and colorful illustrations that are favorites of children and parents alike.

BABY SIGN LANGUAGE

By age 8 months or so, many infants begin to know what they want, need and feel, but they don't necessarily have the verbal skills to express themselves. Baby sign language allows children to use their hands to bridge the communication gap. Slightly older children who have developmental delays may benefit, too. Limited research suggests that using baby sign language may improve a child's ability to communicate and may ease frustration, particularly between ages 8 months and 2 years. Teaching and practicing baby sign language can also be fun and give you and your child an opportunity to bond.

At the same time, don't neglect your baby's verbal skills. Continue to talk to your baby, and encourage baby to use spoken words (or what may only sound like words in the beginning). Voice the meaning of a sign each time you use it.

A variety of books, websites and other resources are available to help you learn baby sign language. You can also use variations of American Sign Language. Start with signs to describe routine requests, activities and objects in your child's life — such as more, drink, eat, mother and father. Keep the following tips in mind:

- *Set realistic expectations.* Feel free to start signing with your child at any age — but remember that most children aren't able to communicate with baby sign language until about 8 or 9 months.
- *Stay patient.* Don't get upset if your child uses signs incorrectly or doesn't start using them right away. The goal is improved communication and reduced frustration — not perfection.
- *Be patient and consistent.* Repetition is the best way to ensure your child's success in using baby sign language.
- *Encourage use by all caregivers.* Encourage all caregivers to use the same signs to ensure consistency.

Sitting up

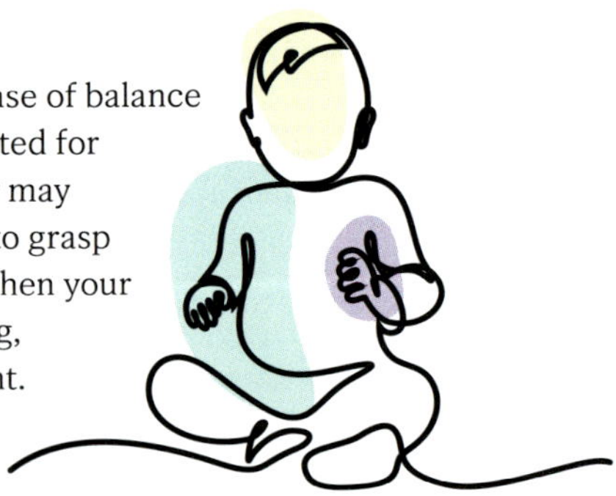

By 8 months, your baby is sitting well. Your baby's sense of balance is improving, and baby will be able to sit up unsupported for longer periods of time without falling over. Your baby may even start to reach with the arms while sitting to try to grasp nearby toys. These exercises will help further strengthen your baby's core muscles, which are important for standing, walking and any kind of forward-propelling movement.

Getting around

After your baby learns to sit up without too much effort, you'll notice other movements that happen before crawling — rolling, twisting, crouching, and rocking back and forth on the knees. In fact, it will be hard for your baby to be still for long. If lying tummy-down, your baby will push up on hands and arms to look around. Lying face-up is an incentive to kick and grab for toes. Your baby also can now flip around at will. Some babies even roll repeatedly as a means of getting from one place to another.

Because your youngster is getting so mobile, it's important to take appropriate safety precautions. Examples include swapping the changing table for the floor or bed to change diapers, making sure tall furniture is anchored to the wall, and installing safety gates at the top and bottom of stairs to avoid a potentially serious tumble. (See more about making your home safer in Chapter 17.)

Hand and finger coordination

Once able to sit well, your baby is also able to maintain upper torso balance while coordinating simultaneous movements of arms and hands. Most babies this age are able to hold a toy in each hand. Eventually they'll develop enough coordination to bring both hands inward and bang the toys against each other.

During this month, your baby probably still uses a raking motion to bring small objects closer. But your baby is also working on coordinating the thumb and first or second finger to pick up small objects (pincer grasp). Baby will practice this technique until achieving this grasp. This usually happens by the first birthday.

Your baby is also learning to let go of items at will. This is clear by baby's enthusiasm for dropping and throwing things — again and again!

SENSORY DEVELOPMENT

During this month, your baby's senses continue to provide lots of information to the brain. This stimulates the development of other skills, such as reaching and crawling, and drawing conclusions about spatial relationships.

Vision

Your baby's vision has improved significantly. Many babies by this age have 20/40 vision. Although baby still sees things better at close range than far away, your baby's vision should be clear enough to recognize people and objects across the room. Increased depth perception helps your baby accurately reach for objects and judge distances correctly when moving forward.

Touch

Between 7 and 8 months old, your budding physicist is learning rapidly about the way matter takes up space, different textures and connections between surfaces. For example, baby may start to realize that balls are round and roll, boxes have flat surfaces, and some toys have a top and a bottom part. Toys with tags, handles and parts that can be manipulated are fascinating to explore.

COGNITIVE DEVELOPMENT

Around this time, your baby is beginning to understand that certain things have meaning beyond the immediate sensory experience. For example, words and gestures, besides being heard and seen, can carry messages. Also, baby is realizing that things that are out of sight aren't gone forever. Your child's brain is starting to make connections between what is seen and what is unseen and is

ENJOYING A RELAXING NIGHT OUT

Because babies react so strongly to separation from their parents, parents are often reluctant to leave their babies with babysitters. You might even wonder if a night out is worth the heartbreak your baby seems to endure when left with a sitter. You can help yourself and your baby through this stage by taking these steps.

Practice

Take advantage of occasions at home to leave your baby alone for a few minutes (in a safe zone, of course) while baby plays. If your baby becomes upset at your absence, call out to baby, but wait a few seconds before coming back. Eventually your baby will learn that it's OK to be away from you and that you always do come back.

Get acquainted

If a babysitter is new, take some time to let the person and your baby become acquainted. Hold your baby on your lap while you and the babysitter talk, and then gradually engage the baby in the conversation. Once your baby seems comfortable with the sitter's presence, put your baby on the floor with a favorite object and the babysitter, and let them get to know each other. Once you're comfortable with your babysitter and you feel assured your baby is getting loving, qualified and competent care, you will be less bothered if your baby should cry when you leave.

Say goodbye

When you're ready to leave, tell your baby goodbye and provide reassurance of your eventual return. Although it's tempting to just sneak out when baby is preoccupied with something else, this approach won't help your baby overcome this anxiety. Instead, baby may become more clingy, never sure when you might leave. At the same time, there's no need to prolong the farewell. Have a distraction ready to go — a bath or new toy — and a few minutes after your departure, your baby's short attention span will be directed elsewhere.

beginning to draw conclusions from repeated experiences. Although it will be a while before your child can actively create and express symbolic thought — such as pretend play, which usually develops in the second year — the very first formations of abstract thought are emerging.

Attaching meaning

By 8 months or so, parents may notice that their baby quiets or perks up at the sound of their name, or even turns toward the person saying it. Your baby doesn't fully understand what this word refers to, but your baby is becoming familiar with hearing that word when you actively seek a face-to-face connection.

Object permanence

Previously, if your baby dropped something, baby likely thought it was gone entirely and made no effort to look for it. Now baby is starting to realize that, in fact, it may still be there, and will look for a hidden toy. Games of peekaboo take on a new significance as your baby realizes that after pulling the blanket away — aha! You are still there! And now that baby knows you're still around even if you leave the room, baby may make more of a fuss to get you to come back.

Language skills

By this time, your baby is likely becoming a proficient babbler, repeating not just single sounds but combining syllables, such as "bah-dah." Some babies are very expressive and jabber away like excited squirrels. Others are a little quieter and may listen more than chatter. But this doesn't mean they're not absorbing what's being said around them. Be sure to talk to your little shy one as much as you might to a little chatterbox, encouraging verbal and nonverbal communication.

SOCIAL DEVELOPMENT

As your baby learns new skills and becomes more mobile, baby navigates between the desire to be with you and the desire to be independent. You may notice this struggle surface in many situations as your baby searches for both predictability and adventure. Living with this new assertiveness may take a bit of adjustment for all parties involved. But understanding it as a typical phase of development helps most parents take the new challenges in stride.

Separation anxiety

At 8 months, most babies are clearly attached to the primary caregiver. Your baby may seem most assertive when you make any attempt to separate, whether it be for a few hours or a few minutes. Your baby may become more clingy — not wanting to let you out of sight — and may grasp at you or cry if you manage to break away. Both parents should understand that this phase is common and will lessen with time. This strong attachment to the primary caregiver can result in a seeming dislike for everyone else, which can be crushing to grandparents, other relatives and friends who feel close to the baby. You can ease feelings of rejection by explaining separation anxiety as a normal phase and helping to create a time of adjustment and transition.

Every baby goes through a stage of separation anxiety, which often begins around this age, peaks between 10 and 18 months, and gradually fades as the second birthday approaches. Some babies pass through this phase fairly quickly, but others remain reluctant to part for quite some time.

Part of baby's frustration stems from not having the motor skills to follow you or keep up with you, coupled with the budding realization that you're still there even if baby can't see you. The positive side of this development is that your baby has clearly established a strong bond with you and wants to make sure you stick around. Eventually, as your baby realizes that you're a permanent part of life despite temporary separations, this anxiety will ease.

If someone approaches your baby quickly, eagerly trying to engage the baby, the baby will probably cling to you even more tightly. Encourage others to spend some time just talking with you while you let your baby watch and listen. Your baby may eventually open up and jabber or want to play.

Peekaboo can be an icebreaker at this age because this game is so tempting for most babies. But don't be surprised if your baby will play this game only when you're close by. Assure others that your baby will outgrow this exclusivity.

8TH MONTH MILESTONES

During the eighth month, your baby is busy:

- Sitting up straight and looking around
- Reaching out with one hand while in a crawling position
- Rocking back and forth on all fours, rolling over repeatedly, scooting on the bottom, or expressing some form of desire to move around
- Using hands to rake up small objects
- Getting better use of thumb and fingers
- Transferring objects from one hand to the other
- Using touch to learn about the physical properties of different objects
- Looking for you or dropped toys (establishing object permanence)
- Attaching meaning to words and gestures, such as no or a farewell wave
- Combining different sounds
- Distinguishing strangers from loved ones
- Cementing the parent-child bond
- Starting to test limits and boundaries

CHAPTER 27

Month 9

Your baby has a lot going on these days. And get ready for a big change! During the ninth month is when most babies learn to crawl, and once your baby is on the move, life changes forever. No longer is your baby content to stay in one spot. There are so many places to go, so many things to see, so much stuff to get into! Daily life with an emerging toddler can be a challenge. But it's also a happy time of having fun and discovering new skills. With a little bit of prep work, you and baby will be all set to enjoy life on the go.

GROWTH AND APPEARANCE

During this month, your baby is growing steadily at about the same rate as the previous month. The average baby at this age tends to gain just under 1 pound a month and grow about 3/8 inch in length. Your baby's head circumference is still increasing slightly every month.

By now, your baby may have a nice head of hair. And now that your baby can flip and turn at will, bald patches are a thing of the past. At 9 months old, most babies still look like little butterballs. But within a few short months of growing, walking and running, your baby will stretch out into a full-blown toddler.

MOVEMENT

It's around this time that many babies catapult forward to a new level of mobility and independence. All that wriggling and fidgeting, rocking and rolling is paying off. Your baby is up and moving!

Crawling

Crawling uses the complex give-and-take movements of all four limbs that are necessary for walking later. It takes some time to understand how to make those little arms and legs work together. The average age at which an infant starts to crawl is 9 months.

At first a baby's arms are stronger than the legs, which makes for some funny crawling variations. Many babies begin crawling by using just their arms, scooting across the floor like a soldier in training. Others may find themselves up on their knees, give their arms a good push and begin moving backward.

Eventually, most babies will become experts at using their legs and arms simultaneously when they crawl. You might look away for a minute, then look back and wonder, "Where did my baby go?"

If your baby isn't interested in crawling, or crawls just for a short time before moving on to something else, remember that moving is the goal. How your baby moves isn't as important as the fact that your baby is interested in getting around.

Standing

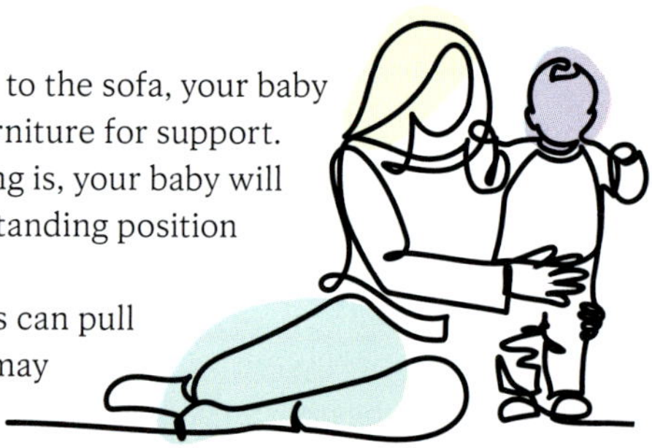

At 9 months old, if you stand up your baby next to the sofa, your baby will probably be able to stay there, using the furniture for support. When your child realizes how much fun standing is, your baby will probably start figuring out how to pull up to a standing position without your help.

At age 9 months, more than half of all babies can pull themselves into a standing position, and some may even begin "cruising" around the room, holding on to furniture for support.

At first your baby may not know how to sit down from a standing position and, instead, may just fall on the bottom. Soon your baby will learn how to lower down without falling. You can show your baby how to do this by gently bending baby's knees into a squat and then a sitting position.

Sitting

By 9 months old, babies love to sit and play and may do so for extended periods of time. Sitting gives your baby a broader perspective to observe and interact with their surroundings, allowing them to fully engage with the world around them. Between ages 8 and 9 months, your child is learning to point to desired objects and lean forward while sitting to reach toward you or an interesting toy.

As a result of improved stability and balance, your baby can now sit unsupported and turn the head to look at things. Your baby may even twist the torso to peer around — although leaning sideways may not be possible quite yet.

Hand skills

Baby is working steadily on the thumb-finger (pincer) grasp. With the pincer grasp, your baby can pick up objects as small as a piece of lint. Self-feeding also is likely to become a popular activity during this month, if it hasn't already. And by now, your baby may have learned to hold a cup or bottle and drink independently. Because almost everything your baby touches goes directly into the mouth for further exploration, be sure to remove anything from baby's reach that could cause choking.

Your baby also is learning to move the fingers individually. Your baby soon will be able to hold a string between finger and thumb and pull a toy along.

SPOT CHECK: WHAT'S GOING ON THIS MONTH

Here's a snapshot of what your baby's basic care looks like in the ninth month.

Eating

During this month, you may start introducing to your baby slightly coarser foods that require more chewing, but keep foods soft. You also might notice that baby is more interested in the food on your plate than what's on baby's plate. During the next few months, you can work your way toward feeding baby what the rest of the family is having. At first, you might try finely chopping the food or making sure it's cooked long enough to be soft. Many parents find using a food processor or blender helpful in achieving the appropriate texture for their baby's current eating abilities.

Breast milk and formula may start to take on a more supplemental role, but they are still irreplaceable sources of nutrition. If you wean your baby from breastfeeding before the first birthday, replace breast milk with iron-fortified formula. Your baby isn't ready for whole milk until that time.

Sleeping

By 9 months old, your baby has probably settled into a regular napping and sleeping schedule. Your baby may take two naps a day and sleep as long as 12 hours at night without waking to feed. But even if your baby has been a good sleeper up until now, you may face some new sleep challenges during this month and the next few months.

As your baby masters crawling and pulling up to a standing position, baby will probably work vigorously on these skills all day. During brief awakenings in the night, baby may automatically start practicing crawling and standing. But early on, your baby may know how to stand up but not get down again. Even after baby learns how to get out of these situations, the physical activity can make it hard to get back to sleep.

Your baby may let you know — loudly — how frustrating this situation is. At this age, your baby can shake the crib and may cry or scream to get your attention. Make sure the crib mattress is set at the lowest level and that there's nothing in the crib your baby could stand on. Once the novelty of the skill wears off, baby is likely to start sleeping better.

BATTLE OF THE SPOONS

Some babies insist on feeding themselves, often turning mealtime into playtime with utensils. Every time you try to slide that spoon in with some food, up comes the little hand to grab it, and splat goes the food. How to get your baby to eat?

If this is the case, provide different ways for your baby to explore food and self-feed. Place some finger foods on the baby's tray, give baby a spoon and use another spoon yourself. You may need to be persistent in finding opportunities to get some food into the baby's mouth.

You can try to teach your baby to eat with a spoon, but if you're not successful, let your baby eat with hands and fingers. For now, these handy utensils are generally faster.

If your baby truly isn't doing any eating, only playing, baby probably isn't hungry at the moment. You can call it quits for this particular meal and try again later.

Letting go voluntarily is becoming easier, allowing baby to set one thing down in order to pick up another. Other impressive hand skills your child may develop during this month include pointing toward desired things, clapping and waving goodbye. These are also forms of communication. Encourage your child's development in this area by using these skills yourself, such as pointing at different objects and naming them, or playing clapping games.

A common milestone achieved during this month is the ability to bang toys together. This is a great achievement. Working both arms simultaneously in this fashion requires an infant to sit upright steadily without support and display a fair amount of balance.

SENSORY DEVELOPMENT

By age 8 to 9 months, your child's sensory skills are fairly evolved and a great help in practicing new motor, mental and social skills. Combined with your child's expanding memory skills and understanding of object permanence, sensory abilities make for easy recognition of recurring sights, sounds and patterns. They're helping your young one gain knowledge of the general order of things.

Vision

Your baby's visual acuity is constantly improving, and baby can see things clearly from across the room. At this age, your baby is quick to recognize familiar faces and objects. Baby may adjust positions to get a better look at something and is more likely to look for a hidden toy.

Crawling and moving about helps develop depth perception, as your baby studies one hand moving forward and then the next, over the varying ground beneath. Better depth perception leads to an increased awareness of heights and a better-timed, more cautious approach to obstacles.

Hearing

Your baby now recognizes sound without difficulty and probably responds when you call baby's name. Your baby may respond to other familiar words as well, such as *bottle*, *mama*, *dada* and *no*.

Touch

Your baby is learning how to wrap hands around a cup or bottle, how to pick up a spoon, and how to handle different toys appropriately.

COGNITIVE DEVELOPMENT

By age 9 months, your infant is sophisticated enough to be bored. This is because the memory is developing and what was once new and interesting isn't so much anymore. Your baby is on the hunt for new stimulation and is keen to try out new games and skills.

This is certainly a fun age, but it can also be frustrating for baby and parents alike if baby moves quickly from one thing to the next, leaving little time for you to get other things done.

FINGER FOODS FOR LITTLE ONES

As your baby develops a better pincer grasp and more advanced chewing skills, you can start offering finger foods. Self-feeding can be great entertainment. What could be more fun than exploring things that actually are supposed to go in the mouth (even if they end up on the floor)? And it helps foster your child's sense of independence and ability to accomplish a task without help.

Keep in mind, however, your baby's ability to handle textures and foods of various sizes. Soft and mushy is the way to go. Small, hard, round, sticky or chewy bits of food can be choking hazards. Here are some suggestions for finger foods to get you started:

- Well-cooked diced vegetables (yams, potatoes, carrots, green beans)
- Soft ripe fruits, cut up into small pieces (berries, mango, peaches, banana)
- Whole-grain breakfast cereals (with no nuts or chunks)
- Teething biscuits or crackers
- Cut-up, well-cooked pasta

Don't worry too much, though. As your child develops further and becomes more mobile and independent, baby will be more capable of creating fun. In the meantime, swap out some of your child's simpler toys for more complex (but still age-appropriate) ones, or fill a basket with board books that your child can easily access. For now, you also might spend a little extra time on the floor each day with your youngster to bridge the gap until self-entertainment becomes easier.

LANGUAGE AND UNDERSTANDING

By 9 months, some babies begin using simple words, such as *mama* and *dada* for their parents. This milestone follows babbling, when they combine syllables into strings of sounds resembling speech.

Your child's understanding of language is increasing as well, even more rapidly than vocal expressions. By now, your baby likely understands the meaning of a number of words, including baby's name, as mentioned previously. Your baby also is starting to understand simple games and rhymes and will laugh and giggle at appropriate parts. For example, about half of babies can play clapping games by age 9 months. You also can try games that involve you showing your baby how to do something and then allowing a chance to do it — "My turn." "Your turn."

GET READY

It's tempting to think that as the months pass, your baby will require less time and attention. But once your baby is on the move, more supervision will be needed. Before, your baby would wait for you to come. Now that your child is mobile, your baby can come to you. You are still your child's primary love and favorite companion, and there is so much your baby wants to share while scooting around and exploring.

Very active or very curious babies may need especially careful supervision. Once they discover their ability to move, they are off and into everything, touching, pulling, tasting, testing. Babies on the go need your presence to ensure that heads don't get bonked, fingers don't get pinched, small objects don't get swallowed and prized possessions remain intact.

This period of intense supervision generally lasts until about 3 years of age, when children are more accustomed to limits and spend more time playing alone or with friends. If you think you'll never make it that long, take heart — you will. This is a time-intensive period of parenting, but it's also one of great joy as you watch your child grow and develop into a walking, talking toddler with some very definite opinions.

With the understanding of object permanence becoming more established, your baby will spend more time searching for something known to be there, such as a key you've folded in your hand. When your baby waves bye-bye as you walk out the door, it's an acknowledgment that you're leaving. But your baby also is coming to expect that you'll be back.

SOCIAL DEVELOPMENT

Once your baby starts to crawl and move around, limits begin to play a larger role in both baby's life and yours. Before, there wasn't much your baby could do without your help. Now that your baby can crawl and climb and discover without you, there are bound to be necessary limits — "No, you can't climb the bookshelf," or "No, don't pull the cat's tail."

Oh, the frustration

Setting limits can be an adjustment for children and parents alike. Not having been stopped from doing much before, a 9-month-old is understandably confused and frustrated when suddenly you are shouting "No!" to prevent a reach for an electrical cord. Your child has no way to differentiate between what's safe and what's not, and won't really understand the reasons behind your rules until much later. In fact, at this age, redirecting your child to a different, acceptable activity is generally the most effective way to stop a behavior.

With an increased capability for expression, your infant is likely to share feelings about these new restrictions, too. At this point, your child has clear likes and dislikes and will communicate them through body language — pointing, clapping, making faces, or stiffening or arching the back. Baby also may use vocalizations such as squealing, howling and jabbering.

This phase can frustrate parents, as the orderly routine is completely turned on its head. Turn your back for a moment, and the basket of folded laundry is now strewn around the dining area and the mail across the living room floor.

Also, it can be difficult to move from being the nurturing parent to being the limit-setter and having to deny some of your child's wishes.

Making life easier

Neither you nor your baby will be happy in a home in which you must constantly keep a close watch and remind baby to keep away from dangerous situations and objects. So many things around the house are tempting, and it's unreasonable to expect much self-control from your child at this age. Instead, try these strategies.

Childproof regularly Maintaining a safe space for your baby to explore independently will make things easier for all. Soon after babies learn to crawl, they also can climb stairs. Monitor your child carefully if stairs are accessible, or properly install and use gates at the top and bottom of stairs. Make sure heavy bookcases and dressers are securely anchored to the wall so that curious climbers can't pull them down. Pad coffee table corners, and remove dangerous items from the reach of little fingers.

Offer safe opportunities for exploration Think about ways you can let your baby explore without getting into trouble. Some parents reserve a low kitchen cabinet for items the baby can safely get into. Or set up an "activity center" with pillows to climb and empty boxes to investigate. If the weather is nice, a small pop-up tent outside can provide lots of fun.

Provide comfort but stay firm When your baby is frustrated, provide some help and comfort but realize that overcoming frustration is a skill that baby will need to develop. Distraction or redirection from a forbidden object or activity

TOYS AND GAMES

Physical games are fun at this stage of your baby's development. They can help baby hone new motor skills. At the same time, your child's communication and language skills are rapidly progressing, so include games that stimulate the mind, too. Try some of these.

Indoor gym

Once your baby learns to crawl, getting through, in and around things is a great source of entertainment. Create your own gym with stuff you have on hand:

- Drape a blanket or a sheet over a table to make a tunnel. Place an unbreakable mirror inside for a visual surprise.
- Create an obstacle course with pillows, laundry baskets and rolled-up towels.
- Use yourself. Lie down with an interesting toy on one side of you and baby on the other. Encourage your baby to climb over your legs to get it.

Walk together

Your baby may not be walking independently just yet. But you can get baby to know the necessary leg movements by holding the hands and helping your child take small steps forward.

Clapping games

To help your baby practice arm coordination and build balance skills, teach clapping games, such as pat-a-cake.

Nursery rhymes

Never underestimate the power of a few silly rhymes to make your child laugh. There are plenty of oldies but goodies, such as "Old MacDonald" and "Little Miss Muffet." If you find yourself a little rusty on some of these, you can look them up on the internet or borrow a book from the library. In fact, chances are there's a mobile app out there to help you learn some songs on the go, whether in a crowded restaurant or on a long drive.

9TH MONTH MILESTONES

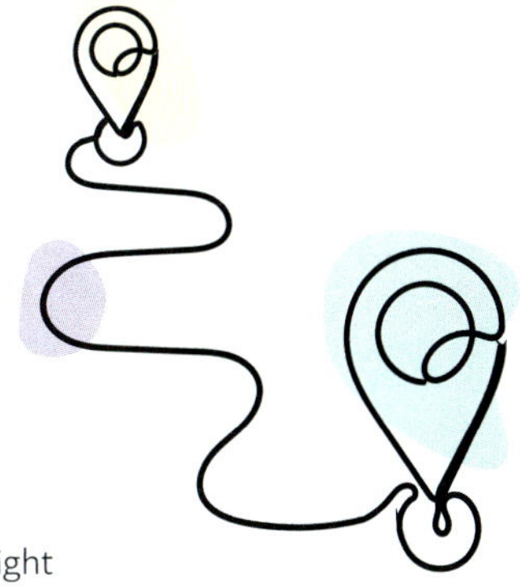

During the ninth month, your baby is busy:

- Learning to crawl
- Standing with support
- Working on pulling up to stand
- Using thumb and first finger together (pincer grasp)
- Banging toys together
- Rattling, shaking, dropping toys
- Looking for toys that have dropped out of sight
- Learning to let go voluntarily
- Learning to point, clap and wave goodbye
- Feeding self
- Recognizing and responding to familiar words
- Babbling, stringing syllables together
- Working on verbalizing familiar words
- Holding toys and objects appropriately
- Testing limits and observing parental reactions
- Avoiding strangers yet interacting more with family

usually works well. Kids need consistency, so stay firm with the safety limits you've set.

Keep your baby busy Most 9-month-olds are active and need a lot of stimulation, but they don't like to be apart from you. It can be difficult to give your baby that attention and get anything else accomplished. One option is to fill a small basket with toys for each room of the house; then take the baby with you as you go from room to room, and let your baby play while you work.

Family life

Although your baby may not feel comfortable around strangers, baby loves to be around you and the rest of the family. Your baby may show affection by patting you on the back or may even start imitating fond gestures such as hugs and kisses. Your baby definitely wants to be a part of the family commotion.

Siblings still love the baby and want to play, but the initial enchantment may largely be over, especially once baby can scoot around and get into their toys. Try to encourage a spirit of cooperation with an older child.

CHAPTER 28

Month 10

Many of the motor skills your baby has been working on since birth are starting to come together this month. These basic skills enable the transition from infancy into toddlerhood. From this point forward, your baby is moving steadily toward an upright view of the world. And even though your baby may still only see knees and legs and the lower half of the world for a while, the ability to maneuver about is a very exciting development.

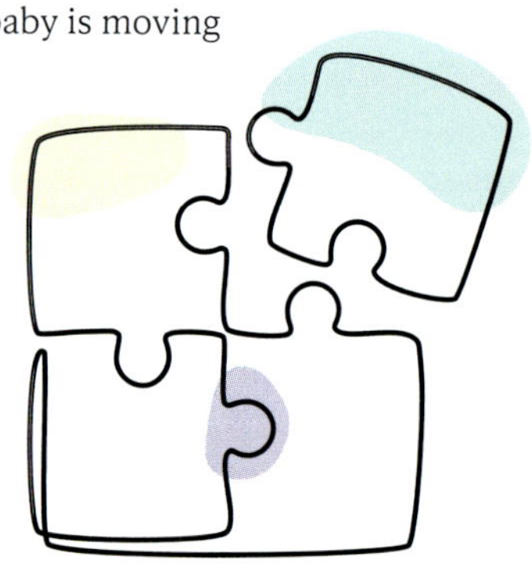

During month 10, many babies practice pulling themselves up to stand with the help of furniture or a parent's leg. By the end of the month, some babies are even able to stand on their own for a few seconds.

Babies also start to be big copycats around this time, which can provide for some enjoyable and amusing moments. Copying the facial expressions, gestures, and vocalizations of adults and older children is one of the primary ways a baby learns how to fit into the family and society at large.

GROWTH AND APPEARANCE

Baby is growing at much the same rate as last month — gaining just under 1 pound a month and growing about $^{3}/_{8}$ inch in length. Your baby's head circumference is still increasing slightly every month.

When your baby first starts to stand and then walk, you might notice that the legs appear slightly bowed. This is typical. In most babies, legs straighten within the next year or so.

MOVEMENT

By month 10, you can really start to see how your baby's early motor accomplishments are building on each other. Good head control plus strong muscles — conditioned by months of pushing up, looking around, wriggling and rolling — allow your baby to become skilled at more advanced motor skills, such as crawling, standing and walking.

At this stage, most babies can sit unsupported with a straight back. For baby, this is a comfortable position from which to play and engage the world. In a matter of weeks, your baby is becoming an efficient crawler, moving with purpose. Your baby also can place weight on the legs, holding on to something to stand upright. You'll see improvements in these basic skills this month.

Switching it up

By the end of month 10, most babies have learned how to pull themselves into a sitting position — bringing the torso up from lying down, flopping over from

SPOT CHECK: WHAT'S GOING ON THIS MONTH

Here's a snapshot of what your baby's basic care looks like in the 10th month.

Eating

During this month, your baby may start eating more of the same foods that the rest of the family is eating. Be sure the food you give to your baby is of manageable size and texture. Soft-cooked or finely chopped foods are still the way to go, or you can use a baby-food grinder to get the food to the right texture.

Breast milk and formula start to take on a more supplemental role but are still irreplaceable sources of nutrition. If you've decided to wean your baby from breastfeeding, replace the breast milk with iron-fortified formula. Your baby isn't ready for whole milk until after the first birthday.

Sleeping

By 10 months, you and your baby have developed a regular napping and sleeping schedule. The general expectation is that your child will take two naps a day and sleep as long as 12 hours at night without waking to feed. But then again, it's still common for babies practicing new skills, such as crawling and standing, to wake up at night and pull themselves into positions they need help getting out of.

If your baby is safe and dry, it's OK to let baby settle back to sleep without help (which might involve some fussing and crying). Once these new skills become routine, your baby is likely to start sleeping better.

crawling or squatting down from a supported standing position. Being able to switch positions at will gives your child a little taste of the mobile freedom and independence ahead.

Pulling to stand

Pulling up to stand becomes a significant focus at this age. Your baby may use any available support — such as crib rails or even a caregiver's clothing — to pull up. While some support might still be needed, this activity is crucial for developing strength and coordination.

Since your baby doesn't know the difference between what's safe to climb and what's not, it's important to keep safety a priority. Make sure the crib mattress is set at the lowest level, and keep out of reach anything that baby might use to climb too high and unintentionally pitch forward out of the crib. Also, keep heavy bookshelves and cabinets anchored to the wall so that baby doesn't accidentally pull down an unsteady structure.

Picking up, pointing and poking

By month 10, most babies are refining their heavy-handed grasp of small objects and graduating to a more delicate thumb-finger grasp. This allows them to manipulate items with precision and become better at releasing things at will. Letting go at this age (and for a while to come), however, tends to mean throwing a toy aside rather than gently laying it down.

Your little one also has discovered the power of the index finger, using it to

PREPARE FOR SOME BUMPS

As your baby starts to stand and move around on two feet, falls and short tumbles naturally become more frequent. This isn't really a big deal, as your baby doesn't have very far to fall and is unlikely to get hurt landing on the bottom.

Often, after a fall, your baby will look at you first to gauge your reaction before making one. Among childhood experts, this is called social referencing. Babies will look to trusted adults for emotional guidance before proceeding with a new experience.

You can help your baby understand that a minor tumble is no obstacle to getting back up by treating it matter-of-factly and offering cheerful reassurance. Some babies will cry no matter what. But if you offer loving encouragement accompanied by positive facial expressions, your baby will quickly learn to shrug off such small setbacks and try again.

At the same time, be sure to provide a forgiving environment for your baby to knock about in. For example, pad sharp coffee table corners and keep loose cords out of sight and reach to avoid accidents.

point, prod and poke at items of interest, including you. Picture books are great for practicing pointing and learning the names of things. Use the same words each time for each picture, and your baby will soon start helping you out. Some books feature different textures, such as furry or rough patches, or foldout flaps, which make them doubly interesting for baby.

SENSORY DEVELOPMENT

As your child approaches the end of the first year, baby is becoming skilled at using the senses to learn and explore.

Hearing

By 10 months, your baby recognizes sounds without difficulty, such as the sound of their name, familiar songs and words, your dog's bark, and even the doorbell. Your child is also becoming more selective about listening. For example, baby can listen to other people talking and pay attention to conversations without being distracted by other noises.

Touch

With the expansion of the mental and fine motor skills — such as increased memory and individual finger skills — your baby now enjoys more control over exploratory activities. By now, for example, your child knows that a maraca can be shaken, a cup goes to the mouth, buttons are pushed and a favorite doll is gently patted (just like you do it).

Your baby also enjoys self-feeding. Let your baby explore with finger foods (see Chapter 4). And even though it's bound to be messy, it's important to let baby practice self-feeding, as this is the only way your baby will get better at it. To make cleanup a little easier, consider spreading a splat mat or newspapers under your baby's high chair.

COGNITIVE DEVELOPMENT

In the last quarter of your baby's first year, language skills really start to blossom. Your baby not only understands more of what is said but may also be close to uttering first words. This is exciting. There's so much to say!

Your child's ability to think as a separate individual is becoming more sophisticated. You may see clues of this expressed through your baby's nonverbal communication as well.

First words

During this month, many new parents start to hear baby sounds bound to warm their hearts. About half of babies use *dada* and *mama* at this point. A few babies even start to use one other word in addition to *dada* and *mama*, such as *baba* for bottle or *mok* for milk. These words are often hard to understand at first, and it may be a while before you figure out that your baby is saying something meaningful. In general, a word at this age is any sound used consistently to refer to the same person, object or event.

When opportunity presents itself, you can reinforce the correct way to say the words your baby is learning. For example, readily acknowledge your child's request for a *baba*, and then say the correct word, *bottle*, when offering it back. As you feed or play with your child, regularly describe what you're doing. Eventually, language skills will develop enough for your baby to use the correct words.

TOYS AND GAMES

Go for toys and games that help enrich your child's growing awareness of the way things work, from toys that stimulate exploration of different functions to ones that allow baby to mimic grown-up behaviors. Games made up of simple actions can be fun, and silly songs with accompanying gestures are sure to be a hit.

Busy toys

As hand skills grow, your child may enjoy toys that feature multiple functions, such as pushing buttons, opening drawers, making noises and lifting lids. Stacking toys and nesting toys are fun for baby to put together and take apart.

Mimic

Offer your child toys that resemble adult accessories, such as a toy phone, plastic keys, a comb, pretend food or a teacup. See what your child does with them. Or make a silly face or gesture and encourage your child to imitate you. Wait to see if your child makes a funny face or odd gesture at you. Return the favor and imitate your child.

Give and take

Many 9- to 10-month-olds enjoy simple games that involve passing an object or toy back and forth. Offer your child a ball. Once your child grasps it, ask for it back. This may sound a bit dull to an adult, but your baby will probably love it. This also helps baby learn the concepts of gameplay and following simple instructions.

Silly songs

Babies at this age delight in silly songs that have accompanying hand gestures. These help stimulate not only your child's funny bone but also hand-eye coordination and fine motor skills. "Itsy Bitsy Spider," "I'm a Little Teapot" and "This Little Piggy" will never go out of style with this crowd.

Conversation

As a result of listening to you talk, your child's own babbling will start to sound more like the ups and downs of a real conversation. Even if most of it makes no sense, join in the conversation and repeat back your baby's sounds. Try to understand any words that might pop up in the middle of all the jabber. Respond positively to your baby's talking, and pause at times to encourage a rhythm like that of real conversation. Your baby will be delighted that you're interested and paying attention.

Nonverbal communication

Although your baby still has few words, this won't get in the way of communicating with you. As your baby starts to discover personal likes or dislikes, baby may point, shake the head no, reach and make sounds, and pull or hold arms out to be picked up.

The nonverbal communication not only shows that your baby is trying to relay ideas to you but also shows an increase in your baby's self-perception. Baby is now able to form thoughts related distinctly to the self, apart from others, and to personal desires. Your child is also developing thinking skills sophisticated enough to communicate those wants and devise ways to achieve them.

Along with simple expressions of thoughts, your baby is beginning to understand brief requests from you. Your child may do what you ask if you use hand gestures with your request and if it involves some sort of interaction with

A TWO-WAY STREET

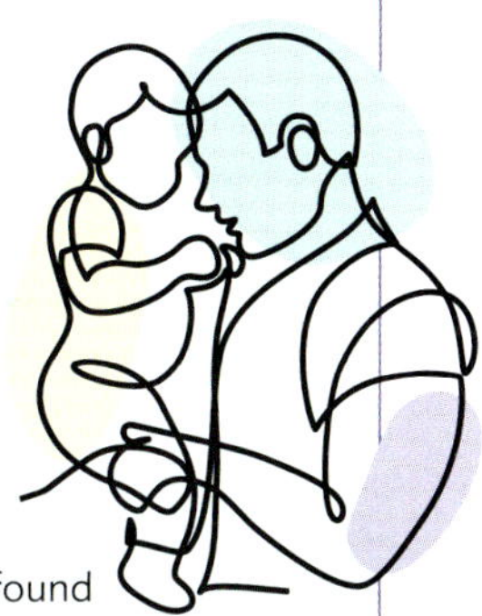

Research underscores the crucial role of early language exposure in a child's development, emphasizing that the quality and quantity of language encountered in the first three years are key to enhancing preschool language skills. Parents are encouraged to engage their children in rich verbal environments through activities like reading and storytelling.

One research study highlighted in the journal *Pediatrics* found that interactive adult-child conversations have the most substantial impact on language development. Chatting has a greater effect than mere exposure to adult speech and the negative influence of TV. These interactions also help parents tailor their communication to their child's growing capabilities. Engaging in dialogue, even through nonverbal means such as gestures and facial expressions, helps build a foundation for future language learning.

Bottom line: Keep on reading and talking to your child, but be sure to include some "conversation" time — such as discussing a picture book — as well!

you. If you ask your child for a cracker and hold out your hand, showing what you want, your child may comply.

SOCIAL DEVELOPMENT

As baby's skills and independence increase, your child will still look to you for safety and security. Even though you have established a solid bond at this point, hugs, kisses and warm affection are still vital to expanding on the trust your baby has placed in you. Giggles, laughter and quiet times together deepen your relationship and further cement the bond you have.

Since birth, your baby has been learning through listening to and watching you. In earlier months, it may have felt like your baby wasn't paying much attention to your day-to-day activities. But soon you'll notice you have a "mini-me" at your heels, imitating many of the activities you thought had gone unnoticed.

Mimicking

Around this age, babies like to mimic the gestures, facial expressions and some of the sounds made by adults and older kids. If your baby gets hold of the remote control, for example, you might find baby pointing it at the TV. Or if baby's older sibling blows a raspberry, the baby will try to do it, too (a scenario that all too often unfolds at the dinner table when you're engaged in the serious business of trying to eat). After a meal, your baby may try to wipe your hands and face.

SHARING

Between months 10 and 12, babies love to be with other babies and watch them play. But they're still not capable of playing with each other. Interactive play usually doesn't take place until around 2 to 3 years of age.

What babies are capable of right now is taking an interest in another child's toy. This can lead to some tussles over toys and other playthings. It would be nice if babies had a natural ability to share and be polite, but at this stage it's all about them and what they want. In general, kids don't understand the concept of sharing or taking turns until the age of 3 or so. And even when they do understand the concept, they may not always put it into practice.

If conflict arises around a toy or other object, your best bet is to distract your baby with something else. Aided by a short attention span, it's fairly easy to engage your baby in a different activity, making the sharing issue unimportant. Eventually you can start showing your child how to share with someone else. For now, though, the lesson is likely to be lost on your baby (especially if it's a long-winded one).

10TH MONTH MILESTONES

During the 10th month, your baby is busy:

- Mastering crawling
- Standing with support
- Pulling up to stand
- Maybe standing alone for a few seconds
- Using thumb and first finger together (pincer grasp)
- Manipulating toys appropriately
- Learning to let go voluntarily
- Using gestures to communicate, such as shaking the head for no
- Feeding self
- Recognizing and responding to familiar words
- Babbling, stringing syllables together
- Saying *mama* and *dada*
- Verbalizing other familiar words
- Looking for hidden toys
- Imitating the activities of adults and older kids
- Testing limits and observing parental reactions
- Avoiding strangers yet interacting more with family

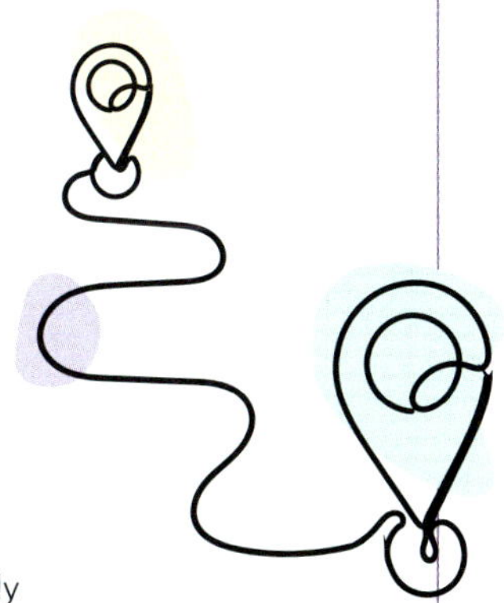

Babies also like to start copycat games, making a sound or gesture and looking to see whether you will do the same thing back.

Mimicking is an important way of learning essential skills. Even adults make use of this form of social learning when they are faced with new cultural situations. Your actions and behaviors as a parent can be powerful teaching tools for your child. For example, if you consistently use please and thank you and if you always treat your partner with kindness and respect, you'll find your child eventually doing the same.

CHAPTER 29

Month 11

Wow. It may seem like just yesterday that you brought your baby home from the hospital. But here your baby is, closing in on the end of a full year. So much has happened since birth that those early months may now start to seem like a blur. And in the eagerness to celebrate your baby's first birthday, month 11 might feel like it gets a little lost in the shuffle.

But there's plenty going on. Your little one is headed toward an upright view of the world, which allows baby to see so much more. This vantage point also places more toys and other objects within easy reach. Your baby will start inching along while holding on to furniture, or cruising, to get to things and places. These are the first steps toward walking without help.

Your child can also see clearly and is learning to listen and look at the same time — a big step forward in the ability to focus and concentrate. Language skills are building as understanding increases, and baby starts using meaningful "words" to refer to people, places and things.

GROWTH AND APPEARANCE

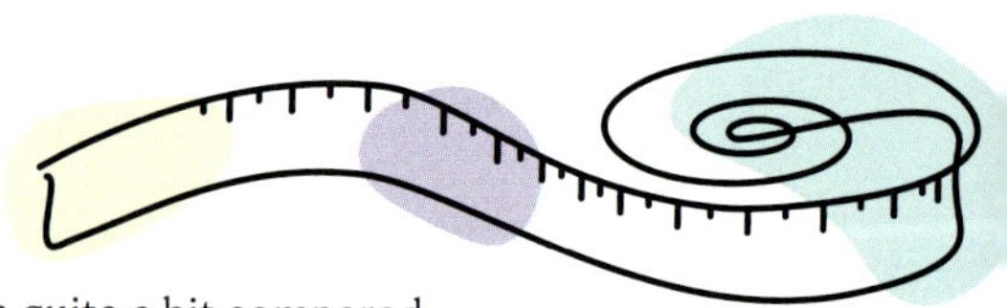

As your child heads into toddlerhood, you can expect the growth rate to slow down quite a bit compared with the first year, which is the period of most rapid growth a person experiences in a lifetime.

For month 11, however, your child's growth rate likely will be the same as last month's. Keep in mind, though, that babies tend to grow in fits and starts, so don't be surprised if a period of very little growth is followed by a big growth spurt.

MOVEMENT

On average, month 11 is when many babies start cruising — moving alongside furniture while holding on, going from one piece to another as they make their way around the room. It doesn't take long for a baby to become quite good at this method of traveling. Although walking without help is just a few steps away, crawling still rules for most babies, affording the most efficient way of getting from point A to point B.

Crawling

With added experience, your baby is getting faster and more confident at crawling (whatever the technique might be). Crawling around helps develop your child's ability to absorb slightly differing views from both eyes, so that the brain can see with three-dimensional capability. This ability provides new depth perception. As your baby's depth perception improves, movements become more controlled. Baby may become more cautious about heading down a slight slope or up a gradual incline.

If cruising has started, your baby will drop down to crawl if there's nothing to hold on to. And many babies continue to crawl even after they start walking. Kids are fairly efficient creatures, though. Once walking becomes the fastest way to get around, they'll mostly stick to walking.

SPOT CHECK: WHAT'S GOING ON THIS MONTH

Here's a snapshot of what your baby's basic care looks like in the 11th month.

Eating

During this month, your baby is probably eating many of the same foods that the rest of the family is eating. Be sure to give your baby food that is manageable in size and texture. Soft-cooked or finely chopped foods are still appropriate, as are small chunks of foods that are easy to chew and swallow. Breast milk and formula take on a more supplemental role but are still necessary sources of nutrition.

Sleeping

Most 11-month-olds sleep as long as 10 to 12 hours at night and take a couple of naps during the day. A few babies may start giving up their morning naps during this month. If that's the case for your baby, try starting the afternoon nap a little earlier and make bedtime a little earlier as well. This will help avoid overtiredness. Pay attention to your child's cues, too, and adjust the sleeping schedule to accommodate the need for sleep.

Standing

Your baby is getting pretty good at staying upright, too. Most babies this age can stand with support, such as while holding your hand, for at least a couple of seconds. Some babies even start to stand alone for a second or two.

Around 11 months, the average baby is also able to get into a sitting position from a standing position without just falling on the bottom. Your baby will probably need to hold on to furniture or your leg, for example, for support while doing this.

Cruising

Some babies walk sooner than do others, and a few babies will start to take their first independent steps during this month. However, most continue to rely on nearby furniture to support their movements. You'll see your baby slide the hands along a piece of furniture, taking small sideways steps to get around. Every so often, baby may pause to examine a toy or a scratch in the wood, or to bang vigorously and happily on the coffee table.

At first, your child likely will keep one arm on one piece of furniture and reach out with the other arm to the next piece — from couch to coffee table to chair, for example. Gradually, baby will become confident enough to move between pieces that are farther and farther away, such as from couch directly to chair if it's close enough. You might even catch your child taking a few quick steps unaided.

DOES YOUR BABY NEED SHOES?

When their babies start standing and cruising, many parents wonder whether shoes are necessary. At this age, your baby doesn't need shoes for standing or walking. You might put shoes on your baby because they look cute, to keep your baby's feet warm or to protect the bottoms of the feet. But your baby doesn't need shoes for any other reason and is probably growing so fast that buying shoes seems impractical.

You may think your baby's feet look flat and seem to be supported by unstable ankles. This is typical. All babies have chubby, thick feet with a fat pad that hides their arches. And they are generally unsteady on their feet. They are just learning to walk, after all. But putting your baby in shoes with special arches, inserts, high backs or reinforced heels won't change your baby's feet or help baby walk more easily. On the contrary, your baby may benefit from being barefoot to get a "feel for the road" when learning to walk.

If you do buy shoes for your baby, make sure they're comfortable and have nonskid soles to avoid slips. You should be able to feel a space as wide as your index finger between your baby's big toes and the tips of the shoes. Shoes should also be wide enough across the front to allow your baby's toes to wiggle.

Finger skills

Passing objects back and forth is a fun game for baby, allowing for lots of practice in using the thumb-finger grasp and in deliberately letting go. Your baby also enjoys pointing at interesting things.

Improved depth perception helps baby to realize that an empty cup has space inside it and that, amazingly enough, things can be put into the cup. By the end of month 11, about half of babies can put things in a container. The new big attraction will be dumping everything out of a basket or a bucket and then putting the things back in again, or at least some of the things.

Having greater depth perception also makes it possible for your baby to take part in simple ball games, such as rolling a ball back and forth.

SENSORY DEVELOPMENT

By month 11, your child's sensory abilities are running in practically full gear.

Vision

Although still nearsighted, your baby can see as clearly as you can, recognizing familiar faces from 20 feet away. Your little one has become a keen observer, watching the movements of others with interest. Baby can visually track moving objects with no problems. And now that your baby knows that things continue to exist even when out of sight, baby is able to look in the right places for play-things and objects that have dropped or rolled out of sight.

Hearing and listening

Hearing and listening abilities — along with an increasing ability to focus attention — are improving to the point where baby is starting to listen and look at the same time. These skills help your child pull in valuable information about the surrounding world.

Touch

During this month, your child is learning about concepts such as "behind" and "inside," which is one of the reasons that checking what's in a bag becomes so much fun at this point. Your child also will probably delight in poking fingers into holes, tearing up paper, or putting fingers into something wet or gooey.

COGNITIVE DEVELOPMENT

Your little one's receptive language skills, what baby understands, are still way ahead of expressive language skills, what baby can say. Around this age, your baby is becoming adept at using body signals to communicate, such as nodding, waving goodbye, pointing and shaking the head for no. But if you pay careful attention, you may notice that amid all the babbling, your baby constantly uses particular sounds ("words") for certain things.

GETTING YOUR CHILD TO LISTEN

During this past year, you've had the luxury of being the center of your baby's universe. It's likely that every time you speak, your baby's ears perk up, and baby turns to you with full attention.

But as your child gets older and interested in more and more things, you might find that it gets harder to capture and keep baby's attention (think about your older kids, or consult any parent of an older child for expert testimony). Getting good at commanding your child's attention in the face of outside forces — such as TV and warring siblings — requires practice. If you start working on your skills now, you'll be one step ahead in helping your child become a better listener, and in making yourself heard:

- *Eliminate background noise.* It's hard for your little one to concentrate if there are a lot of other sounds swirling around.
- *Go to your child.* Don't shout from across the room. Stop what you're doing and go directly to your child. Your child is more likely to hear, understand and respond if you are close.
- *Get down to baby's level.* Being face-to-face helps your child focus attention on you.
- *Say baby's name.* Do this clearly and loudly. Then pause before continuing to allow your child time to shift attention away from current activities to you.
- *Maintain eye contact.* This helps your child stay focused and increases concentration on what you're saying.

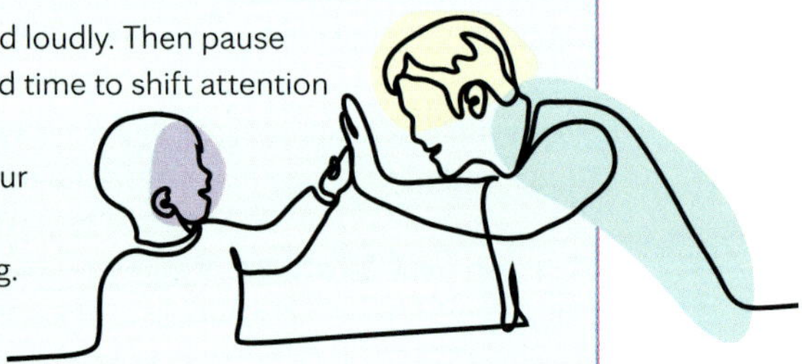

Capitalizing on body language

If you say, "It's time for breakfast!" your child may smile and nod enthusiastically in response. While the two of you are communicating, use signs or hand motions. Doing so will help your youngster communicate immediate needs (and minimize frustration) while learning verbal expression.

Increasing vocabulary

About half of infants have learned their first words by the end of their first year, but it's not unusual for some to wait until their second birthday to really start talking. Boys usually say their first words later than girls.

Other factors affect language development, such as whether your child has a cautious temperament or is the youngest child in a large family. If there's no need to talk, your baby may not view it as a necessary skill just yet.

Also, babies tend to work separately on different skill sets. If walking is a major focus, your child may not have any energy left to work on talking. Once an active toddler is walking well, your child is more likely to devote attention to learning words.

Once first words arrive, vocabulary can increase fairly rapidly in the months that follow. The best way to increase your child's vocabulary is to talk to each other. You want your child not only to hear words but also to hear them as part of an interaction with others. Once you hear your child working on a new word, incorporate it into your conversations. Use it in ways that are easy for your child to understand.

Take the words *mama* and *dada*, for example, which are typically some of the first words a child learns. Hang around parents of young children for any length of time and you'll hear them frequently referring to themselves in the third person: "Do you want mama to help you?" "Can dada put you in the swing?" Doing this accomplishes several things: It reinforces who mama and dada are, places the words in a context that's easy for the child to understand and helps the child learn to vocalize them. So go ahead and do it. It helps!

BILINGUAL BABIES

If you speak a second (or third) language, feel free to use it with your baby. The rule of thumb is that the younger a person is when exposed to a language, the less difficult it will be to learn. A second language is a gift your child can use throughout life.

Some parents are concerned that their child will become confused if presented with two languages at the same time. But there is little evidence to support this concern. In fact, research suggests that the human brain is adaptable enough to learn two languages at the same time just as well as one. Consider also the millions of families around the world who speak more than one language at home and in their communities.

Although bilingual kids may mix words from different languages or attach verb endings from one language to words in another, research shows that eventually they sort it out. If they consistently use one language over another, that language may become the dominant one. For example, if English and French are both spoken at home but English is used everywhere else, English is likely to become the dominant language. Nonetheless, the child can still become skilled in French if the language is used often enough.

Even if your partner doesn't share your second language, you can still expose your baby to it by using it to narrate your day, read books in that language or have the same kinds of "conversations" with your baby that you would have in your family's primary language. It will be worth it when you hear your child say those first words — in each language.

SOCIAL DEVELOPMENT

At birth, your baby had no sense of self as a separate entity from you or the rest of the world. But from about 8 months or so, your child starts to figure it out: "Hey, I'm Sam. I have my own face, hands, fingers and toes. I can wriggle my body when I want, and when my parent makes a funny face, I can make it myself!"

You might notice this when you and your child are in front of a mirror. Before, your baby may have thought the image in the mirror was a different baby. Now your child is starting to recognize the image and may touch the nose or pull a strand of hair to confirm the physical feeling with the actions in the

TOYS AND GAMES

This is often a good month to introduce toys that complement your toddler's growing skills, such as cruising, walking or sorting through objects.

Push toys

These are toys your child can push around while standing upright, such as a toy grocery cart or stroller. Such a toy can help your child practice walking while still offering some support. Stay close, though, to offer a hand when your child gets tired of pushing.

Fill a basket

Place a variety of small, non-hazardous objects in a basket or plastic bowl. Let your child sort through the items, dump them out and put them back in again. You'll be surprised at how entertaining this can be for your little one.

Play catch

Although your child can't catch a ball in midair yet, baby will have fun corralling a rolled ball.

Godzilla

Give your child a chance to unleash some energy and laugh in the process by building a tower of soft blocks for your child to knock down. In a few months, baby will have the skills to build a tower with no help — just to knock it down again, of course.

Create an exploration zone

As your child begins to pull up to stand and cruise, place some interesting objects on a low table. This will give your child extra motivation to stand and move around while holding on to the table.

mirror. When you make a face in the mirror, your baby may try to copy you while watching the reflection.

As this idea of self-concept grows, it affects the way your child interacts with the world. You may notice a growing self-confidence, as well as a newfound wariness of things that may previously have had little to no effect on your child.

Increased assertiveness

The more practiced children become at new skills, the more assertive they are likely to become. This growing independence is good and a sign of healthy development, but it raises the potential for the first power struggles between you and your child. Your child may begin to refuse certain foods, demand more privileges or protest your restrictions more loudly.

With these clear likes and dislikes, your baby's personality starts to shine through. For example, you can now see evidence of your baby's amazing persistence when baby insists on finding that hidden object. Or when your child crawls off to play alone for a while after being surrounded by other people, you realize that baby may need some downtime before interacting with people again.

11TH MONTH MILESTONES

During the 11th month, your baby is busy:

- Mastering crawling
- Standing with support
- Pulling up to stand
- Standing alone for a few seconds, perhaps, or even taking a few steps
- Holding on to furniture to walk around (cruising)
- Using thumb and first finger together (pincer grasp)
- Manipulating toys appropriately
- Learning to let go voluntarily
- Using gestures to communicate
- Feeding self
- Recognizing and responding to familiar words
- Babbling, stringing syllables together
- Saying mama and dada
- Verbalizing other familiar words
- Looking for hidden toys
- Imitating the activities of adults and older kids
- Testing limits and observing parental reactions
- Becoming more assertive
- Avoiding strangers yet interacting more with family

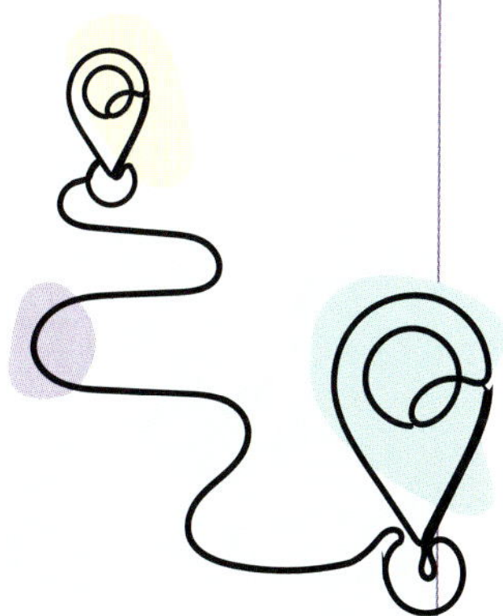

Newfound fears

As your baby's brain continues to develop, so do the perception of danger and the sense of fear. This is a primal step in the development of a child's judgment and ability to recognize unsafe situations. Things that may not have bothered your child before, such as the dark, thunder or loud noises, may now become scary and provoke intense feelings of fear. At this point, it's easier to remove or minimize the sources of fear than to attempt to rationalize them. For example, you might install a night-light in your child's room or leave a closet light on at night. If a scary something is impossible to avoid, stay close and calm. Eventually, based on your reaction and comfort, baby will learn there's nothing to be afraid of in these situations.

CHAPTER 30

Month 12

This month marks the end of your baby's first year. Your baby has changed dramatically in the past 12 months. During those first days and weeks, you may have wondered if you would ever understand each other and work as a team. Now you can read your baby's moods and cues and respond with exactly what's needed. Your baby also understands you and knows how to thrill you, make you smile and even exasperate you.

You've changed, too. While your baby has become more independent and communicative, you've become a more confident and interactive parent. Congratulations! It's not easy becoming a parent, but it's definitely doable. And although this is the last month of year one, it's really only the beginning of many adventures to come.

The confidence you've developed and your ability to understand and communicate with your baby are your best tools in the months ahead. No one knows your child as well as you do. As your little one makes the transition from infant to toddler, your in-depth knowledge of your child will help you provide the challenges, support and assurance that are needed.

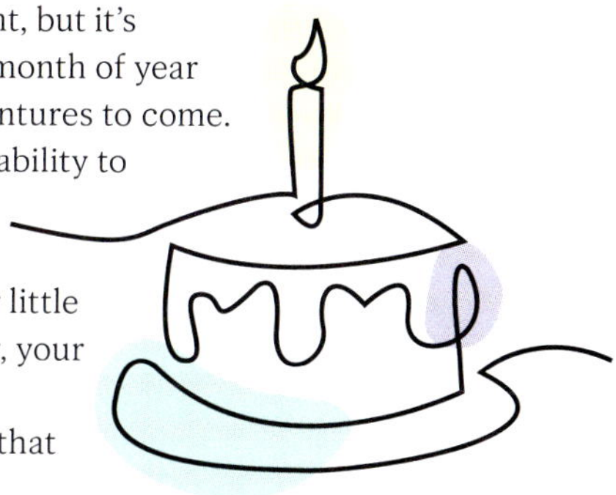

GROWTH AND APPEARANCE

What a difference 12 months can make! For most babies, birth weight has tripled by the end of the first year. So if your baby weighed 7 pounds 8 ounces at birth, your baby now is likely to be between 21 and 23 pounds.

During the first year, most babies grow about 10 inches from birth. The average baby is now between 28 and 32 inches tall. The typical head size at 12 months is about 18 inches, up 4 inches from a newborn size of approximately 14 inches. Some babies may have only one tooth at this stage; others may have up to 12 or more.

SPOT CHECK: WHAT'S GOING ON THIS MONTH

Here's a snapshot of what your baby's basic care looks like in the 12th month.

Eating

By now, your baby's diet probably includes foods with various textures and flavors. But the amount your baby eats at a meal may seem very small. Many parents become concerned that their babies aren't eating enough. Keep in mind that portions for a 12-month-old are pretty small compared with an adult's, perhaps barely ¼ cup from each food group. And as babies transition into the second year, their appetite tends to drop and become more unpredictable. Altogether, this might translate into a meal of a few tablespoons of cooked carrots, two bites of rice, a taste of meat and several bites of pears.

Focus on your baby's signs of hunger and thirst rather than how much is left on the plate. Allow baby to stop eating when full, rather than coaxing or playing tricks to get more food in. If you make a healthy selection of foods available, your child won't starve or lose significant weight.

Keep giving your baby breast milk or formula. Both are important sources of nutrition. If you've decided to wean your baby from breastfeeding, replace the breast milk with iron-fortified formula. After the first birthday, you can gradually transition your baby to drinking whole milk with meals.

Sleeping

Most 11- to 12-month-olds sleep as long as 10 to 12 hours at night and take a couple of naps during the day. Most babies still need two naps a day, but some start giving up their morning naps around this time. If that's the case for your baby, try starting the afternoon nap a little earlier and make bedtime a little earlier as well. This will help avoid overtiredness. Pay attention to your child's cues, too, and adjust the sleeping schedule to accommodate the need for sleep.

By 11 to 12 months, nighttime feedings are generally no longer needed. Nursing or taking a bottle at night is likely to be for comfort, not because of hunger. If your baby is still waking up for feedings and you want to work toward sleeping through the night, try gradually shorter nursing sessions or smaller bottles. Eventually you can cut down to none at all. Also look at your child's bedtime routine. Place your child in bed while tired but still awake so that baby learns how to go to sleep without help.

Childhood experts and medical professionals use a baby's first birthday as a natural benchmark for many milestones, but keep in mind that all babies will continue to grow and develop at their own unique rates. What's important is not that your baby's height and weight numbers match up with national averages but that your child is following a steady growth curve.

In the same way, the typical range for many developmental milestones is quite wide, so don't be concerned if your baby isn't walking or talking yet, or is still very leery of strangers. The first birthday is magical only in the sense that loved ones make it so in celebration of reaching that one-year milestone. However, in terms of measuring development, it's much less significant. Your baby will begin doing all the things that are expected, whether it's a few months before or a few months after the big birthday bash.

MOVEMENT

Your child has learned so much in a year. In a matter of months, your baby has gone from struggling to hold up the head to learning how to sit, crawl, cruise and maybe even walk. Where once your child was able only to bat at large objects with closed fists, baby can now pick up an item as small as a crumb. This is all a result of the rapid development of your baby's nervous system, which is now a much more efficient conductor of messages from brain to muscles and vice versa.

Sitting

Not only can your baby sit for lengthy periods without toppling over, but now baby can pivot while seated to reach a toy or to turn toward you. Your baby also can easily get in and out of a sitting position at will.

IT'S A PARTY!

At the end of this year, the whole family deserves a party — perhaps for the family more so than baby, who likely won't grasp the significance of the event until around age 3. In any case, it's a traditional time to celebrate, and why not? For many families, the baby's first birthday marks the end of a period of labor-intensive parenting. There's more to come, sure, but colicky evenings, breastfeeding struggles and chronic sleep deprivation are now largely behind you. It's time for cake!

Hosting a large party to celebrate your baby's first birthday might seem appealing. Still, consider if a smaller celebration with immediate family may be more fun for baby. At 1 year of age, many babies may not enjoy a large, noisy gathering of friends and neighbors. Even if your little one is the social type, you might still want to limit the party to an hour or so, to avoid meltdowns.

Standing and bending

During this month, about half of babies gain enough balance to stand alone for a few seconds or even longer. This opens up a whole new level of vision and reach, as baby can now play with toys above ground level. At the same time, about a quarter of infants are learning to bend down while standing to recover an item from the floor.

Walking

Between months 11 and 12, some babies achieve another significant milestone — learning to walk. Walking is a complex activity that requires coordination, balance and a good dose of confidence. A key stage in learning how to walk independently is learning to lift first one foot and then the other so that baby is briefly standing on one leg. Your baby practices doing this while cruising around holding on to furniture for support.

When your baby first shows an interest in taking steps, walk with your baby, holding the hands and praising efforts to move forward. Once baby signals readiness to walk alone, crouch down a short distance away with your arms out, and encourage baby to walk toward you. Pretty soon, look out — there goes your toddler! First steps are always exciting. It's good to stand back and let your baby practice, but continue to stay close. It takes a while to get the hang of walking without help.

Don't fret if your baby doesn't seem to be interested in walking just yet. A few babies start walking as early as 9 months, but others wait until 15 months or later to take the plunge.

Getting up and down stairs

Even before walking well, your baby likely will figure out how to get up a set of stairs, which involves a mix of crawling and walking maneuvers. In a few weeks, usually sometime between 12 and 15 months, children learn to go down the stairs, too, most often by sliding down feet first on their tummies.

Getting up and down stairs is an important skill to learn, but you'll want to be close by whenever your child is working on it, to catch any slips and avoid tumbles that are bound to happen.

Hand and finger skills

Your baby's refined pincer grasp at 12 months allows for picking up objects with ease. When reading a book together, your child can turn the pages with a little bit of help. Later, your child will use these same skills to learn to draw, paint, write, and work buttons and zippers.

Most babies can hold an object in each hand by this age and enjoy banging the objects together. Your baby may even have figured out how to hold two objects in one hand and how to put them into a container. Your child also may throw toys to the side when they lose appeal or to pick up something more interesting. But your fickle juggler won't have much control over throwing aim.

Between 11 and 12 months old, many infants are getting a better grasp of their eating and drinking utensils, both literally and figuratively. Your baby may know how to pick up a cup and drink from it but may not be able to set it down just yet, and will probably drop it if you don't take it. Baby is also getting better at using a spoon and has probably discovered that spoons make good toys (especially if they're filled with food).

SENSORY DEVELOPMENT

By the end of the first year, your child's senses are working together in a coordinated fashion to make your child aware of the outside world. As sights and sounds around the house become routine, your child learns to filter out distractions and better focus on things of interest, such as eating a meal or listening to a favorite story.

Looking and listening

Your baby's hearing is sharper now, and baby listens with greater attention. In fact, your baby can look and listen at the same time, making reading books together that much more enjoyable. If you think your baby isn't hearing well, talk to your baby's medical professional about a hearing assessment.

Touch

Babies at this age still enjoy singular sensations, such as feeling different textures or pouring water from one container into another. For some adventure as your baby learns to walk, let baby go barefoot on different surfaces, such as on soft grass or in a puddle of water. Your baby also enjoys human touch and loves to return hugs and kisses, although not always on demand.

At age 1, your baby still explores using fingers and mouth together. Anything your baby picks up will be taste-tested.

SAFETY CHECK

As your baby learns to stand, cruise and walk, the risk of injury increases. Being aware of your baby's ability to move farther and faster is the first step in reducing this risk. It may seem surprising that your baby can get into something that a week earlier was out of reach.

Take time out every few days to get down to the baby's level and look around each room. What new temptations do you see?

Injuries are most common at times when the family is occupied, such as dinnertime. Your baby is active and impulsive. When you're busy and stressed, it's easy to lose sight of the baby for just a second.

For more information on childproofing your home, see Chapter 17.

COGNITIVE DEVELOPMENT

Brain imaging studies of sleeping babies from infancy to 2 years old reveal that the total volume of a baby's brain increases by over 100% during the first year of life. Pretty amazing, isn't it? No wonder a baby's head size grows so much — it has to accommodate all that growth in gray and white matter.

The older your baby gets, the greater the myelination of your baby's nerves — the process where nerves become encased in a fatty sheath called myelin. This makes them stronger and more efficient messengers. Myelination helps bring more and more areas of the brain into use.

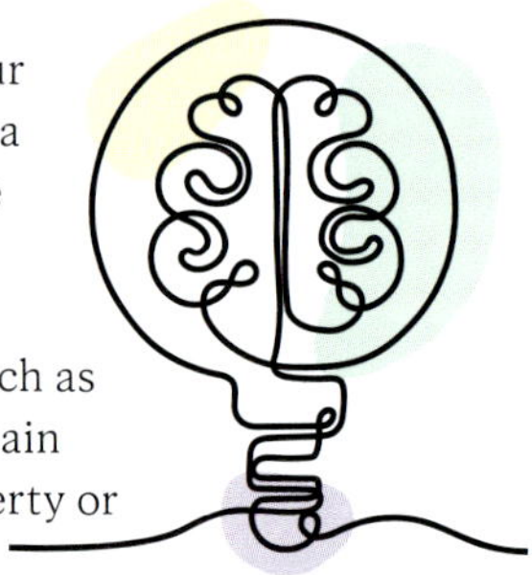

Some areas of the brain don't mature until much later — such as a part known as the reticular formation, which helps you maintain attention. This area doesn't become fully myelinated until puberty or later. The frontal lobes, responsible for executive thinking and judgment, don't become fully myelinated until adulthood (and you thought impulsive teenagers were just out to give a parent gray hair).

TOYS AND GAMES

Through the end of the first year and beyond, your baby will still enjoy toys and games that use and build motor skills. Games that involve picking up and dropping objects will likely be entertaining. At 12 months, your baby's play may range from exercising large muscles to working and mastering fine motor skills. Baby will likely think it's fun to push, throw and knock down everything.

When walking down the toy aisle of your local retail store, it may be easy to get carried away because there's so much to choose from. When purchasing a toy for your child, keep in mind the fun factor, as well as the fact that many objects will still go in your child's mouth. Toys can certainly be educational, but try to stick with something appropriate for your child's level of development. If a toy or game is too difficult for your child to comprehend, your child will quickly lose interest. And while toy manufacturers may think of their products as the perfect developmental aid, there's nothing that beats interaction with you when it comes to helping your baby grow and learn. Here are some ideas to get you started.

Find open space

Often the best thing you can do when your child is learning how to crawl and walk is to allow plenty of space for moving around. This could be at a park if the weather is nice or at a community recreation center or kids' gym. If you have older children who are taking a class in a gym or other open area, such as ballet or karate, take your baby along. There may be an open area for your younger child to practice moving around where you can supervise while also watching your older children.

Increasingly complex thinking

By age 1, your baby is starting to gain control of the limbic system. This is the area of the brain responsible for emotions, appetites and basic urges. It's also responsible for information processing and directing incoming information from the outside world to the appropriate areas of the brain. Thus, a 1-year-old's thinking gains in complexity and starts to contain longer chains of thoughts. If you offer two toys, for example, the child will likely make a choice between the two rather than trying to grab both. Or if there is a toy with a blanket over it, your baby may use knowledge of cause and effect and pull the blanket off to get to the toy.

Understanding

The part of the brain involved with understanding is maturing as well. By the end of the first year, babies are beginning to respond to one-step commands. For example, your child may hold on to you on request when you pull up the child's pants to get dressed. Or your baby may give you a kiss when you ask.

Your baby also may show understanding of simple questions, such as "Is that a puppy?" when pointing at a picture of a puppy in a familiar book.

Walk together

Practice walking together with your baby by holding hands. Gradually baby will move to holding one hand only and then just a finger. Soon you'll be able to take a step back and let your baby walk toward you. Let your baby try out different surfaces, too, such as warm sand, soft grass or a shallow puddle.

Crayons

Some babies start to scribble around 12 months or so. Give your child a crayon and a piece of paper and see what happens. Show baby how it works and see what your child does. Baby may be delighted at the results, and so will you.

Pull toys

As a result of improving hand skills, your child can pull along a toy if it has a string or ribbon attached. Pulling a toy can be just as fun as pushing one around.

Water toys

A book in the bath? Little ones love sitting in the tub and flipping through a waterproof picture book. Your child also might enjoy bathtub paints and crayons that rinse right off with the bath water. Water is fascinating to kids, and many will be content to simply pour it from one cup to another. Just be sure to always supervise your child around water to avoid any possibility of drowning. Remember, if the phone rings or the doorbell sounds, don't leave your child in the bathtub alone.

Language

Speaking develops more slowly than understanding, and it won't be until the second or third year that your child's vocabulary begins to expand dramatically. And it may take even longer for people outside the family to understand what your child is saying.

Still, the beginnings of speech are at hand. More than half of babies can say at least one word, such as *uh-oh* or *doggie*, by the age of 1 in addition to *mama* and *dada*. Some may even know two or three words. Continue to encourage your baby's exploration of words by listening intently and responding to the baby's jabbering. Repeat new words your baby is learning, and verbally name gestures that baby already uses for communication.

If you're concerned about your child's speech development, try to discover what baby is channeling energies toward. Perhaps your child is spending more time standing, cruising and walking. Eventually, once these skills are mastered, speaking will become a priority. Allow your baby to learn these skills in baby's own time frame.

You should also know that how well your baby understands language is a better measure of language development than are the words your baby can say.

SOCIAL DEVELOPMENT

Your baby may be on the road toward independence but still has lots to learn. Some of the fear that accompanies that early independence is starting to fade as your child becomes more sure of a place in the family. However, you and other family members will still be the ones your baby relies on for safety and security.

Veni, vidi, vici

Your baby is starting to take up Julius Caesar's famous motto, "I came, I saw, I conquered." Everything is up for mastery. Early signs of your baby's drive for independence include self-feeding, drinking from a cup and being able to move about without help. For most youngsters, the thrilling part of learning to walk is gaining more control over the world. The world is no longer limited to what comes to them; now they can go out and conquer it. This independence can be both exciting and intimidating.

Tantrums

Although tantrums become more common during a child's second year, you may be noticing the first signs of your baby's temper. Your almost-1-year-old may get upset when something is taken away or when baby doesn't get what baby wants. As a drive for independence and mastery run up against still-limited abilities and your parental limits, your child may feel frustrated and mad. Some children express these feelings more loudly and intensely than do others, depending on their personalities (see Chapter 10 for more on temperament and behavior).

When you see your child becoming irritable, more often than not it's a sign that baby is tired or hungry. This is true even for older children and adults. If your baby is out of sorts or seems increasingly resistant to your efforts at soothing, your best bet may be to head for a nap rather than repeated attempts at discipline. Keep in mind that your baby may need to vent a little before actually falling asleep.

Saying no

By now, your child understands what you mean when you say the word no. It's just that everything in your home is so fascinating — including pot handles, fireplaces, holiday decorations, the way the water swirls in the toilet, and your pet's whiskers, tail and food. Your child's desire to explore is stronger than the desire to listen to your warnings. This isn't a sign of defiance, just your baby's natural, irrepressible curiosity.

As much as possible, remove valuable or dangerous objects that tempt your baby. For the remaining objects, keep a close watch and be prepared to move your persistent baby away from dangerous objects or offer a distraction. If the object remains in the room, expect that your child will likely go right back to what you just said no to. Try hard to reserve the word no for those things that can harm your baby. (Easier said than done!)

For situations that require caution, such as playing with a friend or the family pet, you can also teach your baby the meanings of "be gentle" and "be soft" or give other specific direction.

12TH MONTH MILESTONES

During the 12th month, your baby is busy:

- Standing alone
- Cruising
- Maybe taking first steps
- Using pincer grasp accurately
- Manipulating toys appropriately
- Feeding self
- Learning to let go voluntarily
- Looking and listening simultaneously
- Increasing attention span
- Using gestures to communicate
- Recognizing and responding to familiar words
- Increasing vocabulary
- Responding to one-step commands and simple questions
- Imitating the activities of adults and older kids
- Testing limits and expressing frustration
- Still being wary of strangers but very affectionate with family

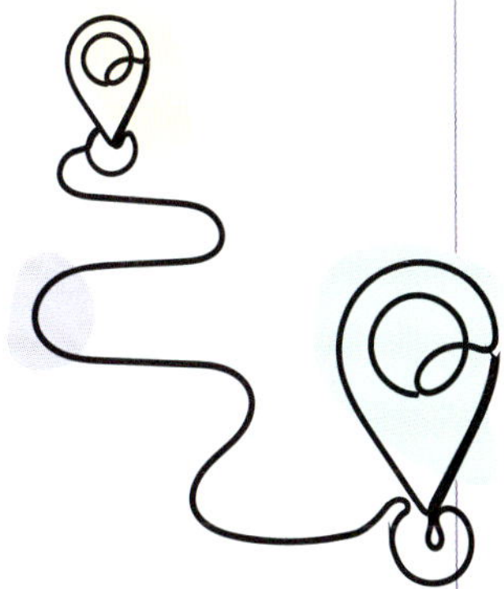

Relating to others

Most children this age are very affectionate with family members and enjoy snuggling and cuddling up for lap time. But don't be surprised if your child's wariness of strangers continues through these months. Many children have a fear of strangers past their first birthdays. Others have shorter stages, and many even have on-and-off periods of stranger anxiety.

CHAPTER 31

Months 13 to 15

Welcome to the toddler years! This phase is often bittersweet. You're proud when your toddler reaches major milestones — taking first steps, building tall towers with favorite blocks, learning new words. But you're also watching your baby grow up and make those first moves toward needing you a little less.

For your toddler, this is a time of feeling torn between two worlds: one in which your child wants to test newfound skills and explore without help; and one in which your child clings to you, not quite ready to be independent.

It can be frustrating for parents as toddlers move back and forth between independence and clinginess. Still, no matter how independent your toddler can be at times, you can bet that when the world feels a little scary, safety and comfort can be found in your arms.

So if it feels like you're back to square one in parenthood, know that all this is just part of raising a toddler. The knowledge and skills you picked up in the first year of your child's life will serve you well as you learn and grow as a parent during the next few years.

As children grow, their development starts to vary more compared to their peers. You may notice your child making lots of progress in one area, such as language, while skills in other areas develop more slowly. As long as your child is making progress, it's likely that other areas will take off next. Still, if you have concerns, talk to your child's medical professional.

GROWTH AND APPEARANCE

Toddlerhood marks a time of major change in your child's appearance. Between 13 and 15 months, most toddlers have a certain look: rounded facial features, short legs and arms that are soft rather than muscular, a long torso and a belly that sticks out when standing up. Over the months ahead, and as your toddler becomes more active, the baby fat will give way to a leaner, more muscular appearance and the limbs will gradually get longer. Brain growth is still substantial, and your toddler's head will increase in size by about 2 centimeters — a little less than 1 inch — over the course of the year ahead.

As you may have noticed, your toddler's growth is much slower now than it was in the first year of life. Moving forward, growth occurs at a steadier pace. On average, toddlers gain 3 to 5 pounds total during the second year. By the end of this period, an average girl will weigh about 23 pounds and measure 30.5 inches in height, while an average boy will weigh about 24.5 pounds and measure 31 inches tall.

Your child's medical professional will keep track of your child's growth and check that it's following a typical growth curve. Compared to the earlier years, what constitutes a typical range is much broader in toddlers.

SPOT CHECK: WHAT'S GOING ON

Here's a snapshot of what your toddler's basic care looks like at this age.

Eating

Your toddler isn't just becoming independent when it comes to movement. Your child also is now becoming better at self-feeding, learning to use sippy cups, and deciding which foods are tastiest. Don't be surprised if this increasing independence goes hand in hand with picky eating and refusal to eat certain foods. Though it can be frustrating, keep offering a variety of healthy options and let your toddler decide which of the foods to eat and how much to eat. This can help your child feel a bit more in control and prevent a mealtime power struggle. See Chapter 4 for more on feeding your toddler.

If you're still breastfeeding and comfortable doing so, continue offering breast milk. Your child still gets the nutritional benefits. Make plans to eliminate bottle-feeding by 18 months, since extended use of the bottle has been linked to obesity and dental cavities. Introduce the use of a spoon at mealtime if you haven't already done so. This can be an exciting step up into toddlerhood.

Sleeping

How much sleep a toddler needs varies, depending on factors such as temperament, health, activity level, and growth. However, most toddlers need between 11 and 14 hours of sleep. Many will still take a nap or sometimes two during the day. If your child decides not to nap, offer quiet time to unwind instead.

As always, keep in mind that height and weight numbers on growth charts are just averages. Your child may fall below or above these; what's important is that your child is thriving and following an established growth curve.

MOVEMENT

A toddler's developing motor skills center on getting around and exploring the environment. Your child may crawl, climb, cruise alongside furniture or walk to accomplish this.

It can be nerve-racking to watch your toddler attempting new feats, but they're essential to development. Restraining children who want to explore or test new skills can leave them doubting their abilities or feeling insecure or frustrated. Instead, recognize that as your child tries new things, there will be inevitable bumps in the road. Learning to walk will lead to a tumble here and there.

Over the course of the months ahead, your child will master the necessary skills to get around without help. In the meantime, stay close by and build confidence by offering support and encouragement — and comfort if there are some bumps or scrapes.

Walking and climbing

If your toddler hasn't already started walking independently, you're no doubt looking forward to those first steps. On average, toddlers start walking between 12 and 15 months, but plenty of children start walking either sooner or later than this age range.

Walking early isn't a yardstick for how intelligent a child is or a measure of future physical abilities. Learning to walk later typically doesn't become a

MILK AND IRON DEFICIENCY

Whole milk is recommended for toddlers from 1 to 2 years old because it's best for a child's brain development. However, drinking too much milk may cause your child to be less interested in eating other nutritious foods, which, in turn, can lead to conditions such as iron deficiency and anemia. Anemia is a medical condition characterized by a low red blood cell count. It interferes with blood's ability to carry oxygen. If your child is drinking 2 to 3 cups (16 to 24 ounces) of whole milk daily, there's no need to be concerned. However, if your child consumes more than this or seems to forgo balanced meals in favor of drinking milk, consider talking with your child's medical provider about whether an iron supplement might be helpful. Children this age should be getting at least 7 milligrams of iron a day.

concern unless your child isn't walking by 18 months old.

Early on, walking is often done with knees bent, feet set wide apart and toes pointed out. Your child may appear to walk "bowlegged." Some toddlers, excited by their newfound abilities, appear to be in frequent danger of plowing headfirst into the ground. This is common and your child will eventually transition to a more confident stride as balance improves.

Until your child is ready to walk, you'll likely find your toddler crawling, cruising along furniture or reaching for your hand. Offering your fingertips to help your child will give just enough support to stabilize those little legs.

Some toddlers get a little cranky as they concentrate on learning to walk independently. Learning a new skill can be stressful for a toddler! But you can generally expect a big improvement in mood once walking starts. Toddlers typically become very happy with their newfound mode of transportation and independence, and they're mighty proud of what they've accomplished.

You'll also need to be extra cautious around stairs — a keen source of interest for many toddlers. At this age, they'll be climbing up them and trying to learn how to get back down. Be prepared to help out. And if you haven't already,

TOYS AND GAMES

Toys are a critical part of development as your child enters toddlerhood. What may look like a simple game of playing with dolls or stuffed animals is actually laying the foundation for communication skills. Encourage the use of words in pretend dialogue and scenarios that help your child practice social engagement. Toys play a significant role in social development, hone fine motor skills and help keep your child physically active.

But your child isn't the only one who gets to have fun. Toys provide the perfect tools for you to bond with your child through play and one-on-one interaction.

Reading

You can help foster your child's language skills by continuing to read together every day. Choose books that encourage your child to touch and point to objects and that have an enjoyable writing style, such as rhyming.

Low-tech

High-tech toys aren't necessarily best, even if they say they're "educational." There's currently no research that backs up the claims that toys such as tablets or apps are as good for a child's cognitive development as traditional toys. In fact, toys with too many features can distract a child and may leave little room for imagination. High-tech toys can also interfere with parent-child bonding, a drawback that's particularly true for digital toys. More often than not, such toys are considered more entertaining than educational.

install safety gates and other childproofing measures to help keep your toddler safe and give you peace of mind. See Chapter 17 for more on home and outdoor safety.

Skilled hands

Those first steps tend to get all the attention. However, your child is also learning to master hand skills. This will allow your child to better grasp and examine objects. The ability to grasp things between the thumb and index finger allows your child to build towers, better use a fork or spoon, and more easily turn the pages of a book — to name just a few skills. In fact, this is a good time to introduce a spoon to mealtimes, if you haven't yet done so.

SENSORY DEVELOPMENT

Your child's interest in exploring the world and playing is helping to fine-tune not only motor skills but also key vision and hearing abilities.

As a low-cost alternative, encourage your child to play with everyday things you can find around the home, such as wooden spoons, cardboard boxes and empty food containers, as well as board books, dolls and simple puzzles. Open-ended toys that have many uses, such as blocks, can test problem-solving skills, introduce math concepts, aid children in understanding how things fit together, and stimulate the imagination to conceive and build things such as bridges, palaces and fortresses. In general, choose toys that help your child hone new skills.

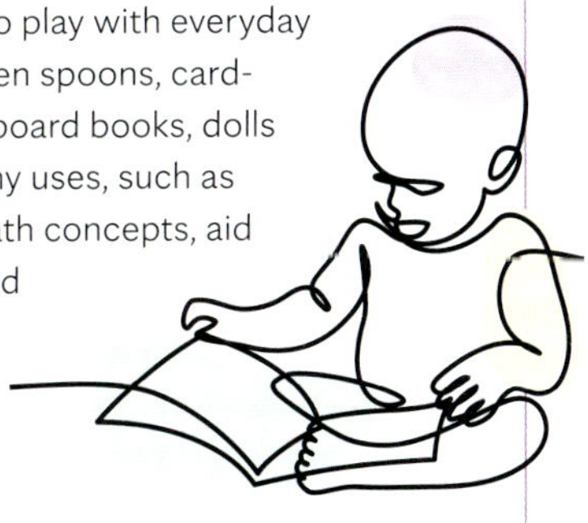

For all ages

Objects that span the various stages of toddlerhood are a good investment, such as toy animals, action figures, dolls, and trucks and cars. As a very young toddler, your child may simply place plastic animals in a box and carry them around as part of a prized collection. When your toddler is older, the figures may be used as characters in an elaborate story your child creates. Crayons, finger paints and paper are sure to provide fun for years to come.

Alphabet

It's not too early to introduce children to letters and written words. Books, magnetic letters and letter crafts can help develop early language skills.

Vision

By this age, your child has an improved sense of distance and can throw objects with a fair degree of accuracy. Activities such as rolling a ball, scribbling with crayons and putting together simple puzzles are laying the groundwork for improved hand-eye coordination later on.

Hearing

At this stage, your child is able to listen and generally follow simple instructions, such as "Bring the ball to me." Your child also can participate in conversations, answering simple yes-or-no questions. Your toddler will enjoy listening and following along as you read stories from a picture book, an activity that can expand your little one's vocabulary.

If your child has difficulties following directions, appears to ignore you or isn't using words in a meaningful way, talk with your child's medical professional. Your child may need to take a screening test for hearing or an audiology exam that checks your child's response to sound.

COGNITIVE DEVELOPMENT

For toddlers, playing is learning, so expect to see your child concentrating on playing like it's a job. Almost everything your child interacts with — whether it be a puzzle or plastic containers with lids — has the potential to sharpen your child's problem-solving skills. These activities also can help your child gather more information about how things work in the world.

Imitation

Your child is no longer content with using objects in random ways. Instead, you'll see your child using them to copy you — for example, pretending to cook by stirring a pot, imitating you drinking coffee using an empty cup or pretending to talk to a grandparent on a toy phone. Your child may invite you to play along. Sometimes your child will want to help you with the household chores. Let your child help you do simple tasks, such as sweeping or wiping cabinets.

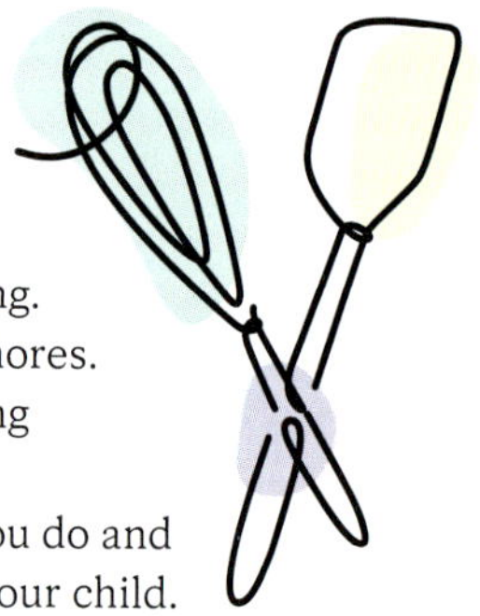

Of course, imitation also means your child is watching what you do and say. Take the opportunity to model behaviors you want to see in your child. Quite often, children learn better by example than by verbal instruction.

Separation

Your toddler is beginning to understand that when you leave, it doesn't mean you're gone for good. Toddlers will still have some separation anxiety, but parents will notice that the amount of time they spend getting upset is decreasing. And most likely you're probably more upset about the separation than your child is. However, try not to let on how much it may bother you. While young, your child is quickly understanding that a good protest might get you to stay.

When you leave, offer an affectionate goodbye and say that you'll be returning. It's best to avoid sneaking out, as this may make your child uncertain or anxious that you might disappear again without notice. When you return home, provide your child with warm, undivided attention. This helps to cement the idea that though you have to leave sometimes, you will return.

Judgment

The relationship between cause and effect is still beyond your toddler's understanding. As a result, your child will continue to depend on your steady guidance to prevent injuries. Your little one may begin to understand that an oven is where you put food to make it hot, but won't necessarily make the connection that touching a hot oven can result in a burn.

Language

Does it seem like your toddler understands most of what you say? That's because your child does! Your child's ability to comprehend language is improving every day, and you'll notice a lot of interest in simple stories, songs and rhymes. It's an exciting time, as a whole new world of communication with your child is opening up. Your child is also listening intently to your conversations, so you'll probably find yourself employing the age-old tactic of spelling out words you don't want your child to hear ("Should we order D-E-S-S-E-R-T?").

Language is another area of child development where a lot of variation exists. Some children start talking and never seem to stop, while others may not say a lot. In general, boys tend to develop language skills at a slower pace than girls. However, understanding what is being said typically outpaces being able to say words at this age. This difference will lessen in the year ahead.

By 15 months, your child may understand 70 or so words, but only use about six meaningfully. In addition to words like *mama* or *dada* that your child may have been saying for a while, your child also may try to identify household pets, relatives and items around the home. Even if your child can't pronounce words and names accurately just yet, the brain is developing the ability to make connections between objects and their names. For example, many toddlers can point to parts of their body or an object in a book when asked.

At the same time, your child won't always be able to let you know about wants or needs through words. This won't stop your child from trying to get requests across in other, not-so-subtle ways, such as banging on the table for more food.

You can build your toddler's vocabulary by using words your child knows to form sentences. For example, if your toddler points and says "car" when a car drives down the street, add some detail, such as "We see a red car." You can also explain everyday events, such as "Here comes the mail carrier. He puts mail in our mailbox." It's also a good time to move away from singsong baby talk. Provide a basis for learning how to speak well by using short sentences containing simple words that your child can understand. Some children also will begin asking very basic questions, such as "Out?" if they want to play outside.

It's likely that you and other close family and friends are the only ones who understand your child right now — and even you may be struggling some of the time. At this age, about 25% of what your child says can be understood. As your child explores the use of language to convey needs and make observations, the inevitable mispronunciations will happen. When your child mispronounces a word, it's OK to correct, but do so gently. For example, if your child says "tuck," you can answer, "Yes, that's a big truck."

SOCIAL DEVELOPMENT

During these early years, a toddler's point of view is primarily self-centered. A 1-year-old's world is instinctively focused on personal needs and wants. Sharing toys with another child at this age, for example, isn't typically voluntary and can create friction if it's forced.

Overriding this natural focus on the self with a growing awareness and accommodation of the thoughts and feelings of others is a key social skill that children develop over time — years, in fact. Understanding this phase of development can help a parent gently guide a young child toward a healthy sense of empathy and the ability to interact with others.

Children this age don't always enjoy playing together. They may observe each other or just like being around other children. However, playtime often involves more parallel play — playing near other children but not really interacting with them.

MILESTONES FOR MONTHS 13 TO 15

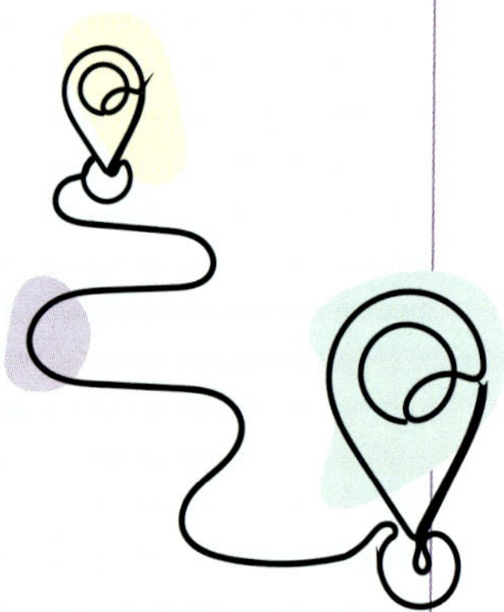

By the end of this period, your toddler is busy:

- Walking without help, or by holding your hand
- Crawling up stairs
- Throwing a ball
- Turning pages of a book
- Stacking two or three blocks
- Making a line with a crayon and scribbling
- Following simple commands
- Responding to their name
- Pointing to show wants or needs
- Imitating your actions, such as stirring an empty bowl with a spoon
- Giving hugs
- Working on language skills, such as naming familiar objects (although it may still sound a little like gibberish) and saying "no" to be independent; they may say 4 to 6 words

IT'S TANTRUM TIME

You've heard of the "terrible twos," right? But what you may not have realized is that this period can start well before the second birthday. One minute you are standing in the frozen food aisle at the supermarket next to your calm child. The next minute your toddler is having a meltdown on the floor because you said no to a box of waffles. And you're standing there feeling more than a little frazzled and avoiding the stares of other shoppers.

Though it can be easier said than done, do your best to stay calm. Even the best-behaved kids have these moments, and they're certainly not a reflection of your parenting skills. Most tantrums are the result of your child's inability to effectively tell you about feelings or needs, or the result of frustration or displaced anger. Being hungry, thirsty or tired can also be a cause for a tantrum.

In most cases, the best way to respond to a tantrum is to ignore it. That includes in public places, though that can be a challenge when others are watching. Often at this age, distracting or steering your child to a different place effectively ends the tantrum. If your child is being particularly disruptive, you may need to move to a private, safe spot for a chance to calm down. Then, when your child is calm, return to the activity. Doing this lets children know that a tantrum is not an effective method to get their way.

Tantrums aren't always preventable. However, there are some ways in which you can head them off before they begin:

- Set a daily routine, including nap time and bedtime, and try to stick to it as much as possible. Routines are especially important for young toddlers.
- Plan ahead, running errands after your child has eaten or taken a nap. Pack toys or other diversions if you expect to spend time waiting.
- If your child isn't communicating clearly yet, show your child how to ask for things — such as more water or food — or express feelings such as being tired through sign language.
- Offer choices. Give your child a couple of options for snacks or what color shirt to wear. This will give your child some sense of control.
- Praise the behavior you want. If your child submits to being buckled into the car seat without a fight, smile and use a happy voice to say how proud you are that you're working together as a team.
- Avoid certain environments. If you know there may be a tantrum risk, avoid the cookie aisle in the grocery store or prioritize quick service when you want to eat out.
- Tantrums tend to happen less often by the age of 3. However, if your child has violent tantrums or you think your child may self-harm or harm others, bring it up with your child's medical professional.

Keeping the peace

When toddlers do interact with each other, it's common for squabbles to break out. The combination of being self-centered and unable to share or take turns often leads to hitting or other aggression. This doesn't mean that play dates are a waste of time, though. Young children need multiple opportunities to develop and practice social skills. You just might need to keep a variety of toys on hand to minimize potential conflicts and be ready to step in as referee.

Remind a child who is possessive with toys that, yes, these toys belong to the child, and playmates are only looking at them or playing with them for a little while. It might help to set aside a few toys your child is particularly fond of for times when other children aren't around. Your toddler may find this an agreeable compromise and be more willing to let children play with other toys.

Physical responses

Even though toddlers are little, they still experience big emotions, and they don't always know what to do with intense feelings. They may scream, hit or kick out of frustration or to get someone's attention. When your child loses control, hold your child to prevent self-harm and harm to others. Show your child how to name emotions. This can help your child better understand feelings and lay the groundwork for future communication and problem-solving skills. For example, you can say, "I see that you're angry because it's time for someone else to take a turn." Mirror your child's facial expression. Then, follow up with "But we don't hit. We use our words." In this way, you help your child identify the emotion but also explain how to handle it.

CHAPTER 32

Months 16 to 18

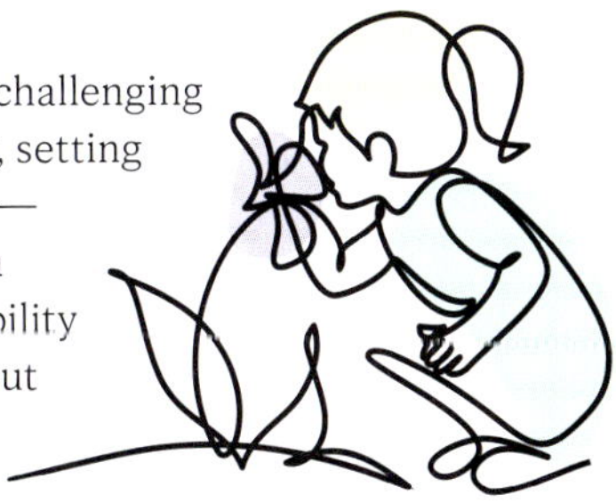

Toddlerhood is a simultaneously rewarding and challenging time. Your child's language skills are blossoming, setting the stage for more interactive — and endearing — conversations. Each day, your toddler becomes a little more independent, eager to show off the ability to run, climb stairs and scribble a drawing without your help.

This is also a time when your child is likely becoming more assertive and isn't afraid to share big feelings — if only you had a dollar for every time you heard the word no come out of your little one's mouth! And those temper tantrums mentioned in Chapter 31 may be on the rise. However, all these are typical and expected developments at this age.

In most cases, it's simply a matter of your child acting as a 1-year-old. Self-control is not something that's developed till well after your child's third birthday. Even then you'll need to help your child cope with emotions and reflexive impulses. Keeping your behavioral expectations in line with your child's age can offer you some comfort when things get a little chaotic.

GROWTH AND APPEARANCE

Slower and steady growth, punctuated by growth spurts, continues during this period as your child slowly sheds the baby look.

On average, toddlers gain about 1½ pounds during this period and about an inch in height. You may notice that as your child's medical professional plots growth on a chart, those lines that used to be straighter or curved now sometimes look more like steps, a pattern that reflects growth spurts.

By 16 months, most kids have their top and bottom front teeth (central incisors), as well as the teeth to the left and right of these (lateral incisors).

SPOT CHECK: WHAT'S GOING ON

Here's a snapshot of what your toddler's basic care looks like this month.

Eating

By 18 months, your child has the hand skills and coordination to use utensils and cups with no problem. Of course, that doesn't mean your child will always want to, and you'll no doubt still find food that's purposely thrown on the floor or used like finger paint on the table. This sort of exploratory food behavior is common and reflects your child's curiosity about how things work.

At this age, picky eating is common. In fact, if you could use one word to describe a toddler's eating habits, it would be *erratic*. Even those who were eager to try almost any food mere months ago may become very selective at mealtime.

Toddlerhood is a time when all the developing senses converge. When it comes to food, that means that taste, appearance, smell and texture all play bigger roles in your child's decisions about what to eat. Patience in the process is crucial. Continue to offer a variety of healthy options and allow your child to choose which and how much of those options to eat. Anticipate that it may take 15 or more tries to get your child to actually eat something new. Offering fun accompaniments, such as dipping sauces, may entice your child to take a bite. For more on toddler nutrition, see Chapter 4.

Sleeping

With so much exploring going on during the day, it can be hard for a toddler to wind down at bedtime. Getting a young child to bed is often one of the most challenging parts of a parent's day. Consistent bedtime routines — such as taking a bath, reading a book and going to bed at the same time every night — can help give your child the structure needed to more easily go to sleep.

Some parents are surprised when their child, who has been sleeping through the night for some time, begins waking again during the night. This can happen for many reasons, including growth spurts, illnesses or changes in routine. However, a regular bedtime routine can help minimize this waking and return your child to a regular sleeping schedule. See Chapter 8 for more on setting up bedtime routines and troubleshooting sleep problems.

MOVEMENT

Between the first and second years, your toddler is gaining physical and movement skills on the double — and learning how to use multiple skills at once!

Multitasking

When children first start walking, they need to keep arms at shoulder level for balance, leaving little room to perform other tasks at the same time, such as carrying a toy. However, after children have been walking for a month or two, they will be able to squat to pick up an object and carry it, as well as push and pull toys, step backward and to the side, and throw a ball overhand without losing their balance. With increased confidence in the ability to get around, your child will begin using physical skills to accomplish desired goals, such as stretching for an object that's out of reach.

Need for speed

Having improved in the mobility department, your child will likely be ready to try running. As with walking, this will take some time to master. Be prepared for a few falls. Early on, your toddler's running style may look pretty stiff and will tend to follow a straight path.

Improved mobility, coupled with a child's natural curiosity, also means your toddler will more easily encounter some unsafe situations. Though it can seem at times that your nerves are being tested on purpose, your child is really just exploring the environment and needs your guidance to stay safe while doing it.

Fingers as tools

At this point, your child is able to pick up very small objects between the thumb and forefinger with ease. Toddlers use this skill to carefully examine objects and perform everyday activities, such as turning doorknobs and book pages.

BYE-BYE BOTTLE

Experts recommend eliminating bottle-feeding after the first year — and no later than 18 months — because of the risk it poses for tooth decay and the potential for overeating and iron deficiency. Drinking from bottles at this age is very often a comfort measure for your child. This is particularly true at bedtime, when the bottle becomes something your child needs to fall asleep. For some children, ditching the bottle is easier said than done. If you're still having difficulty getting your child to give up the bottle, try eliminating bottles one by one. Start with the afternoon bottle, then move on to the evening and morning bottles. Save the bedtime bottle for last. You can also try putting only water in the bottle. However, never leave a bottle in the crib with your baby overnight.

Getting dressed

Putting on clothes becomes a team effort as your child shows off this newly acquired skill. Your child may assist you with pulling a shirt over the head or removing mittens, shoes and socks. With an improved thumb and forefinger grip, some toddlers may be able to unzip their coats.

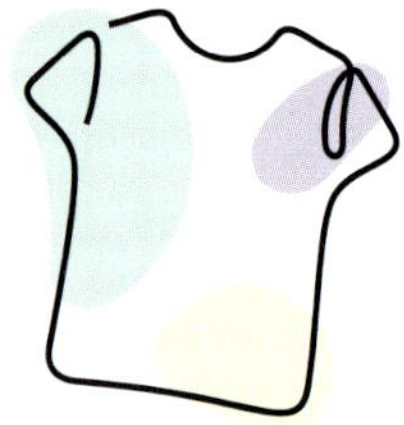

SENSORY DEVELOPMENT

Your child relies greatly on sounds, sights, smells, taste and touch to explore surroundings. Your child may examine an object by turning it over, smelling it and trying to taste it to find out more about it. In addition, improving vision helps your toddler move around, as well as grasp and carry toys, cups and other objects. In a few months, some kids may be ready to start thinking about using a potty chair or the toilet.

Taste test

Understanding that taste is part of how toddlers explore the world is important when it comes to safety. Choking on small objects is a serious risk, and something to keep in mind at home and in new environments. Balloons, small toys or bits of food on the floor are some common choking hazards — and irresistible to toddlers. Make sure floors and easy-to-reach areas are free of choking hazards. This will give you peace of mind and your baby a safe place to explore.

TOYS AND GAMES

It's natural to be attracted to certain toys when you shop for your child. Looking at the toy aisle, you might see trucks and cars marketed to boys and, to girls, dolls and pink toys. However, toddlers are typically attracted to and enjoy all types of toys, if allowed to play with them. By allowing some freedom in toy choice, your child will be able to explore and build self-esteem.

Nesting toys and puzzles

Children this age understand that there are different shapes and are often curious as to how shapes relate to one another. Nesting toys — for example, small boxes that fit inside each other — and puzzles that require your child to put shapes into matching holes help hone cognitive skills.

Pretend play

Pretending to be the host of a fanciful tea party is just one example of how toddlers may create imaginary worlds in which they rule the roost. Pretend play is

Vision

While your child's eyesight is well developed in certain areas — such as the ability to use both eyes to focus on objects — other vision skills, such as depth perception, are still improving. Falls from elevated areas are possible, so keep safety a priority.

Bladder and bowel functions

The muscles that help your child control bowel movements are maturing. By 18 months old, your child can hold urine for up to two hours or longer. It may be some time before you really start toilet training (see Chapter 6), but you can always introduce a potty chair to get your child used to the concept.

COGNITIVE DEVELOPMENT

By 18 months, your child has a firm grasp of many key intellectual (cognitive) concepts — including object permanence. This is the understanding that things don't stop existing even if they're out of sight. As a result, games of hide-and-seek — where you hide things under a blanket or pillow and encourage your child to find them — can be particularly exciting.

Learning through repetition

Experimentation is a key learning tool at this age, helping toddlers better comprehend cause and effect in daily life. Don't be surprised when your child

a great way to develop certain skills, such as ordering events to form a narrative or taking part in conversation. While items such as dress-up clothes can add another layer to your child's play, you don't need to invest much money in the tools of playtime. A large shipping box, for example, can quickly become a house or a race car with a bit of imagination.

Hide-and-seek

Your child now gets the concept of object permanence. A great way to reinforce this is by playing hide-and-seek games, such as hiding a toy under a blanket or pillow and encouraging your child to find it.

Slippery textures

Mediums such as water, paint, clay, soap bubbles and sand are fascinating to toddlers. Exploring them offers children the opportunity to engage in beneficial unstructured play.

performs the same task over and over — say, throwing a cup to the floor — to see how things turn out. This keen interest in experimentation can also lead to trouble. Any items you don't want your child exploring, such as a garbage can, should be childproofed or placed in an area that's inaccessible. See Chapter 17 for more on child safety.

How does it work?

Toddlers love using their fingers to manipulate objects, and you'll probably see your child engaging in activities such as placing and removing tops on containers and placing objects in boxes. This is not only entertaining for your child but also an important part of the learning process. Such activities help toddlers learn about concepts such as "under," "in" and "on."

That's me!

Toddlers this age are becoming increasingly aware of themselves and by 18 months begin to recognize their own reflections in the mirror. Your child may get lots of amusement by making funny faces in the mirror or moving body parts to see if the image in the mirror follows suit.

Language

This is an exciting time of rapid language growth, and you're probably noticing that your child is better able to tell you about personal wants and needs. By 18 months, your child will likely be able to say their own name. Your little one will also be able to combine verbs and gestures to ask you for things, such as extending the arms and saying "up" when they want to be picked up.

As you've probably discovered, the word no is also popular at this age. Saying no is a way for your child to differ from you (see page 378).

With language in particular, it's important to remember that there are variations in when children develop skills. Talk to your child's medical professional if your child doesn't speak at least a dozen or so words by 18 months of age.

Possessiveness

There are few things more important to your child than toys and, well, you. Right around this time you may notice that your child becomes more protective of possessions and family members. Seeing you show attention to another child can lead to a tantrum from your own little one, as can losing a toy to a playmate.

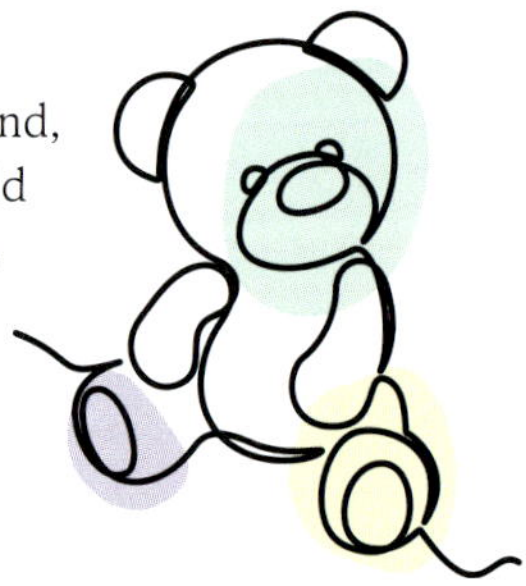

SOCIAL DEVELOPMENT

Play, an important learning and socializing process, continues to be very much a parallel activity, with children playing near each other but not necessarily together. Sharing remains a foreign concept. Still, there are some notable changes.

Everyone has feelings

By 18 months, toddlers are becoming more tuned in to the feelings and reactions of others, and are beginning to develop the foundation for a conscience. In fact, don't be surprised if your child comes over to pat your arm in a comforting way when you're upset, or purposely blows raspberries to make you laugh.

Reading books about feelings can help your child explore personal emotions. You can also help your child understand feelings by naming them, such as feeling sad or happy. See Chapter 10 for more on emotional development in young children.

Renewed separation anxiety

Your child was eager to be independent at the beginning of this period. Now you may find your child going back to being clingy. This results from the growing awareness that your child is very much a separate person from you.

When you go away, or when life throws your child a curveball — for example, going to a new child care center or having a medical test — transitional objects such as blankets and stuffed animals can provide much-needed comfort. These objects serve an important function, so don't be concerned that your child is becoming too dependent on them.

MILESTONES FOR MONTHS 16 TO 18

By the end of month 18, your toddler is busy:

- Walking
- Starting to run (falling down is common)
- Jumping in place with both feet
- Sitting down on a chair with no help
- Exploring inside things, such as drawers or containers
- Pulling and pushing toys
- Stacking as many as four blocks
- Scribbling with a crayon
- Using 10 to 20 words
- Naming body parts and pictures
- Eating with no help
- Looking for help when in trouble
- Being vocal if diaper is soiled or wet
- Understanding simple one-step commands or questions
- Venturing away from you for longer periods

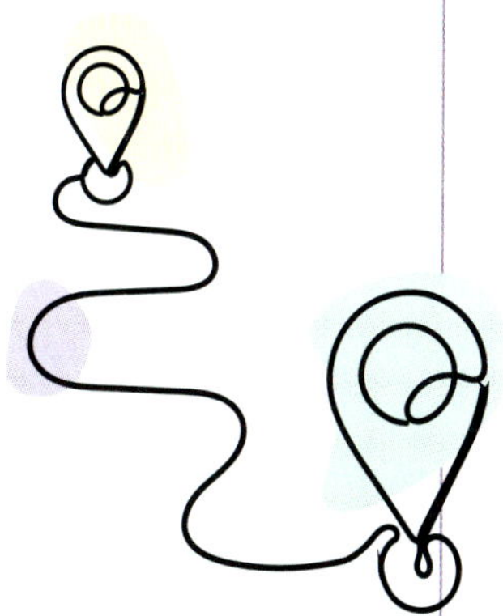

Negative Nellies

For many toddlers, no is a common answer to most questions. This is called negativism and, in this case, doesn't mean that your child is being particularly stubborn or disrespectful. It's more your child's way of exhibiting control and asserting independence. Either way, it can be frustrating. Instead of letting your child know how exasperating it feels, stay calm and avoid asking questions that can be answered with a simple no. Offer choices when possible. For example, if you need to run errands, refrain from asking if your toddler would like to come along. Instead, ask if your child would like to listen to music or look at a book on the way.

CHAPTER 33

Months 19 to 24

Kids approaching age 2 are highly curious about the world around them. Some children will test their parents at every turn with the goal of determining just how much they can get away with. You may hear the word no said to you quite frequently, particularly when you say it's time for bed. You'll probably find yourself uttering it many times as your child pushes against the limits you've set.

But it's also an amazing time of blossoming language skills. Your child is better able to harness words to tell you about needs or wants and to engage you in more understandable conversation. Though temper tantrums certainly still occur with regularity at this age, improved communication skills will eventually help lessen them.

And you'll have a front-row seat to your child's many accomplishments coming soon, such as becoming a master builder of increasingly taller block towers, having the ability to maneuver stairs without holding your hand, and perhaps conquering toilet training and leaving diapers in the dust.

So when you have one of those trying days, remember: You and your child are traveling into unfamiliar territory together. It's an exciting growth process for both of you.

GROWTH AND APPEARANCE

When it comes to growth, boys and girls are fairly even at this stage. By 24 months, girls average 34 inches in height and weigh 27 pounds, while boys average 34½ inches in height and almost 28 pounds. At 24 months, your child's medical professional will also begin keeping track of your child's body mass index (BMI), which is a measurement of weight in relation to height. By tracking growth, the health professional looks for the rate of growth that's right for your child.

By the time your child is 2 years old, 75% of your child's brain growth is completed and the head is about 85% to 90% of its adult size. Your child's height is about half of what it will be as an adult.

Gender and sexuality

At 24 months, toddlers start to recognize the difference between boys and girls, though it will take a while longer for your child to develop a true sense of gender identity. Toddlers also discover that touching their genitalia results in pleasurable feelings. This is typical behavior, and as a parent, you don't need to call attention to it.

Use correct terms for genitalia and avoid using negative descriptions, such as "dirty," for masturbation. This can give your child a faulty impression of sexuality and create unnecessary feelings of shame. If your toddler is touching their genitalia in public, redirect your child to another activity. When your child is older, you can explain the importance of doing such activities in private.

SPOT CHECK: WHAT'S GOING ON

Here's a snapshot of what your toddler's basic care looks like at this age.

Eating

By 24 months, children can use a cup with ease and chew with their mouths closed, and they are pretty good at deciding which foods might require a spoon to eat and which ones can be eaten by picking them up. However, their chewing skills are still rough, so keep looking out for choking hazards.

At this age children generally like to keep their plates simple, usually favoring a few select foods and refusing to try others. Start with small portions, which are less likely to overwhelm your child (see sample plates on page 83). Because this is also a time of growth spurts, be prepared to go through days when your child is intensely hungry, and other times when your child shows little interest in food. See Chapter 4 for more on feeding your toddler.

Sleep

It's not uncommon for children to start to give up naps around this time. Refusing to go to bed and waking up during the night are also hallmarks of toddlerhood — even in children who were previously good sleepers. Factors such as changes in routine, an illness or learning a new skill can cause your child to awaken at night, as can a scary dream. For more information on sleep, see Chapter 8.

Toilet training

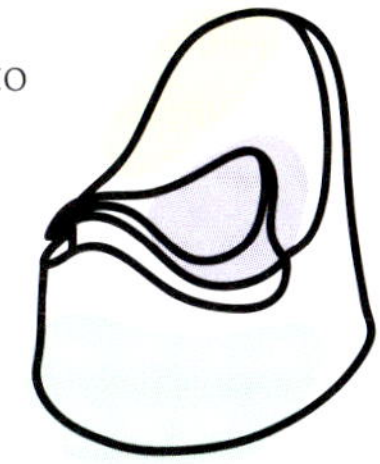

There's no set age for toilet training, but on average, many parents start when their child is between 18 and 24 months old. Learning to use the toilet to have a bowel movement is usually easier for children, as bowel movements tend to follow more of a schedule. Still, it's not always a straightforward process. About 20% of kids will resist having a bowel movement in the toilet initially. Eventually they get the hang of it.

Staying dry at night typically takes longer than mastering daytime control. That's because sleep cycle signals that alert children to wake up and go to the bathroom take a while longer to mature. Bed-wetting isn't unusual in girls up to age 4 and boys up to age 5, and is within the range of typical up to age 7. For more on toilet training — when to start and how to do it — see Chapter 6.

IS IT POTTY TIME?

Aside from first steps and first words, there's probably little that's more highly anticipated — from a parent's perspective — than the day your child no longer needs diapers. But as many parents realize early on, it's often a marathon process. Though the maturing of muscles necessary to control bowel movements and urination gradually occurs by 18 to 24 months, there are also developmental and behavioral elements that are important for toilet training success. Some signs that your child may be ready to use the toilet include when your child:

- Stays dry for two hours, has a decreasing number of wet diapers or wakes up dry from naps
- Wants to be changed immediately when a diaper is soiled
- Has regular bowel movements
- Recognizes the need to go to the bathroom and is able to tell you
- Is able to sit on the toilet for several minutes
- Can perform certain tasks, such as removing pants

Children aren't the only ones who need to be ready. Parents must be, too, by having the time and willingness to invest in toilet training. If things are a little stressful in your child's life at the moment, perhaps due to moving to a new home or having a baby on the way, it may not be the best time to attempt training. For more on toilet training, see Chapter 6.

MOVEMENT

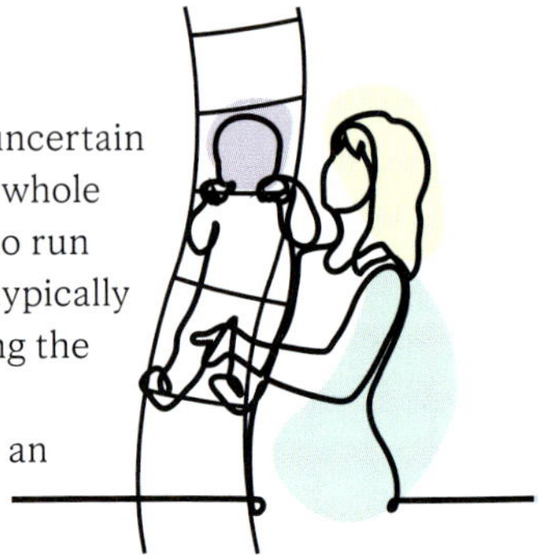

Your child's mobility is rapidly improving, so much so that the uncertain steps taken just a few months ago have probably given way to a whole new level of confidence. By 24 months, most children are able to run fairly well and walk up and down stairs without help. Toddlers typically climb steps by getting both feet on one step and then attempting the next one.

Children at this age are also usually able to stop and pick up an object or kick a ball without toppling over. A new world of exploration — and, often, accompanying hazards — opens up as your child is able to turn doorknobs and navigate steps. Make sure you have childproofing measures in place and that your little explorer is always supervised. See Chapter 17 for more on childproofing and home safety.

Sophisticated skills

Children at this age are able to handle increasingly complex tasks. This might include folding paper, placing puzzle blocks into matching openings, stacking increasingly taller towers of blocks, and dismantling simple toys and putting them back together. You may notice that your child favors one hand over the other when scribbling. Other children can use both hands equally well or may

IS IT TIME FOR A BED?

There's no set age when a child should switch from a crib to a bed. For safety's sake, it would be nice to use a crib until your child is more developmentally ready to stay in bed at bedtime. This keeps your child from wandering the house and potentially finding danger. However, many kids are climbers, and you may find that your child is a regular escape artist, able to get out of the crib even with the mattress set at the lowest possible level. This presents a serious safety hazard, and marks a good time to make the switch.

Some kids transition very early on in toddlerhood, while others may not move to a bed until age 3 or older. Some parents will begin putting their toddlers in beds out of necessity — for example, the crib is needed for a baby on the way, or the toddler has learned to climb out of the crib.

When you decide to make the switch, your child will likely be pretty excited at this newfound freedom. No more crib walls means your child can get up at will. For you, this may mean seeing your child frequently for just one more "good night." When you put your child in bed, be firm about the rules for staying in bed. Also, be prepared to repeat instructions over and over again. Staying consistent now will mean less trouble with bedtime in the years ahead. For more on switching from crib to bed, see page 134.

not show an inclination to right- or left-handedness till much later. With your guidance, your child may be able to brush teeth and wash hands.

"I got this!"

As fine motor skills continue developing, your child is likely able to remove most clothing items independently. Children this age may also be able to put on socks and shoes. However, don't be surprised if your child's outfit displays a lack of understanding of right, left and backward. At this age, shoes are likely to be put on the wrong foot and pants pulled up backward. No worries — your child will figure it out soon enough. Be patient, and compliment their efforts to practice.

COGNITIVE DEVELOPMENT

One of the trickiest things about raising children this age is that while they understand the concept of no, they don't yet grasp the why behind the no. For example, they usually don't understand that jumping repeatedly off the couch not only can damage the furniture but also may cause bodily harm. Even if they get hurt, they may not remember the association between cause and effect the next time the couch beckons. The forethought and judgment required for this type of thinking aren't quite developed yet. It's not that your child is being willfully disobedient so much as it's your child's way of testing the boundaries of what's acceptable and what's not.

Setting limits

Though your little one is intent on testing boundaries, it's important to be consistent in the limits you've set for your child — for the sake of safety and as a way to establish family rules. As your child grows, consider having an ongoing discussion with your spouse, partner or co-parent, and other caregivers as to what's acceptable behavior for your child. Strive to enforce the rules together. Quite often, when your toddler is pushing against limits, distraction and redirection to another activity will resolve the matter. For example, instead of letting your child bang a breakable cup stolen from the table, offer a plastic one instead or a different toy.

Importantly, offer praise and attention as reinforcement for behaviors you want to see in your child. For example, if you see your child cheerfully getting ready for bed, heap praise on your child for the positive behavior. Encouraging desired behavior with your attention is generally more effective than focusing on trying to correct negative behavior (see Chapter 10). Here are some other tips to keep in mind:

- Don't make too many rules. Instead, stick to and enforce what is essential. Another way to look at it: Pick your battles.
- Enable your child to be good. Provide an environment where your child is free to play, not a place filled with items that can't be touched.
- Ignore negative behaviors that aren't potentially harmful or hazardous, such as whining. This is generally the most effective way to eliminate the behavior.

A WORD ABOUT SPANKING

It's been a long day and your toddler is being extra stubborn and acting out. It's tempting to want to smack your child on the bottom to stop the negative behavior. What parent hasn't been there? However, experts agree: There are really no pros to spanking a child. The American Academy of Pediatrics makes the case that spanking sets an unhealthy example for dealing with conflict and can cause injury, even if unintentional. Instead, take a moment to breathe deep and bring yourself under control first — this is a great way to model behavior for your child when it comes to handling frustration. Remember that at this age, redirecting your child's attention to another activity or removing your child from the triggering situation is generally the most effective way to stop disruptive behavior.

Expanding vocabulary

By age 2 years, most children have a vocabulary of 50 to 100 words and can generally understand two-step directions, such as "Put down the puzzle and come get your coat on." *Me*, *you* and *mine* are popular words at this age, as are simple phrases, such as "Daddy go" or "What that?" About two-thirds of a child's speech can be understood at this age. Toddlers will still use gestures to accompany speech and get their points across.

These are rough guides, of course, and the number of words your child uses may be above or below these numbers. Most importantly, keep making conversation with your child and reading together. This is the best way to expand your child's vocabulary.

Bilingual toddlers

If your family speaks more than one language, rest assured that children in bilingual households acquire the same language skills as children who grow up learning one language. The idea that introducing another language into the mix may delay learning the predominant language is a myth. If your child truly has language delays, these will appear in both languages.

Your child may sometimes use words from both languages in the same sentence; this is typical. In fact, now is actually the best time to introduce children to other languages, as they are often quick to pick them up at this age and master the native pronunciation. However, children can certainly learn another language at any age, with effort. Books, music and school programs can help your child become a better bilingual speaker.

Concept of time

Telling time from a clock is a concept that's yet to be learned at this age. But your little one may be getting better at waiting for short periods of time.

Attention spans are still brief, however, so don't expect your child to focus on any one activity too long.

SOCIAL DEVELOPMENT

Toddlers love to imitate those around them, from the way their siblings play pirates to the way parents sip their coffee. It's fun to watch your little one show you how to do something, using your same mannerisms and tone. But it's also a great reminder that imitation is the way your toddler learns to interact with the world. As a result, it's never too early to model the behaviors and attitudes you would like to see in your child. How you react to a spilled cup of milk, for example, will set the stage for how your child learns to handle unexpected stress. Your child is also absorbing how you treat your partner or your pets.

Such keen observation directed your way may feel like a lot of pressure. But keep in mind you're also demonstrating that people aren't flawless — that when

TODDLERS AND SCREENS

For many families, digital devices and electronic entertainment are a part of daily life. But that doesn't mean that screen time is necessary or even helpful to a young child's development. The best kind of entertainment remains the kind that lets a child use the imagination and brings about interaction between parent and child.

Experts agree on the importance of active play and limiting screen time for kids. The American Academy of Pediatrics (AAP) recommends using digital devices only for video chats — with grandparents, for example — for children under 18 months. Both the AAP and the World Health Organization recommend against sedentary screen time for all kids under age 2. There's no benefit to introducing electronic devices early, and some studies demonstrate risk, especially if devices take the place of active play.

Around 2 years of age, kids are more developmentally ready to engage with digital media. If you like, high-quality television programming may be introduced during family time together. Check out PBS Kids, Sesame Workshop or Common Sense Media for suggestions. Limit screen time to an hour or less. To get the most benefit, watch the show with your child and use it as a springboard for further discussion. In general, keep bedrooms, mealtimes and playtimes screen-free for everyone. Turn off screens at least an hour before bedtime and avoid having the television on when not in use. As a parent, you can model healthy moderation in your use of digital devices and show your child how much you value face-to-face interaction. For more background and suggestions around screen time, turn to Chapter 11.

mistakes are made, there are often ways to fix them and that love and warmth persist despite imperfections.

Little helpers

By 2 years old, mealtime is not only nutritional in nature but also a fun time to socialize with the rest of the family. Your child will be able to use a spoon and eat without help, and may show more interest in helping you set the table or put away dishes. Though having your toddler help you with such chores may not save you time, it provides your child with valuable lessons in helping others and being part of a team.

Playtime

Playtime is serious business for children. Free play is the laboratory where they can give curiosity full rein, experiment with how things work and begin to develop problem-solving skills. Being able to play without a lot of rules or structure is key to a child's developing brain and creates rich pathways for cogni-

TOYS AND GAMES

Purchasing a new toy or game is often a fun anticipatory experience, for child and parent alike. When selecting a toy, keep in mind your child's age and developmental stage. Look carefully at the packaging to see if it's appropriate for your child. Some toys have a warning label that the toy may be hazardous to young children — for example, it contains small parts and poses a choking risk to children younger than 3. Others may display a label that recommends a certain developmental age for use. If there are reports that a toy is hazardous, the Consumer Product Safety Commission (CPSC) may issue a recall. For more information about current recalls, visit the CPSC and Safe Kids Worldwide websites.

Keep in mind that you don't always need the latest toys to provide your child with a safe and fun experience. Often you can find household items that fit the bill. Here are some ideas for age-appropriate toys and activities.

Sorting

Toddlers love to sort objects. Have your child help you with the clean laundry by putting socks in one pile and pants in another, or have your child group together plastic containers based on size.

Puzzles

At this age, children usually can match up shapes. Try a shape-sorting game where your child can put different shapes into matching holes.

tive and social development. Around 18 months, toddlers are generally able to engage in symbolic play, where a doll may stand in for a baby or a stuffed animal a pet. Over these next few months, your child may also identify how to solve certain problems, having seen you or another caregiver do it before. For example, your toddler might pretend to soothe a doll by offering a bottle, or you might find a toy dog helpfully placed in front of the family dog's food bowl.

At this age, kids typically still prefer to play independently alongside each other rather than in a coordinated fashion. Sharing is likely to be reluctant at best.

Shy children may cry when encouraged to try a new activity involving people they don't know. At a time when most children are testing out independence, your child may seem to want nothing more than to cling to you. Allow your child to set the pace. Don't pull away when your child looks to you for reassurance in a trying situation. Your support can help your child gain the necessary confidence to venture out.

Arts and crafts

As your child is better able to manipulate the fingers, try complementing your budding artist's talents by providing painting tools, such as brushes and easels.

Hide-and-seek

This classic game is taken up a notch at this age. Now, if you hide something, your child will look in several potential hiding spots to find it.

Reading

By 24 months, your child is developing logic and reasoning. Help develop these skills by reading together and asking your child questions about the story, such as "Why did the person do that?" or "What do you think the dog will do?" You may need to answer your own questions, but practicing now helps your child learn to ask these questions going forward.

Water play

While splashing in water is still likely to be your child's favorite activity, you can also use it to introduce science concepts. You can show your child displacement (dropping a toy into a container filled with water may cause the water to go over the edge) or density (will the rock sink or float?). Water also lends itself to many imaginary activities, such as pretending to wash dishes or sail a boat.

Red light, green light

This and other games that require children to follow directions and "stop and go" are good ways to teach your child about self-control.

MILESTONES FOR MONTHS 19 TO 24

By the end of this period, your toddler is busy:

- Building a tower of six to seven cubes
- Imitating vertical and circular lines when drawing
- Unscrewing a lid
- Developing a vocabulary of 50 to 100 words
- Using simple phrases
- Understanding multiple-step commands
- Knowing his or her own name and using it
- Verbally telling you about needs
- Having fewer temper tantrums (though they still happen!)
- Becoming more independent
- Beginning to understand that other people have their own feelings
- Telling you about something that just happened

Handling aggression

While no one wants to be the parent whose child kicks or hits other children, this sort of behavior isn't uncommon at this age and it doesn't necessarily mean there's a problem. Some children naturally are more intense and may lash out when events don't go their way.

Setting limits is crucial. Let your child know that it's important to be respectful of peers, and offer praise when your child does what you ask. Offer plenty of ways to burn off energy, but keep watch when your child plays with other children. If your child starts acting out, firmly explain that hitting others is never OK and redirect your child to another activity or leave the area. If this doesn't work or the situation worsens, consider introducing timeouts (see page 393). A timely break from the action offers a way for your child to cool off and start over.

CHAPTER 34

Months 25 to 30

"No, I do it!" As the parent of a toddler, you may hear this phrase or one like it from your child on a daily basis. Maybe you made the "mistake" of trying to pick out your child's clothes to help speed along the morning routine or helping your child put food on the dinner plate to avoid creating a mess on the table. You may now get to watch the process in reverse so that your child can do it all over again.

Sometimes toddlers insist on doing tasks they're not quite capable of performing (yet), and their refusal to let you help can be frustrating. But it's important to let your child practice these developing skills, even if it involves some mistakes and a lot of repetition. Increasing independence is the theme for this stage in your child's life, and anything your child sees as hampering it is likely to be met with resistance and some tantrums here and there.

Tantrums are one of the biggest challenges of raising a toddler. Children this age have difficulty dealing with limits, compromise, and disappointment, which often results in angry outbursts and tears. But with time, patience and consistent limits, you'll see tantrums decrease. In the meantime, however, your child still has a great need to see, hear and feel you nearby. You can help your child navigate frustration with plenty of hugs, kisses, praise and attention. Feeling loved and well cared for can help motivate toddlers to behave better.

GROWTH AND APPEARANCE

By 30 months, your little one is looking less and less like a baby and more and more like a big kid. Legs are now getting longer and head growth has slowed. As your child grows and becomes more physically active, muscle tone is improving, which means that so is your child's posture. Better posture helps give children a longer, leaner appearance.

Your toddler's grin also is likely to reveal many more teeth. Most children have about 20 teeth at this age.

Height and weight

By age 2 or so, many toddlers have quadrupled their birth weight while losing baby fat. In fact, by age 5, your child will have only about half the percentage of body fat as at age 1. Some of the areas where this will be most noticeable are in the face, arms and thighs. With the loss of fat pads in the arches of the feet, children will no longer appear to be flat-footed.

In general, you can expect your child to grow about 2½ inches and gain about 4 pounds annually as the preschool years approach. However, if your child's growth seems to have stalled, talk to your child's medical professional to rule out any underlying health issues.

Toilet training

Continue providing encouragement and support as your child works on toileting skills. Even toddlers who are skilled at using the toilet on their own may still need your help with related tasks, such as wiping and dressing.

If your child isn't toilet trained yet, don't worry. Avoid pushing if your child isn't ready. Forcing your child to use the toilet can complicate and lengthen the process. Research has found that starting around the age of 2 typically results in a child who is trained by age 3. In contrast, starting earlier may actually lengthen the process in some kids. For more information on toilet training, see Chapter 6.

MOVEMENT

Children this age are often balls of energy, in constant motion from sunup to sundown. It can be tough to keep up, but think of it this way: All this activity is helping your child strengthen muscles and fine-tune coordination skills.

By age 2½, your child may be able to jump using both feet, balance on one foot for a second or two at a time, start taking some tentative steps on tippy-toes, and walk backward. That once unsure walk is being replaced by a more mature heel-to-toe stride. Stairs are less challenging, as children this age are starting to use alternating feet to climb without holding a grown-up's hand. In the coming months, they'll gain the necessary skills to pedal a tricycle.

Sometimes parents of toddlers worry that their children may be too active (hyperactive). Usually there's nothing to worry about. Most toddlers are constantly on the go, running and climbing from one activity to another in the span of mere minutes. A long attention span is in short supply at this age, so it's generally best to adjust your expectations accordingly. For example, you might want to avoid having an extended meal at a restaurant or engaging in other activities that require staying still and quiet for long periods.

If you think your child has distinct problems with attention span or hyperactivity, especially compared with peers, bring up your concerns with your child's medical professional. A medical professional can reassure you about what's typical for this age and help you determine if further evaluation is needed.

Skilled fingers and hands

Toddlers love to steer objects, and their ability to push things, such as strollers or carts, in the direction they want is improving. Your child is also able to hold a pencil or paintbrush properly and make circular, horizontal and vertical strokes. The more modest block towers of early toddlerhood are giving way to taller, more ambitious projects.

COGNITIVE DEVELOPMENT

To cement patterns of positive behavior, toddlers need lots of praise. Whether your child is well behaved at a play date, using the toilet consistently or going to

WHEN A NEW BABY ARRIVES

Just when your toddler was getting a pretty good idea of how things run in the household, here comes a new sibling. This can be upsetting to a toddler, whose entire routine is being turned upside down. Parental attention is now split, and your child may be upset about losing the crib to the new baby. So it's understandable when children act out at having to welcome a sibling. Keep in mind that there's no ill will in this, just anger about changes in the routine.

If you are expecting, the best time to talk about coming changes is when your child is becoming aware of the pregnancy — for example, your child starts asking questions about a growing belly. Explain what to expect in the coming months, such as decorating a room for the new baby and perhaps staying with a friend or family member when it's time for the baby to be born. Also provide reassurance, such as "I'll need to feed and put diapers on the baby a lot, but I will still read you a bedtime story."

Once the new baby arrives, allow your older child to help out when possible. For example, your child can hand you diapers while you change the baby or help you pick out clothes after the baby's bath. If your child isn't interested in interacting with the new sibling, there's no need to force it. How you word a request may help, too — try asking your older child to help you rather than the baby. With time, the relationship between new siblings will grow. Always supervise a toddler with a young baby.

bed without a struggle, say how proud you are. Praise for positive behavior helps to build competence and confidence, and, in turn, independence and a good foundation for problem-solving and decision-making. Try to be as specific as you can when you give praise. For example, "You did such a great job brushing teeth and putting your toothbrush away!" instead of generalized phrases ("Awesome job!").

You also may notice — with perhaps mixed feelings — that your child is more open to being separated from you. It's yet another sign of your child's growing independence.

Language and association

Gradually, your child is gaining the ability to associate objects with their uses. Your child may recognize that a skillet is used for cooking or that swimsuits are used for swimming. You can see this reflected in imaginative play or excited anticipation when swimsuits and sunscreen come out for a day at the pool.

SPOT CHECK: WHAT'S GOING ON

Here's a snapshot of what your toddler's basic care looks like at this age.

Eating

At this point your child will likely be following a more adult feeding schedule, or three meals a day with two or three snack times sprinkled in. Although your toddler's attention span is limited, it's reasonable to expect your child to sit with the family during meals. Include children even if they aren't interested in eating. This is a formative time when your child learns and benefits from the socialization that occurs at mealtime. During family meals, your child learns good eating habits, such as trying foods that are nutritionally beneficial, and portion control.

Sleeping

Two-year-olds need anywhere from 11 to 14 hours of sleep a day, which includes nighttime sleep and naps. Some children may be giving up naps during this time; others may still be napping for a couple of hours each day.

It's important to keep bedtime the same time every night, and for children to wake up at their regular time — whether it's a weeknight or the weekend. A consistent sleep schedule helps them get enough good-quality sleep.

Regular bedtime routines make it easier to put your child to bed. If bedtime has slipped later than you'd like and you need to hit the reset button, do so gradually. Try setting your child's current bedtime earlier by 15 minutes, then push it up by the same amount again every few days till you reach the ideal bedtime. For more on sleep and sleep issues, see Chapter 8.

Most children this age will proudly be able to say their first and last names and refer to themselves by a pronoun. Children also are learning to use plural nouns and can usually name at least one color. Sentences are becoming more complex. A request to play outdoors may be phrased as "Me and Daddy go to the park?"

Language is an area where children may differ greatly from each other. If your child isn't as talkative as a friend, don't lose too much sleep over it. Some children just talk more than others. It isn't really a reflection of how smart a child is or how well the child is mastering thinking skills. But if your child isn't starting to put words together or can't point to familiar objects or pictures, or if you feel there may be a problem with your child's language development, talk to your child's medical professional.

Read and sing to your child, and with your child, every day. Talk with your child, using simple sentences to describe what you're doing. Introduce new words or names to your child in a familiar setting, and repeat them often. Repeating familiar sounds and words also can expand your child's vocabulary. This prepares your child for more complex speech and reading.

What's that under the bed?

What happened to that very brave toddler of just a few months ago? As you're probably already realizing, some toddlers can develop new anxieties and fears as they get older. Your child may suddenly be afraid of a monster under the bed or

GIVING A TIMEOUT

You may sometimes need to separate your child from an activity when a behavior isn't acceptable — such as for hitting or biting. Toddlers have little self-control and have yet to learn how to effectively regulate their emotions. A timeout can be a tool to help your child learn to accept limits, especially when used calmly and lovingly by the parent or caregiver rather than as a punishment.

Some experts have moved away from recommending timeouts. The idea is that when a child is acting out, a need is not being met. This school of thought encourages supporting the child in regulating their emotions, rather than separating the child, while you enforce the limit (for example, sitting with them to keep them from hitting others). This may help a child feel reassured, grounded and able to learn the self-control skills needed for next time.

If you choose to use timeouts, try to use them infrequently and keep them brief — about about one minute for each year of age. The goal is to help your child calm down and to correct behavior, not to punish. Find a quiet spot, and calmly return your child there if they leave before time is up. Afterward, talk to your child about what happened to cause the timeout and what could be done differently next time.

in the closet and insist on sleeping with every light on. Though it may seem to come out of nowhere, this is typical as toddlers develop better imaginations and memories. You can help your child by explaining what is real and what is pretend, and helping to ease the stress of bad memories. Be mindful of media violence. Even if children are not watching television, the noise that comes from the television can have an impact on them.

Ace problem-solver

Not too long ago, your child had to use trial and error to figure out how things worked. Now, children are developing the ability to work through a problem they're trying to solve in their heads, rather than by acting it out. For example, instead of pulling out a whole drawerful of socks to get to a pair in the back, your child may reach around for the pair. This is good news for parents, as it will likely mean fewer messes in the discovery process!

SOCIAL DEVELOPMENT

Two-year-olds often get excited to see other children, and may even have a couple of friends. This is a great time to meet up with other parents and their kids and give your child a chance to socialize.

What was once a play date that included a few children playing near but not with each other is starting to give way to brief interaction. In some cases, this may be no more than children chasing each other around the room. In others, it may be cooperative play, where one child helps the other complete a block tower. Or it may focus on the developing imagination and involve pretend play, such as taking care of a stuffed animal or driving a pretend car.

For a majority of the time, children this age will still fly solo at playtime, and sharing is still difficult for them.

WHY DOES MY CHILD ONLY ACT UP WITH ME?

Your child has been having a lot of tantrums lately, so you're understandably nervous about hiring a babysitter while you go out. When you get back, however, the sitter reports that your child behaved admirably. Though you may want to keep this sitter's number on speed dial, this contrast with caregivers is common and the explanation is pretty simple: Tantrums are a way of testing limits, and your child feels most comfortable testing limits with you. The same goes for daredevils. Little risk-takers may attempt potentially dangerous things with parents that they wouldn't try with another caregiver. This is because your child feels secure enough with you to try new things.

TOYS AND GAMES

Playing isn't just a way to help your child master important physical skills. It's also a way to develop social skills, expand vocabulary and use critical thinking to solve problems.

Pretend play

Your child may go to the imaginary grocery store or feed a baby doll food from an empty plate. Don't be surprised to see your child's daily routine re-created in this pretend play.

Joke books

Children this age love books that contain jokes or repetition using silly phrases.

Puzzles

Your child is already getting skilled at naming familiar objects. Choose puzzles that contain different colors, shapes or animals. As your child places the pieces, help your child identify these characteristics.

Playing ball

Go out in the backyard or the park and have your child kick a ball with you to practice aim. Once your child masters this skill, have your child run and kick the ball to work on coordination and balance.

Dance party

Toddlers love nothing more than to move. Put on some fast-paced music and let your child wow you with dancing and jumping skills. Join in — your child will feed off your enthusiasm!

Blocks

Building objects with blocks is a great way to encourage cooperative play in children who are just starting to play together. Put out plenty of blocks at the next play date and invite your child and your child's friends to work together building a tall tower.

Walks

Taking a stroll can be stimulating for a child. There's a lot to see, smell, touch and hear. A walk to the park can help your child get to know the neighborhood. Hiking on a nature trail allows your child to explore in a relaxing setting and possibly identify a critter or two.

MILESTONES FOR MONTHS 25 TO 30

By the end of this period, your 2-year-old is busy:

- Walking up the stairs, using one foot at a time
- Walking backward
- Fine-tuning balance, such as standing on one foot
- Climbing
- Turning handles to open doors
- Playing pretend in more elaborate ways
- Learning to make friends
- Unscrewing jar lids
- Following commands with two or three parts
- Identifying common objects
- Saying their name and age
- Using pronouns and learning plurals
- Speaking in a way even strangers can understand
- Learning to take turns
- Showing affection for familiar people

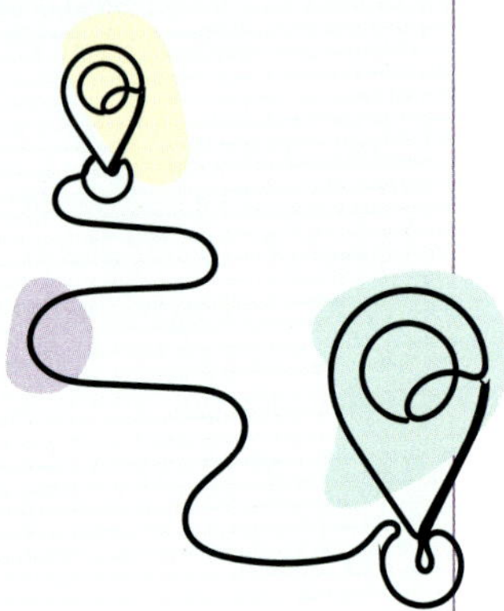

Emerging emotions

Your child's feelings are growing more complex. Your child may express pride, guilt, embarrassment or shame. Guilt in particular comes into play as events happen that, while beyond your child's control, your child may still feel responsible for. Examples include divorce or the death of a loved one. On the flip side, your child's sense of humor is also beginning to emerge. Saying silly things to your child will no doubt produce big laughs.

Handling stress

Though it's sometimes hard for an adult to understand what could be so stressful in a toddler's life, kids this age can and do experience stress. A new child care center, a new sibling or a move to a different home are some of the curveballs life can throw at a young child. While a little bit of stress can help your child learn how to cope with it later on in life, make sure your young child isn't overwhelmed. Look for signs that your child is stressed, such as increased thumb sucking, more tantrums or being aggressive. Ease stress by maintaining consistency in other areas of your routine, offering extra time together or giving your child quiet periods to recover. Periods of free play, in particular, can help release some pent-up emotions.

CHAPTER 35

Months 31 to 36

At nearly 3 years old, your child is steadily gaining an increased understanding of the surrounding world. Your little one is learning new words daily and using them effectively to carry on more in-depth conversations with you. This improved communication is a big part of the reason you'll see tantrums gradually declining. Your child is also figuring out how to better manage behavior and respond to situations appropriately. You'll need to repeat the rules frequently and maintain consistent limits, but your child's brain is rapidly absorbing the lessons of cause and effect.

Your soon-to-be preschooler is also becoming more independent. Your child probably can pedal a tricycle and draw increasingly complex figures. Some children might create and visit imaginary worlds where they get to play hero and save the family from a ferocious fire-breathing dragon.

Although you're moving away from the baby years, there are a whole lot of milestones and good times ahead — think fishing trips, impromptu T-ball games in the park and helping your child build a toy race car. And, of course, there are many things that won't change just yet. Your child, while not requiring the same level of supervision as before, will still need you close by to set limits and offer lots of loving attention.

GROWTH AND APPEARANCE

Your child's arms, legs and upper body are becoming longer and leaner as the body grows and adds more muscle. Slowly, your child's face will mature, too. In the preschool years ahead, the jaw will widen to make room for the eventual arrival of adult teeth.

By the end of this period, the average weight for a toddler is 32 pounds and the average height is 37½ inches. Weight gain slows gradually, with most kids gaining about 5 pounds a year. As tempting as it may be to compare your child to other children, keep in mind that height and weight can vary greatly.

The numbers above provide averages, but plotting your child's height and weight over time is the best way to see if your child is following an individual growth pattern. If you notice that weight is outpacing height, or that your child's height seems stalled, bring it up with your child's medical professional.

MOVEMENT

Running, climbing and jumping are all second nature by now. By the age of 3, toddlers are walking heel to toe with ease and most can pedal a tricycle well.

Children this age are working on mastering other skills, too, such as standing on tippy-toes or balancing on one foot. Two- to 3-year-olds are also working on changing positions more smoothly, such as standing up from a squatting position or catching a ball.

Circles and squares

An exciting new development in fine motor skills is gaining the ability to draw shapes. By the age of 3, children can typically draw squares and circles, as well as a rough outline of a person — minus a few body parts. Your child's drawing technique now includes the ability to create crosses and vertical and horizontal lines. Some children this age may attempt to copy capital letters. Using instruments such as scissors and mastering use of a fork at mealtime are additional accomplishments that your child may achieve.

COGNITIVE DEVELOPMENT

Toddlers have infinite curiosity, and "Why?" is bound to be a favorite question. Short, simple answers generally work best, especially for questions such as "Why can't I have the knife?" or "Why do I have to go to bed?" Sometimes a question can be a good segue for a learning opportunity or further discovery. For example, if your child asks, "What do bugs eat?" take a field trip to the backyard and find a bug to observe. Or look up a book on bugs the next time you go to the library.

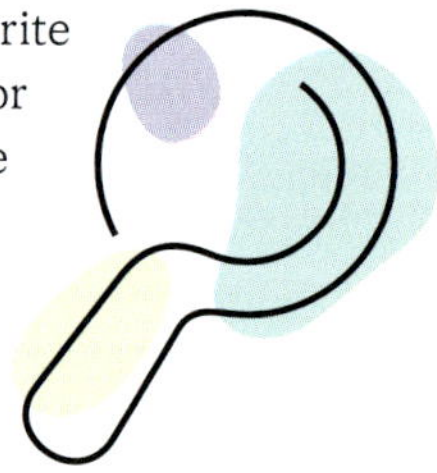

Self-control

By the end of this period, the "terrible twos" are technically behind you. But for some children, the terrible twos may give way to the "terrible threes." That's when it can feel like your child is 3 going on 13, with teenager-like mood swings. Your child may be ecstatic to help you bake chocolate chip cookies one minute, then burst into tears when the cookies look a little bit browner than expected.

Such outbursts will gradually wind down in the months and years ahead, but you may wonder how you'll deal with the behavior until then.

Understanding where the behavior is coming from is a good first step. It's a complicated time, emotionally, for children. For the first time, their supply of feelings has expanded to include embarrassment, guilt and shame — among others — and they're just learning how to cope with them. "Coping" at this age may include yelling, crying, stomping or throwing things.

You can help your child gradually develop the self-control necessary to manage these emotions and impulses by identifying and naming them, and offering better ways to handle them. For example, if your child feels disappointed that the cookies didn't turn out as expected, sympathize: "It's disappointing that they didn't turn out like we thought." Then make a plan to change what you can: "Let's not keep them in the oven as long next time."

In the meantime, be realistic about which situations your child can and can't

SPOT CHECK: WHAT'S GOING ON

Here's a snapshot of what your toddler's basic care looks like at this age.

Eating

Nowadays, your toddler may enjoy the social aspects of meals, such as sitting around the dinner table and talking with family, in addition to the nutritional aspects. Your little one's overall attitude toward food is evolving, which may translate into a certain degree of pickiness. Food preferences can vary from day to day.

At times it may seem that your child hardly eats at all. Often toddlers will eat well at one meal and take only a few bites at others. The most important marker of whether a child eats enough is growth. If you notice weight loss, schedule a visit with your child's medical professional right away. If growth seems slow, schedule a weight check at the medical professional's office.

Sleeping

Children this age still need about 10 to 12 hours of sleep a day. If your child is still taking naps, these may last 1 to 2 hours. Most children this age are ready for bed between 7 and 9 p.m.

Be consistent with bedtime routines. This helps establish healthy sleeping habits and encourages enough rest for your child. Allow your child some time to fall asleep without help. If your child is having trouble falling or staying asleep without your help, read through Chapter 8 for some troubleshooting advice. It's not uncommon for children this age to have nightmares thanks to their developing imaginations. If your child awakens upset from a nightmare, provide comfort and reassure your child that dreams aren't real.

handle. Also, establish consequences for when negative behavior does crop up — for example, taking away a toy for a set number of minutes if your child throws it. It's also important to make sure you're modeling appropriate behavior for your child. While it's understandable to lose your cool when your child repeatedly tests the limits, reacting calmly to the situation sets an example that your child can observe and follow.

As your child moves further along into the third year, better language skills and more experience in dealing with peers, following rules and encountering disappointment will strengthen coping skills. Offering your child other, more appropriate outlets to release frustration or anger also can help. Examples include playing outside in an area where your child can run freely or dancing to music. Sometimes just moving on to other routine activities such as taking a bath or prepping dinner is enough to distract a toddler from disruptive behavior.

Language skills

Chatterbox may only scratch the surface when it comes to describing your child these days. By 3 years of age, most children can tell you their full names and typically have a vocabulary of 900 words or more. Sometimes it can feel like they're trying to use them all at once! Despite an expanding vocabulary, your child likely doesn't understand every word. This can make for some interesting and amusing conversations.

Your child may be eager to tell you stories, and some children speak clearly enough for even strangers to understand most of what they say. Sentences expand to about five or six words and include nouns and verbs. Some children this age still have difficulty with pronouns. Mispronunciation of certain letter sounds is common — for example, replacing "th" with "f," saying "free" instead of "three."

STUTTERING

It's not unusual for children to trip over their words, as their vocabulary expands faster than the words can come out. This is common until age 5 and tends to affect boys more than girls. If your child is stuttering, the best thing to do is to speak slowly yourself. Avoid interrupting or trying to complete your child's sentences. Listen attentively. Pointing out a stutter may only make your child self-conscious and worsen the problem.

If you're concerned that your child may have a speech problem, talk to your child's medical professional about an evaluation. While most children outgrow stuttering by age 5, an evaluation may be recommended sooner if the stuttering has persisted for longer than 3 to 6 months, there is a family history of stuttering or the child is upset about it. Stuttering can be caused by any number of factors, including hearing problems and developmental delays.

SEX ED

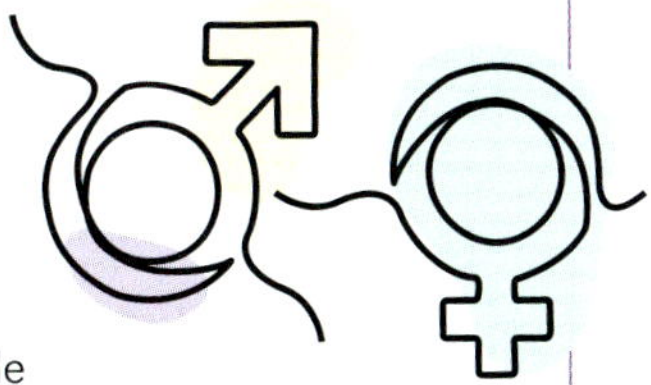

Think questions about sex are reserved for older children? Think again! Children this age are curious and always looking to their parents and caregivers for answers to their questions. So don't be surprised when your child seeks answers to where babies come from or why different people have different body parts. Answer these queries in a simple and straightforward way. Use the correct terms for parts of the body — such as breasts, genitalia, vagina or vulva, and penis — and take your child's questions seriously. Too much detail or an answer that's too complicated may be more than your child bargained for. But if your child wants more details, provide age-appropriate information.

If you're looking for age-appropriate responses to sex-related questions, consider these examples:

- *How do babies get inside the tummy?* You might say, "Parents decide to put a baby in the tummy." If asked how, you can say "By holding each other in a special way." Or you can explain that certain ingredients are needed to make a baby, including sperm and an egg.
- *How are babies born?* For some kids, it might be enough to say, "Doctors and nurses help babies who are ready to be born." If your child wants more details, you might say, "Usually someone who is pregnant pushes the baby out of the vagina."
- *Why doesn't everyone have a penis?* Try a simple explanation, such as "Different bodies are made differently."
- *Why do you have hair down there?* You might say, "Our bodies change as we get older." If your child wants more details, add, "Some people grow hair near their penises, and some people grow hair near their vulvas."

As your child matures and asks more detailed questions, you can provide more detailed responses. At any age, try to answer your child's question, but you can wait for them to ask more questions before offering more detailed answers. Even if you're uncomfortable, forge ahead. Remember, you're setting the stage for open, honest discussions in the years to come.

Sometimes curious children will do some exploring on their own. While masturbation is common at this age, so, too, is wanting to examine the genitals of another child. There's generally nothing sexual about this, and it's typically harmless. However, you may want to set limits on such exploration and provide simple rules on privacy. It's also not too early to teach your child about safety. Explain that vaginas or vulvas and penises are private and that only parents or sometimes a doctor should ask to look at these private parts.

To encourage more vocabulary growth, ask your child to share more details. For example, when your child tells you about seeing the neighbor's dog outside, ask about its color and size, and whether it was barking or quiet.

Pretend play

With a growing imagination, frequently the line between the world of fantasy and reality is blurred for toddlers. Objects such as trees, rocks and cars may take on a life of their own in your child's world of make-believe, which often is populated by imaginary friends.

In fact, your child may float between the real world and pretend play quite frequently. Sometimes it can be hard for your child to tell the difference between the two. This can make it easy for a child to become upset by scary stories, such as tales of monsters or vampires. In these situations, don't poke fun at your child's fears. Instead, provide comfort and reassure your child that these fictional characters aren't real.

Make-believe is an essential part of developing emotions. If your child invites you to play along, do so! You can help your child see new perspectives and ways to deal with emotions. If you don't get invited, don't worry. Your child wants to run the show, and that's perfectly OK.

Concept of time

Though a minute will still feel like an eternity, your child is becoming much more aware of what time involves — particularly as it relates to routines. For example, your child may get excited at a specific time in the afternoon because that's library time.

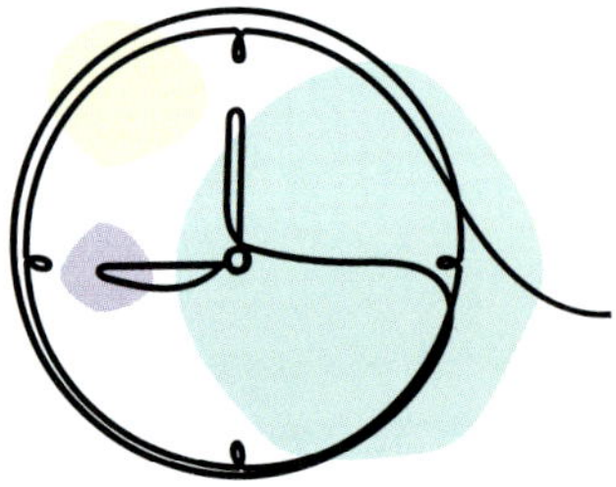

Imaginary friends

You're making dinner when your child asks you to make a little extra food for Sofia. You're taken aback because you have no clue who Sofia is — until your child explains that Sofia is the friend you can't see.

Imaginary friends tend to pop up between the ages of 2½ and 3 years. A child may have only one or many, and these friends may stick around till your child starts school. Pretend playmates serve many critical functions: They can help your child work through emotions, practice their conversation skills, or learn how to make the distinction between fantasy and reality. They may also help your child envision reaching a certain goal. For example, an imaginary friend may reach goals your child dreams about but may not yet be able to achieve, such as riding a horse. It's also OK for a child to not have an imaginary friend. This doesn't mean your child lacks imagination or won't develop certain skills.

So how do you handle Sofia? Acknowledge the friend by name and set out a plate with a little bit of food. However, don't allow your child to blame Sofia for misdeeds. If your child throws a sibling's toy down the stairs and blames Sofia, for example, firmly state that your child is responsible for Sofia's actions.

SOCIAL DEVELOPMENT

By age 3, children are becoming less focused on themselves and more interested in playing and interacting with other children. An increase in empathy and a desire to socialize often lead to more peaceful interactive play and the forging of friendships. These relationships are a great way to help children embrace the differences in playmates, as well as see their own unique qualities and how other children appreciate them ("Brayden says I'm fun!").

Developing empathy

Cooperation with peers is an important theme moving forward. Children may begin moderating their behavior to achieve desired outcomes, such as playing with a toy but also sharing to make a friend happy. Of course, learning to moderate behavior takes time, and unkindness or aggression may flare up every

TOYS AND GAMES

"Not for children under the age of 3" is a common warning label found on toys. These labels alert parents that the toy contains small parts — parts less than 1¼ inches in diameter and 2¼ inches long — and poses a choking risk. So is a 3-year-old ready for these toys? If your child doesn't seem developmentally ready, it's OK to hold off. In the meantime, here are some inexpensive ways to encourage your child's sense of curiosity and learning.

Make-believe

Pretend play with siblings or other children tends to be more cooperative, meaning it's great for keeping the peace. Children learn how to take turns, communicate and respond appropriately to peers.

Craft boxes

Fill a shoe box with craft items such as popsicle sticks, pipe cleaners, foam shapes, glue sticks and construction paper (if you're feeling brave, add glitter). These simple tools help your child develop fine motor skills, as well as provide a vehicle for your little one's imagination.

Matching games

Give your child an object, such as a rectangular box, and have your child find matching shapes throughout your house.

Unstructured play

Having time to play freely, without structure, has been shown to boost cognitive development and social and emotional health in young children.

now and again. You'll still need to step in to redirect your child when necessary. Over the next few years, your child will learn to consider others' emotions, although they may not put others' feelings first just yet. Importantly, compliment empathetic behavior to help build your child's confidence and encourage that behavior again. In addition, keep in mind that you are your child's main example of how to behave and relate to others.

Exploring gender roles

It's common for children this age to explore the concept of gender and where they fit in. For example, your son may want to dress up and play princess. Experimenting with different roles helps children define their own roles. Avoid using stereotypes to control your child's play. Focus instead on highlighting positive character traits found in all genders, such as generosity and determination.

Gearing up for preschool

In the blink of an eye, your baby has gone from diapers and stacking a block or two to speaking a mile a minute and maybe even preparing for preschool.

Many children attend preschool for a year or two before entering kindergarten. There are a variety of programs available, ranging from public to private options. Public school districts often have preschool programs, some of them free of charge, open to local residents. Preschool programs may also be available

MILESTONES FOR MONTHS 31 TO 36

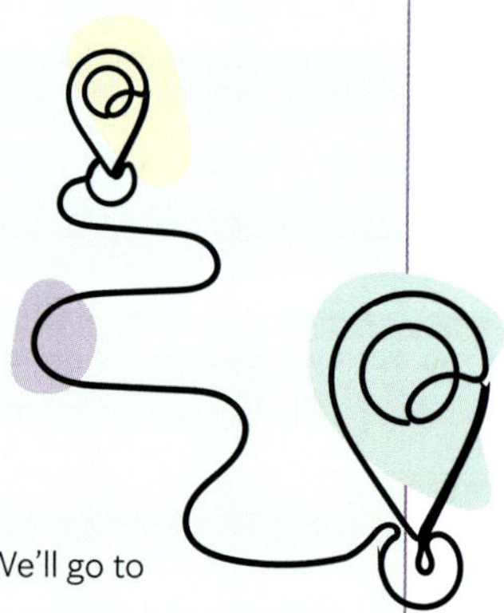

By the end of this period, your toddler is busy:

- Pedaling a tricycle
- Moving with more ease forward and backward, hopping briefly on one foot, and using alternating feet to go up stairs
- Getting dressed, with assistance
- Drawing lines, crosses, shapes; starting to draw people
- Building a tower of 9 or 10 cubes; building bridges
- Using as many as 900 words
- Understanding more complex sentences (such as "We'll go to the park after you eat breakfast")
- Talking and asking questions
- Beginning to understand concepts such as numbers and comparisons
- Recalling events that happened the day before
- Thinking up stories
- Playing with other children and beginning to forge friendships
- Being aware that people look different

through parochial school systems or private organizations. Some child care programs have a built-in preschool curriculum.

Preschool not only helps children prepare for more formal learning but also helps them get used to other school routines. These might include longer separations from you, socialization with classmates and abiding by set rules in a school setting. A good preschool program can help create a smoother transition to kindergarten for your child.

When looking for a preschool, search for certain characteristics, such as:

- *Goals and rules that align with yours.* The focus at this age should be helping children find self-confidence and build independence. It shouldn't be to fast-track academics, such as learning how to read or do advanced math. Make sure you agree with the way discipline is handled.
- *Small class size.* Children up to 3 years old tend to do better with about 8 to 10 classmates.
- *Low turnover.* A high turnover of teachers and other staff can be a sign of a problem keeping good teachers. Teachers and other staff should be trained in early childhood development or education.

If you and your child haven't been separated before, you'll likely have some feelings of sadness or guilt. This is understandable. On the positive side, preschool can help your child become more independent and teach valuable socialization skills. It can also give you and your child some time apart so you can focus on yourself. These are things that can deepen your parent-child relationship.

PART 4

Common illnesses and concerns

One of the many challenges of parenting is caring for your child during illnesses or medical emergencies. Thankfully, true medical emergencies in infants and toddlers are fairly rare. Still, your child can't always tell you when or how much something hurts. So it can be difficult to sort out more serious illnesses from those that are common and easily managed at home.

Illnesses in general are more frequent in the first few years, simply because your child is still developing in many ways. Young children slowly adapt to an environment filled with people, pets and germs. As your child matures and the immune system becomes stronger, illnesses will become less frequent.

As you get to know your child better, it will become easier for you to tell when your child has a minor illness and when you need medical help. You know your child better than anyone else — including details about current and previous illnesses. You will notice, for example, if your little one is suddenly fussier than usual, or has changed eating or sleeping patterns. You'll also be able to tell if your child is less active or clinging to you more.

You're an essential part of the team that cares for your sick child. In most cases, you'll determine when you can handle an illness at home and when it's time to call your child's medical professional or visit an emergency department. You can help the medical professional determine if a problem is present when things just don't seem right with your child.

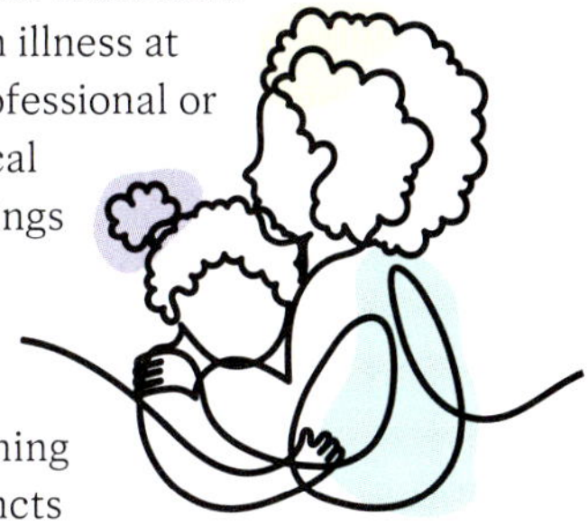

You also play a key role in caring for your sick child. This includes knowing when to give medication, understanding what changes to watch for, and determining when your child can return to child care. Parents' instincts about their sick children are usually very good — trust yours.

INFANTS, TODDLERS AND MEDICATIONS

A question new parents often have when faced with a sick child is whether it's OK to give medication. When you have a headache, for example, you might take a pain reliever. But what about for a child?

When it comes to medications, the benefits must always be weighed against the risks. While some medications play a role in helping infants and children feel better, many others do not. Plus, almost all drugs have potential side effects. So choose wisely when deciding what type of medication to give and when to give it.

The general approach to over-the-counter medications in an otherwise healthy child is that they're rarely needed. If you do use medications when necessary, use only those that are designed for infants or children, and follow the dosage and instructions recommended by your child's healthcare professional.

Fever and pain

If your baby is under 2 months and has a rectal temperature of 100.4 F or higher, call your child's medical professional right away. Don't give your baby any medications unless recommended by the medical professional. Because baby's immune system is still developing, a fever in an infant this age can be a sign of a serious condition and requires a medical evaluation.

Beyond 2 months of age, if your baby has a fever but seems to feel fine, is eating or drinking as usual, and acting like themself, medication isn't necessary, and you may not need to bring your child in to be seen by a medical professional.

If your child seems uncomfortable, acetaminophen (Tylenol, others) can help ease pain and reduce a fever and is safe for babies over 2 months old. Ibuprofen (Advil, Motrin, others), another pain reliever and fever reducer, also is safe for babies older than 6 months, although it may worsen an upset stomach. Check with a medical professional before giving medication to a child with a chronic illness, such as kidney or liver disease or asthma.

Cough and congestion

When your child is coughing or congested, it's tempting to pick up one of the many cough and cold medications available at the drugstore. But these medications aren't safe or effective for children under age 6, and they should generally be avoided until after age 12 unless recommended by a medical professional. The Food and Drug Administration warns that these drugs can have rare but serious side effects.

A safer and more effective alternative for a stuffy nose may be to use saline nasal drops or a saline spray to thin the mucus. Then you can use a suction bulb or other devices — sometimes called nose suckers or snot suckers — to suck the mucus from your child's nose. For children who are over a year old, honey can help soothe a cough (see "Colds" on page 421 and "Cough and cold medications" on page 422).

Precautions

When giving your child medicine, there are certain precautions to follow.

Give the right dose Infant medicines usually come in liquid form but in different strengths based on the individual medicine. Use only the dispenser that came with the medication, and follow the directions on the label carefully. Often, for children under 2 years old, the medicine label will tell you to ask a medical professional for instructions on dosing. If you know your child's weight, use that as a guide (see pages 580-581).

Avoid overdosing Give only medications with a single active ingredient, and write down times when medications are given. This can help prevent an accidental overdose. Some parents alternate between pain relievers such as acetaminophen and ibuprofen, but be cautious about doing this. Each medicine requires a specific time interval between doses (see pages 580-581).

Avoid aspirin Aspirin is not approved for children under 2 years. It's generally not recommended for children under age 18 because of its association with a serious illness called Reye's syndrome, which causes damage to the brain and liver. The risk is mostly associated with using aspirin to treat symptoms of a viral illness, such as the flu or chickenpox. But it's not always easy to accurately distinguish between viral and nonviral illnesses. As a result, experts recommend avoiding aspirin altogether in children under 18, unless specifically prescribed by a medical professional.

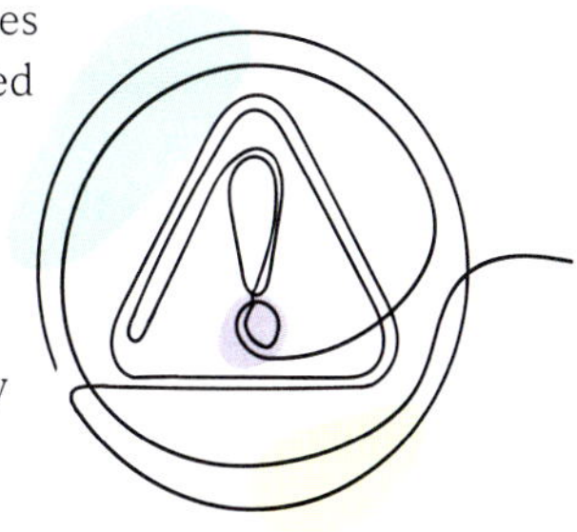

If you have any questions about giving your child a medication, call your child's healthcare team. A nurse or other medical professional may be able to answer your question quickly, and many clinics even have after-hours call services. If your child vomits or develops a rash after taking a medicine, call the care team right away.

How to give medicine

When your child does need medicine, here are some tips to make the job easier:

- A baby is usually more willing to take medicine by mouth before a feeding.
- Some pharmacies may offer flavoring to make medication more appealing.
- Using a syringe, place a small amount of medicine inside the child's cheek, where it's not as easy to spit out and there are no taste buds.
- Try blowing quickly on your child's face after giving liquid medication to trigger a reflexive swallow, before it can be spat out.
- For babies older than 6 months who resist taking oral medication, acetaminophen suppositories are another option for fever or pain relief.
- Avoid chewable medications in children younger than 2 years old.
- Don't refill bottles or use measured droppers for anything other than the original medicine.
- Follow the directions of your child's medical professional for continuing to use a medication, even if it doesn't taste good or your child's symptoms are getting better. A course of antibiotics, for example, needs to be taken in full for it to work as it should and to prevent bacteria from developing resistance to it.

TAKING YOUR CHILD'S TEMPERATURE

If your child feels warm or seems sick, a temperature check can help you identify a fever. When your baby is very young — under 2 months — a fever means your child needs medical care right away. This is because a new baby's immune system is still developing. In older infants and children, however, a fever generally isn't cause for alarm, unless it's combined with other symptoms (see "Fever" on page 434).

Taking your child's temperature sounds simple enough, but if you're new to it, you may have questions. Here's what you need to know.

Thermometer options

There are several types you can choose from:

- *Digital thermometers.* These thermometers use electronic heat sensors to record body temperature. They can be used in the rectum (rectal), mouth (oral) or armpit (axillary). Keep a separate thermometer for rectal use. Rectal temperatures provide the best readings for infants and toddlers. Armpit temperatures are typically the least accurate of the three measures. Digital pacifier thermometers and fever strips aren't recommended due to concerns about accuracy.
- *Temporal artery thermometers.* These thermometers use an infrared scanner to measure the temperature of the temporal artery in the forehead. This type of thermometer can be used even while a child is asleep.
- *Digital ear thermometers (tympanic membrane).* These thermometers use an infrared scanner to measure the temperature inside the ear canal. Keep in mind that earwax or a small, curved ear canal can interfere with the accuracy of an ear thermometer temperature.

Whatever the method, make sure you carefully read the instructions that came with your thermometer. After each use, clean the tip of the thermometer with rubbing alcohol or soap and lukewarm water.

For safety — and to make sure the thermometer stays in place — never leave your child unattended while you're taking a temperature.

Age matters

The best type of thermometer — or the best place to insert the thermometer, in some cases — depends on your child's age.

- *Birth to 2 months.* A rectal temperature is the most accurate method at this age. Use a standard digital thermometer to take a baby's rectal temperature.
- *2 months to 4 years.* In this age range you can use a digital thermometer to take a rectal or an armpit temperature or you can use a temporal artery thermometer. Wait until your child is at least 6 months old to use a digital ear thermometer. If you use another type of thermometer to take a young child's temperature and you're in doubt about the results, take a rectal temperature.
- *4 years and older.* By age 4 or 5 years, most kids can hold a digital thermometer under the tongue long enough to get an oral temperature reading.

How it's done

Here's how to take a temperature using the different methods. Be sure to turn on the thermometer before you start.

- *Rectal temperature.* Turn on the digital thermometer and lubricate the tip of the thermometer with petroleum jelly. Lay your child on their back, lift the thighs, and insert the lubricated thermometer ½ to 1 inch into the rectum. Insert the thermometer slowly, in the direction of the bellybutton, and stop if you feel any resistance. Hold the thermometer in place until the thermometer signals that it's done. Remove the thermometer and read the number.
- *Armpit temperature.* When you place the thermometer under your child's armpit, make sure it touches skin. Avoid touching any clothes. While the device reads your child's temperature, hug your child, keeping the side holding the thermometer against your chest. Keep the thermometer tightly in place until the thermometer signals that it's done. Remove the thermometer and read the number.
- *Ear temperature.* Gently place the thermometer in your child's ear. Follow the directions that come with the thermometer to ensure that you insert the thermometer the proper distance into the ear canal. Hold the thermometer tightly in place until the thermometer signals that it's done. Remove the thermometer and read the number.
- *Temporal artery temperature.* Gently sweep the thermometer across your child's forehead. Remove the thermometer and read the number.
- *Oral temperature.* Place the tip of the thermometer under your child's tongue toward the back of the mouth and ask your child to keep their lips closed. Remove the thermometer when it signals that it's done and read the

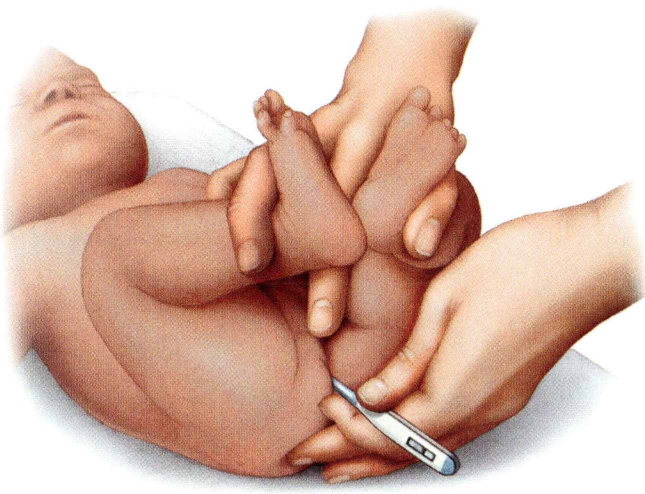

Taking a baby's temperature rectally

number. If your child has been eating or drinking, wait 15 minutes to take a temperature by mouth.

When reporting a child's temperature to a medical professional, give the reading you took and explain which thermometer you used and how the temperature was taken.

CARING FOR A SICK CHILD

Many common childhood illnesses can be treated at home. If you have any questions, seek the help and advice of your child's healthcare team. When you have a sick child at home, a little extra loving care is always in order. To help your child recover quickly and fully, there are some simple steps you can follow.

Encourage rest

Make sure your child has plenty of opportunity to rest. Getting enough sleep will help ease crankiness and lessen irritability and discomfort. Take the opportunity to snuggle up and relax together. A mild illness is often just the excuse you need to pause the family's hectic schedule and spend quality time with your child.

Offer plenty of fluids

One of the biggest risks associated with infections and other common childhood illnesses is dehydration. This happens when children lose more fluids than they're taking in — because of vomiting, diarrhea, difficulty feeding or just the increased demands on the metabolism. If your child is having difficulty eating or keeping fluids down, offer small, frequent sips of breast milk, formula, water or oral rehydration solution (see "Vomiting" on page 464 for more details on getting your child to take in enough fluids). Older babies and toddlers may enjoy sucking on an ice pop.

Make your child comfortable

If your child is congested, adding extra moisture to the air by running a humidifier or vaporizer may help soothe your child's nose. Or have your child breathe the warm, moist air in a steamy bathroom. Saline drops or spray in the nose can help with congestion (see page 423). If your child's room feels hot and stuffy, circulate the air with a fan. Also make sure your child isn't dressed too warmly.

Use medications wisely

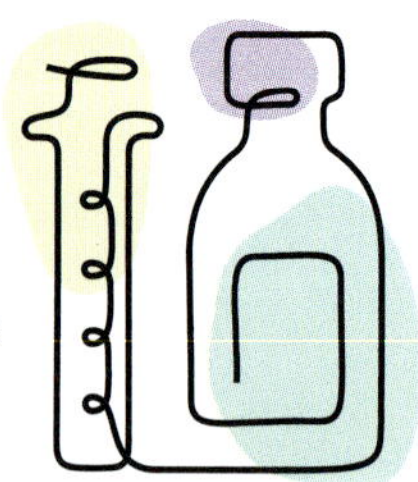

Medication may not be necessary if your child is more than 2 months old and has a fever but is eating and sleeping well and playing as usual. But if your child is fussy and uncomfortable, it's fine to give acetaminophen (Tylenol, others) to relieve the discomfort. Ibuprofen (Advil, Motrin, others) should only be given to babies older than 6 months. Follow the directions on the label, the dosage charts on pages 580-581 or the advice of your child's medical professional. Be sure to wait the appropriate amount of time before giving another dose. If your child's medical professional has prescribed antibiotics or another medication, follow the instructions exactly to maximize the drug's benefits and reduce possible risks.

Call your child's medical professional

When dealing with a sick child, trust your intuition as a parent. If you feel that you should call your child's healthcare team, call. Describe what's worrying you and what you've tried so far. A phone call to a medical professional often can solve a lot of problems and give you reassurance that the steps you've already taken are the right ones. If you feel that you should have your child seen in the medical office, an urgent care clinic or the emergency department, go in.

Prevent the spread of germs

Young babies are especially vulnerable to viruses and bacteria. Take common-sense steps to limit the spread of germs. Above all, wash your hands frequently and thoroughly and make sure other family members do the same. You may want to keep bottles of hand sanitizer in various places around the house.

KEEP GERMS FROM SPREADING

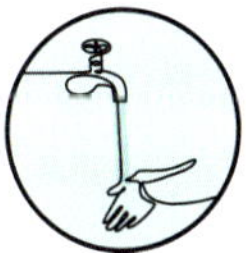

Wash hands frequently for at least 20 seconds with soap. Or, when soap and water aren't available, use hand sanitizer.

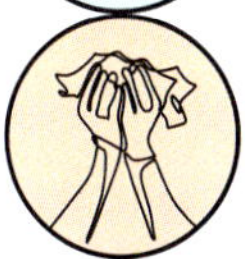

Sneeze or cough into a clean tissue or into your elbow if tissues are unavailable. Toss used tissues promptly.

In general, avoid people who are sick. Stay away from crowded areas in the fall and winter, when more people are indoors and the chances of infection are higher.

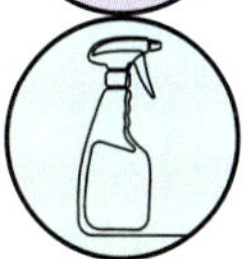

Keep surfaces clean, including pacifiers and toys that your child likes to chew on.

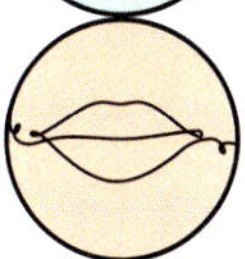

Refrain from kissing a young infant if you have an active cold sore. Cold sores are caused by a type of herpes virus, which can cause serious problems for babies.

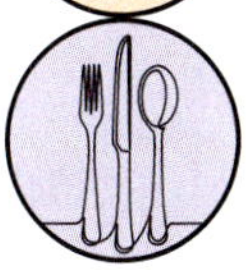

Don't share eating and drinking utensils.

A TO Z ILLNESS GUIDE

Following are some illnesses most common in young children and tips on how to treat them.

ALLERGIES

Allergies occur when your body's natural defense system incorrectly identifies a typically harmless substance as harmful. The body then overreacts in an attempt to protect itself, and the result is an allergic reaction. A tendency to develop allergies is usually inherited.

Food allergies are most common in children, especially toddlers and infants. The top food allergens include eggs, milk, wheat, soy, tree nuts, peanuts, fish and shellfish. Fortunately, most children outgrow allergies to milk, soy, wheat and eggs. Severe allergies and allergies to nuts and shellfish are more likely to be lifelong.

Reactions to pollen and other environmental triggers are less common in infants and toddlers. Pollen allergies, for example, usually don't start until around age 4.

How to recognize it

An allergic reaction to a food typically occurs shortly after eating it. Food allergies often cause symptoms such as:

- Itchy skin
- Rash
- Hives
- Swelling
- Cough, wheezing or shortness of breath
- Diarrhea
- Vomiting
- Irritability or lethargy

Food allergies can be confused with an intolerance or sensitivity to certain foods. Intolerance of a certain food can cause digestive problems — such as a stomachache, gas and diarrhea. But food intolerance isn't related to the immune system. For example, some children don't have enough of the enzyme required to digest milk sugar (lactose), making them lactose intolerant. Also, sometimes the acid found in certain foods, such as tomatoes or oranges, can cause a red rash around the mouth that parents mistake for allergies.

How serious is it?

Food allergies must be taken seriously, as they can cause a life-threatening allergic reaction called anaphylaxis. This reaction requires emergency treatment. However, allergic reactions to pollen, soaps, rough fabric (see page 123), and other environmental factors are typically more annoying than serious.

Anaphylaxis A serious allergic reaction often happens quickly. Symptoms to watch out for include:

- Difficulty breathing
- Facial swelling
- Tongue or throat swelling
- Drooling
- Hives
- Bluish, pale or gray skin color or skin flushing
- Loss of consciousness

When to call

If your child has symptoms of anaphylaxis, call 911 or your local emergency number. After emergency treatment, see your child's medical professional to determine what caused the reaction and to figure out how to avoid another one. Your child might be prescribed an emergency epinephrine autoinjector (EpiPen or Twinject) that you can keep with you at all times. This medication will provide your child relief until you're able to reach the emergency department.

If your child has allergy symptoms such as a constant runny nose, itchy nose, sneezing, itchy red eyes or chronic cough, make an appointment with a medical professional to discuss what's causing it and to learn how to treat it.

What you can do

The best way to prevent any allergic reaction is to avoid the substance that's triggering the reaction. If you're introducing new foods to your child and your child shows signs of a possible food allergy, a medical professional may advise going back to foods you know are safe and holding off on new foods for a week or so. Then introduce new foods one at a time, so that you can monitor which food might be causing problems. Your child's healthcare professional may refer you to an allergy specialist who can conduct tests to identify potential allergens when specific foods are suspected of having caused an allergic reaction. More general food allergy screening is not recommended.

In the past, it was common practice to wait longer to introduce allergenic foods such as peanuts and eggs. But based on newer evidence, experts now advise introducing these foods around 4 to 6 months to help prevent the development of food allergies. If your child is at increased risk of allergies — such as having eczema, an egg allergy or a family history of food allergies — talk to your child's medical professional. An early introduction to peanut-containing foods has been shown to be helpful (see page 79).

ANEMIA

Anemia is a condition in which blood doesn't have enough healthy red blood cells or hemoglobin. Red blood cells carry oxygen to the brain and other organs and tissues, providing energy and giving skin a healthy color. They're also essential to a child's growth and development.

The most common cause of anemia in infants is iron deficiency — too little iron in the body. Iron is needed to create hemoglobin, the substance that enables red blood cells to deliver oxygen throughout the body. Iron deficiency can occur as a result of premature birth or excessive blood loss.

In full-term infants, iron deficiency usually results from a lack of iron in the child's diet. Babies who drink cow's or goat's milk too early, for instance, miss out on iron because these kinds of milk are a poor source of iron. Cow's milk, soy milk, goat's milk and camel's milk can also interfere with iron absorption. Excessive milk intake — especially more than 24 ounces a day — is a common cause of iron deficiency in toddlers.

Most full-term babies are born with a supply of iron that lasts about four months. After that, the supply diminishes and needs to be supplemented with other sources of iron, such as iron-rich foods or an iron supplement. Supplements aren't needed in infants fed fortified formula, as it provides adequate iron. But a supplement may be recommended for breastfed infants.

How to recognize it

Mild symptoms of anemia aren't always easy to recognize. Often children are diagnosed with anemia after a blood test done for a separate reason. In general, though, a child with more severe iron deficiency anemia may:

- Appear pale or yellowish, which might be more obvious on white skin than on Black or brown skin
- Tire easily
- Be persistently irritable
- Have a poor appetite
- Have restless sleep

How serious is it?

If untreated, iron deficiency in children can cause delays in growth and development. Some studies show a long-term association between iron deficiency anemia in infancy and later deficits in intellectual capacity.

Don't try to treat your child on your own. Always talk to your child's medical professional before giving your child any type of vitamins or supplements.

When to call

If your child seems unusually pale or has a change in skin color, if your child is tired, irritable or uninterested in eating, or if you're concerned about the amount of iron in your child's diet, talk to your child's medical professional. In most cases, a simple blood test is all that's needed to diagnose anemia. In many areas, children are routinely screened for anemia before age 2.

Iron deficiency anemia is treated with higher-dose iron supplements, usually in a liquid form for infants. Generally, the supplements are given for about 7 to 9 weeks. Iron medications can change your child's stool to a dark color, so don't be concerned if this happens. Once your child's iron levels are back to a typical level, make sure you provide enough dietary iron through food or supplements.

It is possible to overdose on iron supplements. Too much iron can be harmful or even dangerous in very large doses, so be sure to give supplements to your child exactly as the medical professional recommends. Also, keep this and any other medications away from small children except when you're giving a dose.

What you can do

Iron deficiency anemia can be prevented by making sure your child gets enough dietary iron. Here are some simple steps you can take:

- *Offer milk appropriately.* Wait to give your child milk until at least age 1. Until then, give your child breast milk or formula. After that, limit milk to 2 or 3 cups a day (16 to 24 ounces).
- *Introduce iron at the right time.* If you're breastfeeding, give your child iron-fortified cereal when you start to introduce solid foods. Ground meat, beans, lentils and other iron-rich foods also can be great first foods. If you're breastfeeding exclusively beyond age 4 months, talk to your child's medical professional about giving your child an iron supplement.
- *Use iron-fortified formula.* If your child drinks formula, make sure it has iron added (4 to 12 milligrams of iron per liter). Most standard formulas on the U.S. market contain iron.
- *Offer a balanced diet.* As children get older, you can include iron-rich foods in their diet, such as pureed meat, egg yolks, green beans, peas, squash, spinach, sweet potatoes, tuna, ripe apricots and stewed prunes.
- *Enhance iron absorption.* Offer your child foods rich in vitamin C, which helps the body to absorb iron. Examples include strawberries, cantaloupe, kiwi, raspberries, broccoli, tomatoes, cauliflower, and citrus fruits, including juices.

ASTHMA

Asthma refers to inflammation of the breathing tubes (airways) in the lungs. It is a common condition in children and teenagers. The airways become narrow due to swelling, congestion and constriction of the airway muscle. This makes breathing difficult.

Children with asthma may have episodes of cough, wheezing, noisy breathing, and difficulty breathing that comes and goes. Some children have more nighttime cough. Asthma symptoms can be mild or severe (an asthma attack), and are different from child to child. The symptoms typically appear after exposure to certain triggers.

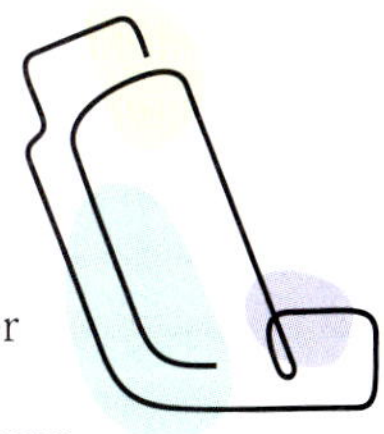

Common triggers are viral infections like the common cold, RSV and flu viruses. Symptoms also can occur with seasonal changes in fall and spring; poor air quality; exposure to cold, dry air or high humidity; and exposure to secondhand smoke, including from cigarettes, marijuana and vaping.

Children with a history of allergies and eczema and with a sibling or parent with asthma or allergies are more prone to develop asthma symptoms.

How to recognize it

Cough spells, along with rapid, labored breathing, especially with a cold, are a common symptom. Wheezing — a high-pitched whistling sound produced when your child breathes out (exhales) — is another sign of asthma, but it can't always be heard. Other symptoms include a cough that gets worse at night, tightness in the chest, and shortness of breath, especially when playing or when exposed to cold or humid temperatures. With asthma, wheezing or coughing episodes tend to happen repeatedly. Some kids may have only one symptom, such as a lingering cough or chest congestion after a cold.

To diagnose asthma, your child's healthcare professional looks for a combination of symptoms, test results, and treatment responses to inhalers or nebulizer medications. However, diagnosing asthma in young children can be challenging, since they may not be able to clearly communicate their symptoms or to perform reliable lung function tests. And other common childhood conditions, such as bronchiolitis and pneumonia, have similar symptoms.

How serious is it?

Asthma symptoms vary from child to child and may get worse or better over time. Some kids outgrow recurrent wheezing when they reach 5 or 6 years old. For others, wheezing episodes may stop and then happen again later in life. Still others have chronic, persistent wheezing that requires management with daily medications.

When to call

Seek emergency medical care if your child has severe trouble breathing or is not able to complete sentences, or if the mouth or fingertips are turning dusky or blue.

Make an appointment right away with your child's medical professional if you notice a fever with persistent coughing or wheezing, or if your child has difficulty sleeping or eating because of wheezing, coughing or troubled breathing.

Asthma is treated with prescription medications. Quick-relief medications work by opening the airways to immediately make breathing easier. Controller medications work to reduce inflammation and open airways. They're used daily by children diagnosed with asthma and have regular symptoms or who have symptoms with colds or other upper respiratory infections.

If your child has asthma symptoms, a medical professional may use a wait-and-watch approach before prescribing medications, depending on the frequency and severity of symptoms. If your child has severe wheezing episodes, a quick-relief medication called albuterol may be prescribed, to help ease your child's symptoms. This medication comes in the form of an inhaler or a nebulizer.

With an inhaler, medical staff can show you how to use a spacer, a plastic tube — with a mask or mouthpiece attached — that makes it easier to deliver the medication to your child's lungs. For younger children, you may also use a nebulizer, a machine that aerosolizes liquid medication. This changes it into fine droplets that your child breathes in. If asthma is severe, a short course of oral medications called corticosteroids may be prescribed. Asthma medications are very safe. All medications carry risks if used inappropriately, but when asthma medications are used correctly, their benefits far outweigh the small risks.

If your child's wheezing continues over time, a medical professional will likely recommend additional evaluation or testing for asthma. If your child does have asthma, your child's medical professional can prescribe medications that control symptoms and help to prevent severe attacks.

Daily asthma medications can sometimes be difficult to remember to use, especially when your child's asthma is well controlled, with no daily symptoms. It may not seem necessary to give medication to a child who isn't ill. But it's very important not to stop asthma medication. Left untreated or undertreated, childhood asthma can lead to permanent lung changes that can result in poor lung function in adulthood.

What you can do

Keep track of your child's wheezing episodes, how often they occur, the triggers, and what medications they typically respond to. Record these details in a log — written or on your smartphone or tablet — if you can. Don't be afraid to call your child's medical professional when symptoms arise. If you're not sure when to call, ask the healthcare team for guidance.

If you notice that certain things tend to trigger your child's wheezing, such as dust or pollen, try your best to avoid them. Clean regularly to eliminate dust, and use air-conditioning during pollen season to keep out airborne allergens. If your child's wheezing is worsened by cold air, bundle your child in a blanket to keep the air around the face warm and moist. However, studies show that allergen avoidance measures are not always effective in controlling asthma. So don't feel that you need to surround your child in a protective bubble at all times.

BRONCHIOLITIS

Bronchiolitis is a common lung infection in babies and young children. It's caused by a virus, often respiratory syncytial virus (RSV). In adults, RSV infection typically causes only mild upper respiratory tract symptoms. In infants, however, the infection sometimes spreads to smaller lung airways (bronchioles), leading to inflamed, narrowed airways (bronchiolitis). RSV infection is very contagious and is most common during the winter months. Other less common viral causes of bronchiolitis include influenza, parainfluenza, measles and adenovirus.

How to recognize it

Bronchiolitis usually starts like a common cold, with symptoms such as a runny nose, mild fever, and cough. As time passes, the cough becomes more severe, and you might notice your child wheezing. If your baby is having trouble breathing due to severe illness, you may see the chest suck in around the ribs with each breath (see illustration, page 453). In addition, since babies primarily breathe through their nose, when excess mucus clogs their nasal passages or flows down their throat, it becomes challenging for them to suck and swallow. As a result, they may find it difficult to eat or drink.

How serious is it?

Symptoms of bronchiolitis can range from mild to severe. Wheezing and coughing typically last for a week to a month or more and then go away on their own.

In some cases, especially if your child has an underlying health problem or is a significantly premature infant, bronchiolitis can become severe and require hospitalization for respiratory support.

During the illness, it's important to encourage your child to drink frequently. Not getting enough fluids creates a risk of dehydration, which can be serious.

When to call

If your child's symptoms are severe — such as marked difficulty breathing, refusal to drink or eat, breathing pauses, or skin that's turning blue or grayish from lack of oxygen (especially around the mouth and fingernails) — call 911 or your local emergency number.

Call your child's medical professional right away (or seek urgent care if after office hours) if your child:

- Is making a high-pitched, whistling sound (wheezing) while breathing out
- Is having trouble eating
- Develops signs of dehydration (three or fewer wet diapers in 24 hours in younger children or reduced urination in older children; dry mouth; crying without tears; taking less fluid)
- Is under 2 months and has a fever, is listless or not waking as you'd expect, or has a fever that lasts more than three days

Also, call your child's medical professional without delay if you suspect bronchiolitis and your child was born prematurely or has an underlying health problem.

If the severity of your child's symptoms requires a hospital stay, your child may need to be given oxygen to maintain sufficient oxygen in the blood. Your child also might need to be given fluids through a vein (intravenously) to prevent dehydration.

What you can do

You can treat most cases of mild bronchiolitis at home with self-care steps. Treat the cold symptoms with a humidifier and perhaps saline nasal drops if your child is very congested (see page 423 for tips on relieving cold symptoms). Encourage plenty of fluids, in small quantities and frequently, as breathing difficulties often cause your child to eat or drink less and more slowly.

Wash your hands frequently to prevent the spread of viruses. When your child is a newborn, avoid close contact with children or adults with any type of respiratory infection — even if the symptoms seem mild.

COLDS

Babies and toddlers are especially susceptible to the common cold — a viral infection of the nose and throat. This is largely due to their developing immune systems and because they're often around other children with colds, either in child care or at home with siblings. In fact, young children have an average of 6 to 8 colds a year. Colds generally last a week or two, but occasionally they last longer. Sometimes it may seem as if your child has a runny nose all winter! This is especially true if a child has older siblings or attends child care.

Colds are most commonly spread when someone who is sick coughs, sneezes or talks, spraying virus-carrying droplets into the air that others inhale. Colds can also be spread through hand-to-hand contact — or, among babies and toddlers, hand-to-nose or hand-to-mouth contact. Some viruses can live on surfaces for a few hours, so toys may be another source of infection.

Once infected by a virus, your child generally becomes immune to that specific virus. But because there are so many viruses that cause colds, your child may have several colds a year and many throughout life.

How to recognize it

During a cold, your child will likely develop a congested or runny nose. Nasal discharge is typically clear at first, then turns yellow, thicker and sometimes even green. After a few days, the discharge again becomes clear and runny.

Cold can appear differently. Some colds seem to settle mainly in a child's nose, and others settle in the chest. Colds also may cause a fever (see page 434) in your child for the first few days. Your child also may sneeze and have a cough, a hoarse voice or red eyes.

If your infant seems to have a lot of sneezing or snorting and is frequently congested, it might not always be due to a cold. Because a baby's nasal passages are quite small, it doesn't take much mucus to cause congestion. Congestion may also result from dry air or from exposure to irritants such as cigarette smoke.

How serious is it?

Colds are mostly annoying and usually don't require a visit to a medical professional. If your child has a cold with no complications, it should go away within 7 to 14 days.

Keep an eye on your child's symptoms, though. Sometimes colds can turn into more serious problems, especially in smaller or younger infants. If your child's symptoms seem to worsen, call your child's healthcare team.

When to call

If your child is younger than 2 months of age, call the healthcare team early in the illness. It's important to check for croup, pneumonia or another more serious illness, which can develop quickly in newborns. Even without such complications, a stuffy nose can make it hard for your child to nurse or drink from a bottle. This can lead to dehydration. As your child gets older, your child's

COUGH AND COLD MEDICATIONS

The Food and Drug Administration (FDA) and the American Academy of Pediatrics (AAP) strongly recommend against giving over-the-counter cough and cold medicines to children younger than 4 to 6 years old. Over-the-counter cough and cold medicines don't effectively treat the underlying cause of a child's cold and won't cure a child's cold or make it go away any sooner. These medications also have potential side effects, including a rapid heart rate and convulsions.

Other remedies have fewer risks and may even be more effective in young children:

- *Warm fluids.* A little soup or broth can have a soothing effect and help loosen nasal congestion.
- *Honey.* For children over 12 months old, ½ to 1 teaspoon of honey as needed is safe to consume and can soothe a cough. It can be given straight or diluted, such as in milk. Due to the risk of infant botulism, a rare but serious form of food poisoning, never give honey to a child younger than age 1.
- *Moist air.* Moistening the air with a cool mist humidifier can help your child breathe easier. So can sitting with your child in a steamy bathroom (see page 423).

Coughing isn't all bad. It helps clear mucus from your child's airway. If your child is otherwise healthy, there's usually no reason to suppress a cough.

healthcare team can guide you on when to seek medical care and when you can treat a cold at home.

If your child is under 2 months and has a temperature of 100.4 F or higher, see a medical professional right away. After age 2 months, call your medical professional if your child:

- Has a fever that lasts more than three days
- Seems to have ear pain
- Has red eyes or develops yellow eye discharge (also see "Pink eye," page 447)
- Has a cough that improves and then worsens, or a cough that interferes with ease of breathing or lasts longer than one month
- Seems lethargic or very irritable or experiences symptoms that worry you

Seek medical help immediately if your child:

- Refuses to nurse or accept fluids and has three or fewer wet diapers in 24 hours, reduced urination, or other signs of dehydration
- Coughs hard enough to cause persistent vomiting or changes in skin color
- Coughs up blood-tinged sputum
- Has difficulty breathing or is bluish or grayish around the lips and mouth

What you can do

Unfortunately, there's no cure for the common cold. Antibiotics kill bacteria but don't work against viruses. Over-the-counter medications generally should be avoided in infants. However, pain relievers may be used — provided you carefully follow dosing directions — if a fever is making your child uncomfortable (see pages 580-581). Acetaminophen (Tylenol, others) is safe in babies age 2 months or older. Ibuprofen (Advil, Motrin, others) is OK to use if your child is age 6 months or older.

Cough and cold medications are not safe for young children. In the meantime, consider the following suggestions for making your child more comfortable.

Offer plenty of fluids Liquids are important to avoid dehydration. Encourage your child to take in the usual amount of fluids. Extra fluids aren't necessary. If you're breastfeeding your child, keep it up.

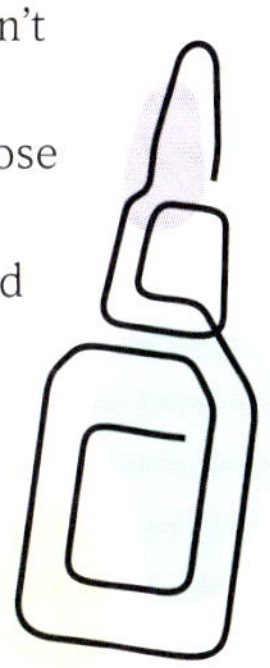

Thin the mucus If your child's nasal discharge is thick, saline nose drops or saltwater nasal sprays may help loosen the mucus. Saline nose drops and sprays are made with the optimal amount of salt and water. They're inexpensive and available without a prescription. To help your child eat better, place a couple of drops in each nostril. In infants, this can be especially helpful if done 15 to 20 minutes before a feeding. This can be followed by using a suction bulb or a nose sucker.

Moisten the air Running a cool mist humidifier in your child's room can help improve a runny nose and nasal congestion. Aim the mist away from your child's crib to keep the bedding from becoming damp. To prevent mold growth, change the water daily and follow the manufacturer's instructions for cleaning the unit. It might also help to sit with your child in a steamy bathroom for a few minutes before bedtime. Avoid the use of hot steam vaporizers because of the risk of burns to infants and children from their use.

Avoid sick people Keep your child away from anyone who's sick, especially during the first few days of an illness. Remind family and friends that the most loving thing they can do when sick is to stay away from young children, especially a new baby. If possible, avoid public transportation and public gatherings with your newborn.

Keep hands clean Wash your hands before feeding or caring for your child. Use hand gels, wipes or soap and water. Ask that everyone who cares for or visits your child do the same.

Don't share Don't share bottles, utensils or sippy cups. If your child attends a child care facility, make sure personal items are clearly labeled. Clean your child's toys and pacifiers often.

Use tissues Teach family members to cough or sneeze into a tissue and then toss it. If you can't reach a tissue in time, cough or sneeze into your elbow.

CONSTIPATION

Parents sometimes worry that their child is constipated because several days go by without a bowel movement. But it's not unusual for an infant who is exclusively breastfed to go for several days — even a week or longer — without a bowel movement. Constipation refers to dry, hard stools that are difficult to pass. As long as the stool is soft and easily passed, constipation likely isn't a problem.

Constipation tends to be more common in toddlers than in infants, especially during toilet training or with changes in diet.

How to recognize it

Constipation may be a problem if your child:

- Is a newborn and hasn't passed the meconium stool one to two days after birth
- Has stools that are hard and dry
- Has painful bowel movements (grunts and grimaces, discomfort, fussiness)
- Has stools streaked with blood
- Appears to have abdominal pain that seems to be relieved after a large bowel movement
- Has frequent soiling accidents after being toilet trained

How serious is it?

Most infant constipation is mild, a result of a change in the child's diet, and eases within a short time. In older children, it can usually be managed by providing extra fluids and more high-fiber foods.

Constipation can interfere with toilet training, especially when bowel movements are difficult or uncomfortable. Treating the constipation can help make toilet training easier.

When to call

Call your child's medical professional if your child seems chronically constipated or if your efforts at home aren't providing any relief. Don't give laxatives, enemas or medication without consulting a medical professional first.

What you can do

Breastfed babies are rarely constipated from changes in the mother's diet. If a change of diet seemed to start the problem, the issue will likely improve with time. For kids who are eating solid foods, these measures may help:

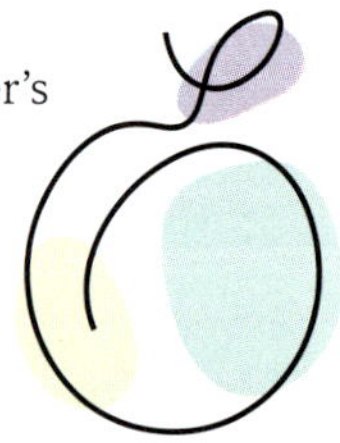

- Offer plenty of fluids.
- Limit your child's intake of milk.
- Offer more fruits and vegetables.
- Gradually add high-fiber foods to your child's diet. This might include apple juice, prunes (or up to 4 ounces of prune juice a day), apricots, plums, peas and beans.

COUGH

Cough is a common symptom in infants and toddlers and often a cause of anxiety in parents. Coughing is a protective mechanism that helps to clear the airways of mucus and other secretions. Most coughs are not serious and are due to viral infections of the upper respiratory tract. A chronic cough that's triggered by exercise, cold air, sleep or allergens may be a sign of asthma. In babies and young children cough could also be due to food or liquids going down the air passages.

How to recognize it

The types and causes of coughing vary, according to the part of the respiratory tract affected. An irritation near the voice box may cause a barking, croupy cough, and an irritation of your child's trachea may cause a raspy cough. Allergies or asthma may cause a dry, unproductive cough that often occurs during the night. Postnasal drip can cause a throat-clearing cough, often seen both during the day and at night. Pneumonia may cause your child to have a deep chest cough that occurs both day and night. Young children with pneumonia usually have a fever and look sick.

How serious is it?

Your child's cough, by itself, may be bothersome but usually isn't serious. The seriousness of the cough depends on the condition that's causing the cough. Treating the underlying problem usually helps the cough.

When to call

Contact your child's medical professional promptly if your child develops a cough and:

- Is younger than 2 months and has a rectal temperature of 100.4 F or higher
- The cough lasts longer than four weeks or worsens after beginning to improve
- Seems to be in pain

Call 911 or your local emergency number if your child:

- Begins turning blue
- Has problems swallowing or difficulty making sounds
- Stops breathing

What you can do

You may be able to ease your child's cough by providing extra fluids and adding moisture to the air with a humidifier. Sitting with your child in a steamy bathroom may help, too. For children who are over a year old, ½ to 1 teaspoon of honey, diluted in some water or milk if desired, can help soothe a cough.

If your child's cough is interfering considerably with eating and sleeping, check with your child's medical professional about measures to take. Cough medicines aren't recommended for young children because of potential side effects. They're also generally not effective in this age group (see "Cough and cold medications" on page 422).

COVID-19

COVID-19 has become a common respiratory infection. It's caused by a virus called severe acute respiratory syndrome coronavirus 2, or SARS-CoV-2. This virus typically spreads through the air in tiny droplets between people in close contact.

Many people with COVID-19 have only a mild illness or no symptoms. Children are less likely than adults to become very sick from COVID. But for older adults and people with certain medical conditions, COVID-19 can lead to severe illness and needing care in the hospital.

How to recognize it

Your child's symptoms could range from mild to serious — or none at all. The most common symptoms are fever and a cough, including a barking cough linked to croup. Other common symptoms include:

- Sore throat
- Stuffy or runny nose
- Headache
- Feeling very tired (fatigue)
- Nausea, vomiting or loose stools (diarrhea)
- Chills
- Muscle aches and pain
- Problems breathing or shortness of breath
- New loss of taste or smell

If your child has symptoms, they may show up from 2 to 14 days after contact with the virus that causes COVID-19.

For many children, symptoms are like those of the common cold, flu or RSV. Testing can help figure out if the virus that causes COVID-19 is the cause. Testing helps you act quickly to prevent serious illness in kids who are at higher risk. It can also help protect others who may be at high risk. Ask your healthcare team about the best way to have your child tested.

How serious is it?

For babies under age 1, the risk of serious illness might be higher than for older children. Babies born prematurely have the highest risk. Certain health conditions, such as diabetes or heart or lung conditions, can increase the risk as well.

Rarely, a child may develop a serious condition called multisystem inflammatory syndrome in children (MIS-C) several weeks after having COVID-19. With MIS-C, children have fever, blood markers of inflammation and serious disease throughout the body. Symptoms include a fever that doesn't go away, along with:

- Vomiting
- Diarrhea
- Belly pain
- Skin rash
- Bloodshot eyes
- Dizziness or lightheadedness

Call 911 or seek emergency care if you notice your child has trouble staying awake or waking up, difficulty breathing, new confusion, or severe belly pain, or if the skin, lips or nails appear gray or blue.

MIS-C symptoms are treated in the hospital as the illness runs its course. Most children get better quickly and don't have any medical issues caused by MIS-C.

When to call

Get emergency help right away if your child is working hard to breathe. Symptoms of breathing trouble include grunting, flaring the nostrils, shortness of breath at rest, rapid breathing, or wheezy, noisy or raspy breathing. In babies, this may show as not being able to cry or feed.

In addition, call or seek medical care right away if your child has other signs of serious illness, including:

- A temperature over 100.4 F in a baby less than 2 months old
- Vomiting or diarrhea that doesn't stop
- Three or fewer wet diapers in 24 hours or other signs of dehydration
- Emergency symptoms of MIS-C (see "How serious is it?")

If your child has a mild to moderate fever and cough or cold symptoms, consider testing for COVID. If your child has a positive COVID-19 test at home, take steps to reduce the spread of the infection to others, especially those at increased risk of serious illness. Most children have a mild infection and can be cared for at home. Call your healthcare team if symptoms get much worse or last longer than 10 days.

However, for children with a higher risk of severe illness, it's important to see a medical professional sooner when COVID symptoms develop.

Anyone who catches the COVID-19 virus can develop post-COVID-19 syndrome, sometimes called long COVID. In young children, persistent cough

HOW CAN I GET MY TODDLER TO WEAR A FACE MASK?

Once your child is 2 years old, you may want to encourage wearing a face mask in certain situations — for example, on a plane ride, when your child has a cold or when you go to the store during peak flu season. Here are some tips for helping toddlers get used to the feeling of wearing a mask so that they might actually keep it on when needed.

- *Model it.* If you want your child to wear a mask, wear yours, too.
- *Find a mask that is easy to breathe through and fits your child well.* You may need to adjust the ear loops so it stays in place.
- *Practice wearing a mask at home for short activities your child enjoys.* Do a puzzle, read a book, build something with magnetic tiles or have screen time together.

and respiratory symptoms appear to be the most common symptoms of long COVID. If your child isn't getting better, talk with your healthcare professional.

What you can do

A COVID-19 vaccine is recommended for all children starting at 6 months of age to help lower the risk of severe infection from the virus that causes COVID-19. It also may prevent your child from becoming seriously ill. Children from 6 months to 4 years old should get all doses from the same vaccine maker. Talk with your healthcare professional about any questions you have.

Pregnant people can help lower an infant's risk by getting the COVID-19 vaccine during pregnancy. Some evidence suggests that protection can pass to the baby and continue after birth. Protective antibodies also are present in breastmilk after mRNA COVID vaccines.

If your child is sick with COVID-19, keep them away from others, especially those at higher risk for severe illness, as much as possible for as long as they're ill. Encourage resting and drinking fluids, and monitor symptoms. Medicines such as acetaminophen (Tylenol, others) or ibuprofen (Advil, others), depending on your child's age, can lower a fever to help your child feel more comfortable.

You can take steps to stop the spread of the virus. Have your child frequently wash hands with soap for 20 seconds. When that's not an option, use an alcohol-based hand sanitizer that contains at least 60% alcohol. Clean high-touch surfaces and objects regularly, including your child's changing table. Use fans, open windows and filters to keep air moving through indoor spaces. Keep some distance from others, especially in crowded indoor spaces, and wear a face mask in public if many people in your area are sick. However, don't place a face mask on a child younger than age 2 or a child with a disability who can't safely wear a mask.

CROSSED EYES

Crossed eyes (strabismus) is one of the most common eye problems in young children. It occurs as a result of an imbalance in the muscles controlling the eye.

It's typical for a newborn's eyes to wander or appear cross-eyed because the brain cells haven't yet learned how to control eye movements. But by 4 months of age your child's nervous system should be developed enough that the eyes work together to focus on the same point at the same time. If they continue to cross or wander, then it's time to see your child's medical professional.

How to recognize it

You may notice that one of your child's eyes turns in, out, up or down. This misalignment may be present all the time, or it may come and go.

Some babies have what's referred to as false strabismus (pseudostrabismus). Although their eyes are perfectly aligned, they appear cross-eyed because of the way their face is shaped. They might have extra skin around the inner folds of the eyes or a wide bridge of the nose. As your child gets older, the appearance of being cross-eyed should fade.

How serious is it?

A child can't outgrow true strabismus, and the condition typically gets worse if left untreated. At first, a misaligned eye can lead to double vision. But eventually the brain will learn to ignore the image from the turned eye, and the eye may become "lazy" (amblyopic). This may result in permanently reduced vision.

When to call

If by 4 months of age your baby's eyes appear crossed, even if only sometimes, make an appointment with your child's medical professional. Your child may need to see a pediatric eye doctor for an evaluation. It's important to get an accurate diagnosis as soon as possible. The earlier treatment is started, the better the outcome for your child.

Rarely, a child's eyes may suddenly become misaligned after having been straight. If this happens, call your child's medical professional right away, as it may signal a more serious problem.

To treat strabismus, your child may need prescription eyeglasses, eyedrops, eye patches or surgery on the eye muscle. Surgery is usually reserved for when other treatments aren't working. It's safe and effective, but a second procedure is sometimes required to get the eyes exactly aligned.

What you can do

You can't treat strabismus at home, but you can monitor your child's eyes. Request an evaluation as soon as you suspect any problems with your child's eyes. If your child needs treatment, make sure your child wears prescribed glasses or that you give your child eyedrops exactly as recommended. Sometimes surgery is necessary. An eye surgeon will explain what you need to know about the procedure if it is recommended.

CROUP

The most common characteristic of croup, a viral infection of the upper respiratory tract, is a harsh, repetitive cough that's often likened to a seal barking. Because the cough is so harsh, it can be scary for children and their parents. But croup usually isn't serious, and most cases can be treated at home.

The barking cough of croup is the result of inflammation around the vocal cords and windpipe. When the cough reflex forces air through this narrowed passage, the vocal cords vibrate with a barking noise. Because young children have small airways to begin with, they tend to have more marked symptoms.

As with a cold, croup is contagious until the fever is gone, or a few days into the illness. The virus is passed by respiratory secretions or droplets in the air.

How to recognize it

The classic sign of croup is a loud, harsh, barking cough — which often comes in bursts at night. Your child might have noisy or difficult breathing. Other cold-like symptoms — such as a runny nose, fever and hoarse voice — are common, too.

How serious is it?

Most cases of croup are mild, and your child likely won't need to see a medical professional unless symptoms are severe. Croup generally lasts three to seven days (plan on at least a couple of difficult nights) and then goes away on its own.

Rarely, the airway swells enough to interfere with breathing, warranting a trip to an urgent care clinic or emergency department. Pneumonia is a rare but potentially serious complication.

When to call

If your child's skin is turning blue or grayish around the nose, mouth or fingernails, or your child is struggling to breathe, dial 911 or your local emergency number.

Call immediately or seek medical care immediately if your child:

- Makes noisy, high-pitched breathing sounds when inhaling or exhaling (stridor)
- Begins drooling or has difficulty swallowing
- Seems agitated or extremely irritable
- Becomes unusually sleepy or lethargic

Call as soon as you're able if you're concerned that your child:

- Has a fever for more than 3 to 5 days
- Can't sleep or settle
- Is getting worse night after night, despite home treatment
- Isn't taking fluids well for 24 hours or shows signs of dehydration

What you can do

While your child is sick, there are a few things you can do.

Stay calm Comfort or distract your child — cuddle, read a book or play a quiet game. Crying makes breathing more difficult.

Spend some time in cold air Cool outdoor air has been shown to help improve breathing in children with croup. In one study, 30 minutes in outdoor air cooler than 50 F helped with symptoms. If it's cool outdoors, you can open a window to get fresh air or wrap your child in a blanket and walk outside to see if that helps your child breathe more comfortably. If your child has asthma or a history of wheezing, watch to make sure that cold air doesn't make symptoms worse.

Alternatively, there's no evidence of benefit from warm, humid air, but some feel it is helpful. Bring your child into a steamy bathroom to breathe the warm, moist air.

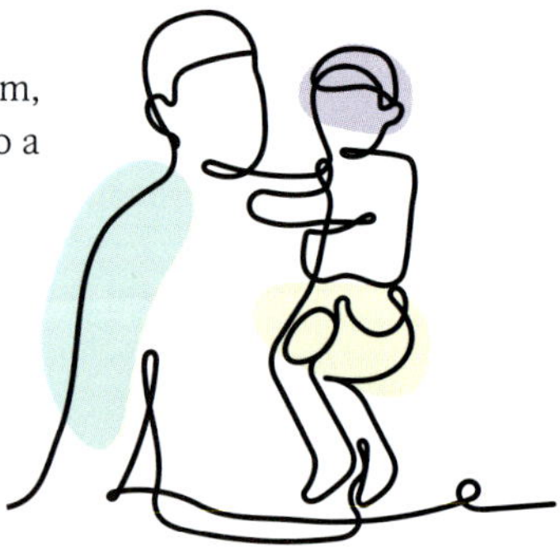

Hold your child in an upright position Sitting upright can help make breathing easier. Hold your child on your lap, or place your child in a favorite chair or infant seat.

Offer fluids For babies, breast milk or formula is fine. For older children, soup or ice pops may be soothing.

Encourage rest Sleep can help your child fight the infection.

DIARRHEA

Diarrhea in a young infant is a common concern for new parents. Bowel movement patterns can vary widely among young infants — from a single bowel movement once a week or so to over 10 a day, especially in breastfed babies. So it can be tricky to tell when diarrhea is a problem. A "blowout" every so often is nothing to worry about, but if you notice stools that are more frequent than usual and have a watery consistency, your child may have diarrhea.

Once your child is regularly eating solid food, when diarrhea does hit, you'll most likely know.

Diarrhea is most often caused by an infection of your child's stomach and intestines (gastroenteritis), usually by a virus. Sometimes bacteria or parasites may cause diarrhea. Although it's rare for a child to have diarrhea from a specific food allergy, diarrhea can be caused by certain dietary factors. Examples include drinking more juice, lactose intolerance or the addition of new foods. Antibiotics also may cause diarrhea.

How to recognize it

If you're changing more dirty diapers than usual and the contents in the diaper (or the potty) are consistently thin and watery, your child likely has diarrhea. Diarrhea caused by an infection may also be accompanied by vomiting, belly pain and fever. You may see blood in the stool as well. That could be caused by a bacterial infection, skin irritation from frequent stools or irritation of the intestinal lining.

How serious is it?

Dehydration is the main complication that can result from diarrhea, especially if your child has also been vomiting or isn't drinking fluids as well as usual. Your child has a much smaller reserve of fluids than you do.

When to call

Contact your child's medical professional immediately if your child:

- Passes more than eight diarrheal stools in eight hours or has blood in the stool
- Seems to have belly pain and a temperature of more than 102 F, or other obvious signs of illness (or just a temperature of 100.4 F or higher for a child less than 2 months old)
- Can't keep any fluids down
- Shows signs of dehydration (reduced urination for older children, or three or fewer wet diapers in 24 hours for younger children; no tears when crying; dry mouth; or sunken eyes or fontanels — the soft spots in the head of young babies)
- Seems unusually sleepy or noticeably less active than usual

You might also contact your child's medical professional if your child has mild diarrhea for more than a week and you're concerned.

What you can do

If your child has mild diarrhea and is hungry, there's no need for dietary restrictions. Continue feeding your baby as you typically would with breast milk or formula. If your child is eating solid foods, offer bland foods if that's what your child prefers. Offering yogurt may help, but there's no consensus that probiotics — found in fermented foods such as yogurt and in supplements — can help with diarrhea due to infection. Offer frequent, small feedings, meals or snacks rather than large ones. Aim to get your child back to a typical diet within a few days to ensure adequate nutrition.

If your child has moderate diarrhea, use a commercially prepared oral rehydration solution (Pedialyte, others) to replace the sodium and electrolytes lost in your child's stool. These solutions are available without a prescription and can be used until your child's symptoms improve.

Call your child's medical professional if diarrhea is severe or symptoms get worse. Call right away if you notice signs of dehydration (see "When to call" on page 431).

EAR INFECTION

An ear infection (acute otitis media) is a common reason children need medical care. An ear infection is caused by a bacteria or virus that affects the middle ear, the air-filled space behind the eardrum that contains the tiny vibrating bones of the ear. Children are more likely than adults to get ear infections.

Ear infections often occur after a cold or other respiratory infection. These illnesses set the stage for inflammation and buildup of fluids in the middle ear.

How to recognize it

Infants with an ear infection usually develop the infection after an upper respiratory tract infection, such as a cold. Here are some signs and symptoms to look for.

- Ear pain, especially when lying down
- Tugging or pulling at an ear
- Unusual crying or fussiness
- Difficulty sleeping or irritability, especially after a cold or other upper respiratory infection
- Fever that returns after initial cold symptoms seem to be improving
- Difficulty hearing or responding to sounds
- Drainage of fluid from the ear
- Loss of appetite

How serious is it?

Mild ear infections may improve within the first couple of days. Symptoms that are severe or persist are often treated with antibiotics.

Long-term problems related to chronic ear infections — persistent fluids in the ear, long-lasting infections or frequent infections — can cause hearing problems and other serious complications. So it's important to bring ear infections, especially recurring ones, to the attention of your child's medical professional.

When to call

If your child is less than 2 years old and you suspect an ear infection, have them seen by a medical professional. For a child age 2 or older, contact your health-care team if:

- Symptoms last for more than two days
- Ear pain is severe
- Your child has a fever over 102 F. (See page 434.)
- You see fluid, pus or bloody fluid coming from the ear

In babies, most ear infections are treated with antibiotics. For older children, a medical professional may wait to see if the condition improves on its own before prescribing antibiotics.

Ear tubes are tiny tubes that are surgically placed through the eardrum to help ventilate the middle ear and prevent the accumulation of fluid. They are usually reserved for children who have many ear infections and persistent fluid behind the eardrum, or hearing problems.

What you can do

Whether or not an antibiotic is recommended, pain management with medications can improve comfort. Consider giving acetaminophen, if your child is more than 2 months old, or ibuprofen after 6 months of age. In addition, placing a warm (not hot), damp washcloth over the affected ear may lessen pain.

To reduce your child's risk of ear infections, practice good infection prevention habits. Wash hands frequently, don't share eating and drinking utensils, and avoid contact with others who are sick. Secondhand smoke also may contribute to frequent ear infections. When giving a bottle, hold your child upright to avoid blocking the passage between the middle ear and the throat (eustachian tube).

EARWAX BLOCKAGE

Earwax blockage occurs when earwax (cerumen) accumulates in the ear or becomes too hard to be washed away naturally.

Earwax is a helpful and natural part of the body's defenses. It protects the ear canal by trapping dirt and slowing the growth of bacteria. Typically, it will dry up and tumble out of the ear on its own. But occasionally wax buildup occurs. This might happen because of a narrow ear canal, an excess production of earwax or even well-meaning attempts to clean out the ear, which can push the wax farther into the ear and cause a blockage.

How to recognize it

Although it may not be easy to identify in your child, symptoms of earwax blockage are likely to resemble some of those related to an ear infection. Your child may pull or tug at the ear, cough, or be unusually fussy or irritable. You may also notice that your child doesn't hear quite as well or doesn't respond to sounds.

How serious is it?

A buildup of earwax is unlikely to cause serious problems, unless you try to dig it out yourself. Trying to remove earwax with a cotton swab or other instrument may push the wax farther into your child's ear and cause serious damage to the lining of the ear canal or eardrum.

When to call

Make an appointment to have your child's ears checked if your child is tugging at the ears or you notice hearing problems.

A medical professional can determine if there's excess earwax by looking in your child's ear with an otoscope, a special instrument that lights and magnifies the eardrum. The medical professional often can remove excess wax using a small instrument called a curette. Wax also might be flushed out using a water-filled syringe or other tools.

What you can do

Avoid cleaning your child's ears with cotton swabs, your finger or anything else. If your child doesn't have tubes or holes in the eardrum, a medical professional may recommend eardrops to soften the wax. The medical professional can show you how to wash out the softened wax with warm water and a bulb syringe.

FEVER

Body temperatures vary for different people. Your newborn's temperature will vary by about 1 degree throughout the day. It's usually lowest in the morning and highest late in the afternoon. In general, infants and young children have a higher body temperature than do older children and adults.

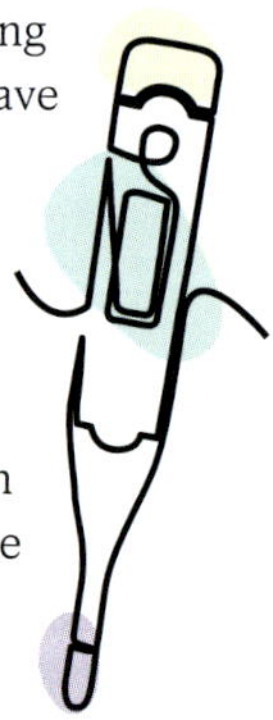

When faced with an infection or other illness, however, your child's central nervous system cranks up the internal "thermostat" to help fight the infection. This results in a fever. In newborns and infants less than 2 months of age, a fever warrants an immediate call to your child's medical professional. In older infants and children, the need for medical evaluation of a fever depends more on how your child is feeling and whether there are other accompanying symptoms of illness.

How to recognize it

If your child feels unusually warm to you, take their temperature with a thermometer (see page 410). Although laying your hand or your cheek on your child's forehead may give you a suspicion of fever, it won't tell you the difference between 99 F and 101 F. A temperature of 100.4 F or higher signals a fever. See page 411 for tips on getting an accurate temperature reading.

How serious is it?

A fever itself usually isn't harmful. Any potential harm would come from the cause of the fever. Often, a child with a fever is fighting an infection; a fever is a sign of the immune system at work.

In young infants, especially those under 2 months, an infection signaled by a fever can quickly become serious. Their immune systems are not yet up to the task of fighting off bacteria and other germs, making them particularly vulnerable to an infection that can easily spread throughout the body.

An elevated temperature after being in a hot environment is different from a fever caused by an infection. A temperature in response to an infection rarely

FEBRILE SEIZURES

Some children experience convulsions as a result of a rapid rise in body temperature, often from an infection. Watching your baby have a febrile seizure can be alarming, but the good news is that it's usually harmless and typically doesn't indicate a long-term or ongoing problem. Studies suggest there also isn't much that can be done to prevent a febrile seizure. Most of the time, a febrile seizure happens on the first day of an illness, sometimes even before parents realize that their child is ill.

A febrile seizure causes repeated rhythmic jerking of the arms and legs. Children aren't responsive to you or aware of their surroundings while this movement occurs.

If your child has a febrile seizure, stay calm and follow these tips to help your child during the seizure:

- Place your child on their side, somewhere where your child won't fall.
- Watch and comfort your child.
- Remove any hard or sharp objects near your child.
- Loosen any tight or restrictive clothing.
- Don't restrain your child or interfere with your child's movements.
- Don't attempt to put anything in your child's mouth.

Have a first-time febrile seizure evaluated by your child's medical professional as soon as possible, even if it lasts only a few seconds. If the seizure ends quickly, call the medical professional as soon as it's over and ask when and where your child can be examined. Note how long the seizure lasted and what the movements looked like. If the seizure lasts longer than five minutes or is accompanied by vomiting, a stiff neck, problems with breathing or extreme sleepiness, call for an ambulance to take your child to the emergency department.

By staying calm, observing your child and knowing when to call for medical help, you're doing everything that's needed to take care of your child.

climbs high enough to be dangerous. But a high temperature from being in a hot car, for example, can be deadly.

When to call

Always call your child's medical professional right away if your child is under 2 months of age and has a rectal temperature of 100.4 F or higher, even if your child seems otherwise fine. This is important because your child's immune system is still developing and may not be able to fight off an infection as well as an older child.

For older infants and children, call if you have concerns or if your child's fever lasts more than three days. Seek urgent care if your child experiences:

- Repeated vomiting or diarrhea
- Unusual fussiness or irritability
- Dehydration — three or fewer wet or soiled diapers in 24 hours, dry mouth, crying without tears, sunken eyes and, in young babies, sunken fontanels (the soft spots in the head)
- Unusual drowsiness and unresponsiveness

If your child seems feverish after spending time in a hot area, such as on a beach or in a hot car, seek medical help immediately. Overheating (heatstroke) is an emergency and needs to be treated quickly.

What you can do

If your child has a fever, monitor their behavior closely. Look for other symptoms. Call your child's medical professional if you have any concerns. The most common reason for a fever in young children is a viral infection. For the majority of viral infections, no specific treatment is required; the fever and the illness that caused it will resolve with time. In the meantime, there are several steps you can take.

Provide plenty of fluids Continue breastfeeding or formula-feeding as usual. For infants over 6 months, you can also offer water or an oral rehydration solution (Pedialyte, others). For toddlers, offer water, Pedialyte or ice pops. Prioritize drinking fluids over eating solid foods. Sick toddlers often don't eat well. Let your child decide whether and how much solid food to eat.

Encourage adequate rest Provide extra opportunities for rest and quiet play until the fever improves or stops.

Keep cool If your child seems hot, keep your child's room comfortably cool. Dress your child lightly.

Use medication for discomfort If your child seems uncomfortable, is older than 2 months and weighs 6 pounds or more, you can give oral acetaminophen (Tylenol, others). If your child is 6 months or older, acetaminophen suppositories are another option, and giving ibuprofen (Advil, Motrin, others) is OK. Read the label carefully for proper dosage (see pages 580-581). Don't use aspirin to treat a fever in anyone age 18 years or younger, as it can cause a rare but serious disorder called Reye's syndrome. Keep in mind that it's generally not a good idea to give fever-reducing medication for more than three days without consulting your child's medical professional.

FIFTH DISEASE

Fifth disease (erythema infectiosum) is a highly contagious and common childhood illness caused by a virus called parvovirus B19. It's sometimes called slapped-cheek disease because of the red rash that appears on the cheeks. In most children, the infection is mild and requires no specific treatment.

How to recognize it

A child with fifth disease will develop bright red, warm patches on both cheeks. During the next few days, there will be a pink, lacy, slightly raised rash on the arms, trunk, thighs and buttocks. On darker skin, these symptoms may be harder to see. The rash is usually itchy.

Generally, the lacy rash occurs near the end of the illness when the child is no longer contagious. A few days before the rash begins, some children develop flu-like symptoms such as muscle aches, fever, headache, upset stomach and fatigue.

It's possible to mistake the rash for other viral rashes or a medicine-related rash. The rash may come and go for several weeks, becoming more visible when your child is exposed to extreme temperatures or spends time in the sun.

How serious is it?

For most children who are otherwise healthy, fifth disease is a mild illness. Rarely, it can cause more serious problems, especially in children with a weakened immune system or sickle cell disease or other blood disorders.

Parvovirus infection can be a concern during pregnancy, too. Keep a sick child away from anyone who's pregnant, particularly in the first trimester. If a person develops a parvovirus infection during pregnancy, the fetus may be affected.

When to call

Call your child's medical professional if your child is under 2 months old and has a rectal temperature of 100.4 F or higher. Your child may need to be examined to rule out more serious causes of fever (see page 434).

Typically, once the rash appears, the illness has mostly run its course and no treatment is needed. However, call your healthcare team if your child has a fifth disease-like rash and another condition such as sickle cell anemia or a weak immune system.

What you can do

Make sure your child gets plenty of rest and drinks lots of fluids. You can use acetaminophen (Tylenol, others) or ibuprofen (Motrin, others) if appropriate to relieve fever or minor aches and pains (see pages 580-581).

It's not always practical or necessary to isolate a child with fifth disease. You likely won't know your child has parvovirus infection until the rash appears, and by that time, the illness is no longer contagious.

FLU (INFLUENZA)

Influenza, commonly called the flu, is a frequent fall and wintertime viral illness that affects the upper respiratory system. It's often confused with the common cold, although the flu may leave your child feeling more achy and miserable than a cold does.

Several types of viruses can cause influenza (types A and B are the most common), with each type having several strains. Influenza viruses change over time, with new strains appearing regularly. This is why it's important to receive an annual flu vaccine — each year's vaccine is developed to prevent the three or four strains most likely to appear that year. The Centers for Disease Control and Prevention (CDC) recommends annual flu vaccination for everyone age 6 months or older (see page 191). It's typically available as an injection. Some years it's available as a nasal spray. Ask your child's medical professional about the best type of vaccination for your child.

How to recognize it

Having the flu usually causes:

- A sudden fever, although not everyone gets a fever
- Chills
- Achy muscles
- Extreme tiredness
- Dry cough

How serious is it?

Influenza can be a serious illness for your otherwise healthy child, although most babies recover without major problems. The main complications of influenza are ear infections and pneumonia; both require treatment from your child's medical professional. Children with underlying health problems are at greater risk of complications.

Influenza infections are contagious a day or so before and while your child is sick.

When to call

Children under age 2 are at higher risk of complications from the flu. Call your child's medical professional for advice if you notice flu-like symptoms, especially if your child has a fever for more than a couple of days or is getting worse, or if you are concerned about dehydration. If your child has flu-like symptoms and trouble breathing, seek medical care immediately. If you know your infant has been exposed to influenza, contact your child's medical professional.

What you can do

The best way to prevent the flu is to receive the flu vaccine, recommended to everyone 6 months of age or older. This includes people who are pregnant or breastfeeding, as antibodies can pass to the baby and provide some protection during the first few months of life.

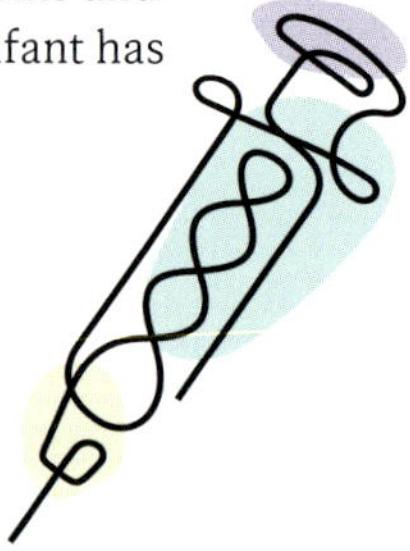

If your whole family receives the vaccine, you're less likely to get the flu and pass it to each other.

If your child is under 6 months of age, it's especially important to take commonsense precautions against infections:

- Wash your hands frequently.
- Keep heavily used surfaces clean.
- Cough or sneeze into a tissue or the crook of your elbow. Discard used tissues promptly.
- Don't share eating or drinking utensils or toothbrushes.
- Avoid cross-contamination between sick family members by not kissing each other on the hands or mouth.
- Avoid people who have the flu.
- Avoid crowds at peak flu season.

If your child does develop influenza, encourage plenty of rest, fluids and hugs. If your child seems fussy and uncomfortable, acetaminophen or ibuprofen, depending on your child's age, can help ease aches and pains, as well as reduce fever (see pages 580-581). Don't give aspirin, which can cause serious side effects in children. Keep your child out of child care for at least 24 hours after the fever has passed.

HAND, FOOT AND MOUTH DISEASE

Hand, foot and mouth disease is a usually mild, contagious viral infection that's common in young children. Symptoms include sores in the mouth and a rash on the hands and feet, including the palms and soles. Hand, foot and mouth disease is caused by viruses in the enterovirus family, such as coxsackieviruses.

Once exposed to the virus that caused hand, foot and mouth disease, your child will build up immunity to it. However, there are multiple viruses that can cause this illness. A different one could cause another round of hand, foot and mouth disease in the future.

How to recognize it

A fever is often the first sign of hand, foot and mouth disease, followed by a sore throat, irritability and sometimes pain with eating or a refusal to eat. Painful mouth sores are found inside the mouth. Most children will also get a rash on the hands and feet and sometimes on the buttocks or genitals. This mostly looks like small red dots, circles, bumps or blisters. The illness typically lasts about a week.

How serious is it?

Hand, foot and mouth disease is usually a minor illness causing only a few days of fever and relatively mild symptoms.

The sores in the mouth and throat can make swallowing painful and difficult for your child, however, increasing the risk of dehydration. Watch closely to make sure your child sips fluids frequently during the illness.

Infected people are most contagious during the first week of illness.

When to call

Contact your child's medical professional if mouth sores or a sore throat keeps your child from drinking fluids. Call also if your child's symptoms worsen after a few days.

What you can do

There's no specific treatment, but you can help speed healing by encouraging plenty of fluids and rest. Acetaminophen or ibuprofen, depending on your child's age, can help relieve discomfort and fever (see page 408 for more on medications).

For kids eating solid foods, certain foods may irritate blisters on the tongue or in the mouth or throat. You can help make blisters less bothersome and eating more tolerable by:

- Offering frequent feedings of breast milk or formula (drinking is more important than eating solids)
- Offering ice pops or a small amount of sherbet to soothe the mouth and throat
- Avoiding acidic foods and beverages, such as citrus fruits and fruit drinks
- Offering soft foods that don't require much chewing

HIVES

Hives is the name for a skin reaction that causes itchy welts. The medical term for the condition is urticaria. Often there's no clear explanation for what triggers hives, but viral infections are a common cause, especially when the hives last

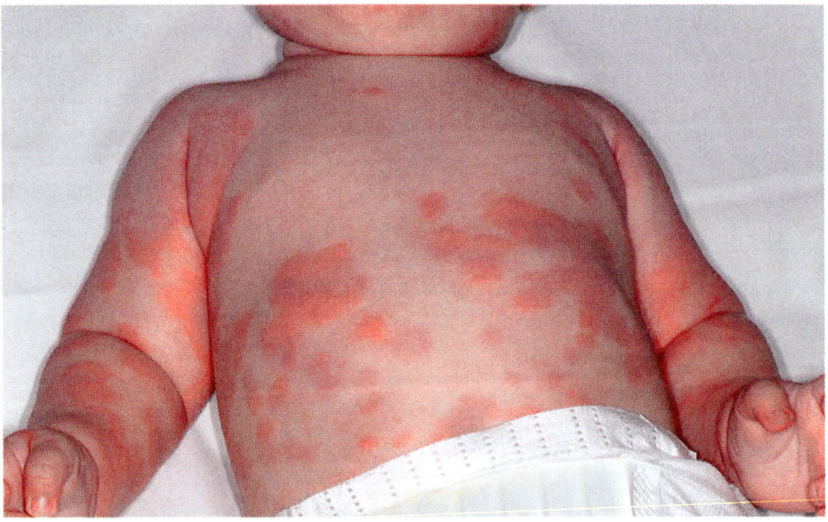

Hives causes itchy welts that may appear anywhere on the body.

more than 24 hours. Hives also can occur as an allergic reaction to a food, drug, airborne allergen, insect bite or sting.

How to recognize it

Symptoms of hives include batches of welts that can arise anywhere on your child's body. The welts may be red, purple or skin-colored. The welts usually cause itchiness, which can be intense. They can be irregularly shaped and can change locations. Some areas may enlarge and merge into each other. Hives may come and go for a few days or a few weeks.

How serious is it?

Hives usually isn't serious unless swelling develops around your child's throat area and windpipe. If this happens, it can make it difficult for your child to breathe and swallow.

When to call

If your child has difficulty breathing or swallowing or develops a swollen tongue with hives, call 911 for emergency care.

Otherwise, ask your medical professional about the proper treatment if your child develops hives.

Call right away if your child:

- Develops hives while taking medication
- Seems to have sore joints
- Has hives for more than a few days

What you can do

Kids with hives often look much worse than they feel. To keep your child as comfortable as possible, give an antihistamine as indicated by your child's medical professional. Keep your child dressed in light clothing and avoid bathing your child in hot water. Lukewarm water is less likely to aggravate the itching. Trim your child's fingernails to minimize irritation from scratching.

If you notice a pattern in when hives appear, try to determine what may be triggering it so you can avoid the trigger.

IMPETIGO

Impetigo is a common and highly contagious skin infection that mainly affects infants and young children. It is typically caused by the bacteria *Staphylococcus aureus* (staph) and group A streptococcus. It usually appears as reddish sores covered in a flaking, honey-colored crust (see the photo on page 121). The redness may be harder to see in darker skin. Less commonly it can also look like thin blisters filled with yellow fluid, which leave crusts on the skin when they break open.

Impetigo tends to develop on the face, especially around the nose and mouth. The kind that causes blisters is often found on the trunk or extremities.

Impetigo occurs when bacteria enter the skin through cuts or cracks, though it can develop in skin that's intact.

Keeping the skin clean and intact is the best way to prevent infection. Treat cuts, scrapes, insect bites and other wounds right away by washing the affected areas with gentle soap and water. Children with sensitive skin or eczema may be more prone to skin infections. Talk to your child's medical professional about the best ways to keep the skin healthy.

How to recognize it

Your child might have impetigo if you notice:

- Red, purple, brown or gray sores that quickly rupture, ooze for a few days and then form a yellowish-brown crust
- Itching of the sores
- Painless, fluid-filled blisters, usually on the trunk, arms and legs (more common in children under 2 years old)
- Painful fluid- or pus-filled sores that turn into deep ulcers (a more serious form that's less common)

How serious is it?

Mild impetigo usually clears on its own in two to three weeks. But because impetigo is very contagious and can sometimes lead to more severe infection, your child's medical professional will usually choose to treat impetigo with an antibiotic ointment or oral antibiotics.

When to call

If you suspect that your child has impetigo, ask your child's medical professional for advice on treatment. For mild cases, an antibiotic ointment may be recommended. This can be applied to the affected areas. If your child is uncomfortable, or if the sores are oozing or widespread, make an appointment to have the sores examined. Severe or widespread cases may be treated with antibiotics taken by mouth.

What you can do

For minor infections that haven't spread, an over-the-counter antibiotic cream or ointment may help. Try the following steps:

- Wash or soak the affected areas of skin with warm, soapy water. This helps the crust detach so that the antibiotic can penetrate the skin.
- After washing the area, apply the antibiotic ointment three times daily. Wash the skin before each application, and pat it dry.

To help keep the infection from spreading to others:

- Wash your hands frequently, especially after treating the sore.
- Trim your child's nails to prevent scratching and spreading the infection. Applying a nonstick dressing to the infected area can help, too.
- Avoid touching the sores as much as possible until they heal.
- Wash your child's towels and washcloths every day. Don't share them or other items, such as blankets or toys, with family members.

To prevent the infection from spreading, keep your child home from child care or preschool and ask your medical professional about the best strategy for a safe return. Often your child can return to childcare after starting antibiotic treatment if the sores can be covered. Once the sores heal, your child will not be able to spread the bacteria to others.

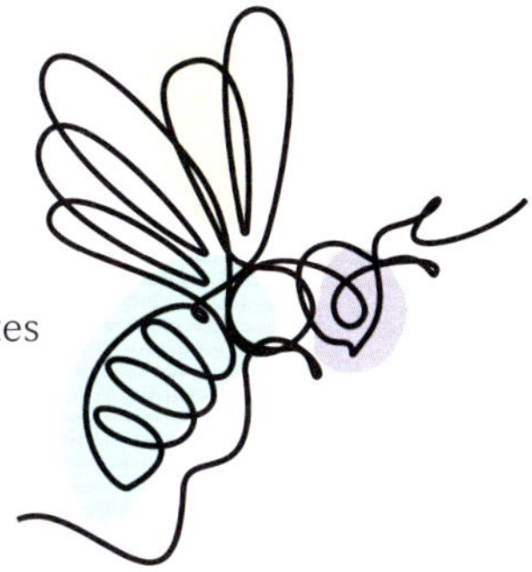

INSECT BITES AND STINGS

Stings from bees, wasps, hornets and yellow jackets and bites from fire ants are typically the most troublesome. Bites from mosquitoes, ticks, biting flies and some spiders also can cause reactions, but these are generally milder.

How to recognize it

Bites and stings may come from:

- *Bees, yellow jackets and hornets.* In most children, stings cause initial pain, changes in skin color and swelling within the first several hours. But in a few kids, stings can cause severe symptoms of anaphylaxis, including vomiting, diarrhea, dizziness and sometimes trouble breathing (see "When to call").
- *Mosquitoes.* Usually the site simply itches and swells. In some children, the swelling can be substantial.
- *Deerflies, horseflies, fire ants, harvester ants, beetles and centipedes.* These may cause painful bumps and changes in skin color. The bumps may blister.

How serious is it?

Most children will have only a mild reaction to bites and stings. But some children are more sensitive than others to insect venom, especially from stinging insects. These children can have a severe allergic reaction (anaphylaxis) that requires emergency treatment.

When to call

Call 911 or your local emergency number if your child:

- Has difficulty breathing
- Vomits
- Shows signs of shock (rapid breathing, dizziness, clammy skin)
- Has received multiple bee, wasp or hornet stings
- Develops extreme facial swelling
- Develops hives all over the body or in an area separate from the sting itself
- Has increased swelling and redness around the sting or bite after the first six to eight hours

What you can do

If a stinger is noticeable, remove it from your child's skin as soon as possible. Use a fingernail, credit card or other thin, dull edge to scrape the stinger away. Avoid pinching or squeezing the stinger, as this may release more venom into the skin. Once the stinger is gone, apply a cool washcloth or ice pack to relieve pain and swelling. Cool compresses can also help relieve itching associated with other insect bites.

Ask your child's medical professional about ways to relieve itching, such as applying calamine lotion, hydrocortisone cream or baking soda paste. If itching is severe, the medical professional may recommend giving your child an oral antihistamine.

To decrease the likelihood of bites, take these steps:

- Cover your child's skin with lightweight clothing when you spend time outdoors.
- Help your child avoid areas where insects are commonly found, such as garbage cans, stagnant water (breeding ground for mosquitoes) and blooming flowers.
- Don't use strong perfumes or scented soaps and lotions on yourself or your child.
- Cover all picnic food, and seal picnic garbage in plastic bags.
- Keep garbage cans securely covered.
- Don't allow pools of stagnant water to sit in your yard.

DEET is the most widely used chemical in insect repellents. Products that contain DEET aren't recommended for babies under 2 months old. However, for older infants and toddlers, the AAP recommends choosing an insect repellent with a 10% to 30% concentration of DEET.

Apply DEET only once a day and wash it off at the end of the day to avoid toxicity. The higher the concentration of DEET in a product, the longer the duration of protection it supplies. The AAP recommends using the lowest effective concentration for the amount of time your child spends outside. A 10% DEET product provides about two hours of protection; a 30% DEET product protects for about five hours.

To apply repellent to your child, put it on your hands first and then rub it on your child's skin. Avoid your child's eyes and the hands, which children often put in the mouth.

There are alternatives to DEET products. Picaridin in 5% to 10% concentrations is safe for young children. Oil of lemon eucalyptus is a plant-based repellent, but some products based on oil of lemon eucalyptus should not be used for children under 3 years of age. Check labels to be sure a product is intended for use with young children.

JAUNDICE

Jaundice is a yellow discoloration of the skin and eyes. Newborn jaundice is a common condition, particularly in babies born before 38 weeks gestation and breastfed babies. It develops when a child's liver isn't mature enough to filter out bilirubin, a yellow-colored pigment of red blood cells, from the bloodstream. Jaundice after the neonatal period is rare.

How to recognize it

The main signs of newborn jaundice are yellowing of the skin and eyes. These usually appear between the second and fourth day after birth. You'll usually notice jaundice first in your child's face. If the condition gets worse, you may notice the yellow color in the eyes and on the chest, abdomen, arms, and legs.

The best way to check for newborn jaundice is to press your finger gently on your child's forehead or nose. If the skin looks yellow where you pressed, it's likely that your child has jaundice. If your child doesn't have jaundice, the skin color should simply look slightly lighter than its usual color for a moment.

It's best to examine your child in good lighting conditions, preferably in natural daylight.

How serious is it?

Mild newborn jaundice often disappears on its own within two or three weeks. If jaundice is moderate or severe, your child may need to stay longer in the newborn nursery or be readmitted to the hospital for phototherapy. This is a special blue light that helps the body clear the bilirubin.

Although complications are rare, severe infant jaundice can lead to cerebral palsy, deafness and brain damage.

When to call

Most hospitals have a policy of checking babies regularly for jaundice while they are hospitalized after birth and before they're discharged. The American Academy of Pediatrics recommends that your newborn be examined for jaundice whenever a routine medical check is done.

Your child should be checked for jaundice before being discharged from the birth hospital, and again between 3 and 7 days of age, when bilirubin levels usually peak.

The following symptoms may indicate severe jaundice or complications from jaundice. Call your child's medical professional if:

- Your child seems listless, sick or difficult to wake
- Your child isn't gaining weight or is feeding poorly
- Your child makes high-pitched cries
- Your child develops any other symptoms that concern you
- Diagnosed jaundice lasts more than three weeks

What you can do

Feeding more frequently will provide your child with more breastmilk or formula and cause more bowel movements, increasing the amount of bilirubin eliminated in your child's stool. Breastfed infants should have 8 to 12 feedings a day for the first several days of life. Formula-fed infants usually should have 1 to 2 ounces of formula every 2 to 3 hours for the first week.

If your child is having trouble breastfeeding, is losing weight or is dehydrated, your child's medical professional may suggest giving infant formula or expressed milk in addition to breastfeeding. In some cases, a medical professional may recommend giving only infant formula for a couple of days, pumping and storing breastmilk in this time, and then resuming breastfeeding. Ask your child's medical professional what feeding options are right for your child.

LAZY EYE

Lazy eye (amblyopia) develops when nerve pathways between the brain and the eye aren't properly stimulated. This can lead to a condition in which the brain favors one eye, usually due to poor vision in the other eye. The weaker eye, commonly referred to as the lazy eye, tends not to track with the stronger eye. Eventually, the brain may ignore the signals received from the weaker (lazy) eye.

Treatments such as corrective eyewear, eyedrops or eye patches can often correct lazy eye. Sometimes lazy eye requires surgical treatment.

How to recognize it

Lazy eye usually affects just one eye, but it may affect both eyes. With lazy eye, there's no apparent damage to or difference in the eye. Symptoms to look for include:

- An eye that wanders inward or outward
- Eyes that may not appear to work together
- Poor depth perception

How serious is it?

Left untreated, lazy eye can cause permanent vision loss. In fact, lazy eye is the most common cause of decreased vision in children, according to the National Eye Institute.

Depending on the cause and the degree to which your child's vision is affected, a number of treatment options may be possible.

Corrective eyewear If a condition such as nearsightedness, farsightedness or astigmatism is contributing to lazy eye, a medical professional likely will prescribe corrective glasses. Sometimes corrective eyewear is all that's needed.

Eye patches To stimulate vision in the weaker eye, your child may wear an eye patch over the stronger eye — possibly for two or more hours a day, depending on the severity of the condition. This helps train the brain to use both eyes to see.

Eyedrops An eyedrop medication that temporarily blurs vision in the stronger eye is used daily or twice weekly to encourage use of the weaker eye. It offers an alternative to wearing a patch.

Surgery If your child has crossed or outwardly deviating eyes (strabismus), the eye muscles may benefit from surgical repair. Droopy eyelids or cataracts also may need surgical intervention.

For most children with lazy eye, proper treatment improves vision within weeks to several months. And the earlier treatment begins, the better. Research suggests that the treatment window extends through at least age 17, but results are better when treatment begins before age 7.

When to call

If you notice your child's eye wandering at any time beyond the first few weeks of life, consult your child's medical professional for an evaluation. Depending on the circumstances, your child may be referred to an eye specialist (ophthalmologist or optometrist).

What you can do

There's really nothing you can do at home to treat lazy eye. However, you can monitor your child's eyes closely in the first few months of life to make sure they are in proper alignment and to make sure your child's vision seems to be consistently improving. The sooner treatment for lazy eye begins, generally the better the outcome for your child.

PINK EYE (CONJUNCTIVITIS)

Pink eye is an inflammation or infection of the transparent membrane (conjunctiva) that lines your eyelid and part of your eyeball. It's frequently caused by a viral infection — usually the same virus that causes the common cold. In fact, pink eye may develop after a cold. But conjunctivitis can also result from bacteria or allergies.

How to recognize it

You might suspect that your child has pink eye if you notice that the white part of the eye and the eyelid are reddened in one or both eyes. Allergic conjunctivitis — pink eye due to allergies — typically affects both eyes at once.

Pink eye can also cause mucus, or "matter," to form in your child's eye, varying from thin and watery to thick and yellowish green. With viral conjunctivitis, eye matter is usually worse in the morning. You may find your child's eyelids stuck together on awakening, needing you to wash them clean.

Also suspect pink eye if your child experiences discomfort with exposure to bright lights or if your child does a lot of blinking.

How serious is it?

Pink eye generally lasts about as long as a cold, usually a week or so, but sometimes up to two or three weeks. If infectious, pink eye is contagious by contact.

Viral infections, which account for most cases of pink eye, just need time to run their course. Bacterial infections may or may not be treated with antibiotic drops. Mild bacterial conjunctivitis often gets better on its own in a few days.

If pink eye is due to allergies, your child's medical professional may recommend specific eyedrops for people with allergies.

When to call

Make a call if your child:

- Develops a red and swollen eyelid
- Develops a fever or starts acting ill

- Has the symptoms of an ear infection
- Doesn't seem to improve after starting treatment

What you can do

Wash the outside of your child's eyelid, using clean cotton balls (a new one for each eye) and warm water. You also can use washcloths and warm water. Wipe from the inner to the outer part of the eye to prevent spreading infection to the uninfected eye. Because pink eye is usually contagious, you and others who care for your child should take precautions to avoid spreading it. A child with pink eye should have a separate towel and washcloth that no one else uses, both at home and away. Wash your hands carefully after you come into contact with secretions from your child's eyes.

In some cases of bacterial infection, your child's medical professional may recommend antibiotic drops or ointment. Some parents find ointment easier to use than eyedrops, although ointment can blur your child's vision for 20 minutes or so after application. In either case, the discharge should improve within a day or two, although the redness may persist a few days more. Follow the instructions of your child's medical professional and use the antibiotics until the prescription runs out to prevent the return of the infection.

Applying the drops or ointment in your child's eye is sometimes easier with two people. Wash your hands before applying ointment or drops. (The other person should do the same.) To prevent contamination of the medication, don't let the applicator tip touch any surface, including the child's eye. When you finish, wipe the tip of the tube with a clean tissue and tightly close it. Wash your hands after touching your child's eyes. Follow these application tips:

- *Eyedrops.* Lay your child on the back. Gently pull the lower eyelid down to form a little pouch, and place the drops in the pouch. The drops will disperse over the eye as your child blinks.
- *Ointment.* Pull your child's lower eyelid away from the affected eye to form a pouch. Unless your child's medical professional tells you otherwise, squeeze a thin strip of ointment into the pouch. Release your child's lower eyelid, and then ease the upper eyelid down to cover your child's eye. Hold the lid closed for just a moment or two.

PNEUMONIA

Pneumonia is an infection that inflames the air sacs in the lungs. Young children who get pneumonia are usually sick first with a cold or other viral upper respiratory tract infection. Some viral infections can then affect the lungs, resulting in viral pneumonia. Pneumonia can also stem from a bacterial infection, perhaps after a cold.

In children under 5, bacterial pneumonia is less common than the viral kind. Bacterial pneumonia may be helped by antibiotics.

How to recognize it

Pneumonia is usually worse than a bad cold. A child with pneumonia may cough and have a fever. Breathing may become fast and labored. Your child may also appear pale, develop a fever, lose appetite, and become either more listless or fussier than usual.

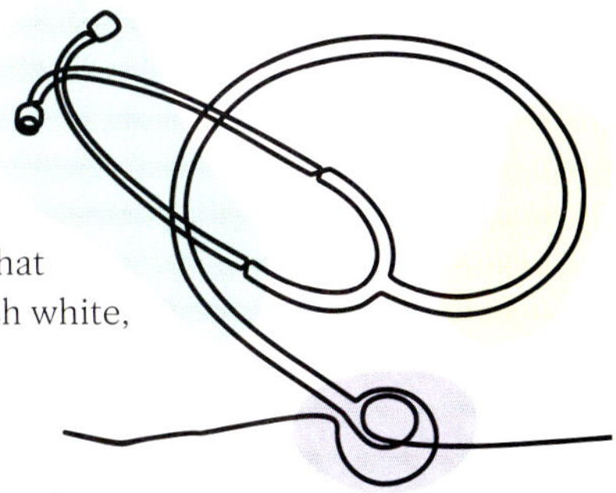

How serious is it?

In the past, pneumonia could be a dangerous illness. Now, most babies recover well if they receive prompt medical attention. If you notice that your child's lips or tongue appear bluish or grayish white, this is a sign that the illness may be more severe.

When to call

Call immediately if you suspect that your child may have pneumonia or your child is less than 2 months old and has a rectal temperature of 100.4 F or higher. Be sure to check back with your child's medical professional if:

- Your child's fever continues for more than two or three days, despite taking an antibiotic
- Your child has difficulty breathing

What you can do

If your child's medical professional suspects bacterial pneumonia, a course of antibiotics may be prescribed. Antibiotics don't help viral infections, but sometimes it's difficult to distinguish between viral and bacterial pneumonia. Be sure to give the full course of antibiotics, even if your child starts to feel better. This helps reduce the recurrence of the infection and minimizes the chances that the bacteria will become resistant to the drug.

Viral pneumonia typically doesn't require anything other than home treatment. Encourage quiet activities so that your child gets plenty of rest. Your child may need extra holding and cuddling. Your child also needs plenty of fluids. Coughing is usually beneficial for children with pneumonia because it helps to clear the mucus and secretions associated with the infection. You can help prevent bacterial pneumonia in many cases by making sure your child is up to date with all vaccinations.

REFLUX

Spitting up is common in new babies. Often it stops after the first few months. But in some babies spitting up continues throughout the first year or so. The medical term for this condition is gastroesophageal reflux.

The causes of infant reflux are generally simple. Usually the ring of muscle between the esophagus and the stomach (lower esophageal sphincter) relaxes and opens only when you swallow. Otherwise it's tightly closed — keeping stomach contents where they belong. Until this muscle matures, stomach contents may sometimes flow up the esophagus and out of your child's mouth. Sometimes air bubbles in the esophagus may push liquid out of your child's mouth. In other cases, your child may simply drink too much too fast.

How to recognize it

Although infant reflux most often occurs after a feeding, your child also may spit up when coughing, crying or straining. You also may notice your child becomes more irritable during or after feedings, or coughs, wheezes or cries when you lay your child on the back, especially after feeding.

How serious is it?

Infant reflux typically goes away by the time your child is around 12 months old. Unless it is severe, infant reflux doesn't interfere with a child's growth or well-being. Gastroesophageal reflux disease (GERD) is a severe version of reflux that can cause pain, vomiting and poor weight gain.

When to call

Call your child's medical professional if your child:

- Isn't gaining weight
- Is projectile vomiting (spits up forcefully and in a large quantity)
- Spits up green fluid, blood or a material that looks like coffee grounds (call immediately if this happens)
- Resists feedings
- Has blood in the stool
- Has other signs of illness, such as fever, diarrhea or difficulty breathing
- Begins persistent vomiting at age 6 months or older

What you can do

Infant reflux is usually not a cause for concern. Until your child outgrows the condition, you may have to keep burp cloths nearby and an extra supply of spit-up cloths on hand (for both you and baby). To minimize reflux in the meantime, try the following:

Offer smaller, more frequent feedings Feed your child slightly less than usual if you're bottle-feeding, or cut back a little on the amount of time you breastfeed. Feed more often.

Burp your child Frequent burps during and after each feeding can keep air from building up in your child's stomach. Sit your child upright, supporting the head with your hand, and rub the back (see page 72).

Check the nipple If you're using a bottle, make sure the hole in the nipple is the right size. If it's too large, the milk will flow too fast. If it's too small, your child may get frustrated and gulp air. A nipple hole that's the right size will allow about a drop of milk to fall per second when you hold the bottle upside down.

Thicken the formula or breast milk If your child's medical professional approves, add a small amount, such as 1 teaspoon, of rice cereal to your child's formula or expressed breast milk. You may need to enlarge the hole in the nipple to make sure your child can drink the thickened liquid.

Make a change Occasionally some babies respond better to a more hydrolyzed version of infant formula. Other babies develop an allergy to cow's milk protein. If you're breastfeeding, that means you may have to eliminate milk products from your diet. If you're formula-feeding your child and there's a concern your baby may have a milk allergy or may benefit from a hydrolyzed formula, your child's medical professional may suggest switching to a different formula.

RESPIRATORY SYNCYTIAL VIRUS (RSV)

Respiratory syncytial virus (RSV) causes infections of the upper respiratory tract, such as a cold, or the lower respiratory tract, such as bronchiolitis and pneumonia. It's so common that most children are infected with RSV before age 2. Reinfections with RSV are common, but as a child gets older, symptoms usually become less severe.

In many cases, the symptoms of an RSV infection resolve on their own. Self-care measures are usually all that's needed to relieve any discomfort.

In a few cases, the infection can be severe enough to require a stay at the hospital. Premature babies and infants with underlying health conditions are at greater risk of severe illness.

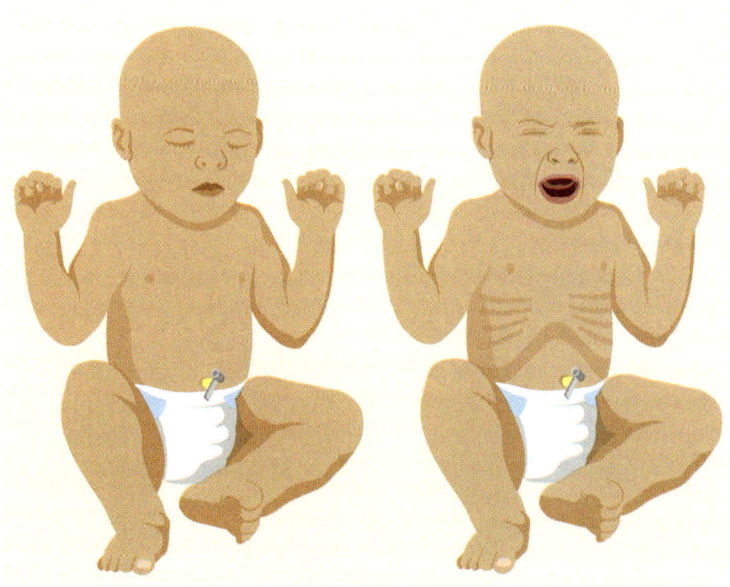

Typical breathing (left) vs. chest wall retractions RSV can cause serious breathing difficulty in infants. Seek medical attention if your child has very fast and shallow breaths, or if you see the ribs suck inward when breathing in (right), as these are signs of trouble breathing.

How to recognize it

Initially, infection with RSV may cause a runny nose, a decrease in appetite and perhaps a fever. Over the next few days, the infection may spread to the lower airways and lungs. Your child may start coughing, wheezing and breathing fast. Ear infections are occasionally associated with RSV infections.

In babies who are only a few weeks old, infection with RSV may cause more general symptoms, such as coughing, wheezing, extreme tiredness, irritability and poor feeding.

How serious is it?

Children who are otherwise healthy generally recover from the illness in one to two weeks without medical treatment.

Young babies are at greater risk of serious infection. Babies who are finding it difficult to breathe may need to stay at a hospital to receive supportive care, such as supplemental oxygen and suctioning of mucus from their airways. Even among babies who need to be hospitalized, most have a full recovery within a few weeks.

When to call

Seek urgent care if your child:

- Is less than 2 months old and has a fever (100.4 F or above), even if no other symptoms are present
- Is struggling to breathe (your child's chest muscles and skin pull inward with each breath)
- Turns bluish or dusky, particularly on the lips and in the nail beds
- Shows signs of dehydration (dry mouth, reduced urination, sunken eyes and fontanels, extreme fussiness or sleepiness)
- Breathing or poor eating seems to be getting worse

What you can do

Mild symptoms can be treated at home, although be ready to call your child's medical professional promptly if symptoms worsen. Keeping your child upright and the air moist with a humidifier may help ease congestion.

Have your child drink plenty of fluids to prevent dehydration. Continue breastfeeding or bottle-feeding your infant as usual. Wash hands frequently and avoid sharing eating and drinking utensils to prevent spreading the infection.

If your child is older than 2 months, you can give acetaminophen (Tylenol, others) if needed to soothe discomfort. Children 6 months or older also can take ibuprofen (Advil, Motrin, others). See page 408 for more on medications.

Babies up to 8 months old can receive a monoclonal antibody immunization known as nirsevimab to protect against RSV. This single dose should be given during or at the start of their first RSV season. However, if an RSV vaccination was given during pregnancy, most babies don't need this shot.

Some babies and toddlers age 8 to 19 months may benefit from another dose of nirsevimab before their second RSV season. Your pediatrician may recommend this second dose if your child is at risk of severe RSV. Additionally, some children under the age of 2 who are at risk of severe RSV are eligible for a different monoclonal antibody immunization, called palivizumab, which is given monthly during the RSV season.

ROSEOLA

Roseola is a generally mild infection that commonly affects children by 2 years of age. It is sometimes referred to as sixth disease, exanthem subitum or roseola infantum. It's caused by a virus that spreads from person to person. The condition usually causes several days of fever followed by a rash.

How to recognize it

Roseola typically starts with a sudden, high fever. Some children have a sore throat, runny nose or cough along with or before the fever. Your child may also develop swollen lymph nodes in the neck. The fever lasts for three to five days.

Once the fever goes away, a rash typically appears — but not always. The rash consists of many small spots or patches, mainly on the child's chest, back and belly. Although not itchy or uncomfortable, the rash can last from several hours to several days before fading.

How serious is it?

Roseola typically isn't serious. If otherwise healthy, your child will most likely recover quickly and completely. Treatment includes rest, fluids and, if your child is uncomfortable, medications to reduce fever.

When to call

Call your child's medical professional if your child is under 2 months old and has a rectal temperature of 100.4 F or higher, or if your child has a fever and appears sick or unusually fussy (see "Fever" on page 434). The medical professional may want to examine your child to rule out more serious causes of fever.

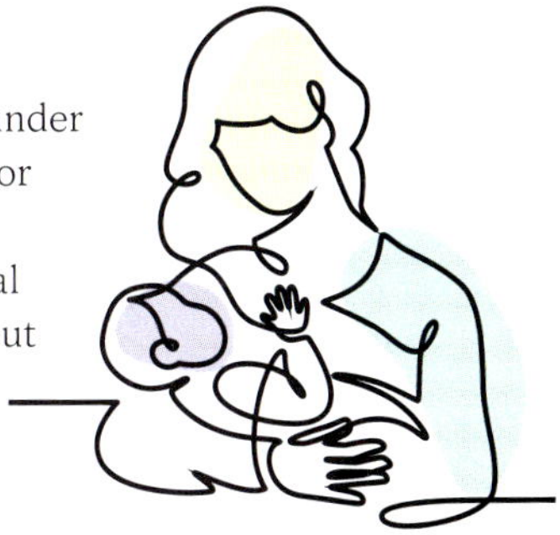

If your child is diagnosed with roseola, call if the fever lasts more than five days or if the rash doesn't improve after three days.

What you can do

Like most viral illnesses, roseola needs to run its course. Encourage plenty of rest and plenty of fluids. A cool washcloth applied to your child's head can soothe the discomfort of a fever. Once the fever subsides, your child should feel better soon. Most children recover fully from roseola within a week of the onset of the fever. The rash should fade on its own in a short time.

If the fever is causing discomfort, you can give acetaminophen (Tylenol, others) if your child is over 2 months old. Once your child is older than 6 months, you can give ibuprofen (Advil, Motrin, others). See page 408 for more on giving medications. Don't give aspirin to a child who has a viral illness because aspirin has been associated with the development of Reye's syndrome, which can be serious.

A child who is sick with roseola should be kept home until the fever has broken.

STOMACH FLU (GASTROENTERITIS)

Although it's commonly called stomach flu, gastroenteritis isn't the same as the flu. Influenza affects your child's nose, throat and lungs. Gastroenteritis, on the other hand, attacks the intestines.

Rotavirus and noroviruses are two common causes of gastroenteritis. Children usually become infected when they put their fingers or other objects contaminated with a virus into their mouths.

A vaccine against rotaviral gastroenteritis is available in some countries, including the United States. It has dramatically reduced the rate of rotavirus infection and its complications.

How to recognize it

Gastroenteritis often causes these symptoms:

- Watery, usually non-bloody diarrhea (bloody diarrhea typically means a different, more severe infection)
- Abdominal cramps and pain
- Vomiting
- Loss of appetite
- Irritability
- Low-grade fever

Depending on the cause, viral gastroenteritis symptoms may appear within one to three days after your child is infected and can range from mild to severe. Symptoms usually last just a day or two, but occasionally they may last as long as 10 days.

How serious is it?

A bout of viral gastroenteritis usually goes away within a week or two (although it can often include a miserable few days). Antibiotics offer no help for viral infections.

The main complication of viral gastroenteritis is dehydration. Your child might not be able to take in enough fluids — through breast milk, formula or an oral rehydration solution — to replace the fluids being lost through diarrhea or vomiting. As a result, your child could become dehydrated and may need to go to a hospital to receive fluids through a vein (intravenously).

If your child has severe or prolonged diarrhea, especially if accompanied by vomiting, watch carefully for signs of dehydration. These include extreme thirst, dry mouth, crying without tears and less urination than usual. Babies who are dehydrated often change from fussy to quiet to unusually sleepy.

Call your child's medical professional promptly if you notice signs of dehydration.

When to call

Call right away if your child:

- Is less than 2 months old and has a fever (100.4 F or above)
- Seems very irritable
- Is in a lot of discomfort or pain
- Has bloody diarrhea
- Has vomiting that lasts more than several hours
- Can't keep fluids down
- Has no wet diapers in 6 to 12 hours or three or fewer wet diapers in 24 hours
- Has a sunken fontanel — the soft spot on the top of your child's head
- Has a dry mouth or cries without tears
- Is unusually sleepy, drowsy or unresponsive

What you can do

When your child has an intestinal infection, the most important goal is to replace lost fluids and salts. After vomiting or a bout of diarrhea, let your child's stomach rest for 30 to 60 minutes. Then offer small amounts of liquid, 1 to 2 teaspoonfuls at a time.

Infants If you're breastfeeding, offer just one breast and let your child nurse for five minutes. If you're bottle-feeding, offer small amounts of regular formula. Don't dilute your child's already-prepared formula. After 15 to 30 minutes, if the liquid stays down, offer it again. If you're concerned about possible dehydration, ask your child's medical professional about giving your child a small amount of an oral rehydration solution.

Toddlers If your child is eating solids, these tips may help ease discomfort and avoid complications of dehydration:

- *Help your child rehydrate.* Give your child an oral rehydration solution (Pedialyte, others). Don't give only water. In children with gastroenteritis, water isn't absorbed well and it won't adequately replace lost electrolytes. You can find oral rehydration solutions in most grocery stores. Talk to your child's healthcare team if you have questions about how to use them.
- *Return to a typical diet slowly.* Drinking is more important than eating in the short term. When your child seems ready to eat, there's generally no need to restrict eating. But bland foods — such as toast, rice, bananas and potatoes — may be easier to digest than foods that are high in fat. Milk and sugary foods or beverages can make diarrhea worse.
- *Make sure your child rests.* The illness and dehydration may have made your child weak and tired.
- *Avoid certain products.* Don't give children aspirin. It may cause Reye's syndrome, a rare, potentially fatal disease. Also don't give your child anti-diarrheal medications, unless advised to do so by your child's medical professional. These medications can make it more difficult for your child's body to get rid of the virus.

STYE

If you notice a red, painful-looking lump appear suddenly near the edge of your child's eyelid, it may be a bacterial eyelid infection called a stye. The redness may be harder to see on brown and Black skin. A stye may develop when your child rubs or scratches the eyes with dirty hands or fingernails, bringing bacteria to the eyelids.

In most cases, a stye will disappear on its own in a few days to a week. In the meantime, you may be able to relieve the pain or discomfort of a stye by applying a warm washcloth to the eyelid.

How to recognize it

A red lump on your child's eyelid that looks similar to a pimple is usually an indication of a stye. A stye often contains pus. Your child's eyelid also may be swollen and the eye may be teary.

How serious is it?

Most styes are harmless and don't need treatment. A stye typically resolves on its own in a few days to a week.

When to call

Contact your child's medical professional if the stye doesn't go away in a week, or if the redness and swelling extend beyond your child's eyelid, involving the cheek or other parts of the face. For a stye that doesn't go away, your child's medical professional may recommend antibiotic ointment or drops to help clear the infection.

What you can do

Don't try to pop the stye or squeeze the pus from a stye, and keep your child's face and hands clean. To relieve discomfort, apply warm compresses to your child's eyelid. Run warm water over a clean washcloth. Wring out the washcloth and place it over the closed eye. Re-wet the washcloth when it loses heat. Continue this for 5 to 10 minutes. Applying a warm compress several times each day may encourage the stye to drain more quickly.

SUNBURN

A young child's skin is quite susceptible to sunburn, even with only 10 to 15 minutes of exposure, and even on a cloudy or cool day. It's not the visible light or the heat from the sun that burns but the invisible ultraviolet (UV) light. The lighter the color of your child's skin, the more sensitive it is to UV rays. But that doesn't mean darker skin is immune to sun damage.

Significant sun damage can occur in the childhood years. While you don't want to minimize the fun your child has outdoors, it's important to be sun smart. You can help prevent sun damage by setting up in shady areas (or using an umbrella or sun shelter), using sunscreen appropriately, and dressing your child in hats and lightweight protective clothing. For swimming, look for rash guards and suits with long sleeves and more coverage.

How to recognize it

You may not realize that your child is getting sunburned because the pain and redness may not appear for several hours. Sunburn may cause red, tender, swollen or blistered skin that is usually hot to the touch and makes your child feel uncomfortable. Redness may be harder to see on brown or Black skin.

How serious is it?

It's a good idea to be cautious about the possibility of your child getting a sunburn. Babies and young children can develop blisters, fever, chills and nausea with an amount of sun exposure that may not affect an older child or adult.

When to call

Contact your child's medical professional if the sunburn blisters or if your child begins vomiting or acts ill.

What you can do

Treat sunburn by gently applying cool compresses every few hours, taking care not to allow your child to become chilled. Encourage plenty of fluids. Give your child acetaminophen (Tylenol, others) or ibuprofen to relieve the pain. Avoid using anesthetic lotions or sprays on a child's skin. Some sting, and a child's skin may react to anesthetic sprays. Benzocaine in particular can have rare but serious side effects in children under 2 years old. Don't use it without talking to your child's medical professional first. It's also important that you take steps to prevent sunburn.

In babies under 6 months Keep your child out of direct sunlight as much as possible, especially between 10 a.m. and 4 p.m., when the sun's rays are strongest. This precaution includes cloudy days, when the clouds don't block but simply scatter UV rays. Routinely dress your child in a brimmed hat for outings during the middle of the day. If you can't avoid sun exposure, use sunscreen just on areas of the body that will be exposed, such as the face and backs of the hands.

In babies older than 6 months Use a broad-spectrum sunscreen, which protects against UVA and UVB rays, with a sun protection factor (SPF) of at least 30. Ideally, apply sunscreen 15 to 30 minutes before going outside to maximize absorption. Don't forget the back of the neck, ears, nose, cheeks and tops of the feet. Reapply it every two hours or after the child has played in the water, even if the sunscreen is labeled as waterproof.

If you think your child might have sensitive skin, do a patch test. Apply a small amount of sunscreen to your child's forearm and watch for the next 48 hours for any reaction. If your child is sensitive to one sunscreen, try a sunscreen without chemical sunblock components. Sunscreens containing the minerals zinc or titanium are less likely to irritate skin. If at any time you notice your child turning pink, take your child out of the sun. Pink now can mean red and sunburned later.

SWOLLEN SCROTUM (FROM A HYDROCELE)

A hydrocele is a type of swelling in the scrotum, the pouch that holds the testicles. This swelling happens when fluid collects in the thin sac that surrounds a testicle. Hydroceles are common in newborns. Before birth, your child's testicles develop in the abdomen and move through a passage into the scrotum. When the opening to the abdomen doesn't fully close, fluid in the abdomen can pass into the scrotum and cause swelling.

A hydrocele is usually painless. By the time a child is a year old, the fluid typically has been absorbed and the hydrocele goes away on its own.

How to recognize it

You may notice that your child's scrotum seems swollen on one side. It may seem more swollen when your child is crying or active and less swollen when your child is lying down.

How serious is it?

Generally, a hydrocele doesn't cause your child any discomfort. It usually goes away on its own by the time your child is a year old.

However, if the area becomes very large and tender, part of the intestine may have moved into the scrotum, causing an inguinal hernia. In this case, surgery may be needed to move the intestine back into the abdominal cavity and close the opening between the abdomen and the scrotum.

When to call

If your child develops a sudden swelling of the scrotum that appears painful, call your child's medical professional immediately. These symptoms can happen with certain health problems, including blocked blood flow in a twisted testicle. This problem is called testicular torsion. This requires immediate surgery.

If your child's medical professional didn't notice the hydrocele when your child was born, mention it at your office visit. Your child's medical professional will likely continue to examine it regularly for changes.

In the meantime, call your child's medical professional promptly if your child has tenderness, redness or other color change in the scrotum, or starts vomiting or showing signs of nausea for no other apparent reason, as these can be signs of pain and possible torsion.

What you can do

Share any concerns you may have with your child's medical professional and watch for any change in your child's condition.

TEARY EYES

Teary, or watery, eyes in a newborn are usually caused by a blocked tear duct. Typically, tear fluid flows down the surface of the eye to lubricate and protect the eye. It then drains through a system of holes and canals into the nose, where the fluid evaporates or is reabsorbed. This system typically takes time to fully develop. Babies under 8 months of age produce enough tear fluid to coat the eye, but not necessarily to cry "real tears."

Quite a few babies have a blocked tear duct at birth. Often a thin membrane remains over the opening (duct) that empties into the nose. This blockage causes tear fluid to well up in your child's eyes, leaving them watery.

How to recognize it

One or both of your child's eyes may appear to be continuously watery, with tears occasionally running down the cheeks, even though your child isn't crying. However, the eye usually doesn't look red or swollen unless it's infected.

How serious is it?

A blocked tear duct generally isn't serious. In most babies, it resolves by about 6 to 9 months of age. Because the tear fluid isn't draining as it should, however, infections (pink eye, or conjunctivitis) are slightly more common when a tear duct is blocked. In the morning, your child's eyes may be crusted over with dried-up discharge.

When to call

Call your child's medical professional if your child's eye is red or swollen or looks infected.

What you can do

Your child's medical professional may show you how to massage the lower inner corner of your child's eye, where the tears collect. This is the lacrimal sac. Use a clean finger to gently press upward from the inner corner. This may or may not help open the duct, but it can help empty the lacrimal sac.

Use moist compresses to wipe away the fluids from your child's eyes. Keeping your child's face and hands clean will help prevent infections.

TEETHING

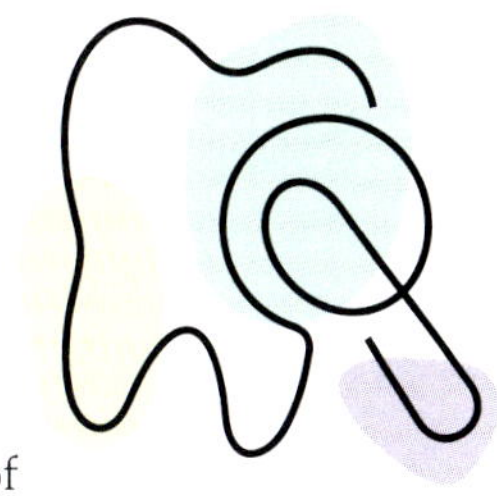

Your child may have a first tooth by 6 months or may not begin teething until much later. Often the two bottom center teeth (incisors) appear first, but not always. When they've both come in, a tooth may appear on the top. Your child will probably get four top teeth before a matching set of four is completed on the bottom. Between ages 2 and 3 years, your child will have all or most of the baby teeth, including the second molars.

Your child's baby teeth were formed during pregnancy. As these teeth come in, your child's body will begin preparing adult teeth to take their place in a few years.

How to recognize it

Drooling is a classic sign of teething. However, it may take about two months after the drooling starts before the first tooth pops up. For some babies, teething causes pain or discomfort. So your child might be crankier than usual. You also might notice swollen gums and a drive to chew on solid objects. Many parents suspect that teething causes fever and diarrhea, but research hasn't proven this. Teething most often causes symptoms in the mouth and gums.

How serious is it?

Teething is part of your child's development. But where there are teeth, there's the possibility for tooth decay. Help your toddler get in the habit of brushing teeth now to prevent problems later.

When to call

Contact your child's medical professional if your child seems particularly uncomfortable, or has other symptoms of illness — including fever or diarrhea.

The American Dental Association and the American Academy of Pediatric Dentistry recommend scheduling a child's first dental visit after the first tooth erupts. Ask what your dentist recommends. All children should see a dentist by age 3 at the latest. Your child's teeth and gums also will be examined at well-child checkups with your medical professional. At some clinics, fluoride varnish can be applied during well-child visits for children who haven't yet seen a dentist.

What you can do

Sometimes you may not even notice your child is teething until you see the new tooth! But if teething is making your child uncomfortable, here are some steps you can try:

- *Offer something to chew on.* Try a teething ring. Some are made from firm rubber and others are plastic with liquid inside. Keep in mind that the liquid-filled variety may break under the pressure of your child's chewing. A pacifier may help. Avoid giving a bottle of formula, milk or juice for comfort. Prolonged exposure to the sugar in these may cause tooth decay.
- *Keep it cool.* A cold washcloth or chilled teething ring can be soothing. If your child is eating solid foods, you can try a homemade teething ring such as a frozen bagel. Make sure you offer a frozen food that will turn soft so that your child can safely swallow any pieces that might break loose, and monitor your child closely anytime they have food. When giving your child something frozen, it's also possible that the extreme cold may hurt the gums. Refrigerated, cold soft foods such as applesauce or yogurt may feel soothing to your child's gums.
- *Rub your child's gums.* Use a clean finger, a moistened gauze pad or a clean, damp washcloth to gently massage your child's gums. The pressure may help ease your child's sore gums, at least for a short while.

- *Dry the drool.* Excessive drooling is part of the teething process. To prevent skin irritation, keep a clean cloth handy to dry your child's chin.
- *Try an over-the-counter remedy.* If your child is especially cranky, acetaminophen (Tylenol, others) — or ibuprofen (Advil, Motrin, others) if your child is more than 6 months old — may help reduce gum irritation and discomfort.
- *Avoid certain products.* Teething necklaces shouldn't be given to children without close supervision due to the risk of strangulation or choking. Don't give your child products that contain aspirin, and be cautious about teething medications that can be rubbed directly on a child's gums. Avoid teething medications that contain benzocaine. Benzocaine has been linked to a rare but serious and sometimes deadly condition that decreases the amount of oxygen that the blood can carry, especially in children under 2 years old.

Tooth brushing When your child's first teeth appear, brush them with a small, soft-bristled toothbrush, a tiny amount (the size of a grain of rice) of fluoride-containing toothpaste and some water. Some parents find it easier to use a soft finger toothbrush that fits over the parent's finger. As your child gets older, allow your child to use the toothbrush. Show your child how to clean each tooth, making sure to get those teeth that may be out of direct sight. Do this with your child twice a day. As your child approaches 3 years of age, you can gradually increase the amount of toothpaste to the size of a pea.

THRUSH

Thrush is a fungal infection that can occur in your child's mouth. It's caused by the same fungus that causes yeast infections, *Candida albicans*. This fungus is usually found in the mouth, skin and other mucous membranes. If the mouth's natural bacterial balance is upset, an overgrowth of candida may result, producing thrush. This commonly occurs in otherwise healthy babies. If a baby with thrush is breastfeeding, the infection can affect the nursing parent's breasts.

How to recognize it

When your child has thrush, it looks like there are patches of milk on the inside of the cheeks and on the tongue that won't wash off (see image on page 462). Occasionally thrush causes discomfort, and your child may have trouble feeding or be fussy and irritable.

If your child's tongue looks white all over but there are no white patches inside the lips or cheeks, this may not be thrush. Milk can make your child's tongue have a white coating.

How serious is it?

Thrush can be painful in severe cases, but it doesn't generally cause discomfort or serious problems. It can lead to a diaper rash in your child as the yeast travels through the child's gastrointestinal tract.

Infants can pass the infection to a nursing parent during breastfeeding. The infection may then pass back and forth between the breasts and the child's mouth. People whose breasts are infected with candida may have the following symptoms:

- Red, sensitive or itchy nipples (redness may be harder to see on darker skin)
- Shiny or flaky skin on the darker, circular area around the nipple (areola)
- Unusual pain during nursing or painful nipples between feedings
- Stabbing pains deep within the breast

When to call

If you notice white patches inside your child's mouth, call your child's medical professional during office hours. Check back if your child's mouth becomes increasingly coated and causes discomfort, or if your child has difficulty swallowing.

If you are breastfeeding and you think your breasts have become infected, talk to either your medical professional or your child's medical professional.

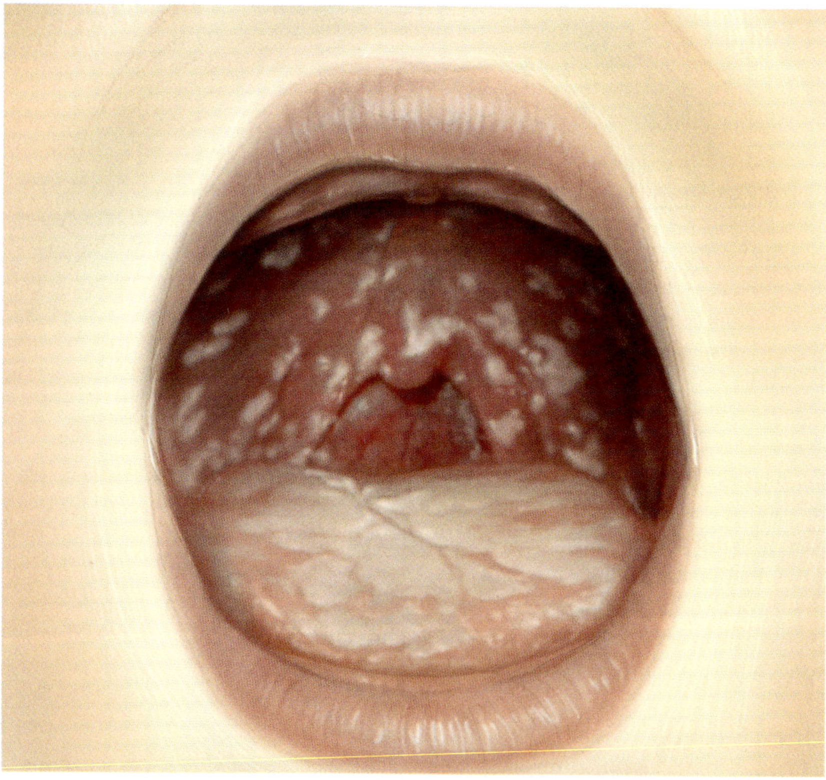

Thrush typically produces white patches on the tongue and the inside of the cheeks.

What you can do

Your child's medical professional may prescribe a liquid antifungal medication, which you apply to the patches of thrush in the mouth. During treatment, you'll want to sterilize bottle parts, pacifiers and toys that go in baby's mouth (as well as breast pump parts if pumping). Ask your healthcare team about the best way to do this. If your child is having recurring infections, it's probably a good idea to replace your child's pacifiers and bottle nipples. They could be harboring the fungus.

If you're breastfeeding an infant who has oral thrush, you and your baby will do best if you both are treated. Otherwise, the infection is likely to be passed back and forth. For you and your baby:

- A mild antifungal medication may be prescribed for your child and an antifungal cream may be prescribed for your breasts. You can also use a nonprescription antifungal cream, such as clotrimazole (Lotrimin AF). Apply it to the breasts four times a day after feedings.
- If you use a breast pump, after each use, clean and sterilize all parts that touch the milk.
- If you develop a fungal infection on your breasts, using pads will help prevent the fungus from spreading to your clothes. Look for pads that don't have a plastic barrier, which can encourage the growth of candida. Wash reusable pads and your bras in hot water with bleach.

URINARY TRACT INFECTION

Urinary tract infections are fairly common in young children, especially girls. The tube that carries urine out of the bladder (urethra) is shorter in girls than in boys, making it easier for bacteria to travel to the bladder. When bacteria enter the bladder or kidneys, an infection may result. Most often, the bacteria come from stool and the anal or genital area.

How to recognize it

In children younger than 2 years old, a urinary tract infection can be hard to identify. Often the only sign is a fever with no clear cause. Sometimes fever is accompanied by symptoms such as irritability or poor feeding. An older toddler might be able to describe urinary symptoms such as painful or difficult urination or abdominal pain. Infections of the kidneys can also cause back pain.

How serious is it?

A urinary tract infection requires prompt treatment. Left untreated, the infection can cause permanent damage to the kidneys.

When to call

Call anytime your child has an unexplained fever that lasts for more than 24 hours. Call your child's medical professional right away if your child is under 2 months of age and has a rectal temperature of 100.4 F or higher.

What you can do

Be alert to unexplained, lasting fever in your child, and don't be afraid to call your child's medical professional when necessary. A urinary tract infection can be diagnosed with a urine sample. In infants and young children who aren't toilet trained, a urine sample is usually obtained by briefly inserting a catheter into the urethra to withdraw a small amount of urine. Your child's medical professional can give you tips on how to collect a sample from a toilet-trained child.

If your child has a urinary tract infection, a course of antibiotics will be prescribed. Make sure to give your child the medication exactly as directed. An ultrasound or other testing may be done to rule out a urinary system problem.

VOMITING

In the first few months of life, it's common for babies to spit up or regurgitate their food from time to time. Vomiting is different. It's the forceful ejection of a large portion of the stomach's contents through the mouth and sometimes even the nose. Because your child won't understand what is happening, vomiting can be a frightening experience. And as a parent, it can be very stressful when your child begins to vomit without warning.

Most vomiting in early childhood is caused by viral infections that affect the stomach and intestines (gastroenteritis; see page 454). Your child also may have fever and diarrhea in addition to vomiting.

How to recognize it

Typical infant spit-up seems to dribble out of your child's mouth without much of a disturbance. In contrast, vomit comes out like a projectile, fast and furious. Generally, there's more of it, too.

How serious is it?

Most of the time, vomiting is due to a viral infection and stops on its own within 12 to 24 hours. The greatest risk your child faces is dehydration from losing too much fluid and not ingesting enough.

In a few cases, vomiting can be a symptom of a more serious problem, such as an intestinal obstruction, anatomical or stomach disorder or infection.

When to call

If your child is very young — between 2 and 6 weeks — and vomits forcefully within 30 minutes after every feeding for 6 to 12 hours, call your child's medical professional right away. This may be a sign of a stomach disorder called pyloric stenosis. In this disorder, a narrowing of the stomach's outlet to the intestines prevents food from passing. This requires prompt attention so that your child can get the nutrition needed to grow.

Also, call immediately if your child seems to be getting worse, you're concerned about possible poisoning or your child has any of the following symptoms:

- Blood or green matter (bile) in the vomit
- Vomiting for 12 hours in newborns, 24 hours in older infants and toddlers
- Forceful, repeated vomiting
- Dehydration — reduced urination or three or fewer wet diapers in 24 hours, dry mouth, no tears (although young infants don't usually show tears), or sunken soft spots (fontanels) in the head
- Unusually sleepy or unresponsive
- Inability to keep liquids down
- Seems to have persistent abdominal pain

What you can do

To prevent dehydration in your child:

- *Wait a little after a vomiting episode.* After your child vomits, let the stomach settle for a while. Wait 30 to 60 minutes before offering more fluids. Sleep may ease your child's nausea.
- *Offer small amounts of liquid.* Start out with a teaspoon or two. Breastfed babies usually tolerate breast milk fairly well and digest it quickly. Offer just one breast and nurse for only five minutes or so. Small amounts of regular formula for bottle-fed babies are OK, too. After 15 to 30 minutes, if the liquid stays down, offer it again.
- *Offer an oral rehydration solution.* For older toddlers or babies who continue to vomit, offer a teaspoon or two of oral rehydration solution (Pedialyte, others). Gradually increase the amount as your child keeps it down. If your child can't keep anything down, call your child's medical professional.
- *Gradually return to a typical diet.* After eight hours without vomiting, gradually return to feeding your child the usual amounts of breast milk or formula. If your child is eating solids, slowly return to a typical diet. You might want to start out with easily digested foods, such as cooked cereal, bananas, crackers, toast or plain pasta.

WHOOPING COUGH

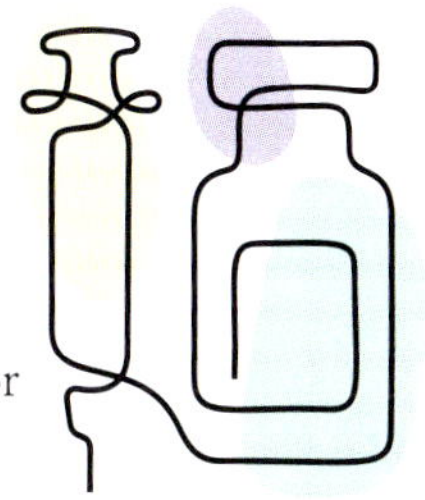

Whooping cough (pertussis) is a highly contagious bacterial infection of the respiratory tract. It's transmitted from person to person through airborne droplets from coughing or sneezing.

A vaccine against whooping cough is part of your child's recommended vaccinations. It's usually given as a series of five injections at 2 months, 4 months, 6 months, 12 to 18 months and 4 to 6 years. Because babies under 6 months haven't been fully vaccinated, they're at greater risk of getting the infection and of developing significant complications. Vaccination during pregnancy against whooping cough will protect infants during these first six months.

The protection offered by the vaccine wears off after several years, meaning that older children and adults who haven't updated their vaccinations may become infected and pass the infection to infants and younger children.

How to recognize it

At first it may seem as if your child has a mild upper respiratory tract infection — a runny nose, congestion, and cough, but no fever. However, the cough worsens throughout the first week, until your child experiences exhausting coughing fits consisting of 10 to 30 forceful, abrupt coughs. Sometimes this will be followed by a "whoop" sound, as your child inhales forcefully. Many children don't develop the "whoop" sound. Some vomit after a coughing fit.

In infants under 3 months of age, the initial phase of mild symptoms may not always be obvious. The first sign of whooping cough may be a sudden fit of coughing, difficulty breathing or a period of not breathing, especially after coughing. In between episodes of coughing or trouble breathing, the child may appear well.

How serious is it?

In infants — especially those under 6 months of age — complications from whooping cough are more severe than in older children and adults. Complications may include ear infections, pneumonia, dehydration, respiratory failure and seizures. Pneumonia can be life-threatening in new babies.

Young infants diagnosed with whooping cough are often kept at a hospital to receive supportive care and to be closely monitored for potentially serious complications. If your child is older and has mild symptoms, hospitalization may not be necessary. Antibiotics can decrease the chances of transmitting the infection to others.

When to call

Contact your child's medical professional right away if your child:

- Is under 6 months old or hasn't been fully immunized, and has been exposed to someone with a chronic cough or whooping cough
- Has severe coughing fits
- Has spells of difficulty breathing, turning bluish or gagging
- Has had a bad cough for more than five to seven days
- Vomits after a coughing fit, eats poorly or seems ill

What you can do

If you're caring for your child at home, these steps may ease discomfort.

Avoid cough medicine Over-the-counter cough medicines don't usually help and aren't recommended in children under 4 years old (see page 422).

Encourage plenty of rest A cool, quiet and dark bedroom may help your child relax and rest better.

Offer plenty of fluids Keep up your baby's regular feedings of breast milk and formula. Smaller, more frequent feedings may be helpful. Water, 100% fruit juices and soups are good choices for toddlers. If your child is having trouble consuming enough fluids, offer small amounts of an oral rehydrating solution (Pedialyte, others). Call your child's medical professional right away if you notice signs of dehydration, such as decreased urination and increased irritability or sleepiness.

Use a humidifier Use a cool mist humidifier to help soothe irritated lungs and to help loosen respiratory secretions. If you use a humidifier, follow directions for keeping it clean. If you don't have a humidifier, sitting with your child in a steamy bathroom also can help temporarily clear the lungs and ease breathing.

Clean the air Keep your home free of irritants that can trigger coughing spells, such as tobacco smoke and fumes from fireplaces.

Prevent transmission Cover your cough and wash your hands often; keep your sick child away from others. Ask your family's medical professional about getting your whole family's vaccinations up to date.

PART 5

Managing and enjoying parenthood

CHAPTER 36

Adapting to your new lifestyle

Adding a baby to your family brings some of the most profound changes you'll ever experience. These include the mundane (finding your groove with diapers) as well as the magical (learning what makes your baby smile). No matter how much you've read or how careful you've been about getting everything in place, nothing can fully prepare you for the first weeks and months after your baby's birth. Even if you're already a parent, adding a baby brings big changes to your family's routine and relationships.

This time of transition can be exciting — and sometimes overwhelming, difficult or uncertain. There are many physical, social and emotional issues to deal with all at once. You're trying to get a handle on your baby's needs and habits while you adjust to a new role and identity. Relationships, possibly with your partner, other children, family and friends, are shifting. And round-the-clock newborn care can make even simple tasks such as showering a challenge.

The first few weeks after you bring your baby home are likely to be some of the most challenging times of your life. The changes in the daily rhythms of your life may feel chaotic and foreign.

And more challenges often come later on. If you have family and friends for support, most are ready to help with meals, gifts and advice when you have a new baby. As weeks and months go on, sometimes it feels like the help and enthusiasm wane, and some new parents feel increasingly isolated. This can be even more difficult if parents routinely don't get enough sleep. All these challenges can turn into sadness, withdrawal and even depression. Make sure you're checking in on your mental health well beyond the newborn phase.

Amid the challenges, this also is a time of great growth. A few practical strategies can help you adapt as the transition unfolds and help you create a nurturing, loving home for all members of your family.

LIVING ON LESS SLEEP

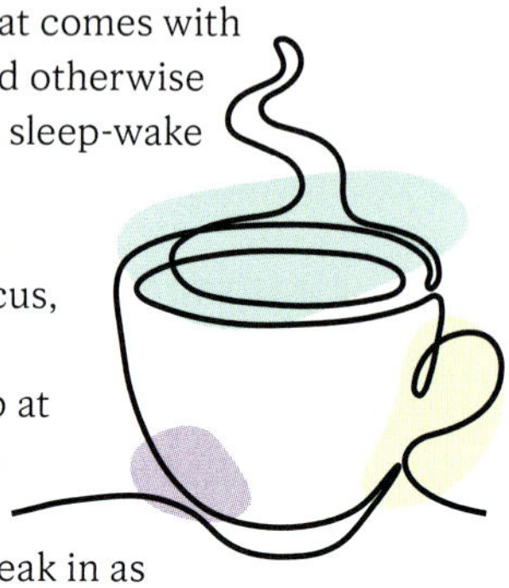

If there's any issue all parents can relate to, it's the fatigue that comes with caring for a baby. You're up at all hours feeding, diapering and otherwise tending to your newborn, who needs time to develop regular sleep-wake cycles. Parents' sleep is often disturbed nightly for weeks to months after a baby's birth. Lack of sleep not only leaves you exhausted but also can make you irritable and less able to focus, remember details and solve problems.

But it gets better. By age 3 months, many babies can sleep at least five hours at a stretch. By 6 months, many infants sleep through the night, and 70% to 80% of babies are doing so by 9 months. In the meantime, hang in there — and try to sneak in as much sleep as possible.

While there's no magical formula for getting enough sleep, here are some tips that may help (also see Chapter 8).

Rest whenever you can

"Sleep when the baby sleeps" is a common piece of advice, but sometimes it feels wildly unrealistic. Some babies doze off for just 15 or 20 minutes at a time, and you may need to seize that time to shower, eat a meal or just go to the bathroom.

WHEN SLEEP BECOMES A STRUGGLE

The rigors of caring for a newborn may leave you so exhausted that you feel you could fall asleep anytime, anywhere — but that's not always the case. Some new parents experience insomnia.

Prolonged sleep deprivation can set the stage for depression and other health problems. If you're having trouble sleeping even when you have the opportunity, try these suggestions:

- Make sure your environment is suited for sleep. Turn off digital devices, including TV, ideally an hour before bed, and store them outside the bedroom if possible. Keep the room cool and dark. If it seems cool for your baby in the same room, try warmer pajamas and a swaddle or sleep sack.
- Avoid nicotine, caffeine and alcohol late in the day or at night.
- If you don't nod off within 30 minutes, get up and do something else, such as read a book. But avoid digital devices. When you begin to feel drowsy, try going back to bed.

If you think you have a sleep problem, consult your medical professional. Identifying and treating any underlying conditions can help you get the rest you need.

A HOUSE BECOMES A HOME

Children's book writer Christopher Harder describes the way his house changed after he and his wife had a child:

We had renovated the house by getting rid of our dining room, living room and den and replacing them with one, house-sized playroom. We had scarred the new furniture, stained baseboards and repainted walls. . . . Half our books were in the attic. The hardwood floors had skid marks. And it felt like home.

Still, even an hour or two of extra sleep can make a difference, so try to make it a priority. Turn off the ringer on your phone, shut down your computer, hide the laundry basket and ignore the dishes in the kitchen sink. These things can wait.

Avoid bed sharing during sleep

It's OK to bring your baby into your bed for nursing or comforting, but return your baby to the crib or bassinet when you and your baby are ready to go back to sleep.

Share nighttime duties

If you have a partner, work out a schedule that allows both of you to rest and care for the baby. If you're breastfeeding, perhaps your partner can bring you the baby and handle nighttime diaper changes. If you're using a bottle, take turns feeding the baby. You could also split the night into two shifts or trade nights to be on duty.

If you're trading shifts or nights with a partner, you may want to use a guest room or separate sleep space, if available. That way, the parent who is supposed to be resting isn't woken by baby noises or by the sounds of feeding and changing.

Wait a few minutes

Sometimes middle-of-the-night fussing or crying is simply a sign that your baby is settling down. Unless you suspect that your baby is hungry or uncomfortable, or the crying is escalating, wait a few minutes before responding.

Go easy on yourself

If you're not getting enough sleep, you may feel cranky and disoriented. Try not to beat yourself up about it. Set aside nonessential tasks for a time when you're feeling more rested or when you have help.

GETTING COMFORTABLE WITH CHAOS

In the first weeks after you bring home your baby, you might feel like you're in a fog. Your day-to-day routine goes out the window. Yet somehow you still have to find time to feed yourself and do essential chores. And if you have older children, you may be caring for their needs and continuing daily activities with them, too.

Although your days will likely include moments of awe and enjoyment, you still might long for the comfort of your old routines. A structured workday or a cup of coffee — enjoyed while it's hot — may never have sounded so luxurious.

Over time, you'll adjust to the new normal, revive old routines and create new ones. In the meantime, you can bring a little bit of order to the chaos and learn to embrace it.

Decide what's important

Determine the tasks and activities you want to keep from your pre-baby days, and prioritize them. If you have a partner, you might each have a list. Then decide where you can cut, compromise or take shortcuts for other tasks, at least for a while. You might keep clean clothes in a laundry basket instead of putting them away, for example, or buy healthy heat-and-serve options or use meal delivery services that bring meals to your door.

BALANCING AND ESTABLISHING FAMILY ROLES

If you're experiencing new parenthood with a partner, the balance of your new roles and responsibilities is among the many things you're figuring out together. Several decades ago, it was expected that moms assumed most or all of the responsibility of raising the children. Today, as dual-earner households are the norm, partners typically share responsibilities at home.

The ideal balance is different for every couple and family. But however evenly you divided your roles and chores before becoming parents, your system may need an overhaul once you bring a newborn home.

Talk with your partner about your new roles. What do you each want for your role as a parent? How can each of you nurture a physically and emotionally close relationship with your child? How can you support your partner in meeting baby's basic needs? How can you meet each other's needs?

For example, if one partner is breastfeeding the baby and pumping, can the other person take charge of washing bottles every day? If one partner returns to work outside the home before the other, what share of responsibilities at home seems fair to both of you? Some chores may need to shift from one partner to the other, and you'll want to stay flexible as baby grows and your routines evolve. Consider planning times to check in and reassess the balance of responsibilities.

Parenting babies and toddlers can put more stress on a relationship than ever before. Keep the conversation open, and try to give each other grace as you navigate your new roles.

Check your expectations

Many new parents start out with unrealistic expectations, perhaps shaped by social media or nostalgic memories. The gap between expectations and reality can lead to stress and disappointment, or even a feeling that you're failing. Throw out any ideas about what life with a new baby should be like, and be realistic about the increased demands you face.

Go with the flow

It's never too early to establish a routine — but let your newborn set the pace. Allow plenty of time each day for feeding sessions, naps and crying spells. Keep scheduled activities to a minimum. When you need to head out, plan for extra time to pack your supplies and pause for an inevitable last-minute feeding or diaper change. As your baby's routine develops and changes over time, you'll find a new rhythm.

Establish visiting rules

When friends and loved ones want to meet your newborn, let them know which days work best and how much time you have for a visit. Insist that visitors wash their hands before holding the baby, and ask anyone who's ill to wait for a better time to visit. Your loved ones should understand that your goal is to keep your baby healthy.

Accept help

When family members and friends ask if there's anything they can do, give them a job. It can be as simple as watching the baby while you take an unhurried shower or a nap. If you have other children, let someone take them so you can have some alone time with the new baby. Or let them care for baby while you take time with your older children. If someone is staying with you, let that person help (or ask them to!) as much as possible. You deserve it and need it, and it will probably make your guest feel special as well.

Keep your perspective

The newborn days won't last long. Before you know it, your infant will be a toddler, walking and talking. Try to step back and appreciate the moment, even amid the chaos.

ADJUSTING TO YOUR NEW ROLE

Taking care of a new baby is an awesome responsibility. You may frequently have a moment of feeling amazed followed by a moment of "What am I doing?" Infants depend on their parents to meet all their physical and emotional needs. Even if you've dreamed about being a parent since you were a kid, the realities of dressing, feeding, bathing and other child care routines take time to learn. Along with the joy, excitement and fulfillment parenthood brings, don't be surprised to experience doubts and uncertainties in your new role.

Feelings of incompetence are common. Like many new parents, you may be going from a working life where you feel confident and successful to a job for which you lack experience and won't get instructions from your new "boss." You're acquiring a whole new skill set at a rapid pace. Although many people think that their instincts are supposed to kick in, new parents don't automatically know exactly what their babies need. You may feel anxious, helpless or lost as you try to figure out why your baby is crying or not sleeping. Does the baby need to be fed, entertained or simply comforted while taking in the new surroundings?

If you have older children, you may feel confident performing baby routines but find that it's a whole new game with siblings also requiring your time and love.

Becoming a parent, for the first time, or with a new baby, is a process. As you gain experience, you'll learn to read your baby's cues and master the tasks of child care. In turn, your sense of competence and satisfaction will increase. As one mom remarked six weeks after giving birth, "I know how to put him back down to sleep. And I can tell if he's hungry when he's crying or he's just tired. . . . I have my little tricks now that I feel like I know him a little more."

FOCUS ON RELATIONSHIPS, NOT GUILT

Opinions on whether child care is good for kids can run strong. Some people want to be home with their child through the first years, even if it means taking a break from a successful career. For others, the income from work may be necessary, or they simply may not want to pause a job they enjoy. But there's no evidence that a parent staying home is better for children. And good-quality, stimulating and nurturing child care offers some benefits. Spending time in child care can improve social competence, language development, independence, school readiness and peer interaction skills. See Chapter 15 for more on child care.

The most influential factor in parenting is not the quantity of time you spend with your child but that you have a loving, nurturing relationship. For example, studies have found no difference between working mothers and stay-at-home mothers in the quality of mother-child interactions or their influence on children. And both moms and dads are spending more hours a week on child care than they have in the past, in addition to more combined hours spent working. What's important is that when you're with your child, the time you spend together is quality time.

Whatever your choice, if you feel happy and fulfilled, your child will enjoy the happiness as well. If you resent your current arrangement or feel cheated by it, you'll likely pass on these feelings to your child.

Believe in yourself

Parenting brings a seemingly endless list of decisions. Where will baby sleep? Cloth or disposable diapers? What about child care? Ultimately, you'll have to trust that you do know what's best for you and your family. There are some answers you can learn from research. Other questions may not have one right answer, or will have an answer that is different for each parent and child. Your parenting is now and always will be a work in progress. You'll learn as you go.

Let go of being perfect

These days, you may experience a new level of anxiety, as parenting often feels like a competition, posted for all to see on social media. You may find yourself searching online for the "best" way to care for your child or painstakingly following the latest trend in baby care. Well-meaning friends and family may offer advice or criticize your methods in an attempt to be helpful.

All this input can be exhausting. Try to filter the "noise" around you as best you can. Rely on a medical professional you trust, as well as evidence-based information from reputable sources, to help answer your parenting questions. Quite often, you'll find there are multiple ways of doing things that are acceptable. You have your child's best interests at heart, and that's what matters most.

Tune in to your baby

Your baby will also help build your confidence. As you respond to your child's needs, you'll see your baby's response — a contented gaze, a grasp of your finger, a fleeting smile and, soon enough, an excited babble. Spending time alone with your baby, away from distractions, can be ideal for fostering this relationship. Bonding and learning your child's habits and rhythms takes time.

Build a network of social support

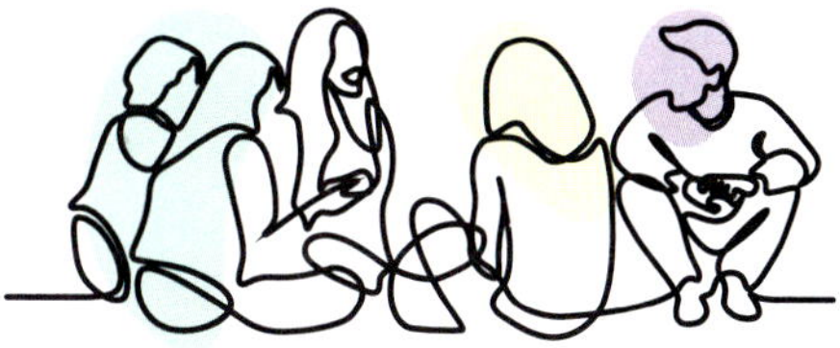

Social support is one of the most important buffers against stress. Take time to seek out and appreciate individuals who can give you encouragement and practical help. This may include a partner, friends, parents, siblings or neighbors. The quality of friendships is more important than the quantity of them.

Talking with other new parents can help you realize you're not alone. Other parents can offer support and empathy. Find ways to connect with other parents in your neighborhood or community, such as a new-parents group organized by a hospital, place of worship, community center or school district. You can also reach out to other new parents through online support groups or at the park. By sharing stories, not only will you realize that you're dealing with similar issues but you might also form strong, lasting friendships. Having friends who can really relate makes your journey easier and more fun.

Minimize stress

Your bundle of joy also brings a bundle of stress, which typically accompanies any major life change. Besides the disrupted sleep, new responsibilities and changes in your lifestyle, other sources of stress may include financial strain, hormonal fluctuations, changes in your identity, less time with your partner and for yourself, and loss of sexual activity (at least temporarily).

Realistically, you won't be able to avoid stress altogether as a parent. But feeling stressed doesn't make you a bad parent. Learning to handle the new challenges in your life can spur personal growth and help you enjoy the riches parenting has to offer. With each new phase as your child gets older, you'll find a new rhythm that works for your family.

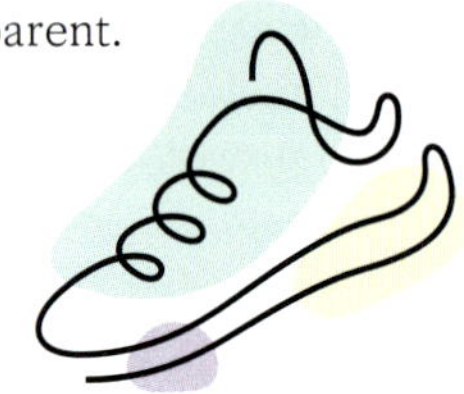

Eat well and get some exercise every day, even if it's just a couple of stretches or a short walk. Remember to do things you enjoy, whether it's reading, lounging in the backyard or going for a bike ride.

If you have a partner, offer support for their new role. Be an active listener. Whether your partner just wants to talk about new feelings or needs to vent — even if it's not baby-related — provide your undivided attention. Laugh together at your mistakes and remind each other that things will get smoother. Experiencing this life transition together can ease stress and make you stronger friends in the long run.

Grow with your child

Many parents find that they have plenty of help with their newborn but less assistance as the baby grows and then becomes a toddler. While you're sure to have more confidence in steering your toddler, still consider accepting help when it is offered.

The connections with other parents that you developed when your child was a young baby may develop into deeper friendships and play dates with active toddlers. Sometimes connections fade, and that's OK, too. You'll likely form a variety of social links as your child's needs and preferences — as well as your own — change over time.

YOUR VIRTUAL COMMUNITY: SOCIAL MEDIA AND NEW PARENTHOOD

When you have a question about getting your nocturnal baby on a regular nighttime sleep schedule or want tips for less painful breastfeeding, where do you turn first? If you're like many parents, your first inclination might be to go online to social media apps, sites or message boards. A recent national survey found that 80% of parents with young children take to social media to tackle parenting. These sources are widely accessible and may offer support from like-minded peers.

Social media can offer a sense of community during what may seem like an isolating time in your life. You can connect with other parents, exchange tips and even get some much-needed laughs over videos and memes that embrace the funny side of raising children. But it's also important to recognize the risks and decide how — and how much — you'll use social media.

Seeing a social media influencer who seems to have it all, including a spotless house and a happy baby, can be inspiring. However, most new parents know that this likely isn't a realistic depiction of parenthood. Still, you may find yourself feeling envious or depressed that your version of parenthood looks drastically different. Careful social media use can help you gain reassurance and confidence in your parenting journey while being aware of online pitfalls.

Weighing the pros and cons of social media

The early parenting years present significant emotional, psychological and social challenges. In some ways, social media can help address them. But that same new-parent vulnerability can make people more susceptible to fake news, judgment and unhealthy comparisons.

Consider these pros and cons of social media:

Pro: It helps you maintain important connections You live in one part of the country, and your family is in another. You don't get to see each other often. At its most basic level, social media allows you to keep loved ones in the loop. But it goes beyond that. Posting pictures and videos of your baby's milestones can help you and your family and friends feel closer and more connected, bridging the physical distance. You might even find that you're frequently sharing funny videos or activity ideas with local friends to stay connected when you can't hang out in person as much as you used to.

Con: You might be sharing too much What you post about your child or family may inadvertently reveal personal information. Some information shared online now may embarrass your child when they're older. And artificial intelligence (AI) may gather data from text and photos that could be used in ways you never planned. If your online posts include photos of other people's children, ask for permission before posting. If your child spends time with other relatives, talk to them ahead of time about whether it's OK to post pictures of your child to social media. Evaluate your data privacy settings on social media sites to limit others' access to your personal information.

Pro: You find support The journey into parenthood can be a solitary one. Engaging in conversations and sharing common experiences with other parents on social media — whether on comment threads or in online parent groups — can offer much-needed emotional support.

For example, if your baby has a challenging health condition, you may feel more educated and empowered about your child's care after connecting with parents in the same position. You might even feel more confident in your parenting moving forward. Or maybe postpartum depression has you doubting your ability to be a good parent. Interacting online with others dealing with the condition can help you feel less lonely and reassure you that you have a lot of love and guidance to offer your baby.

Con: It's not all warm and fuzzy It's infamously common to face criticism, personal attacks and bullying if your viewpoint differs from that of others online. Parents may be labeled "bad" for nearly any aspect of raising a child. At a time when you may already feel unsure of your parenting skills, this can be devastating for self-esteem.

Con: You might be leaning too heavily on social media for support One in 10 parents in a recent survey thought social media was instrumental in helping decide when their child should see a healthcare professional. However, especially when dealing with very young children, your child's healthcare team is best equipped to help make that determination. They are skilled at handling a wide range of questions and concerns.

If you need help between your child's regular checkups, call the clinic office to speak to a nurse, schedule a telehealth visit, or send a message to your child's healthcare professional through a patient portal, if available, for guidance tailored to your child. Your child's healthcare team may also be able to recommend in-person, supportive parenting groups, classes or other resources to help you.

Pro: Information is available at your fingertips At 2 a.m., you have a burning question about getting your reluctant baby to take a bottle when you return to work. So you go online to find your answer.

Access to easy-to-digest information at any hour is one of the perks of the internet and social media. Often you can find what you're looking for among different ideas and fresh perspectives. That can quickly help ease minor worries and anxiety about your baby.

Con: The internet is teeming with misinformation Reputable sources such as government sites and professional organizations have rigorous fact-checking and review processes, making them the most reliable sources of information. However, information from official sources can sometimes be difficult to understand, or those sources are not as "flashy" as other sources. Because of this, you may find yourself turning to less reliable sites.

However, the information there might be solely the viewpoint of the person posting. It may not be identified as an opinion or may not be based on scientific evidence. Also, comment sections often contain information that's not backed by science or express views contrary to what medical professionals might recommend.

Is technology affecting your parenting?

A recent survey found that more than two-thirds of parents feel distracted at some point by their smartphones when they're with their kids, which gets in the way of spending quality time with their children. More than a third of parents surveyed felt they spend too much time on social media.

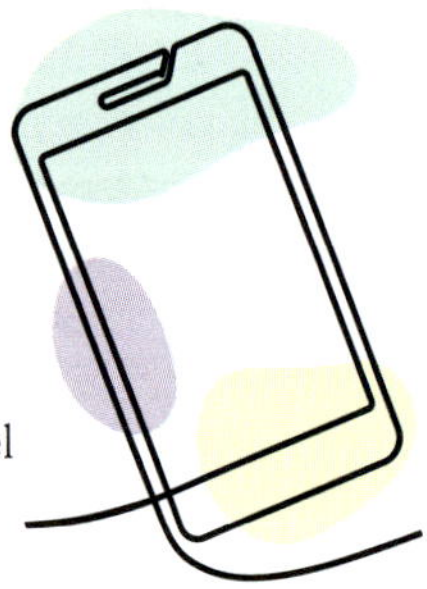

When parents engage with their phones, children may feel they need to compete for attention. Other research has found that spending too much time on smartphones actually made parents feel less connected to their children. Mothers who used cellphones while with their infants, such as during breastfeeding, were less likely to interact with their babies through eye contact. Interactions such as gazing, talking and touch between a parent and child are important to the development of a baby's brain. Putting down the phone and being more responsive can help strengthen the feeling of being connected to your child and help with development.

The American Academy of Pediatrics offers tips for disconnecting and creating customizable family media plans to put into action. (Search for "family media plan" at www.healthychildren.org.) You'll want to set boundaries early on, such as establishing screen-free times before bed and creating screen-free zones in your home, such as at the dining table. Remember that these apply to everyone — including grown-ups. And as your child grows, you can revisit and revise these accordingly.

JUGGLING WORK AND FAMILY

Working a full- or part-time job is a fact of life for many parents. While there's no wrong or right way to mix work outside the home with parenthood, most parents would like to find a good balance between their jobs and their families.

Both moms and dads struggle with work-life balance. According to surveys, both are equally likely to say that parenting is a big part of their identity, but a good number also feel "rushed" or constantly pressed for time. Despite the challenges, it is possible to manage and even thrive with the juggling routine. Here are some suggestions for creating balance.

Embrace "good enough"

Let go of perfectionism. Balance requires being good enough rather than perfect. You might not have time to cook all your meals from scratch anymore. Maybe you can't work as many hours a day or get as much done. Focus on the positives, and let go of guilt about what you're doing or not doing.

Seek flexibility

If possible, talk to your employer about creating a work schedule where you can be both productive and in tune with your family. Following the COVID-19 pandemic, more family-friendly work options — such as flexible hours or working from home — are often available.

If you have a partner and both of you are employed, consider who might have more flexibility at the moment. For example, who will take time off to care for a sick child? Work together to create an arrangement that is positive for the whole family.

Get organized

Make a to-do list. Divide the list into tasks for work and tasks for home, or divvy up tasks between you and your partner. Identify what you need to do, what can wait — and what you can skip entirely.

Seek support

Accept help from others, including your partner, loved ones, friends and co-workers. Keep up your friendships. Speak up if you're feeling guilty, sad or overwhelmed. If you can afford it, consider paying for some housekeeping to have extra time for your family or yourself.

LONG DAYS, SHORT YEARS

These first few years are full of ups and downs. Chances are you'll experience a deep sense of accomplishment and joy along with the long days and nights, the fatigue, and the worries. As your baby grows and changes, you'll grow and change, too. You'll create new routines, discover your parenting quirks and learn from missteps. You may even discover a new sense of meaning in life, greater self-esteem, and a deeper connection to your family and community.

CHAPTER 37

Caring for your mental health

Parenting triggers a whirlwind of emotions and challenges, often catching new parents off guard despite all the preparation and anticipation. One second, you're basking in the glow of your beautiful baby. The next, you're juggling the demands of parenthood with other responsibilities and feeling overwhelmed, anxious or even depressed.

These feelings are common as your life shifts to the realities of caring for a baby. Then just when you think you've gotten the hang of it, your baby becomes a toddler, and you may feel like you're back at square one as you face a whole new set of challenges.

But you're not alone in your feelings and obstacles, as the numbers show. As many as 1 in 5 people experience postpartum depression or an anxiety disorder after giving birth. Some groups, such as Black women in the United States, contend with higher rates of postpartum depression, anxiety and birth trauma than others.

And the stress, depression and mental health concerns aren't limited to the postpartum period. A recent survey found that more than half of parents with children up to the age of 5 thought parenting was tiring and stressful all or most of the time, while more than a third of parents with older and preteen children felt the same.

As you navigate through your child's first years, know that it's very common to feel these times are really hard — even if you also find them precious and fleeting. These months and years are filled with many sacrifices, highs and lows. It's not just you! It's OK to struggle, and it's OK to seek support at any stage of the journey. Doing so doesn't make you less of a loving or capable parent.

It's also important to remember that caring for your mental health is not selfish. In fact, it's key to your child's health and development. Recognizing when you may need help is an important first step. There is a wide range of treatment options to address parental mental health, from therapy and medication to self-care and social support. Prioritizing your well-being is beneficial both for you and for your baby's health.

MAINTAINING MENTAL HEALTH: WHAT YOU CAN DO

When making the giant leap into parenthood, a successful transition is closely linked to the support you receive. Parents with access to a support system tend to have greater self-esteem and more confidence in their parenting.

Of course, you may have already noticed in these early days of being a parent that the support system you had before children may not look the same now. While some friendships will not waver, others were not built to last through this new chapter in your life. Childless friends or those with adult children may not understand your inability to drop everything and attend a spur-of-the-moment concert. As your priorities change, so too will these relationships.

To help you stay connected to yourself and others, consider these tips:

- *Find local parent meetups.* You're all in the same boat, so you get each other. This can be a great venue to swap tips for getting your baby to sleep at night, or vent about the challenges of breastfeeding or getting onesies clean after a diaper blowout.
- *Sign up for a class.* Local music or movement classes are a great way to meet other parents and involve your little one, too.
- *Search for online support groups.* Sometimes it's just easier to "get together" with fellow newbie parents without pressure to shower or leave the house. These groups also have the benefit of being available 24/7. To ensure groups provide a safe space, consider seeking out one with a moderator. Mayo Clinic Connect (https://connect.MayoClinic.org) offers free moderated support groups on a wide range of topics. You can also check with your healthcare provider for local in-person support groups.

Equally crucial for new parents is to make time for themselves:

- *Relish the chores.* You probably never thought that errands could be so rewarding. But getting your grocery shopping done or running to the post office to mail a package — alone — puts you back into the world and can restore some sense of normalcy. Arrange for the baby to be with your partner or another trusted adult while you run out.
- *Ask for help.* It can initially feel awkward to ask a friend or family member to watch your baby or help clean your house. However, most people want to help. They don't know what they can do. Offer some suggestions.
- *Find "me" time.* Many new parents feel guilty or selfish for wanting some adult time. However, getting even just an hour to yourself to read a book or have a quick lunch date with your partner is valuable decompression time. And that's beneficial for both you and your baby.
- *Be realistic.* Eyeing that stack of dishes in the sink while your baby sleeps? Don't. Time is precious, and while it would be nice to have a magazine-

worthy house, sleep is more important right now. Make a beeline for your bed when the baby goes down for a nap or at night.

- *Compromise.* You want to meet up with an old friend, but going to the local cafe isn't in the cards. Instead of going out, invite your friend to chat over coffee and takeout.

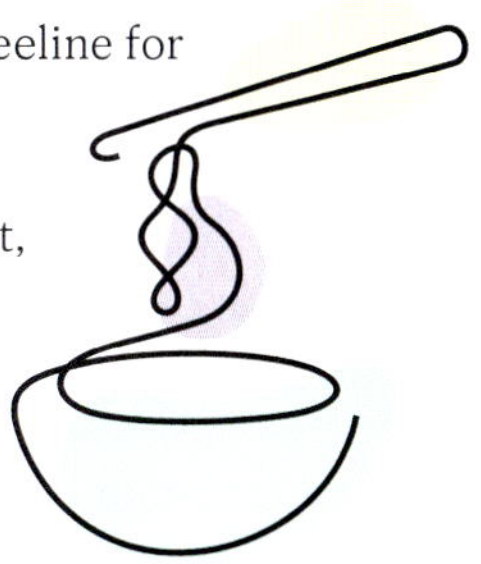

Remember that self-compassion and understanding are vital components of the parenting journey. Acknowledging the sacrifices made and the emotional roller coaster that comes with parenting while also celebrating the joys and milestones along the way is essential.

IDENTIFYING DEPRESSION AND OTHER MENTAL HEALTH ISSUES

You may have heard the term baby blues. This describes the worry, sadness and tiredness many parents experience in the first couple of weeks after having a baby. These feelings are usually mild and go away without treatment. But sometimes these feelings are more intense and last longer — or they start later.

It's important to note that mental health conditions can develop for the first time in parents well beyond the postpartum period. If you think you may be experiencing a new mental health issue, speak to your healthcare professional.

Postpartum depression

If your mood changes and feelings of worry or sadness last longer than two weeks after giving birth, you may have postpartum depression (PPD). PPD can develop any time in the first year after giving birth, though it's more common in the first few months.

The exact cause of PPD isn't known. Several factors may likely be at play. These include a rapid decline in hormones to pre-pregnancy levels and declining thyroid hormones. You may also be more likely to develop PPD if you have a high level of life stress, poor support, or a history of depression, including during pregnancy. The risk also may be higher if you're Black, single or younger than 25.

Symptoms of PPD can vary in intensity, from mild to severe:

- Mood swings
- Intense irritability or anger
- Losing interest in activities you used to enjoy
- Trouble sleeping
- Changes in appetite or weight
- Feeling anxious, restless or nervous
- Severe panic or anxiety attacks
- A lack of energy or fatigue
- Problems concentrating or making decisions
- Feeling guilty, hopeless, worthless, shameful, inadequate or that you're not a good parent
- Frequent crying
- Difficulty bonding with your baby

- Withdrawing from family and friends
- Thoughts of suicide, death or harming your baby

A parent with mild to moderate PPD may have five or six of these symptoms, while someone with severe PPD may have seven or more. Thoughts of suicide and apparent problems with functioning and judgment are more common with severe PPD.

Postpartum depression in partners

Partners can experience many of the same symptoms of postpartum depression, including sadness, irritability, anger, sleep problems, changes in appetite and weight, and issues with concentration and decision-making. This affects up to 5% of new fathers, referred to as paternal postpartum depression (paternal PPD). Female non-birthing partners also are at risk.

Postpartum depression in partners may be linked to hormonal changes. Other possible contributing factors include:

- Relationship strains from sleep deprivation and all the other stressors that often come with a new baby.
- Feeling left out or not as connected to a baby, especially if their birthing partners spend more time with the baby than they do.
- Feeling disconnected from friends and that pre-baby life.

For all new parents, having support from one's family and partner is strongly linked to a lower risk of depression. Less social support, on the other hand, increases the risk. Other risk factors include a history of depression, poor overall health and stress such as unemployment or breakup with a partner.

New parents who identify as LGBTQ+ may be at higher risk of depression. While more research is needed, studies suggest that LGBTQ+ women — both birthing and non-birthing mothers — experience PPD at higher rates than others. Gay fathers of babies born through third-party pregnancy may also be at higher risk, compared with fathers in the general population.

Perinatal anxiety

Perinatal anxiety is excessive stress or worry that's usually focused on your baby. It can make it difficult to function or be a parent to your child. If you have perinatal anxiety, you may notice that you:

- Constantly worry about the health or well-being of your baby, and you can't control that worry
- Have thoughts that are racing and are regularly negative
- Feel irritable or on edge and have sudden mood swings
- Lose interest in things you enjoy or consider important, such as intimacy
- Don't want to be around friends and family
- Feel sad and cry a lot and don't know why

Perinatal anxiety can also present as panic attacks — racing heartbeats, problems breathing, shaking, muscle discomfort and stomach tightness — sleeping too much or not enough, feeling tired, high blood pressure and dizziness.

Multiple factors contribute to perinatal anxiety, including questioning yourself and your parenting abilities, as well as environmental and social factors related to race, gender, age or disability, and hormonal or chemical imbalances.

Birth-related post-traumatic stress disorder

Childbirth can be a traumatic event for some, resulting in birth complications or threatening the life of the birthing parent. People with birth-related PTSD have symptoms such as obsessive thoughts and flashbacks, nightmares, sadness, fear and anxiety. Up to 6 percent of parents are affected by birth-related PTSD.

Postpartum obsessive-compulsive disorder

Though it may begin in pregnancy, postpartum obsessive-compulsive disorder (OCD) occurs most often in the first few months after having a baby and can last for months or longer. Parents with postpartum OCD have repeated, frightening thoughts, such as harm coming to their babies, either from themselves or another source. This can trigger compulsive behavior, such as constantly checking on the baby to make sure nothing is wrong. There may also be rituals such as excessive cleaning, handwashing and counting. Postpartum OCD occurs in up to 4% of women.

THE IMPORTANCE OF GETTING HELP

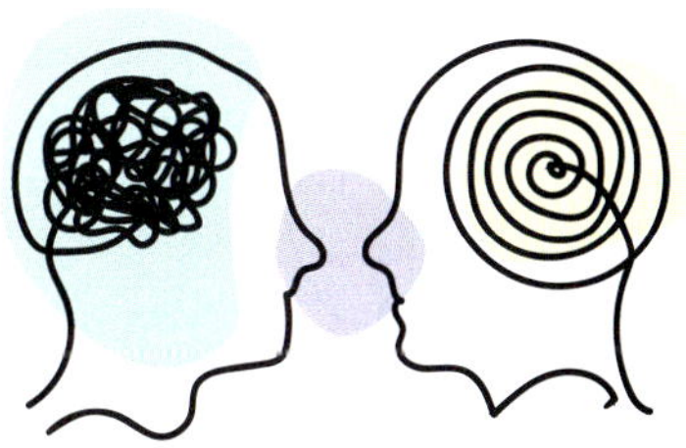

When you're dealing with a mental health condition, it's important to remember that it doesn't define you. You can be a great parent and struggle with mental health issues. They are not a personal failure or a parenting failure. And getting help in caring for your mental health, when needed, doesn't mean you couldn't handle parenthood on your own. In fact, acknowledging you need help and getting it is the most important thing you can do for you and for your child's health.

Research has shown that when left untreated, postpartum mental health conditions can affect a parent and baby in multiple ways. Depending on the condition, this can mean:

- *Issues with infant bonding.* Research suggests that postpartum mental health issues can make it harder to interact and form a relationship with your baby. Parents might be less likely to engage in activities that help with development, such as reading stories or playing games like peekaboo.
- *Problems with partners.* Mental health issues can put a strain on relationships, which, in turn, can negatively affect a child's health.
- *Thoughts of suicide.* It's estimated that about 7% of all postpartum mothers have contemplated suicide. Attempting suicide or dying from suicide is rarer.
- *Thoughts about harming the baby.* Some parents have thoughts of hurting the baby, although most have no intention of doing so.
- *Less breastfeeding.* This includes fewer attempts to start breastfeeding and not breastfeeding for as long overall.

- *Health issues for the baby.* Though not likely the sole factor, conditions such as PPD in a parent may be linked to developmental issues in children, including social skills and language development, illnesses, and problems with emotions and behavior.

It's not easy to talk with a healthcare provider about your mental health concerns. You may be afraid that you'll be judged or even have your concerns dismissed. But remember, the sooner you bring up the subject, the sooner you can get help. Schedule an appointment with your provider and be prepared to discuss how you've been feeling and any concerns about your current mood. Sometimes you may need to ask your provider directly for a referral to speak to a mental health specialist.

Effective treatments are available

Consideration for how best to treat postpartum mental health relies on many things. Your provider will need to assess your health history and the severity of your condition and consider factors such as whether you are breastfeeding, treatment availability and your preferences.

Mindfulness Mindfulness is a form of meditation that's used to help manage stress, anxiety and depression. During a mindfulness exercise, you focus on being fully present and aware of your senses and feelings in the moment, without interpretation or judgment. Exercises may focus on breath going in and out of your body or on concentrating on a familiar object to notice new details about the object. Mindfulness can help improve clarity of thought and decrease tension.

Psychotherapy Talking to a mental health professional can help identify your stress and anxiety triggers. Different types of talk therapy have been used successfully to treat mild to moderate PPD, as well as perinatal anxiety and post-birth PTSD:

- *Cognitive behavioral therapy.* During cognitive behavioral therapy (CBT), you focus on your thoughts, feelings and behaviors, working to unlock negative patterns of thinking, how they may be related to your feelings of depression, stress or anxiety, and how this might be causing unhealthy behavior. CBT teaches you to think of problems differently and reframe them to reduce those negative thoughts. It also teaches you how to better respond to what's happening around you. Those with OCD may receive a specific type of CBT called exposure and response prevention (ERP). This therapy involves having the person confront the fears or discomfort they obsess about — the "exposure"— and teaches them how to resist performing compulsions, or "response prevention." Ultimately, the goal is for people with OCD to learn that what they fear is safe.
- *Interpersonal therapy.* This form of psychotherapy focuses on improving relationships or circumstances your condition has negatively impacted. The goal is to identify negative social patterns, such as isolation, and teach you how to better interact with others.

While talk therapy is often the first choice for parents with milder forms of PPD and anxiety and for parents who don't want to take medication while breastfeeding, it might not be readily available in your area. If this is the case, an antidepressant can be used.

Medications Antidepressants are an effective way to treat mild, moderate and severe PPD and paternal PPD, as well as anxiety. Selective serotonin reuptake inhibitors (SSRIs) are the most commonly prescribed antidepressants. SSRIs have been extensively researched and are considered safe for parents who breastfeed and their babies. SSRIs pass into breast milk at less than 10% of the dose the parent took. If SSRIs don't help your depression, another antidepressant may be used.

Severe PPD and other, rarer postpartum mental health conditions may require other types of medicine or treatments. Discuss any concerns you may have about your mental health with your healthcare provider to help identify the right treatment for you.

MANAGING YOUR EMOTIONS

Though we tend to think of our children as the ones needing guidance to keep emotions from boiling over, the truth is parents do, too. It's not always easy to quickly shift gears from the joy of pushing a delighted toddler on the swings to the epic meltdown that follows when you tell your child it's time to leave the playground.

But how you manage your response to these challenges can set the tone moving forward. In these early years, before your child can properly regulate emotions, you will serve as the model for how to remain calm and to cope when difficulties arise.

As part of this self-regulation process, it's important to acknowledge your feelings and know that they're not right or wrong. Doing so can help you make a more conscious decision about how to respond to your child.

It's also crucial to look at your child's behavior developmentally. Seeing that playground temper tantrum for what it is — a normal part of development — can help put things in perspective and allow you to respond more calmly. It can also foster empathy. Imagine being a toddler and not being able to express your wants and needs in a more rational way. Acknowledging your child's feelings and disappointment alongside your own can often help defuse meltdowns and minimize frustration for everyone.

Managing your emotions helps put you in control. And when you're in control, you're more likely to react to challenging behavior in a way that shows your child how best to deal with life's difficulties.

Of course, there will be times when your child tests your patience and you respond with frustration. It's important to be kind to yourself and know that there's no such thing as "the perfect parent." Every parent faces similar challenges. Take comfort in this during the more difficult times. Meanwhile, your efforts to model self-regulation — whenever you can — will help your child learn to do the same.

CHAPTER 38

Parenting as a team

As new parents, you're busy keeping your child fed, clean, safe, loved and nurtured. But parenting also means getting dinner on the table, doing laundry, keeping up with housework and earning money to support the family.

If you're part of a couple, along with sharing the joys and pleasures of parenthood, you and your partner must also juggle a never-ending set of tasks and responsibilities. The stepped-up demands of life with a child require you to negotiate new arrangements for dividing up duties. At the same time, your relationship as a couple is changing as your focus shifts to your child and you have less time and energy for each other.

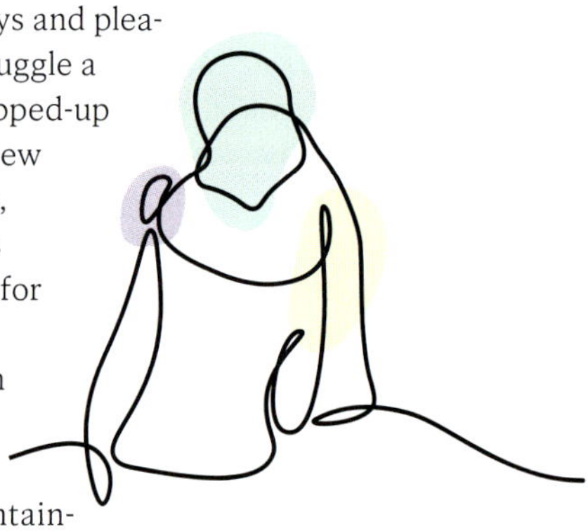

Sometimes these new stresses — especially when layered on top of sleepless nights and new routines — can set the stage for strife and uncertainty. Yet it's possible to learn to adapt to family life while maintaining a positive view of your relationship with your partner.

What makes the difference? Creating practical strategies to share decisions, responsibilities and rewards. Staying alert to potential pitfalls as well as new opportunities for closeness. Remaining committed to preserving a deep connection with your partner. The goal is to work as a team toward your shared goal.

As you and your partner develop complementary roles and support, you may be surprised at the strengths you uncover in both of you. And the stronger your bond is, the more effective you'll be as parents. A supportive, mutually satisfying relationship serves as the foundation for a healthy, happy family.

A NEW BOND

Many couples say that having a child brought them closer than ever and that it gave them a new and powerful point of connection. Watching your partner cuddle with the baby, lying next to each other with the baby nestled between you, joining hands with your child during those first wobbly steps — sharing these moments bonds you and your partner in new ways.

Many people also appreciate the feelings of closeness and belonging that come with being in a family. You and your partner may feel a sense of achievement and fulfillment, especially if you've both longed for a baby or if your journey to parenthood included a few bumps in the road. A baby can be a powerful symbol of your love and commitment. And then there's the fun and humor you enjoy together, from the silly stuff you do to entertain your baby to the sight of your child covered in pureed peas or carrots. You can even bond over your tales from the trenches, such as surviving a week of the flu.

NEW CHALLENGES

The rewarding moments are interspersed with the day-to-day stresses of child care and housework. The first year or so of parenthood can be especially hard on a couple's relationship. No matter how well you got along before the baby arrived, you may find yourselves disagreeing and becoming annoyed with each other now. As one new mom says, "We bickered. We said crazy things to each other that we never did before."

Part of the problem in the first year is the unique demands of caring for an infant, including the lack of a regular schedule, the crying and the nighttime feedings. Infant care adds an estimated 35 to 40 hours of work each week to the average household. Many new parents say they didn't realize how difficult and time-consuming caring for a baby would be. Of course, it's hard for most people to find an extra 35 to 40 hours each week to accommodate this new load. So asking for help and splitting up duties is essential.

In addition, disagreements that might have lived in the background — about life goals, for example, or how to handle finances — may be brought to the forefront. Other issues also may put a strain on your relationship.

Division of labor

Along with sex and money, the issue of "who does what" is one of the most common arguments among couples. How partners divide up their responsibilities both inside and outside the home is an ongoing source of discussion and debate, not only in individual couples but also in books, social media posts and articles about parenting.

Less time as a couple

After your baby arrives, your couple time may seem to vanish overnight. Gone are the leisurely meals, evenings snuggling in front of the TV and impromptu nights out. Now that you're a family, you have less time, energy and attention to devote to your partner. Even your identity as a couple may seem threatened at first. "It was always about the baby," notes one parent. You may feel less like a couple and more like business partners checking items off your endless to-do list.

Fatigue and exhaustion

Lack of sleep adds to stress. Sleep deprivation can make you irritable toward anyone, but perhaps especially toward someone who shares your living space and who very likely is also sleep-deprived. You might find it harder to share your needs and goals in an effective way. It may also be harder to consider your partner's point of view. Both skills are essential for healthy communication.

Decline in disposable income

The financial squeeze of increased costs, along with a possible dip in income if one or both parents reduce work hours or choose to stay home full-time, can leave you with little money to spend on a babysitter or outings as a couple.

Changing roles

Most parents struggle with the competing demands of work, parenting and their relationship. In dual-earner families, which account for the majority of two-parent families with children these days, balancing the competing demands can be challenging. In families of different-sex couples, even though men are taking a more active role in caring for children and doing housework, studies have shown that working moms typically spend more time handling child care and household chores than dads.

SHARING THE LOAD

Who will do the baby's bath? Who's responsible for planning meals, buying the groceries and cooking? Will you or your partner be the one to work more hours or spend more time at home with the baby?

As the saying goes, "The devil is in the details." Working out the nitty-gritty of the day-to-day duties causes many of the conflicts among parents. Before childbirth, most parents-to-be share the ideal of participating equally in family life, household management and child rearing. After childbirth, traditional gender patterns may reassert themselves, even among nontraditional parents. Although both partners may have similar workloads overall, one may spend more time doing paid work, while the other puts in more hours on the home front. The difference between expectations and reality can sometimes come as a surprise and a disappointment to both partners.

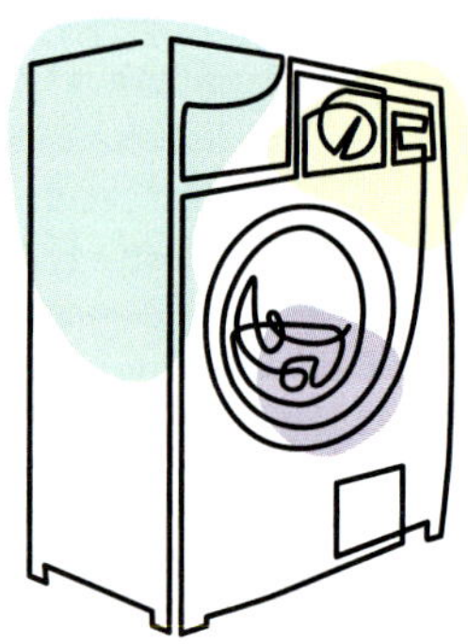

To avoid this scenario, jointly work out a division of labor that distributes the stresses — and the rewards — of parenthood. It's not that you have to split all the responsibilities of life 50-50, but you want to come up with a plan that both of you can embrace — one that allows you to work as a team in caring for your child and sharing decisions and tasks.

How much responsibility should you each take on? Negotiate. Make a list and talk about what you can do, want to do, enjoy doing and are good at. Structure the arrangement as an experiment, and tweak it as you go. Keep communicating about what's working and what's not. One dad comments, "It's a lot of give and take. In the morning I wake the baby up, get her dressed, and I get her out the door. My wife picks her up, she takes care of her while she's cooking, and when I get home we feed her together. Then my wife takes care of her while I do the dishes and then we play for a while. I put her to bed."

Acknowledge different priorities

Discuss what matters most to each of you in terms of your child, your career, your free time and the household chores. You and your partner aren't going to agree on everything — and you probably won't find a perfect balance. Be willing to negotiate some compromises. When you're dividing up household chores, take into account your preferences and strengths and the most efficient use of your time.

Account for the mental load

The mental load is the work involved in planning and coordinating a task before the actual execution. It's remembering to schedule medical appointments. It's

ADDED STRESSES

Some couples may be more prone than others to relationship problems after the birth of a baby. You may be more at risk of stress during this transition if you:

- Haven't been in the relationship for very long
- Have limited social support
- Have limited financial means
- Have an unplanned or unwanted pregnancy
- Are experiencing depression or another mental health disorder
- Are going through other stressful life events
- Grew up with parents who had a poor relationship
- Had a poor relationship with your parents during your childhood
- Have an infant with a difficult temperament or a serious medical condition

If you're dealing with one or more of these issues, the first step is to be aware of the risk, and take steps proactively to bolster your relationship. Seek support from family, friends or a counselor if you're struggling.

planning meals and making grocery lists. It's noticing when baby is growing out of clothes and making sure you have the next size up. It's the mental note to keep an eye on baby's temperature, feeding patterns and diapers when sleep or behavior is unusual. As you divide responsibilities, make sure you're including the mental work as well as the execution step.

Stay flexible about how things get done

Your partner won't do chores and child care the same way you do. Agree that it's OK for each of you to have different ways of doing things, as long as you're providing consistency for your child.

Avoid scorekeeping

You and your partner are on the same team — you don't need to keep score. Instead of taking inventory of everything your partner is (or isn't) doing, trust that you're both committed to your family's success. Work together to solve problems, and show gratitude for what your partner does. Pitting yourselves against each other shortchanges everyone.

Watch out for gatekeeping

Your partner always dresses the kids wrong, constantly leaves the house a mess or can't seem to soothe a crying baby. Does this sound familiar? You may be falling into the trap of thinking that only you know how to do things the "right" way.

This phenomenon, known as "gatekeeping," happens when one parent assumes they have more knowledge about child rearing than the other parent or criticizes the other parent's efforts. You can positively influence your partner's involvement by providing encouragement and ensuring that each of you has opportunities to gain experience.

Consider alternatives

If you can afford it, think about hiring someone to help with the housework or yardwork. But be clear whose responsibility it is to make those arrangements. Join a babysitting co-op, if available, or start one yourself.

Remember that the balance will sometimes shift. There will be times when you need to do more and other times when you can do less. Needs for each person in the relationship will change based on other demands. Understand at the outset that even the best plans will need some adjustment, so flexibility and understanding will be key to continuing a successful family partnership.

NURTURING YOUR TEAM

To parent together as a team, you have to nurture your own relationship as well as your child. You and your partner depend on each other for support, both physically and emotionally. By tending to your relationship, you'll feel more satisfied as a couple. In turn, this improves your parenting ability. Studies show that couples who experience ongoing conflict are less responsive and sensitive to their infants in their first year of life. Negativity in a couple's relationship expands to family interactions.

On the other hand, supportive, mutually satisfying couple relationships enhance the well-being of the whole family. Making a special effort to see yourself not just as a parent but also as a partner is good for both of you — and your child. Here are some other ways you can nurture your team.

Communicate openly

Discuss issues and difficult situations as they arise. Express your feelings, and be specific and honest about your concerns. Don't use this as an opportunity to blame or criticize your partner. Make sure you both have time to talk.

Set realistic expectations

Couples do better when they share realistic expectations about their relationship and parenting. Discuss what you expect of each other and your family life. Acknowledge that the first years of parenting are challenging and that your relationship requires maintenance.

Encourage each other

Both of you need support and encouragement in handling the challenges of parenting. Be sure to talk about what's positive as well as what's more difficult. Tell your partner what you need to feel supported, and listen to your partner's needs. Discuss how well your needs are being met.

Be courteous and considerate

When you're feeling depleted or overwhelmed, you're more prone to lash out at your partner and to be less forgiving. Try not to let courtesy and caring go by the wayside. Cut yourself and your partner some slack by not overreacting if one of you is irritable. Try to see situations from your partner's point of view.

Be adventurous

Plan something small but special for your family each month, and look forward to it together.

REKINDLING ROMANCE

Sex after pregnancy happens. Honestly. But it might not happen very soon, or very often — romance usually isn't a priority for new parents. Many factors contribute to a decrease in sexual activity in the first year after childbirth. These may include vaginal soreness, exhaustion, postpartum blues, an unpredictable schedule, changes in libido and body image, and the adjustment of going from partners to parents. Your bedroom may have turned into a nursery, pumping station and diaper storage center — not exactly conducive to romance.

Some people feel ready to resume sex within a few weeks of giving birth, while others need a few months or longer. In surveys of new parents, most say they're having sex by six weeks after the baby is born. Most also say that sleep is more important than sex, and that they're not having sex as often as they did before.

The body needs time to heal after pregnancy, whether the birth occurred vaginally or by C-section. Many medical professionals recommend waiting six weeks before having sex. This allows time for the cervix to close, postpartum bleeding to stop, and any tears or repaired lacerations to heal. After a vaginal delivery, decreased muscle tone in the vagina may reduce pleasurable friction during sex — which can influence arousal. This is usually temporary. Due to hormonal changes, the vagina may be dry and tender, especially during breast-feeding. If this is bothersome, talk to a medical professional about estrogen cream to alleviate some of the dryness.

Until you're ready to have sex, you can maintain intimacy in other ways. Spend time together without the baby, even if it's just a few minutes in the morning and after the baby goes to sleep at night. Share short phone calls throughout the day or occasional soaks in the tub. Rekindle the spark that brought you together in the first place.

Most sexual problems that occur after pregnancy resolve within a year. In the meantime, concentrate on promoting your physical and mental health, be patient, and ease back into intimacy and sex.

AGREEING ON CHILD REARING

From infancy on, child rearing brings countless decisions about a range of issues — rules and expectations, discipline, structure and routines, time with grandparents, and exposure to TV, apps and other media, to name a few. Granted, during your baby's first year or so, discipline won't be a major issue. But by the time your child is a toddler, you'll be dealing with misbehavior as your child tests the limits. You may not know exactly what those limits are yet, but commit to talking them over with your partner. Parents should agree on general principles and present consistent guidelines for your child.

New parents tend to copy their parents in their child-rearing beliefs and behavior — though some people make a point of doing the opposite of what their parents did. What's important is for you and your partner to discuss your parenting beliefs and agree on the strategies you'll use. For example, what type of consequences will you set when your toddler breaks a rule? How will you handle tantrums or requests to sleep in your bed? How will you encourage cooperation? Research over the past several decades has shaped experts' recommended strategies for behavioral parenting, mealtimes, and more. So it's worth looking to reliable resources before defaulting to the model you grew up with.

You and your partner may not agree on everything. Acknowledge any differences, and compromise to maintain a united front. Make sure you and your partner (and other adults who care for your child) follow the same rules and discipline guidelines. This reduces your child's confusion and need to test you. Work together to provide love, attention, praise, encouragement and a degree of routine.

Both you and your partner come to parenthood with inner visions of what you hope it will be. To build a life that satisfies both of you and nurtures your child, share your core values and choose goals that matter to both of you. Some partners don't want to discuss their hopes and anxieties because they're afraid that they'll reveal unbridgeable differences or start major conflicts. But confiding what you hope will happen and what you're concerned about strengthens the bond between you.

A FIRM FOUNDATION

Your relationship with your partner serves as the foundation for your family. You make your foundation stronger by engaging with each other with respect and mutual appreciation, sharing tasks and responsibilities, and regularly tending to your relationship. Parents in satisfying relationships report feeling more confident in their parenting and more resilient in the face of challenges. They're less worried and stressed.

Your parenting patterns are the least stable during your baby's first year. Over time, you'll establish patterns that work for you, and the stress on your relationship will ease. Practice does makes perfect — handling the initial challenges together will help you and your partner weather future stresses better.

By approaching parenting as a team, you create an optimal environment for your baby to grow and form a secure attachment to you. You'll set the tone for an affectionate, communicative family life. For all the challenges parenting brings, you and your partner are also in for a lot of fun, love, surprises and deep satisfaction.

CHAPTER 39

Single parenting

If you're raising your baby on your own, you're not alone. Single-parent families are more common than ever — 1 in 3 children in the United States live with one parent, according to the U.S. Census Bureau. Although most single-parent households are headed by mothers, the number of single fathers is increasing. Close to a quarter of single parents today are fathers, compared with 14% in 1960.

Whether by choice or otherwise, parenting without a partner brings special challenges. The responsibility for all aspects of daily child care may fall squarely on your shoulders. Juggling work and child care can be financially difficult and socially isolating.

But single parenting can also be rewarding, and it can result in an especially strong bond between you and your child. Yes, you can raise a healthy, happy child while tending to your own needs and happiness as well.

One of the keys to raising a child on your own is to develop a solid support network. Other strategies can help you manage the challenges that come with the territory.

HARD WORK, ADDED PRESSURE

All new parents face many of the same challenges in taking care of a baby and raising a child. But parenting without a partner puts more pressure on you. Along with handling the day-to-day duties and decisions, it's up to you to support your family. One woman who chose to become a single parent felt panicked after she came down with a severe bout of flu: "What if anything happens to me?" Another single mom worried, "What happens if my baby gets sick, and I have to go to work? Will I lose my job because I'm on my own?"

Many single parents can relate to these fears. You may face several specific challenges as you adjust to your new role and raise your child.

Financial and work issues

Single parents often are the sole providers for their families. For some, being the only earner can make it hard to make ends meet. Single parents may also find it more difficult to build a safety net for emergencies. In general, single parents tend to have fewer financial resources than partnered parents.

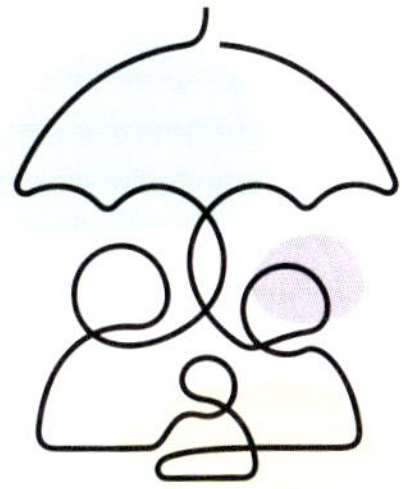

To juggle their work and caregiving roles, some single parents find that they may need to reduce their work hours, turn down promotions or take less-demanding jobs. For many single parents, it can be difficult to find ideal employment opportunities, family support programs and subsidized child care centers.

Still, single parents can find creative ways to make their financial situations work for them. Here are some suggestions to consider.

Assess your finances Make a list of your income and expenses so that you can budget your money. Will you receive child support? Pay for child care? Now that you have a child, your expenses will likely increase, and your income may change if you shift to fewer hours or change jobs. If necessary, seek financial advice from a trusted source. Some communities, local libraries or banks regularly offer free financial workshops.

Cut down on spending If you need to make the most of money coming in, figure out where you can minimize money going out. Some expenses are have-to's, but others may be decreased or cut. Take advantage of free or low-cost activities, and eat out less often. Buying used baby gear can save you money.

Prepare for emergencies Even if money is tight, try to build up an emergency fund. Ideally, you'd have enough to cover several months' expenses.

Find out if you qualify for assistance Public programs offer supplemental nutrition assistance and subsidized child care and housing. In addition to receiving federal benefits, you may qualify for grants, scholarships and other assistance from state governments, private foundations and faith-based organizations.

Check into employment resources If you need help with finding a job or getting a better job, contact your state employment office.

Consider additional training or education Getting special training or an additional degree may boost your chances of finding a job.

Getting it all done

The advantage of being a single parent is that you automatically have final say in all household and child-rearing decisions. You don't have to worry about fighting over where your baby will go for child care or what foods are best for your toddler. On the other hand, you bear the entire burden of child care and housework, including the logistics, organizing and planning. As one single mother notes, "There is a constancy of parenting on your own that you don't understand until you've had to do it. Nothing ever stops. The minute you wake up in the morning, you hit the ground running, and needs don't stop until you pass out. That's when things go right."

Support issues

In the first weeks and months after having a baby, you'll likely be feeling more physically and emotionally vulnerable. As a single parent, it's important to reach out for support — see the suggestions below, under "Seek and accept support."

Being a single parent in itself doesn't increase your risk of depression or other mental health problems. But single parents are more likely to have other risk factors for depression, such as financial hardship and unemployment. Keep in mind that having a partner doesn't help much if your partner isn't supportive. A relationship with an unsupportive partner may be worse for your mental health than is single parenting.

Emotional challenges

Many single parents say that the emotional challenges of single parenting can be as difficult as the practical ones. It's hard to feel exhausted and not have someone at home to hand your child off to for a break when you need one. You might feel guilty about raising a child without another parent. If your relationship with the other parent has ended, you may be grieving the loss of your partner, as well as your vision of how your life would be as you raised your child together.

Acknowledge your feelings and mourn any losses, even if you don't regret your choices. If you've recently lost a partner or are going through a divorce or separation, recognize that it can take months or even years to resolve the emotional ups and downs that follow. Consider seeking professional support as you work through these transitions. See Chapter 37 for more guidance on caring for your mental health as a parent.

FROM SURVIVING TO THRIVING

Some days it may feel like you're doing all you can just to survive. It will get better. As one mother says, "I learned that regardless of whether or not this is the life I planned, this is my life and I need to embrace it. I love being a mom and wouldn't trade it for the world. My son makes all of the difficult times worthwhile."

Several strategies have been shown to improve outcomes for single-parent families. With these in mind, you can create an environment that helps you and your baby thrive and grow.

Seek and accept support

Probably the most important thing you can do as a single parent is to develop a strong support network. Practical and emotional support from others can not only help you handle your responsibilities but also boost your well-being. Asking for help can be hard on your pride, since many people are brought up to believe they should and must do everything by themselves. But it's better to lean on others a little than to become so overwhelmed or stressed that you can't parent effectively.

Many single moms say their own mothers are their best sources of both practical and emotional support. You can also turn to other trusted family members, friends or co-workers. Ask for what you need, whether it's someone to babysit while you run errands, a friend to call when you need to talk, or someone who's willing to provide backup child care if your baby is sick or your regular arrangement falls through.

In addition to seeking help from family and friends, look for a support group for single parents, or seek social services. Faith communities can be helpful resources, too. A support group, whether in person or online, offers a great opportunity to share feelings and get advice.

Find quality child care

Good child care is crucial for your baby's well-being and your peace of mind. If you need regular child care, look for a qualified caregiver who can provide stimulation in a safe environment. See Chapter 15 for more information. Many single parents say they view their child care providers as valued partners in raising their children.

Be careful about asking a new friend or partner to watch your little one. Anyone who cares for your child should be someone you know and trust and should have some experience with young children.

To learn more about child care in your area, contact your local child care resource and referral (CCR&R) agency. The agency can help you find out if you qualify for free or subsidized child care. Links to state CCR&R agencies are available through Child Care Aware of America (www.childcareaware.org). You can also find child care resources by state at the Office of Child Care (https://childcare.gov). The federally funded Head Start program serves infants and toddlers in low-income families. Local government, United Way agencies and

SINGLE DADS

One of the first hurdles single fathers must face is their invisibility in society. When people hear the words "single parent," they usually think of a mother. But in the United States, close to 2 million fathers are raising kids on their own.

Finding support and a peer group for single dads can be a challenge. Many parenting classes, support groups, play groups and books are geared toward women. As a single father, you might feel like you stick out in some situations. You might not appreciate the unsolicited advice you get. Eventually you're likely to meet other single dads. And if you don't, make an effort to seek out — or create — a support group in your community.

other community or faith-based organizations sometimes provide child care scholarships. Some employers may provide child care benefits or discounts.

Aim for a stable family life

Changes in family structure, such as one parent leaving or a new adult entering the family, can be hard on kids. Try to ensure consistency in your family and your child's caretakers and, if possible, keep moves and major changes to a minimum. For example, if you're dating, carefully consider when you would like to introduce a new significant other to your child. There's no right answer, but it may be challenging for your child to meet and become attached to a new significant other and then have that person step out of the picture. It may be better to wait until a relationship lasts at least several months. If there are custody negotiations with another parent, talk to your lawyer about how dating and introducing significant others to your children could impact a court decision.

Create routines

Family routines — such as regular bedtimes, mealtimes, naps and reading — promote good health and cognitive development in children. A lack of bedtime and mealtime routines, for example, increases the risk that children will have sleep problems, eat a less healthy diet and become overweight.

Single-parent families may be less likely to keep daily routines for young children than two-parent families. Some of the reasons include time constraints, financial pressure, fatigue and lack of support. Do the best you can to establish routines — but also be kind to yourself in those instances where the routine goes out the window.

During your baby's first months, you're still helping your child develop regular sleep habits, and the feeding schedule might vary from one day to the next. As your child gets older, create a regular schedule for meals, naps and bedtime. If you're having trouble establishing daily routines, figure out what's in your way and brainstorm solutions. You can also seek assistance from your child's medical professional.

Take care of yourself

To take good care of your child, you must take good care of yourself. Include physical activity in your daily routine, eat a healthy diet and get plenty of sleep. Make sure you get some "me time" regularly. Time away from your child will help replenish your energy and spirit, helping you be a better parent. Even taking 15 or 20 minutes to relax can be helpful.

Of course, this is all easier said than done. Sometimes it can feel selfish to take time to yourself, but it shouldn't. Try to let go of any guilt about caring for yourself. Here are some tips:

- Arrange for a babysitter for a few hours once a week so you can get out of the house and do something you like, either by yourself or with friends.
- Find a gym membership that includes child care.
- Take naps when you can.

- Read or walk on your lunch break.
- Work out or read after your child is in bed.
- Once your child is sleeping regularly, get up a little early to enjoy a quiet cup of coffee or do some yoga stretches.
- Reduce stress with relaxation techniques.
- Accept your limits, and don't be too hard on yourself.

Prioritize family time

Throughout your child's life, and particularly in the early years, time with parents is important to health and development. Single parenting can put the squeeze on your time with your child. Make it a priority — even if it means having a messier house or not getting something else done that day. Set aside time each day to cuddle, play with or simply hold your child. Find out if you can modify your work schedule to have more time with your child.

Get organized

Being organized can help reduce stress. Try these tips:

- Stock up on basic household supplies, such as toilet paper and diapers, as well as easy-to-prepare foods and meals that can be frozen and reheated.
- Eliminate clutter.
- Plan your week on a calendar.
- Develop a list of timesavers.
- Keep a list of babysitters.
- Prioritize. Figure out what's most important for your child's needs and your needs, and focus on those.

Stay positive

Make a conscious decision to focus on the positive and not dwell on the negative aspects of single parenthood. Try to keep your sense of humor when dealing with everyday challenges, and don't forget to have fun. Take a break from the routine and plan a fun activity you can do with your child, such as a hike in the park, trip to the zoo or picnic with friends.

One single mother advises recognizing your accomplishments and blessings: "Give yourself a pat on the back daily. What worked out well and what made you smile today? There is no question that being a new single mom is one of the hardest challenges life will throw your way, but you will get through it and it will get better."

If you're feeling down much of the time or find yourself stuck in a pattern of negative thinking, talk to your doctor, a counselor or a psychologist.

REWARDS AND STRENGTHS

Despite the challenges, being a single parent can bring great rewards, including a deep parent-child bond. In this relationship, the parent and child depend on each other, and they may become more communicative and supportive. Over time, you may create special routines and rituals together or discover places you like to go and things you like to do.

Children growing up in single-parent families often learn to take on more responsibility at home and develop self-reliance. As for the parents, many say they find a strength they never knew they had. Some also appreciate the freedom to make child-rearing decisions on their own, without constant negotiation and compromise. You may find yourself with a welcome clarity about what's important and learn to let go of what's not. As a single parent, you can take pride in your accomplishments and feel good about what you're giving your child.

If at first you feel overwhelmed and alone as a single parent, overcoming such feelings can foster a sense of inner strength. As one parent comments, "I have done things I never thought I was capable of all by myself. I am in control of my own happiness."

CHAPTER 40

Siblings and grandparents

Bringing home a new baby can be an exciting experience for your family. If you already have one child or more, your baby is a new sibling. Your older child or children will likely play with, laugh with and share a lifelong relationship with your new baby. If this is your first baby, your parents might be more eager than you expected to dote on and help care for your newborn. You also might begin to view your parents and your relationships with them differently.

Bringing a newborn home can require some adjustments within a family. Babies need a lot of attention — which can cut into the amount of time you spend with your older child or children and cause jealousy. Grandparents, on the other hand, may be so excited about your new baby that they unknowingly overstep certain boundaries, such as by giving unwanted parenting advice.

Don't underestimate the impact your tiny newborn might have on your family. Consider your personal family dynamics, and understand how you can help your older child or children, as well as your parents, adjust to their new roles.

SIBLINGS

The experience of bringing a newborn home is a little different the second time around. With your first child, you were probably focused on the transition to parenting and figuring out how to care for a baby. With the second — or third or subsequent — baby, you're more likely wondering how your older child or children are going to react to having a new sibling and how you're going to juggle and meet all their needs. Help set the tone for your children's early interactions by preparing your older child or children for what's ahead.

Introducing your new baby

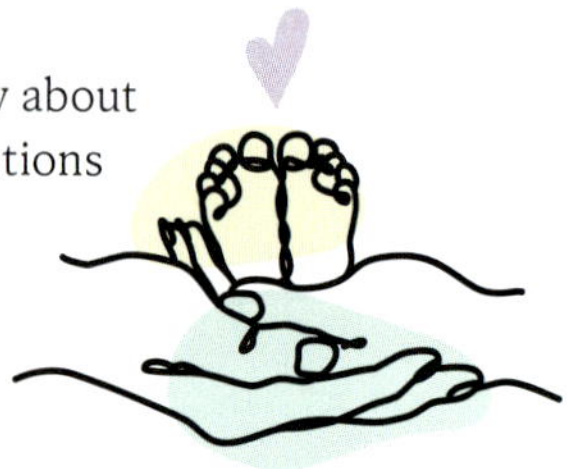

You've probably been talking to your older child for a while now about the arrival of your new baby. Perhaps your child has asked questions about your growing stomach, gone along to prenatal checkups or helped set up the nursery. Or maybe your child attended a sibling preparation class at your hospital. But it may still be difficult to know how your child will react to an addition to the family and the changes a new baby will bring.

While older children are typically eager to meet a new sibling, young children may be confused or upset and have a hard time adjusting — especially as the new baby sleeps less and demands more of your attention. Explain to your child that your newborn will probably cry, sleep and eat most of the time. The baby won't be a playmate right away.

To lessen the stress your child might experience once the new baby comes, think ahead. If your child will need to change rooms or move out of the crib so that your new baby can use it, do this before the baby is born. It will give your older child a chance to get used to the new setup before dealing with the other changes associated with the new baby's arrival. Arrange for your child's care during labor and delivery, and explain the plan to your child.

When the baby arrives, arrange to bring your older child to the hospital for a brief visit. This is a great way to introduce your child to the new baby and spend special time together. Ask another family member to hold the baby for a while so that you can give your older child plenty of cuddles. Consider giving your older child a gift that's from the baby to celebrate the new baby's arrival.

SIBLING REACTIONS

Age and development will play a role in your older child's reaction to having a new sibling.

TEACHING GENTLENESS

Sometimes older children, stressed by the changes happening around them, take out their frustrations on a new baby. If your older child tries to pull your baby's hair, take away the baby's bottle or harm the baby in any way, it's time for a serious talk. Calmly explain to your older child that it's not OK to hurt the baby. In addition, make an effort to give your older child some extra attention. Also, include your child in activities that involve the baby, such as singing, bathing or changing diapers, to encourage positive interaction between the siblings. Keep in mind that, for safety reasons, you shouldn't leave your newborn alone with a child who is younger than age 12.

SIBLING SAFETY HAZARDS

If you have an older child, you probably have toys in your home with small pieces that an exploring baby could easily choke on or swallow. Round up games and toys that have small parts, and keep them out of your baby's reach. When your older child wants to play with these toys, keep them in an enclosed area. This will give your older child a chance to play without little hands getting in the way — an increasingly challenging task as younger siblings grow into toddlers. Encouraging your children to play separately with their own toys may also help you sidestep a few battles — especially if your older child is younger than age 3 and isn't eager to share. For more information on childproofing your home, see Chapter 17.

Children under age 2

Young children likely won't understand yet what it means to have a new sibling. Try talking to your child about the new addition to your family and looking at picture books about babies and families.

Children ages 2 to 4

Children at this age may feel uncomfortable sharing your attention with a newborn. Explain to your child that the baby will need lots of attention. And encourage your child's involvement by shopping together for baby items. Read to your child about babies and siblings. Give your child a doll to take care of. Look at your child's baby pictures together. Share your child's birth story.

If there's time, finish your child's toilet training before the baby is born. Otherwise, wait until a few months after you bring your baby home to start the process. Keep in mind that siblings sometimes take a step backward in behavior after the arrival of a new baby — such as by having potty accidents or asking to drink from a bottle or be carried to bed. They want to be sure they still have your attention. There's no need to punish such behavior. Instead, give your child plenty of love and assurance. Don't forget to praise your child for good behavior.

School-age children

Children age 5 and older generally are pretty excited about having a new baby in the house. But they also may feel jealous of how much attention the baby gets. Talk to your child about your newborn's needs. Encourage your child to get involved by helping to decorate the baby's room with handmade artwork and participating in taking care of the baby. Explain the importance of being gentle with the new baby. Point out to your child the advantages of being older, such as being able to go to bed later or play with certain toys. Show your appreciation for your child's help in caring for and entertaining the baby and share your delight in the baby's behaviors.

MANAGING SIBLINGS DURING BREASTFEEDING

If you're breastfeeding your baby, you may wonder how your older child will react to your nursing sessions — or how to keep your older child busy while you nurse. Try not to worry. Your child will likely express curiosity and may hover upon first seeing you breastfeed. Simply explain what you're doing, and answer any questions your child might have. If you breastfed your older child, explain that you did the same thing when your child was a baby. To keep your child entertained while you nurse, consider setting out a couple of toys, picture books or even a special new item to play with only while baby is nursing. You might also play music or audio versions of children's books.

All children

Make sure that your older child gets plenty of individual attention from you and other family members once your baby arrives. Grandparents can be particularly helpful during this time. Watching parents coo over a new baby can be frustrating for an older child. If you're taking lots of pictures or videos, include your older child, too. Take some pictures or videos of your child alone, as well as with the new baby. During your newborn's feedings, include your older child by talking or reading stories together. Provide reassurance that you love your older child and your new baby. Explain that your older child has an important role to play now, too — that of big sibling.

SIBLING RIVALRY

Right now, sibling rivalry may not be a concern. But it can become an issue as your youngest gets older and competes with other children for parents' love and respect. Signs of sibling rivalry might include hitting, name-calling, bickering and regressive behavior. This kind of behavior is common after the birth of a new baby — but it can also happen anytime one child in the family gets extra attention.

While sibling rivalry is a natural part of growing up, many factors can affect how well your children might get along with each other, including their genders, ages and personalities, as well as the size of your family and each child's position in it. For example, younger children might be more likely to fight physically, while older children might argue instead.

Children who have less than a two-year age difference might battle each other more than children who have bigger age gaps between them. Although children of the same sex might share more of the same interests, they might also be more likely to compete against each other. Middle children might feel less secure and be more likely to seek affection because they may believe they don't get the same privileges or attention as the oldest or youngest child in the family.

Although all siblings are bound to fight, tease and tattle on one another at some point, there are things you can do as a parent to encourage healthy sibling relationships now and as your children get older. Consider these tips.

Respect each child's unique needs

Treating your children the same isn't always practical — and the harder you try, the more your children may look for signs of unfairness. Instead, focus on trying to meet each child's unique needs.

Avoid comparisons

Comparing your children's abilities can cause them to feel hurt and insecure. While it's natural to notice your children's differences, avoid discussing them out loud in front of your children. When praising one of your children, stick to describing the action or accomplishment — rather than comparing it with how a sibling does things.

Set the ground rules

Make sure your children understand what you consider acceptable and unacceptable behavior when it comes to interacting with each other, as well as the consequences of their misbehavior. Consistently follow through with consequences, such as a loss of certain privileges or a timeout, when your children break the rules.

Listen to your children

Being a sibling can be frustrating. Let your children vent their negative feelings about each other, and listen. Respond by showing your child that you understand. If your child is old enough, you can ask for help creating an acceptable solution to the problem. If you have siblings, share stories of conflicts you had when you were a child. Holding regular family meetings can give your children a chance to talk about and work out sibling issues.

WHEN YOUR NEWBORN IS SICK

If your new baby has health problems, try to answer your older children's questions about the new baby in simple terms. You might explain that the baby is sick, and you're worried. Reassure your children that the baby's illness isn't their fault. If your baby needs to stay in the hospital after birth, ask about the sibling visitation policy. You also might take pictures of the baby and show them to your older children.

Even if you don't talk to your older children about the baby's illness, they will sense that something is wrong and may act out to get your attention. Rather than being secretive, give your older children some basic information about the situation. Do your best to show that you are there for them.

Don't take sides

Try to avoid being drawn into your children's battles, unless physical aggression is involved or safety is in jeopardy. Encourage your children to settle their own differences. While you may need to help younger children resolve disputes, don't take sides. In addition, avoid using teasing or insulting nicknames for your children that might encourage sibling rivalry.

Give praise

When you see your children playing well together or working as a team, compliment them. A little praise and encouragement can go a long way.

IF YOU HAVE MULTIPLES

Sibling rivalry often isn't an issue for twins and other multiples. While the children may compete against each other, multiples typically also depend on each other and develop close relationships early on. However, they may have problems maintaining their individuality. For example, twins are often treated as a unit, rather than as two children with unique personalities. As a result, twins are often dressed alike and given the same toys. If you have multiples, pay attention to their different needs and try to foster individuality.

Multiples can also cause other children in the family to feel left out or jealous — since they are not part of this unique relationship. If you have multiple babies and an older child, spend plenty of special one-on-one time with your older child. Also, encourage your multiples to play separately with other children. For example, arrange a play date for one of your twins while the other twin plays with a sibling or has one-on-one time with a parent. Your multiples may resist separation, but being apart without anxiety is a skill your children will benefit from as they get older. For more information on multiples, see Chapter 43.

GRANDPARENTS

Grandparents can play a major role in your newly expanded family. Your parents will likely give you emotional support and encouragement, and calm first-time parent jitters as you figure out life with a baby (and soon enough, a toddler).

They may share their experiences as well as helpful tips. If they live nearby or visit, they may be great babysitters and helpful in a pinch. Grandparents can serve as role models for the kinds of parents you want to become. Best of all, they can provide your child with a special kind of love and affection that can only come from grandparents.

Changing relationships

The arrival of a baby often causes new parents to reexamine their relationships with their own parents. As you prepare for your future as parents, it's only natural that you think about the ways in which you were raised — what you would like to carry forward from the past or would like to change. In the process, you might find that you have questions for your parents about how they handled becoming a parent and why they made certain decisions. Your parents will likely be able to share advice, discuss some of the ups and downs they experienced as new parents, and reassure you that you'll be able to handle your new role.

Typically, the birth of a new baby brings families closer together, giving new parents and their parents a chance to renew and strengthen their bonds. But the shift in your role and your parents' roles may not always go as smoothly as you might hope. You and your parents might unknowingly have different understandings and expectations of your new roles. Make an effort to talk to your parents about how you feel about becoming a parent and your parents becoming grandparents — and listen to their feelings on the subject, too. Keep the conversation going as your child gets older.

Receiving help

As you navigate the early years of parenthood, your parents will likely want to provide help and support. Sometimes, however, the support you get isn't the support you need. For example, excited new grandparents might want to come to stay for a few days once the baby is born. While some new parents might find this helpful, others might find it stressful. Or grandparents may have views that are different from yours — and sometimes pretty strong opinions — on when to introduce solid foods, how to dress your child or how to handle toddler tantrums.

Think about what might work best for you and your family, and discuss your needs with your parents. Would you like to spend a few days on your own with your new baby before relatives visit? Would it be helpful for your parents to have a standing "date" with your child so you can have an occasional night out? Would you like to have your parents and in-laws visit at different times so that each set of grandparents can have time with their grandchild?

Tell your parents what they can do to be most helpful — household chores included. This may help prevent misunderstandings and tension, as well as help you make the most of your parents' desire to be there for you.

Like it or not, your parents might go a little overboard on getting gifts for your child. While you might not be able to stop your eager parents from buying

GIVING GRANDPARENTS TIME

Sometimes new grandparents aren't quite ready for their new role. They may still have careers and life plans, and the idea of being grandparents may make them feel old. If your parents are uncertain about becoming grandparents, give them an honorable out. Don't push grandparent language or traditional grandparent duties or tasks. With time and sensitivity, things may change.

the gifts, tell your parents what your child needs. Also, remind your parents that for a child, nothing really rivals spending quality time with grandparents. Doing an activity together, such as taking a walk in the park or going to the zoo, can be a fun way for grandparents and new babies to begin bonding.

And don't forget that as much as your parents want to help you during this time, they likely also want to spend some time cuddling with your child and building that special connection. This is especially important if your parents don't live nearby or won't be able to visit your baby frequently. Offer your parents as much time with your child as you're comfortable giving them. Remember, this is a precious and exciting time for them, too.

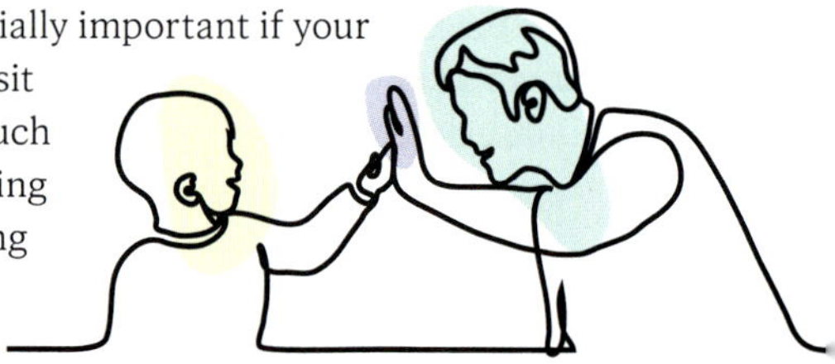

Conflicting opinions

You likely have some ideas about how you plan to care for your child — and they might be different from your parents' ideas. For example, while your parents may have fed you formula, you might plan to breastfeed. One of your parents may have stayed home to take care of you, while you and your partner both plan to continue working. As your baby gets older, you and your parents may also have different opinions about the toys your child should play with — wood or plastic? — or the amount of television that's OK to watch. This can be tricky territory.

If your and your parents' parenting styles differ, it might be difficult for your parents to keep their opinions to themselves. Consider explaining to your parents that what you could really use is support or help around the house, not advice. You have the final say over the way your child is raised and the rules in your home. However, try not to dwell on these issues. Keep in mind that your parents are probably trying to help and may still be working through the transition from being your parents to being grandparents. And expect that if your parents babysit your child, they will likely handle things slightly differently than you would. These little differences may even help your child learn to be more flexible.

LETTING GO OF THE PAST

If you and your parents aren't close or have a difficult relationship, the birth of your baby might serve as motivation to work through your problems — especially if you want your parents and your child to have a strong connection. During your pregnancy or after your baby is born, consider making an effort to work on your relationship with your parents. In addition, remember that your child will have a separate and different relationship with your parents than you do. If couples divorce, the grandparents on both sides of the family will still want to spend time with their grandchild.

GRANDPARENTING FROM A DISTANCE

If your parents don't live nearby, they might miss out on your baby's first smile, first steps or first words. Consider helping your parents keep in touch with your child through regular phone calls or video chats — perhaps at the same time each week — or by frequently sending videos or pictures. While it might still be a while before your little one can talk much, your baby will likely enjoy listening to your parents' voices and grabbing the phone or computer. If your parents aren't up on current technology, regularly mailing printed pictures might be your best option. To help your child get to know your parents and other family members, make a photo album with their pictures and look at it with your child during playtime or before bed. Tell your child the names of the people in the photos.

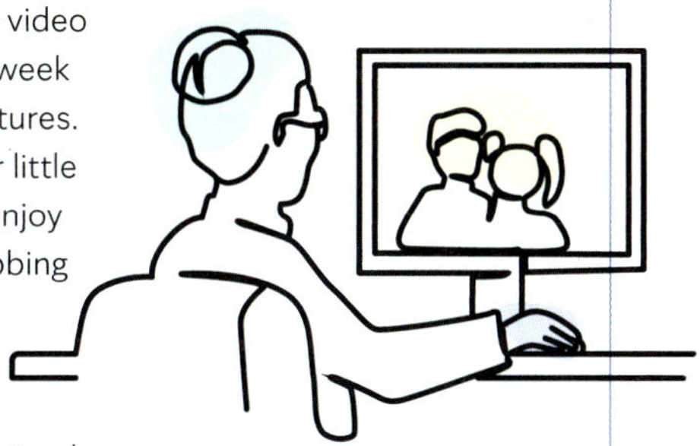

In addition, just as you and your partner have your own thoughts about what kind of parents you'd like to be, your parents might have thoughts about what kind of grandparents they'd like to be. Some grandparents aren't comfortable babysitting and prefer a more formal relationship with their grandchildren. Others are playful and enjoy engaging their grandchildren in activities. And still others want to be a part of their grandchildren's daily lives, serving as surrogate parents. Consider talking to your parents about what kinds of roles they'd like to play in your child's life. Do they want to babysit? How available do they plan to be? Are they willing to help out in case of a crisis?

When making requests for help in taking care of your child, keep in mind your parents' ages, abilities and any other limitations. To avoid unnecessary misunderstandings or resentment, ask your parents what they can handle and if you're expecting too much from them.

Holidays

Holidays and birthdays will likely be important events that grandparents will want to help celebrate. But while big family parties can be fun, they're not always possible. Chances are that you'll end up alternating holidays with different grandparents. Or perhaps you'll have multiple celebrations, with different sets of grandparents, on different days.

Either way, if holidays are particularly important to your parents, talk to them ahead of time about your plans and your desire to make sure everyone feels included in your child's big days. If your parents are having a hard time understanding the situation, explain that alternating holidays will allow each set of grandparents to spend more quality time with your child in a relaxed setting. You might also encourage your parents to focus on new or different traditions, such as taking your child out for a half-birthday.

GRANDPARENTS AS CHILD CARE PROVIDERS

Some couples rely on grandparents to provide part-time or full-time care for their children. Having someone you know and trust take care of your child can be comforting. Grandparents are often flexible with their hours, may be able to watch your child in your home and may not ask for payment. However, grandparents might not have any training in car seat use, CPR or other emergency care. These types of arrangements can also cause tension, especially if you don't feel comfortable communicating expectations to your parents about how you want your child cared for, or if you don't want unsolicited parenting advice.

Think about the pros and cons before asking your parents to provide child care. If you have concerns — whether for safety reasons or differences in opinion about feeding or discipline, for example — consider hiring a sitter, asking another close friend or family member to babysit, or seeking out another child care option instead.

If you decide to have grandparents provide regular child care, ask them to take a CPR class if necessary. Be sure to discuss the details and come to an agreement beforehand about how the arrangement will work. For more information on child care, see Chapter 15.

If your parents will be watching your child in their home, consider asking them to purchase their own crib or high chair — or offer to get one for them. This will make meals and naps easier on your child, as well as on your parents. You might also consider providing your parents with their own stroller, car seat, potty chair and basic medications, such as for a fever or diaper rash.

If it's been a while since your parents took care of a young child, they might need a refresher on the basics — especially in areas where the rules have changed over the years, such as in car seat safety and baby sleeping positions. Before you leave your child in your parents' care, discuss safety topics. Make sure your parents are aware of all safety precautions discussed in Chapters 16 to 18. If

NAME PREFERENCES

Your parents may have their own ideas about what they would like to be called — beyond grandma or grandpa. For some grandparents, these traditional titles just don't fit with the way they see themselves. Consider talking to your parents about what names they might have in mind for themselves. Remind your parents, however, that your baby might come up with names, too.

your baby is going to be at their house, the house needs to be childproofed. It's also important that they not leave medications and other dangerous items within a child's reach, and that they take precautions around hot liquids and other items that could lead to a burn. These are just some of the safety issues that need to be addressed.

Car seats

Make sure your parents have a reliable car seat and know how to install and use it properly when transporting your child. You might offer to check or re-install a car seat as often as is needed. Explain the importance of having your child ride rear-facing or forward-facing as appropriate until your child reaches the maximum weight or height allowed by the car seat manufacturer. For more information about car seat safety, see Chapter 16.

Sleep positions

Insist that your parents put your baby to sleep resting on the back, rather than on the stomach or side, until your baby can roll over both ways without help. Remind your parents that adult beds aren't safe for infants. Make sure your baby is put to sleep on a firm mattress in a crib, without blankets or soft toys. Let grandparents know when your child reaches milestones that allow these rules to change, such as when your child can sleep with a special blanket or stuffed animal. For more information about sleep safety, see Chapter 8.

CHAPTER 41

When to have another child

As your first baby approaches toddlerhood, family, friends and strangers might feel free to ask if you're going to have another child. (Often it's "when" and not "if.") And the question may be on your mind as well.

Like other parenting decisions, figuring out how many children you want is a personal process, though you may receive plenty of advice and opinions. Deciding whether or not to have another child is one of the most important decisions you'll make for your family, and it may be even harder than deciding to have the first one. It's common to worry about how another child will affect your family, relationships, lifestyle, finances and work and to wonder whether you're making the right choice.

If you think you want another child, when might be the best time? Again, only you can answer that question. Pregnancy spacing affects how close your children are in age and may have an impact on your health and your baby's health. There are many factors to weigh when planning your next pregnancy.

As you and your partner consider the possibility of having another child, approach each other with compassion, respect and a willingness to listen. Talk about the issues with an eye toward strengthening your relationship and your family.

DECIDING ON ANOTHER CHILD

Maybe you've always dreamed of having three kids, each spaced three years apart. Or you're agonizing over whether you can really handle another baby. Whatever your hopes, fears and dreams, there are a number of issues to consider as you think about expanding your family.

Added responsibilities

Caring for a growing family can be physically, mentally and emotionally taxing, despite its many rewards. Most parents say that adding a second child more than doubles the work. You need plenty of time and energy to care for an infant, while your older child also needs your attention. With two kids, your life will be more hectic — and your house will no doubt be messier. But you'll also find that you grow to meet the challenges.

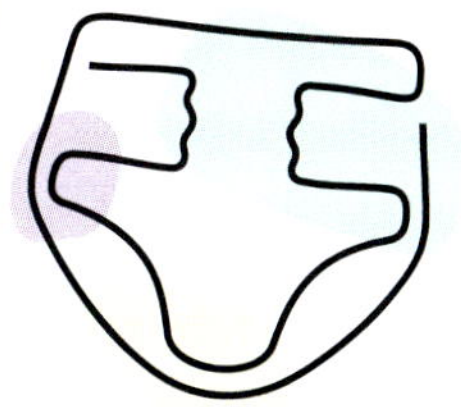

"I felt like my life as a parent finally had a rhythm to it (my child finally slept at night, I didn't need to lug around all the baby paraphernalia anymore, etc.) and I wasn't sure how I'd do once a second child came along," writes one parent. "Taking care of the needs of two little people can definitely be more stressful, but you get progressively more creative to get everything done." With a second baby, you'll realize how much you learned the first time around. You'll have increased confidence in your abilities and knowledge, and you'll find it easier to handle things that might have seemed daunting the first time around, such as breastfeeding and taking care of a sick baby.

Your preferences

Sometimes one partner is ready for another baby and the other isn't. It's important to understand each other's concerns. Sit down together and talk about your points of view and your differences. What does having a second child mean for each of you? What are your goals and dreams? Explore ways to resolve concerns and conflicts. If your partner is worried that your relationship will suffer, make specific plans for keeping date night alive. Work together to come up with ways to lessen the financial burden.

Both of you need to be on board with the decision. If you remain at odds, perhaps you can agree to revisit the issue in a year or two. It might also be helpful to talk to other couples who've been in the same position or to consult a marriage and family therapist.

Family finances

A new child adds to your family's expenses. You'll want some extra money in the budget before you conceive another child. Think about what your financial picture will look like with a new baby. Will you or your partner need to reduce your work hours or stay home to care for your children? Can you afford to pay for the new baby's child care if you keep your job? Are you willing to sacrifice certain things in order to cover baby costs? Will you have enough money to save for college tuition? If you're living paycheck to paycheck or fear a layoff, you may decide to hold off on having the next baby.

In the longer term, having babies close together frees you from child care costs sooner. On the flip side, spacing children further apart can give you more time between kids to recover from the financial impact of pregnancy and early child care.

Impact on your career

It might be harder to juggle your job and child care responsibilities when you add another baby to the mix. If you have a partner, how will you divide the work disruption of caring for another infant? Is it important for you to reach another level in your career path before you take on newborn care again? Then again, it might be easier to focus on careers later if your kids are in school at the same time.

Family dynamics

Many people have more than one child because they don't want their firstborn to be an only child. Providing a sibling for your child may be part of your motivation, but it's also important to want to raise another baby in general. You can't predict how well siblings will get along, and there are pros and cons to having siblings or not. (See "Deciding one is enough," page 518.)

Another common concern is that you'll disrupt the smoothly functioning, happy family structure you've created. Change of any sort can bring up fears, and a second child will change the dynamic and logistics of your family life. However, most parents say that soon after expanding their family, they can't imagine life without a second baby.

Sharing the love

Probably most parents have wondered how they could possibly love their second child as much as they love their first. You may worry that you'll lose your special relationship with your first child and shortchange the second child by having to share your attention and time. It's common to worry that the second child will feel less wanted and loved and that the first one will feel resentful. Rest assured that your relationship with each child will be unique, like the children themselves, and that you'll have plenty of love to go around.

As writer Lisa Belkin notes, "I remember the moment I said goodbye to Evan as I left for the hospital to deliver Alex. I had the overwhelming feeling that I was about to ruin his life. I tried to remember what I try to remember in all tough parenting situations — that I am giving them something, not taking it away. . . . And when I brought home a baby brother, I gave each of them proof that neither of them was alone in the world, and that neither was the center of the universe."

Social pressures

Although one-child families are increasingly common, couples still face cultural and family pressure to have a second child. If your friends are all having a second or third child, you may feel left out. You may feel pressure from your partner or feel guilty if your partner wants another baby and you don't. Be honest with yourself about what's right for you. Parenting another child is a big responsibility to take on because someone else thinks it's a good idea.

Thinking in reverse

If you're having trouble making a decision about having another child, you might try turning the question on its head. How would you feel if you were told you couldn't have another child? Your sadness or your relief may give you insight into what you really want.

Until you make a decision about when to have another child, use a reliable method of birth control — even if you're breastfeeding. If you're still thinking about another pregnancy, you may want a method that's easily stopped or quickly reversible. Examples include an oral contraceptive or a barrier method, such as a condom. If you and your partner agree that your family is complete, or complete for now, or if you are undecided, you can switch to something longer lasting but still reversible, such as an intrauterine device (IUD) or implantable rod. You also might opt for something permanent, such as a vasectomy or tubal sterilization.

Remember that a decision this big takes time and thought. Do your research and discuss any concerns with your medical professional. Make sure you have the information you need — and the time you need to process it — before going through with a permanent plan.

PREGNANCY TIMING

Once you've said yes to another baby, the next decision is when to start trying. There's no perfect time to have another baby, and if you wait until the circumstances are just right, you might never do it. Even with careful planning, you can't always control when conception happens. You might get pregnant sooner than you thought or long after you hoped you would. In the end, pregnancy spacing is often based on a combination of personal preference and luck.

You can make an informed decision about when to grow your family by understanding the health issues associated with timing your pregnancies too close together or too far apart, as well as the advantages and disadvantages of different pregnancy intervals for parents and children.

Health issues

Some studies show that spacing pregnancies too close together or too far apart can pose some health risks for both the birthing person and the baby.

Short interval Closely spaced pregnancies may not give the birthing person enough time to recover from the physical stress of one pregnancy before moving on to the next. It can take a year or longer to develop stores of essential nutrients that may have been depleted during pregnancy and breastfeeding. If you become pregnant before replacing those stores, it could affect your health or your baby's health.

Getting pregnant within 18 months of giving birth may slightly increase the risk of low birth weight, small size for gestational age and preterm birth. If you had a cesarean birth and allow for less than an 18-month interval before your next child is born, you may increase your risk of uterine rupture if you decide to try a vaginal birth.

Limited research suggests that a pregnancy within 12 months of giving birth is also associated with an increased risk of placental problems. One study reported a link between pregnancy intervals of less than 12 months and an increased risk of autism in second-born children.

It's possible that behavioral risk factors, such as smoking, substance misuse or lack of prenatal care, as well as stress and poverty, are more common in people who have closely spaced pregnancies. These risk factors — rather than the short interval itself — might explain the link between closely spaced pregnancies and health problems for mothers and babies.

Long interval Spacing pregnancies many years apart also may pose some health concerns for birthing persons and babies. A pregnancy five years or more after giving birth is associated with an increased risk of:

- High blood pressure and excess protein in your urine after 20 weeks of pregnancy (preeclampsia)
- Slow or difficult labor or delivery
- Preterm birth
- Low birth weight
- Small size for gestational age

It's not clear why long pregnancy intervals are linked to these potential problems. Researchers speculate that people who wait five years or more to have another baby may lose some of the protective effects generated by the first pregnancy. Age or factors such as illnesses also may play a role.

To reduce the risk of pregnancy complications and other health problems, wait at least 18 to 24 months but no more than five years before attempting your next pregnancy. Balancing concerns about infertility, people older than 35 might consider waiting 12 months before becoming pregnant again.

The risks and recommendations don't apply to couples who have had a miscarriage. If you're healthy and feel ready, there's no need to wait to conceive after a miscarriage.

DECIDING ONE IS ENOUGH

The number of families with one child has nearly doubled since the 1960s, as more people are starting families later in life and facing financial pressures. But negative stereotypes about only children — that they're spoiled, selfish, lonely and bossy — still persist. Such beliefs may prompt couples to have more than one child.

Years of studies in several countries have found no evidence to support these stereotypes. Only children are no different from their peers in terms of character, sociability, adjustment or personal control. One way they are different is that they score consistently higher in intelligence and motivation compared to children with siblings. Interestingly, some research suggests that parents of only children are happier than parents with more than one child. When you have just one child, you spend a lot of time with that child, which can make for a close relationship. However, parents with multiple children also are close to their children.

If you do get pregnant while breastfeeding and decide not to wean your baby, you'll need to take extra care with your diet. You may want to meet with a dietitian to be sure you're meeting your nutritional needs.

SPACING PROS AND CONS

Is there an ideal spacing between children for their sake and yours? Probably not. Many families settle on an interval of two to three years, but various types of spacing all have advantages and disadvantages.

1 to 2 years apart

Having children 1 to 2 years apart can be the ultimate test of your endurance. But that doesn't mean it can't work.

Pros Some of the benefits are:

- Your children will be close in age as they grow up. They may share many of the same interests and activities, making it easier to juggle family schedules. Parents often hope that siblings close in age will be close companions and play together.
- You condense the time when you're dealing with carrying, feeding, diaper changing, sleep deprivation and toilet training. Also, you may not need to childproof your home as many times as you would if you had your children further apart.
- You can double up on some tasks, such as reading to your older child while nursing the baby or having them nap at the same time.
- Your first child may have an easier time adjusting to a sibling and will barely remember what life was like before.

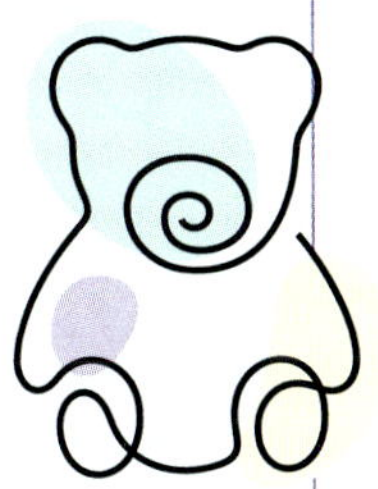

If you're struggling with the idea that a childhood without siblings will damage or shortchange your child, you can let go of that fear. Yes, having siblings can be a positive experience and help kids learn skills such as dealing with conflict. As a parent of one child, you'll want to make an effort to give your child opportunities to interact with other children.

What's most important is to know what's right for your family. "I am being honest with myself when I admit that I will be a much happier and better parent to one child than more," says one parent. "Some people thrive in a busy, spirited environment. . . . I fall apart. I think the worst thing about deciding to have an only child is dealing with my own feelings of needing validation." Another says, "By having a second child, we would stretch ourselves way too thin mentally, emotionally, financially, physically, and we know we would end up in pure misery."

Cons Some possible drawbacks are:

- Caring for two in diapers is likely to leave you exhausted much of the time and with little personal space for a few years. Life with two little ones can feel like constant chaos.
- Stress and fatigue can take their toll on your relationship with your partner. You'll need to work together as a team to meet the challenges ahead. And you'll need to set aside some quality time for each other.
- Supplies for two young children can be costly.
- Sibling rivalry may be a problem as your children grow up.

2 to 5 years apart

A spacing of 2 to 5 years is what most experts recommend. Your first child is a little more independent, and you and your partner have had some time to regain strength and energy.

Pros Some of the benefits are:

- During the time between pregnancies, you'll bond with your first child and share your undivided attention.
- Your first child will have the opportunity to be the baby of the family without any competition.
- When the new baby arrives, the older sibling will be more likely to play independently at times, giving you some one-on-one time with the baby.
- Your children will still be close enough in age to bond easily.
- You're only paying for diapers for one. Some baby supplies, such as a crib or stroller, can be reused.
- Your body has time to restore its nutritional supply to prepare for the next pregnancy.
- You've fine-tuned your parenting skills, but it hasn't been so long that they're rusty.

Cons Some possible drawbacks are:

- Your first child may feel jealous of the new baby. It's not uncommon for 3- and 4-year-olds to revert to baby-like behavior when faced with competition for a parent's attention. This usually goes away with time, though.
- Rivalry issues regarding toys and activities may occur as the baby gets older and starts getting around independently.
- Your older child may be outgrowing naps just as your baby is settling into a regular nap schedule.
- The further apart your children are, the more different each child's activities are. Coordinating schedules may be stressful and involve a lot of planning.

5 years or more apart

Some parents liken having kids who are five years or more apart to having an only child twice.

Pros Some of the benefits are:

- You get a big break between babies. This may give you some time to go back to doing things you enjoyed before having an infant, such as going out for dinner or a movie or taking adventurous vacations. It may also give you a chance to refocus on your career or your marriage. Waiting five years or more can also give you a financial break and allow you to save money for the next baby.

- Each child gets plenty of individual attention in infancy and beyond.
- You get to enjoy and focus on specific stages of growth and development with each child.
- Because of the difference in age, sibling rivalry tends to be less intense. Instead, your younger child may see an older sibling as more of a hero, while the older child may assume a more protective or guardian-like role. Depending on the age of your first child, you may even have a built-in babysitter.

Cons Some possible drawbacks are:

- After several years of being out of baby mode, you may have a hard time getting back into it. You tend to forget how much work caring for an infant can be and how exhausted you become at the end of the day.
- It may be a challenge to keep up with your older children while caring for a baby.
- You'll probably need new baby gear, because your car seat and stroller will likely be out of date.
- Schedules in your household may vary widely. It can be stressful to keep them all coordinated.
- Due to the age difference, your children may not share many of the same interests. They may not be as close as children who are more similar in age.

Other issues

Other factors also can influence the timing of a second baby:

- *Your age.* Couples who start a family when they are older sometimes must race against the biological clock. If you're in your late 30s and you would like two more kids, you may not have the luxury of spacing your children three years apart.
- *Your age when you had a first child.* Especially for younger women who had their first child at an earlier age than planned, a longer pregnancy interval will allow time to catch up on education, stabilize finances, or address other things that may have been impacted by pregnancy.
- *Your fertility.* If it took you a long time to conceive the first time, or if you used fertility procedures, you may not want to wait long before trying to conceive again.
- *How many children you want.* If you would like to have a large family, you may need to space your children closer together.

Most important, listen to what your heart says. Whatever the pros and cons of various pregnancy intervals, if you want another baby, this might be just the right time.

PART 6

Special circumstances

CHAPTER 42

Adoption

One way to become a parent is through adoption. Adoption is an active process, often involving a great deal of paperwork to be filled out, personal information to be shared, home studies to complete and agency fees to work into the budget. And unlike a nine-month pregnancy, adopting a child can take anywhere from several months to several years. The wait can be difficult and adoptions can sometimes fall through.

For prospective parents pursuing adoption, the level of self-examination and outside scrutiny required can be considerably greater than for others making the transition into parenting. In short, those who undertake adoption are some of the best-prepared parents around! This can be a great strength when it comes to facing the challenges and opportunities ahead.

Most of what you need to know about caring for a young child is already in this book: All children require love, nurturing, guidance and medical care. But because you may have no control over the prenatal and postnatal care of the child you adopt, you may have some unique concerns. This chapter offers basic advice on adoption and addresses medical and emotional issues that may be on your mind.

SUPPORTING YOUR CHILD'S HEALTH

One of your jobs as a parent is to keep your child as healthy as possible. Since you may not know ahead of time what your child's health status or medical history is, you may need to take a few extra steps to ensure that your child gets on the right track. Here are key tasks to add to your checklist so you can help your child thrive.

Find a medical professional

The best time to choose a medical professional is before your child arrives, if possible. Although many professionals who care for children's health have experience with adoption, you may need to shop around a bit to find one who suits your needs. Talk to other parents who have adopted and ask for recommendations. Call a few of those medical professionals to say you're planning to adopt, and ask if there's any specific medical information you should request from the agency concerning your child. If you'll be adopting internationally, ask the medical professionals if they've had experience with international adoptions.

Once you've selected a healthcare team, you may want to ask if they typically schedule a pre-adoption visit. Not all clinics do, but it may be an option so you can ask questions and discuss general developmental expectations before your child arrives.

Some international adoption clinics offer physician services, such as reviewing a child's medical information before a prospective parent accepts a referral, travel consultations for parents traveling abroad to pick up their child, and post-adoption checkups.

Update family immunizations

Adults and children who will be in close contact with the child being adopted may need to catch up on immunizations, including vaccines against measles, hepatitis A and B, tetanus, diphtheria, and pertussis. If you're traveling to a different country to bring your child home, your medical professional can give you advice on travel safety and any necessary vaccines or medications you'll need to receive before or during your trip, depending on your child's country of origin.

Try to track down a medical history

If possible, try to get any records of your child's medical, genetic and social history in writing from the birth parents or adoption agency. There might not be much information, but it will be easier to track down now rather than years later.

It's important to gain full disclosure from the agency before you adopt so that you get a more accurate representation of any medical conditions your child may have. This is where having a medical professional for your child already selected may come in handy. The medical professional may be able to help you make sense of medical reports you obtain, explain the implications of a medical condition or alert you to what might be missing from the records.

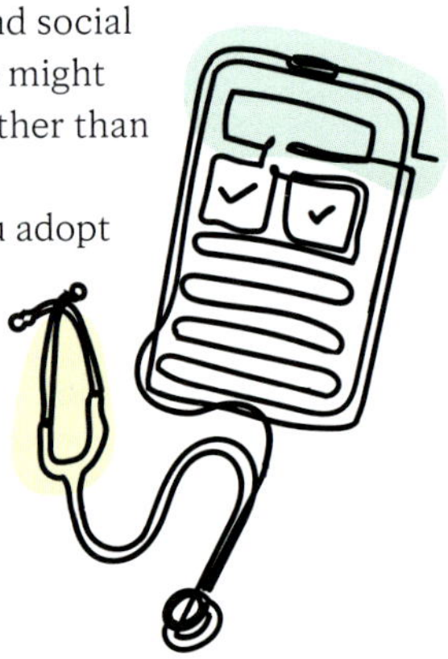

Get post-adoption care

If your child has a known medical condition or arrives ill, you may need to visit your child's medical professional soon after arrival. But if your child appears healthy after joining your family, you might wait a couple of weeks or even a month. This gives your child a chance to adjust and you a chance to get to know your new little one. After this period, you may be better able to answer a medical professional's questions about your child's "usual" behavior.

If you had an open adoption, you might be able to follow the same well-child schedule as any child. (For more on well-child care, see Chapter 13.) First-time parents, especially if they did not have a pre-placement visit, may want to consult their child's medical professional sooner if they need information and support.

For children arriving from overseas, the Centers for Disease Control and Prevention recommends a medical exam within two weeks of arrival in the United States, or sooner if your child has a fever, difficulty eating, vomiting or

INTERNATIONAL ADOPTIONS

Immigration laws in the United States require that all immigrants seeking permanent residence in the United States show proof of having received the vaccines recommended by the Advisory Committee on Immunization Practices (ACIP). Internationally adopted children under 10 years of age are exempted from this law, however, if the parents sign a waiver declaring their intention to comply with immunization requirements within 30 days of the child's arrival in the United States. Over 90% of children adopted from abroad need catch-up vaccinations when they arrive.

Certain countries also have high rates of infectious diseases or parasites that prompt testing and treatment, if necessary, both for the care of the child and for the protection of the rest of the family. In addition to a complete physical examination, including vision and hearing screenings, your child's medical professional may recommend screening for the following:

- Hepatitis B
- Syphilis
- HIV
- Intestinal parasites
- Stool pathogens
- Tuberculosis
- Anemia and blood disorders
- Vitamin and mineral deficiencies
- Thyroid disorders
- High lead levels in the blood

Depending on your child's country of origin, the medical professional may also recommend testing for:

- Hepatitis A
- Hepatitis C
- Chagas disease
- Malaria

Treatment exists for many of these conditions. The sooner a health concern is found, the more effectively it can be treated.

diarrhea. In addition to a comprehensive exam, your child's medical professional may also recommend certain screening tests and vaccinations, depending on your child's country of origin.

At the first appointment, your child's medical professional will review the child's immunization status and perform any age-appropriate screening tests, as well as any further tests indicated by the exam. If your child has no written record of immunizations or has missing or ineffective vaccines, the medical professional may recommend starting a new schedule. The risk of side effects from repeating a vaccination is lower than the risk of getting an infection. If your child is older than 6 months, the medical professional may recommend checking antibody levels in your child's blood before recommending certain vaccines. These tests can show if your child has already had certain infections.

A few children have no official birth date. Determining their age can be difficult if their growth is delayed because of prematurity, problems at birth, malnutrition or neglect. Your child's medical professional will try to make an educated guess based on the information available.

After your child's first medical examination, it's important to follow the schedule of examinations and immunizations recommended by your medical professional.

Give it time

It's not uncommon for children adopted internationally to show delays in development when they arrive. However, most are able to catch up within the first 12 months of arrival, after being on a nutritious diet coupled with a stimulating, nurturing environment. For example, a baby who may not have had the opportunity to learn to crawl because of previous conditions may quickly learn by being placed on a blanket on the floor and given a toy just out of reach.

Get support

If you're adopting an older child, especially one who has had a difficult past or a child with special needs, your child's medical professional may refer you to a counselor or mental health professional who has experience with adoption. A therapist can help ease the transition for the whole family and provide help in working through issues of loss and change. Support groups for families created through adoption also can be helpful.

BONDING

Some parents bond immediately with their baby the first time they meet. It seems as if the family they've created was always meant to be. But for others it takes a little longer. Don't worry too much if the first time you meet your baby, both you and your child feel more bewildered than smitten. As with any relationship, it takes time and commitment to establish a deep, solid connection.

The longer you're there to provide consistent, loving care, the more your child will feel safe and secure, and realize that you're in this for the long haul. With time and consistent effort, both of you will become more confident and comfortable with each other and in the way you interact.

The same activities can foster the attachment process for both biological and adoptive parents: holding your baby close, cuddling, feeding, laughing, serenading, playing games, going through the daily activities of living.

Allow time for adjustment

Parents who adopt have sometimes waited so long for a child that they cannot wait to smother the child with love and attention. But your child may have just been separated from everything that was familiar and need time to warm up to you and take in a new environment.

Holding children close is important because it helps them get accustomed to your scent, to hear your heartbeat and to feel your body warmth. But pay attention to their signals. Some children prefer to be held more than others do.

In general, the best way to nurture a healthy attachment is by observing closely your child's needs and determining how best to make your child feel supported, safe and loved in any situation. This may call for different strategies in a young infant when compared with an older child. Older children are more likely to have difficulties with attachment. Parents of these children may wish to

MAKING ROOM FOR GRIEF

Adoption is a wonderful event and most people rightly want to focus on the joy and fulfillment that comes from uniting parent and child. But while a family formed by adoption has many things to celebrate, it's important to acknowledge that those involved often experience some sense of loss during the process. For the children, this may include loss of the opportunity to be raised by birth parents or to be raised in their birth culture. For the birth parent, there may be loss of an intimate connection with the child. An adoptive parent may grieve the loss of a biological connection. It's important to create time and space for each party to grieve the loss. Glossing over the loss to meet happiness expectations, whether within yourself or those around you, can cause problems later.

Sometimes just acknowledging the loss and accompanying grief is enough to allow you to move forward. Doing the groundwork now can help set the foundation for a healthy relationship with your child over time. But if you're having difficulty or just want advice, don't hesitate to reach out to a mental health professional. Your child may struggle with emotional or behavioral issues or both and may benefit from talking with a behavioral health specialist such as a child and adolescent psychiatrist. These experts will be able to determine whether further help is needed.

connect with specialists in post-adoption services either through their adoption agency or through their medical professional.

Talk, sing and read to your child

These activities allow the child to get used to the sound of your voice. This is especially important for children who come from a country where a different language is spoken, because it helps them learn to understand and ultimately communicate in a new language. Consider narrating everyday events, for example, as a way to increase the number of words your child hears.

BREASTFEEDING AN ADOPTED BABY

Many adoptive parents are surprised to learn that nursing their babies may be an option for them. Because lactation, or the production of breast milk, can sometimes be induced (with a combination of medication, pumping and nipple stimulation), it's possible to breastfeed without ever having been pregnant.

Non-birthing mothers who seek to nurse young infants usually do so to enhance their relationships with their children. Although most non-birthing mothers can't produce all the milk their infants need, even limited breastfeeding allows them the opportunity for physical and emotional attachment with their babies.

When the baby's arrival can be anticipated, some women try to establish a milk supply in advance by using an electric breast pump at regular intervals.

Others wait until the baby arrives, because the baby's sucking will stimulate lactation better than any pump on the market. These mothers use a supplemental nursing device that allows infants to receive formula through a soft tube inserted in their mouths while nursing. Even after their milk comes in, many mothers continue to use supplemental nursing devices if they need to increase their breast milk volume.

Babies are usually more willing to breastfeed if they are younger than 8 weeks of age, but some adoptive mothers have reported success with older infants, too.

If you try breastfeeding but can't produce milk, don't worry. There are plenty of other ways to foster attachment with your baby, including holding your baby close with skin-to-skin contact during feedings, and at other times, too.

If you think you might like to nurse your adopted infant, discuss the advantages, disadvantages and techniques with your medical professional or a lactation consultant well ahead of the time you anticipate your child's arrival. There may be a lactation consultant on staff at your hospital, or you may contact the International Lactation Consultant Association or La Leche League International. Check their websites for more information.

Respond to your child's needs

Be quick to find out why your child is crying. Tending promptly to your child in the first few months won't spoil the child but will provide reassurance and comfort. Eventually your child will become more secure in the family and less clingy or demanding. In fact, this is advice for every parent.

Also keep in mind that your child may not yet be open about discomfort. Children who have spent time in an institution or have been neglected may internalize feelings of abandonment and insecurity by withdrawing from others and failing to make their needs known. Keeping a quiet eye on your child and maintaining a regular schedule for meals, naps and bedtime will help promote health and provide a sense of security and well-being.

Learn about your child

Ask about the child's previous environment and routine so that you can help smooth the transition. For instance:

- A child who shared a crib or a mat with other children or family members may be frightened at night in a room alone. You may want to bring the child into your bedroom and keep the crib or bed in your room for a while until your child gets used to the new environment and has had time to adjust. After a while, the child likely will establish more independence and be able to sleep alone. You might also consider giving your child a soft blanket or stuffed animal (see safe sleep precautions in Chapter 8). Having a loved object to hang on to while everything seems to be in transition may help your child feel more secure.
- A child who was carried everywhere on the back of a caregiver, as is the custom in some cultures, may feel right at home in a back carrier. Even a child who isn't used to it may enjoy the security of being carried close to you in a front or back carrier.
- A child who is used to falling asleep with the room light on may be extremely attached to that simple routine. Be sensitive to any routines that seem important to your child and allow some time before gradually trying to change habits.
- A child may experience sensory overload with a nursery full of toys, unable to decide what to play with first. Introduce one toy at a time, as the child is ready.

Identify your child's developmental stage

On joining your family, your child's developmental stage can affect your interactions. For instance, in the first four months, babies cry mostly when they need something and they'll bond most easily with the person who responds to their cries. Later, they begin learning cause and effect and may cry just to see what happens. This behavior could frustrate parents meeting their child for the first time at this stage. At around nine months, separation anxiety can be very intense for a child who's been attached to another caregiver.

Read through the chapters in Part 3 of this book that correspond to your baby's developmental stage. You'll find that some of your child's behaviors indicate the developmental phase they are in rather than their personality.

If you're adopting a child who's 6 months or older, keep in mind that your child may have already learned certain cultural behaviors. For instance, a child from a culture where passivity is encouraged may appear unresponsive. If you're adopting a child of 12 months or older, it may take more time and understanding to get acquainted and develop mutual trust. You may find reassurance in reading about parenting, talking to someone from the adoption agency or a counselor familiar with the adoption process, and doing what you can to help your child feel loved, secure and wanted. Eventually, most children — especially those who arrive most needy — make great gains in their social and behavioral skills. This is a testament to the resilience of human nature.

Take care of yourself

It's tempting to let everything else fall by the wayside — including yourself — when focusing on your newest family member. But becoming worn down and stressed out isn't helpful to anyone and may in fact undermine the attachment process.

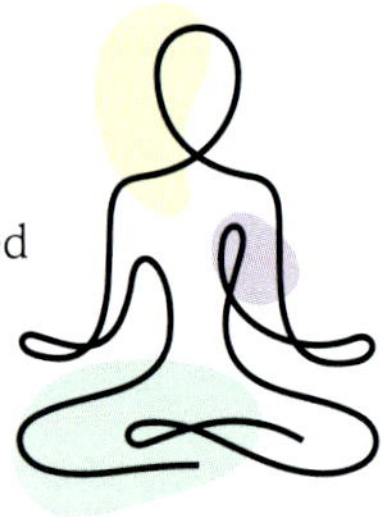

For any new parent, it's common to feel overwhelmed when faced with the intense demands of parenting. Accept help from family members and friends with housecleaning and other chores, spend some time on your own, get some exercise (even if it's just a walk around the block) and eat regular, healthy meals. If you take care of yourself, you'll be better equipped to care for your new child and your family.

Get help when needed

All children are individuals with definite likes, dislikes and inborn personality traits. Some adjust quickly and respond with joy to their new families, but others might have a longer and more difficult adjustment period.

Many families benefit from talking to an outside party who has seen and talked to other adoptive families. This can help you work through the necessary steps to achieve mental and emotional wellness and to bond as a family.

If you're feeling discouraged or lost, or if your child exhibits behavior problems or doesn't seem to be building a relationship with you, seek professional help. Your child's medical professional, your adoption agency, a social worker or a mental health professional may be able to help you understand and resolve the challenges you're facing.

SIBLINGS AND ADOPTED CHILDREN

If you have other children in addition to your adopted child, you'll probably face some of the same issues any parent has when introducing a child to siblings (see Chapter 40).

Help your other children with the transition by including them in plans for welcoming your newest addition and in daily family activities. Children typically love new babies and children, and will be thrilled to help. Even after the novelty wears off, older siblings continue to bond with your adopted child, even when conflicts arise. Try to find some time to spend with each child individually, even if it means running a quick errand together or snuggling for a few minutes before bedtime.

The younger the siblings and the adopted child, the more likely they are to bond with little trouble. Most children under the age of 4 generally don't notice differences among themselves and like to hear the adoption story. Older children are more likely to ask questions and feel some differences.

In some cases, an older adopted child may have developed certain behaviors before joining a permanent family that persist for weeks or months after adoption. This might include survival behaviors, such as hoarding food or sleeping with the back against a wall. Other siblings may see this as "weird." But it's important to realize that these behaviors are likely there for a reason. Over time, as your new child continues to receive consistent loving care, these behaviors are likely to fade. In the meantime, encourage your children to focus on the positive aspects of their relationship with their new sibling. Younger children, for example, are usually easily distracted by a new topic of conversation or by the suggestion of a game. Older children may be able to better understand the possible reasons for unusual behaviors and may be able to help you in providing consistent support to their sibling.

Sibling relationships can be a lifelong gift, continuing to be a source of strength even after parents are gone. Look for opportunities to promote bonding between your children. If you have doubts or questions, or if you feel your family needs help in bonding together, talk to someone who is knowledgeable in the matter. This may be someone from your adoption agency, your medical professional, a social worker, or a family counselor or therapist.

SHARING YOUR FAMILY STORY

A renewed focus on an adoptive child's well-being has paved the way for increased openness when it comes to telling the adoption story. More adoptions are now carried through as open adoptions, where the birth parents are in contact with the adoptive family during the adoption process and possibly beyond. This avoids the scenario of previous generations when parents didn't always tell their children they were adopted and the news might be revealed by a relative or come as a surprise later on, leaving the children feeling puzzled, angry or betrayed.

But even with open adoptions, it's not always easy for a child to understand the relationship between the two sets of parents. Right now your adoptive child may be too young to understand, but when your child is older and the time is right, look for natural opportunities to weave your family's story into your daily life. If you start early and simply, the transition to more complex discussions down the road may be that much smoother. Keep in mind that this is your own family story; how you share it with others outside your immediate family is up to you.

Be positive

Experts agree that if parents demonstrate they are comfortable talking about adoption as a positive experience, their children will be much more likely to feel comfortable with it themselves. They will also be more willing to share their questions and concerns about adoption as issues arise.

Use books

Even before your child is old enough to ask questions, you can begin to introduce age-appropriate books that explain adoption through simple concepts and words (see below).

Tell your story

Many experts recommend that parents develop their own story of how their family was created and tell it to children from the very beginning. Children won't understand everything at first, but the words and phrases will become a natural part of their vocabulary. And all children love hearing stories about themselves.

Use the story to introduce your child's birth parents in an understanding way, explain why you chose adoption to build your family, and give your child a sense of personal history and belonging. You can say, for example, "Just as you were growing in your birth mommy's tummy, you were also growing in my heart." Any details you can add to such a story about the joy of your first encounter will make it more delightful to your child.

Creating a "life book" for your child is another way to celebrate the unique way your child joined your family. Save any mementos such as letters, toys, hospital name tags or documents that came with your child at the time of placement; they can serve as a source of "roots" later. Include pictures, too. Save

BOOKS ABOUT ADOPTION TO READ WITH YOUR CHILD

Reading age-appropriate books about adoption together with your child is a great way to jump-start a conversation about your family's adoption story. Here are some suggestions:

- *The Story of You* by Lindsay McKenzie
- *The Mulberry Bird: An Adoption Story* by Anne Braff Brodzinsky
- *Why Was I Adopted?* by Carole Livingston
- *When You Joined Our Family* by Harriet Evans
- *Adoption Is Both* by Elena S Hall
- *We Belong Together* by Todd Parr
- *The Baby with Three Families, Two Countries, and One Promise* by Julie Gianelloni Connor
- *The Little Green Goose* by Adele Sansone

any information or mementos that are directly from your child's birth parents, no matter how small they may appear to be. Even a slip of paper with the birth parent's handwriting may ultimately become a treasured possession for your child. If your child is from another country, pictures, trinkets and other mementos from your trip there can provide a sense of background.

Tell the truth

Be factual about your child's story, while keeping in mind what's age appropriate. It's important not to embellish or add details that you don't know to be true. You may feel uncomfortable with the fact that there are holes in the story, and you may wish you knew all the answers. Your child may ultimately grieve the loss of those details, too. However, it's healthier to acknowledge the missing information and deal with not knowing than it is to make up details that you don't know to be true. You don't need to share all the information with your child right away. There may be some details better saved until your child is mature enough to handle them.

Use positive language

Let your language reflect your own positive values toward adoption. Be open and honest about the adoption, but don't use it as a label. Say "my child" and not "my adopted child." Phrases such as "given up for adoption" may leave children

ONE MOM'S STORY

We have an open relationship with my 4-year-old daughter's birth mother. My daughter knows her birth mother's name, and a picture of the two of them hangs above her bed. Her birth mother and I exchange emails and pictures, and we all talk on the phone on holidays and birthdays. When my daughter and I discuss our family story, it goes something like this:

I feel so lucky that your birth mom (we use her first name) chose me to be your mommy! I remember the day that you were born . . . when I first held you, I couldn't believe how small you were! I'd been waiting for you and seeing you made me smile so big. You had tiny little fingers, and you wrapped them around my little finger right away — I think maybe that's why we like to hold hands today. Your birth mom and I took turns holding you and feeding you. We talked about how cute you were and about what we hoped you'd do when you got older. We both want you to be happy and to do good in school and be nice to your friends. We want you to have lots of adventures and to go to college when you're bigger. Most importantly, we want you to know that you're loved. You grew in your birth mom's tummy and you grew in my heart and that means that you get two people to love you.

feeling there was something wrong with them that made their parents give them away. Instead, talk about the decision made by the birth parents to make an adoption plan or arrange for an adoption so that their child could be well cared for.

Celebrate your family

Some families make a tradition of doing something special on the day their family was created, such as having a family anniversary party or doing something special for the birth parents. This is a great way to get your other children involved as well.

Seek out other families like yours

Look to make connections with other families that have been touched by adoption. Both the children and parents will find this type of peer group helpful as a source of friendship and support. Transracially adopted children will get the added benefit of spending time with children — and other families — who resemble them.

It is also important for parents and families who might be part of a majority community where they live to educate themselves about issues that their child who is of a different racial or ethnic background might face. This is an important part of adoption preparation and something that can be an opportunity for ongoing discussion and bonding within the family.

HANDLING DIFFICULT REMARKS

At one time or another, parents and children may be faced with ignorant or even hurtful remarks from others. It isn't always easy to speak up when someone says something naive or offensive, but it is important to keep your child's well-being in mind. You don't have to answer every question, and you don't have to let everyone know you adopted your child. Instead, your response may be more for your child's benefit than to educate the person asking the question or making the comment.

You'll likely develop your own responses to things people might say. But here are some approaches suggested by adoptive parents to frequently asked questions:

- *Who are the real parents?* We are — we're not imaginary. We are the ones who do the parenting. (There's no need to explain any further. Information about the birth parents is the child's to give.)
- *Are they really brother and sister?* Yes, they have the same parents. (Whether they are biologically related is also the child's information to share or not.)
- *I don't know how anybody could give up a child.* The decision to place a child for adoption is a painful, difficult decision for anyone, but it's always made in the best interests of the child. It's not because the birth parents don't care but because they couldn't provide for any child at that time in their lives.

- *Too bad you couldn't experience pregnancy.* You don't get to experience everything in life. I may never get to travel around the world, either. But my adoption experience has been wonderful, and I wouldn't trade it for anything.

PARENTING IS PARENTING

Becoming a parent opens up opportunities for amazing fulfillment and incredible challenges, no matter how you come into that role.

In the end, parenting is parenting. In order to move successfully from dependent infant to independent adult, every child requires consistent, loving care in a warm and nurturing environment. Providing this to your child makes you a parent, and research indicates that parents through adoption are keenly aware of their parental responsibilities. Together, you and your child make a family that is abundantly prepared for the adventures ahead.

CHAPTER 43

Caring for multiples

Congratulations on not one but two (or more) babies! Your first years together will likely be busy ones, filled with chaos and, yes, delight. Like any new parent, you may have times when you wonder if you'll ever make it through, and times when you feel that it's all more than worth the effort.

Raising multiples, especially in the early months, can seem truly overwhelming, simply because of the extra logistical and physical demands involved. Daily parenting tasks may be doubled or tripled, and the amount of time left to yourself may very well be minuscule. But most parents of multiples are able to rise to the occasion and find inner reserves of energy and strength they never imagined they had.

You already have plenty of helpful information in other sections of this book. This chapter aims to give you some practical tips on caring for multiple infants and finding time to care for yourself. If your babies were born prematurely, you may also find Chapter 44 to be helpful.

FEEDING

Nursing parents of multiples often say that feeding the babies is stressful. Newborns and young infants need to eat frequently — generally between 8 and 12 times a day. When you're feeding more than one child that many times, you may feel as if all you do is sleep, eat and feed your babies. Even formula-feeding, which many assume would be the most efficient method, takes a surprising amount of time and technique — not to mention a lot of bottles that require washing and storing! And when it's time to introduce solids, the mess may double or more.

Feeding multiples may seem to be an enormous task at times, but there are a couple of things to keep in mind.

Regardless of which method you choose to feed your babies — breastfeeding or formula-feeding — a source of support and help is invaluable. This may come through your partner, grandparents, support groups or a hired caregiver. No one says you must do this alone.

This stage doesn't last forever (even though it may feel that way). As one experienced parent said, "The days are long, but the years are short." In a few months, as your children begin eating other foods and become more independent, the demands placed on you will become less intense.

A quick note: Don't let others pressure you into one form of feeding or another. This is a personal decision, based on sound advice from your children's medical professional or another specialist. The most important things are that your children grow and thrive and that you are able to enjoy the process (at least some of the time).

Breastfeeding

Most experts agree that breast milk is the ideal source of nutrition for infants. Breast milk's nutritional value is also one of the biggest reasons that parents of multiples seek to breastfeed. While it takes a certain amount of dedication, it is possible to do, as shown by so many mothers who have successfully breastfed multiples. Some parents even say that breastfeeding is easier and less time-consuming, once lactation is established, than is bottle-feeding. And research studies indicate that most women will generally produce as much milk as is demanded, so it's possible to produce enough milk for multiple children.

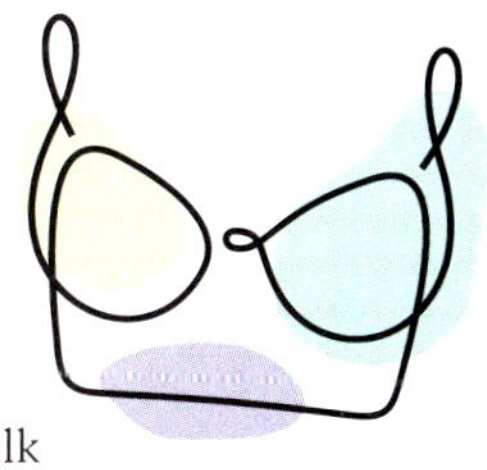

If you decide to breastfeed, it's helpful to find a mentor who can give you insights and tips. This may be an experienced mother of multiples, a medical professional or a lactation consultant. Support groups for parents of multiples, such as local chapters of Multiples of America, are another way to meet experienced parents of multiples.

At first most women breastfeed one infant at a time. This allows time to get the hang of breastfeeding and spend time with each infant. You can find out more about breastfeeding basics in Chapter 3.

Simultaneous breastfeeding Many mothers find that once their milk supply is established and breastfeeding is going well for all involved, they're able to feed their babies at the same time. This may or may not be for you, but it's worth a try because it can save time and energy. As with feeding one baby, get comfortable. Use pillows to support yourself and your infants. Some manufacturers make breastfeeding pillows designed specifically for multiples.

Here are some commonly used positions for breastfeeding twins:

- ***Double clutch, or double football, hold.*** In this position, you hold each baby in a clutch, or football, hold. Place a pillow on each side of your body. You might also want to place another pillow on your lap. Place each baby on a pillow beside your body — almost under your arm — so that the babies' legs point toward the back of your chair. Make sure each baby lies on the back with the head at the level of your nipple. Place the palm of one hand at the base of each baby's head to provide support. Alternatively, you can place both babies — head to head — on pillows directly in front of you. Be sure to keep your babies' bodies turned toward you, rather than facing up. Use the palms of your hands to provide support for each baby's head.

- ***Cradle-clutch combination.*** In this position, you hold one baby in the cradle position — with the head on your forearm and the whole body facing yours — and the other baby in the clutch position. If one of your babies has an easier time latching onto your breast or staying latched, place that baby in the cradle position.
- ***Double cradle hold.*** To use the double cradle position, place both of your babies in the cradle position in front of you. Position your babies so that their legs overlap and make an X across your lap.

Rather than assign one baby to each breast, try to alternate them. This way, if one infant sucks less vigorously, the other may make up the demand and balance out the supply in each breast. If you have three or more babies, use a rotation system so that each one gets milk from both breasts. For example, if you have triplets, you might breastfeed one on each breast simultaneously and then the third on both breasts. At the next feeding, rotate their positions.

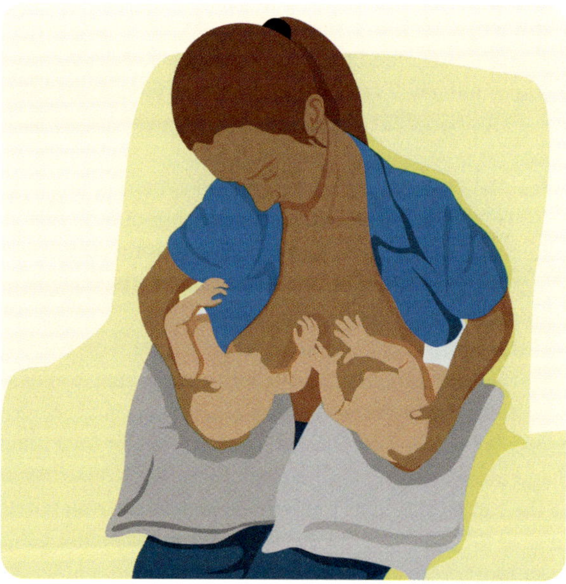

To breastfeed two babies at once, you might use the double clutch, or double football, hold. In this position, you hold each baby in a clutch, or football, hold under your arms. Make sure each baby lies on the back with the head at the level of your nipple. Place the palm of one hand at the base of each baby's head to provide support.

Combined breastfeeding and bottle-feeding Breastfeeding doesn't have to be all or nothing. While frequent breastfeeding helps establish and maintain your milk supply, any amount of breast milk you can give to your children is beneficial.

Many parents find that a combination of breastfeeding and bottle-feeding (pumped breast milk or formula) works well because it allows them to breastfeed their babies but also share the job of feeding with a partner or other caregivers. For example, you might breastfeed one baby while your partner bottle-feeds the other one, then swap at the next feeding. Or your partner might take over a double bottle-feeding session while you get some rest. Ideally, you want to establish a milk supply before supplementing regularly with formula.

Some parents of triplets prefer to set up a rotation where they breastfeed two infants supported by pillows while bottle-feeding the third sitting in an elevated infant seat. This is usually easier when babies are a little older and can hold up their heads well.

If you give your babies formula, keep in mind that your milk production might begin to decrease if you breastfeed or pump fewer than 8 to 10 times within 24 hours.

Pumping If one or more of your babies are preemies or require an extended stay at the hospital, you can still establish a milk supply by renting a hospital-grade breast pump and pumping milk until you're able to nurse. A breast pump may also be beneficial if you have a baby at home and one at the hospital, or if one or more babies have difficulty latching on or sucking. Pumping is also helpful if you need to return to work but would like to continue feeding your babies breast milk. See Chapter 3 for how-tos on pumping.

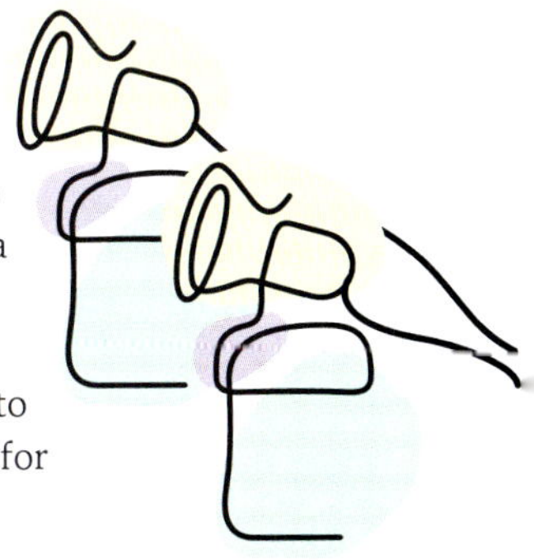

Formula-feeding

Parents decide to feed their babies formula for a variety of reasons — illness on the part of the nursing person or one of the babies, difficulty sustaining an adequate milk supply, the ability of both parents to feed their babies, or simply because it feels more convenient. Ultimately, it comes down to the babies' needs — getting adequate nutrition is the ultimate goal.

As with breastfeeding, it may be best to start out feeding one infant at a time. Chapter 3 will tell you what you need to know about formula-feeding basics. Once your babies are feeding well, you can save time and bottle-feed them simultaneously with the right techniques. One thing to avoid is propping up bottles and leaving a baby unattended, as this can increase the risk of aspiration and choking.

Two pediatricians who are also parents of twins offer some different ways to bottle-feed twins simultaneously:

- Sit on the floor with your legs extended in a V shape. Place the babies between your knees with their feet toward you and heads propped on a pillow. Hold a bottle in each hand and use your thighs as armrests.

- Sit in a comfortable armchair with your left elbow propped on the armrest. Hold both babies with their heads resting against your left arm and their bodies supported in your lap. Hold one bottle with your right hand and lean the other bottle against your chest.
- Cradle one infant in your left arm and curl your left wrist and hand around the baby to offer this baby's bottle. Support the other baby's head in your lap with the feet extended away from you and offer this baby's bottle with your right hand.
- Lean back in an armchair or against pillows and put both babies on your lap facing away from you with their heads supported against your chest. Offer a bottle from each hand.
- Place one baby in an elevated infant seat next to you on the floor and hold the other baby in your lap. Offer a bottle from each hand.
- Use two infant seats and sit between them on the floor. Offer a bottle from each hand.

Are my babies getting enough?

If your babies are growing adequately, then they're getting enough milk. Your babies' medical professional may recommend some extra office visits early on to make sure each is gaining weight properly. Knowing your babies are getting enough to eat and they're gaining weight properly may help you feel more confident in breastfeeding. As a general rule, after the first week of life, weight gain should be ½ to 1 ounce a day.

During the first few weeks, you might find it helpful to maintain a daily chart to record feedings, wet diapers and bowel movements for each child. In general,

TIPS TO OPTIMIZE MILK PRODUCTION

Taking care of your body will help you make the most of breastfeeding:

- *Rest when you can.* Although a solid night's sleep may be a thing of the past, take every chance you get to rest. Extreme fatigue can interfere with breast milk production.
- *Eat a healthy and adequate diet.* Breastfeeding requires good nutrition. Eat a well-balanced diet with regular meals and plenty of liquids.
- *Continue taking prenatal vitamins.* Your prenatal vitamins provide nutrients that may be missing from your daily diet.
- *Drink plenty of fluids.* Although extra intake of fluids hasn't been proved to increase milk production, nursing does tend to make you thirsty. Have a glass of water or juice before you sit down to nurse and keep water handy while nursing. Some nursing pillows even have pockets for just such a purpose.

a baby who is getting adequate nutrition will eat 8 to 12 times a day, and produce at least four to six wet diapers (and at least one that's really soaked) and one bowel movement a day. There may be slight differences between babies who are breastfed and babies who are bottle-fed. If you have any questions or concerns, don't hesitate to ask your babies' medical professional.

RAISING STRONG INDIVIDUALS

Multiples are born with a strong connection to each other. They have similar genetic material. They're usually delivered within minutes of each other. And they go through each phase of development around the same time. They come into the world with a ready-made companion and playmate at hand. They're likely to share bedrooms, toys and even attention from others.

When you have twins or other sets of multiples, it can be easy to slide into a mode where you treat them as a pair or a set. For example, you may dress them alike or others may refer to them as "the twins." This isn't necessarily harmful, but it can sometimes get in the way of each child's ability to develop separately. Also, if you treat your multiples as alike in every way, you may be missing out on some effective parenting strategies.

One-on-one time

Research shows that, overall, multiples grow and develop in much the same way as single-born children — unless they were born prematurely. Prematurity may impact growth and development.

Some studies indicate that children who are multiples tend to display a slight delay in language development compared with singletons. One study concluded that one of the reasons for this delay may have to do with the level of parent-child interaction. In this study, mothers of twins were less likely to engage each child in back-and-forth "conversations" and less likely to report regular book sharing — looking at books together and talking about pictures or pointing at them and investigating the story further.

This seems fairly natural, as parents of twins tend to have more demands placed on them on a day-to-day basis than do parents of single babies, who may have more time to actively engage one-on-one with a child. Although the study was limited to studying mother-child interaction, in real life parents and caregivers also can play major roles in a child's daily care. In the long run, being a twin doesn't appear to affect academic performance once children reach school age.

So, while studies like these don't mean that multiples are permanently disadvantaged, they do show the value of spending interactive one-on-one time with each child when possible.

Parenting strategies

Another reason to look at each child as an individual — one who just happened to be born at the same time as a sibling — is that you can learn to recognize different temperamental qualities in each one. Especially as your children get older, you can use your understanding of their different temperaments to target your parenting strategies more effectively.

For example, you may notice that one child is more flexible when it comes to transitioning from one activity to another, but the other may need ample warning that a change is coming. Knowing this difference between the two may help you plan your day and avoid meltdowns. However, as you come to recognize their differences, avoid labeling your twins, such as referring to one of them as the "quiet one" and the other as the "outgoing one."

LOGISTICS

In addition to the physical demands of raising multiples, there are logistical challenges. You don't just need one crib, stroller, high chair and car seat. You need two or more. Here are some practical tips that may help you save money and get the job done.

Buy in bulk

If you're near a wholesale club that sells items in bulk, it may be worth considering a membership. These places offer formula, baby food, diapers and wipes in large volumes and at a discount. Another option is to purchase bulk items online and have them delivered right to your door.

Check out supply stores

Preschool and child care supply stores carry equipment that's specifically designed for handling multiple children of the same age at once. Some examples include feeding tables with multiple seats built in, diaper storage units, activity tables built to accommodate multiple children and stackable toddler chairs. Plus, these items are generally built to withstand a fair amount of use.

Join a parent group

Groups for parents of multiples not only provide regular gatherings and emotional support but members of the group also may hold resale events where families can buy and sell gently used baby equipment.

Explore your options

It's helpful to assess your needs and know what's available when it comes to equipment:

- *Gates and locks.* Thoroughly childproofing your home — placing gates in bathroom and kitchen doorways and in front of stairs and putting childproof locks on cabinet doors — allows you to relax more easily when you are busy with one toddler and don't have a hand on the other.
- *Strollers.* Double strollers for twins come in a few variations. Side-by-side ones are nice for walks in the park and jogging with your infants. Front-to-back models are easier to navigate in and out of doorways and in tight spaces.

You can also clamp two lightweight umbrella strollers together to make a double stroller.

All the equipment and supplies you acquire may seem to overwhelm your house, car and every other area of your life in the first few years. But as your children get older, you'll find that some things are no longer necessary, such as infant swings, playpens, and eventually high chairs and cribs. Hang in there!

TAKING CARE OF YOURSELF

During your first few years together with your little ones, you're likely to find yourself so wrapped up in caring for them that a life apart from your babies may seem almost surreal. Although it may come as small comfort, rest assured that your parenting job will become less labor-intensive and easier to manage as time goes by.

In the meantime, it's important to carve out time for yourself. Extreme fatigue and lack of personal time can understandably lead to depression and isolation. If you feel overwhelmed or unable to enjoy your kids, it's important to seek professional help from your children's medical professional or from a counselor, therapist or other mental health professional — someone who can help you get back on track.

Taking care of yourself may seem like it should come last on your to-do list, but in fact it is the first step toward taking care of your family. If your energy supply is depleted, it will be much harder for you to accomplish the daily tasks required to care for your children.

The demands of early parenthood are especially high for parents of multiples, and real life rarely falls together as neatly as advice found in a book. Here are some practical reminders and suggestions of what can help make this season of life easier.

Get enough rest

When others tell you to get more sleep, it may feel like a joke. How? you ask. Two nurses conducted a survey of parents of twins, published in *Applied Nursing Research*, to see if they could find any consistent answers to this dilemma. Their question was simple: What strategies did parents of twins use to get sleep in the first six months after taking their babies home?

Although no single answer emerged as completely effective, common strategies used by the parents included:

- Assigning shifts or taking turns with nighttime caregiving
- Getting help from relatives
- Sleeping while the babies slept, although some parents reported taking advantage of this time to complete other tasks
- Getting the twins on the same sleeping and eating schedules
- Using white noise and dimming the lights to help the babies sleep

During the first few weeks, it will likely be difficult to get enough sleep as everyone adjusts to the transition. But eventually you'll develop a routine, and your days and nights will even out a bit. If you have difficulties or concerns about getting enough sleep or getting your children to sleep, talk to your children's medical professional for advice.

Get help and support

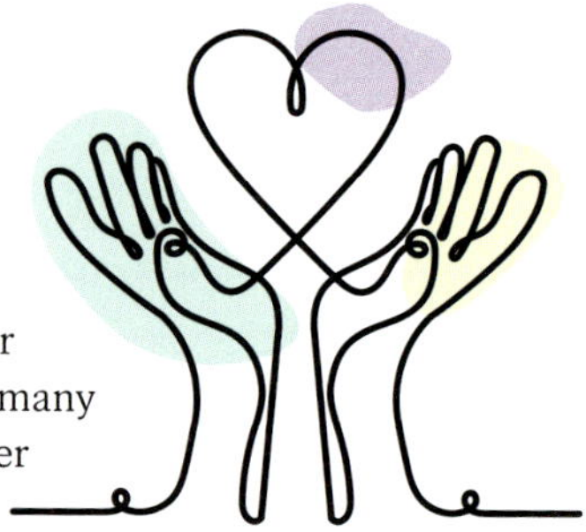

Getting help can make a big difference. Some families hire help, some rely on extended family, and some get help from friends, neighbors, their religious community or other organizations.

Also consider attending a local support group for parents of twins or other multiples. You'll likely get many invaluable ideas and practical suggestions from other parents. Online communities dedicated to supporting parents of multiples are another option.

Let go of guilt

Some parents, after experiencing infertility and then having multiples, feel guilty when they become stressed or exhausted by the demands of caregiving. They may believe that they should only have feelings of happiness and joy after finally achieving their wish for children.

This is a false and unrealistic proposition. There's no doubt that having children when you may have felt you couldn't is a great source of pleasure. But this doesn't mean you won't feel tired and out of sorts at times, wondering what you've gotten yourself into. These are typical feelings for any parent. It's important to set realistic expectations for your situation.

These parents sometimes feel as if they should be able to bear the full load of caregiving because "they got what they were asking for." This is an emotional trap to avoid. Accepting help doesn't make you a bad parent. In fact, as demonstrated earlier, it can help you be a better one.

Take outside attention in stride

Twins, triplets and greater numbers of multiples frequently attract attention in public, which can be positive or negative. Regardless of what others say about you or your family, remember to keep your eye on the prize — raising happy, healthy and well-adjusted children who will eventually contribute to society in their own right.

Take time to replenish

The stresses and demands of early parenting can take a toll on your personal life, your relationship with your partner and other relationships. It's important to remain flexible about your changing roles in the family and maintain open communication so that each knows what the other is thinking.

Try to carve out time for yourself. Take periodic breaks to nurture and sustain yourself with exercise, relaxation or time with friends — whatever you need to recharge your batteries.

In addition, find time to nurture your relationship with your partner. This doesn't have to be anything complicated — it might be as simple as watching a favorite TV show together or making a decent dinner for yourselves after the kids are in bed. (Turn to Chapter 38 for more tips for weathering the early parenting years together.) Look for ways to support each other as new parents and compliment one another on a job well done.

CHAPTER 44

Premature baby

Most babies are born full-term — at or after 39 weeks of pregnancy — and without medical problems. However, some are born early. A premature or preterm birth — a birth that occurs before 37 weeks — gives a baby less time to develop and mature in the womb. As a result, premature babies may need specialized treatment in the neonatal intensive care unit (NICU). Sometimes, even after leaving the hospital, the baby may continue to need special medical care.

If your baby was born prematurely, the marvel of birth might be overshadowed by health concerns and the possible long-term effects. It can be a very stressful time as you learn to manage expectations, cope with an unexpected reality and find time to be with your baby. But there's much you can do to take care of your premature baby — and yourself — as you look toward the future. Understand what to expect after your baby is born, the health problems that premature babies may face and how to best care for your premature baby.

WHY PREMATURE BIRTH HAPPENS

Many factors can increase the risk of premature birth. A multiple pregnancy is one cause. Chronic conditions experienced by a pregnant person, such as diabetes, high blood pressure, and heart and kidney disease, also can lead to premature birth. However, a specific cause is often unclear. And a premature birth can happen to anyone, including pregnant people who have no risk factors.

As the parent of a premature newborn, you might feel that you did something to cause the preterm birth or that you could have done more to prevent it. Parents especially might think about how they might have changed the outcome by making different decisions during pregnancy. Try to let go of any feelings of guilt about your baby's premature birth by talking about them with your baby's medical professionals. Your partner also might be able to provide comfort. Focus your energy on caring for and getting to know your child.

Definitions

If your baby was born prematurely, you're not alone. It's estimated that premature births occur in about 10% of pregnancies in the United States and that nearly 60% of multiple deliveries result in premature births. While all babies born before 37 weeks' gestation are considered preterm, there are a few specific types of preterm birth, including:

- *Late preterm.* A baby who is born at 34 through 36 weeks of pregnancy.
- *Moderately preterm.* A baby who is born between 32 and 34 weeks of pregnancy.
- *Very preterm.* A baby who is born between 28 and 32 weeks of pregnancy.
- *Extremely preterm.* A baby who is born at less than 28 weeks of pregnancy.
- *Low birth weight.* A baby who is born weighing less than 5 pounds, 8 ounces.
- *Very low birth weight.* A baby who is born weighing less than 3 pounds, 5 ounces.
- *Extremely low birth weight.* A baby who is born weighing less than 2 pounds, 3 ounces.

The NICU

Your first close-up look at your baby might be in the hospital's NICU, which is designed to provide round-the-clock care for premature babies as well as full-term babies who develop problems after birth. You'll probably be amazed, overwhelmed and perhaps a little shocked by this first look at your newborn.

Your baby may be lying in an insulated enclosure called an incubator. An incubator provides warmth, which is important because premature babies have less protective body fat than do full-term babies and may get cold in typical room temperatures. The incubator may have a round porthole through which you and the NICU staff can reach in and touch your little one. You may also notice tubes, catheters and electrical wires taped to your baby. For example, your baby may be placed on a cardiorespiratory monitor, which tracks the heart rate and rate of breathing. Seeing this equipment may be intimidating. It's important to remember that these are tools to help keep your baby healthy and inform the medical staff about your baby's condition.

In the NICU, your baby will receive specialized care, including a specialized feeding plan. Some premature babies may initially need to have fluids given to them intravenously or through a feeding tube that passes through the mouth or nose into the stomach. If you plan to breastfeed but your baby is unable to nurse at first, you can pump your breast milk. Your milk can then be given to your baby via a feeding tube or bottle. The antibodies in breast milk are especially important to support a premature baby's immune system. Your milk is designed especially for your baby, and it is something that only you can provide for your baby.

CARING FOR A PREMATURE NEWBORN

Premature newborns require specialized care. The medical team caring for your baby will do everything they can to help your baby thrive. Your role as a parent is essential, too. Consider ways to get involved in your baby's care and begin bonding with your newborn.

In the NICU, medical teams care for babies from many diverse backgrounds, and it is common to have families that will prefer communicating in a language other than English. If you prefer a different language, talk to someone from your

THE NICU TEAM

In the NICU, your baby may be cared for by many specialists and other healthcare professionals. The team attending your baby may include the following:

- *Neonatal nurse.* A neonatal nurse is a registered nurse who has special training in caring for premature and high-risk newborns.
- *Neonatologist.* A neonatologist is a pediatrician who specializes in the diagnosis and treatment of newborn health problems.
- *Neonatal nurse practitioner.* This is a neonatal nurse who has completed additional training in the treatment of newborns, particularly babies in the NICU.
- *Neonatal medicine fellow.* A neonatal fellow is a pediatrician who is receiving specialized training in the diagnosis and treatment of newborn health problems.
- *Pediatric resident.* A pediatric resident is a physician who has completed medical school and is receiving training in treating children.
- *Lactation specialist.* A lactation specialist can help birthing persons who want to breastfeed establish a milk supply, learn the ins and outs of pumping, and introduce breastfeeding when baby is ready.
- *Neonatal dietitian.* The dedicated nutrition team works with the team to ensure that the baby is receiving the right nutrition to grow well.
- *Respiratory therapist.* A respiratory therapist or respiratory care practitioner assesses respiratory problems in newborns and manages respiratory equipment.
- *Neonatal pharmacist.* A pharmacist helps provide the right doses for the medications your baby may receive in the NICU.
- *Social worker.* A social worker can provide support and resources for parents.

Keep in mind that your baby's medical team may also call on other specialists, such as a pediatric surgeon or pediatric cardiologist or neurologist, for help in providing care for your child.

child's medical team. Some NICUs have in-person interpreters, while others have interpreters available via phone or video calls. Being in the NICU can be difficult, and it is important that you have access to the resources you need to fully be part of your child's care. If there are other accessibility concerns, talk to your child's medical team about this as well.

Appearance

A premature baby may look a little or a lot different from a full-term baby. The earlier a baby is born, the smaller the baby may be and the larger the head will be in relation to the rest of the body. Your baby's features may appear sharper and less rounded than a full-term baby's.

A preemie's skin may be covered with more fine body hair (lanugo) than is common in full-term babies, and the skin may look thin, fragile and transparent. These characteristics will be easy to see because most premature babies aren't dressed or wrapped in blankets. This is so NICU staff can closely observe a preemie's breathing and general appearance. The medical team will likely treat your baby's skin with care, avoiding lotions and ointments and using special tape that's gentle to the skin.

Your baby has a lot of growing to do in the coming weeks. In time, the baby will begin to look more like a full-term baby.

Condition and care

Uncertainty can be frightening — as can seeing and hearing monitors, respirators and other types of equipment in the NICU. Ask questions about your baby's condition and care, or write them down and seek answers when you're ready. Read material provided by the hospital, or ask for other recommended sources. If you prefer to be present during a procedure, let the NICU team know. If necessary, make an appointment to discuss your baby's progress. The more you know, the better you'll be able to handle the situation. If you're concerned about changes in your preemie's condition, talk to your child's medical team.

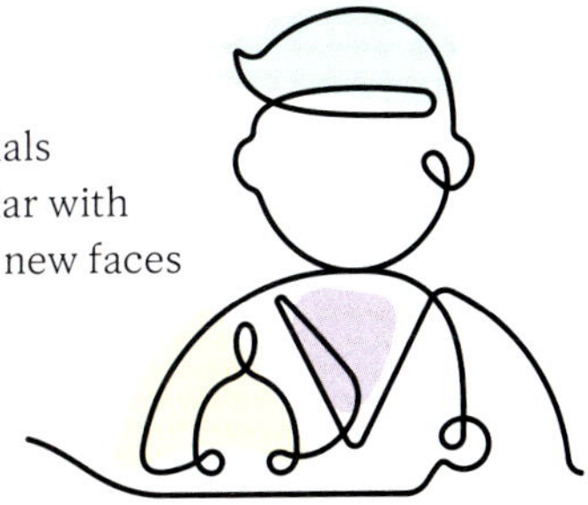

Medical team

You may see a dizzying number of medical professionals providing care for your baby. Until you become familiar with staff rotations, introduce yourself every time you see new faces and ask about their role in caring for your baby.

Nutrition

Breast milk contains many unique components that help fight infection and promote growth. Although your preemie might not be able to feed from your breast or a bottle at first, breast milk can be given in other ways — or frozen for later use. Begin pumping as soon after birth as possible, generally within 2 hours. Aim to pump at least eight times a day, round-the-clock.

Keep in mind that it will take time to establish your milk supply but that every drop of breast milk is precious to your baby, whose first feedings will be small anyway. Give the milk in a container — clearly labeled with your baby's name and the date and time you pumped — to one of your baby's nurses, who can refrigerate or freeze it and use it as your baby needs it.

Preemies typically require additional calories to grow and develop, as well as additional minerals for bone health. Consequently, your baby may be given a supplement in addition to breast milk.

Once nursing is possible, your baby might need more time getting used to the process than does a full-term baby. Give yourself and your baby time to learn and ask for help from the NICU team when you need it.

Growth and development

Become physically involved with your baby as early as possible. Gentle, loving contact can help your premature baby thrive. Your touch, presence and soothing voice will also support your baby's brain development.

For extremely premature babies, ask the NICU nurses about the most helpful ways to comfort your baby. Even before a baby is healthy enough to be held, you may be able to provide comfort with a steady, calm touch. For the youngest babies, patting or stroking may be overwhelming at first. Speak to your baby in loving tones or quietly hum a lullaby. Reading to your baby also can help you feel closer.

NICU nurses can help you hold your baby to allow skin-to-skin contact by placing the baby on your bare chest, covered loosely with a blanket. This type of contact, sometimes called kangaroo care, can be a powerful way for you to bond with your baby. Eventually you'll become very comfortable feeding, changing, bathing and soothing your little one. A NICU nurse can help you with these activities and teach you how to deal with equipment such as breathing tubes, intravenous tubes or monitor wiring.

Don't hesitate to ask the NICU staff how you can become more involved in your baby's care. Being hands-on with your baby can give you confidence as a new parent, as well as make the transition home a little easier when your child is ready to leave the hospital. While this may not be the way you imagined your baby's first days or weeks, your time with the baby is special. Focus on enjoying your firsts together, such as the first time you feed or bathe your baby, and your baby's progress.

DONOR BREAST MILK

For premature babies whose mothers are unable to provide sufficient breast milk, many NICUs may arrange for donated breast milk as a source of nutrition. The source of donated breast milk in a NICU is taken very seriously, with the milk generally coming from established milk banks. Donor breast milk is not always feasible, partly due to the expense of ensuring a safe supply.

HEALTH ISSUES

Due to medical progress, the outlook for premature newborns is much more hopeful than it was years ago. In fact, infants as young as 22 to 24 weeks of completed gestation may survive. A premature baby who is born after 28 weeks of pregnancy and weighs more than 2 pounds, 3 ounces has nearly a full chance of survival.

While not all premature babies experience complications, being born too early can cause short-term and long-term health problems for babies. Generally, the earlier a baby is born, the higher the risk. Birth weight plays an important role, too. Some problems may be apparent at birth, while others may not develop for weeks or months. The likelihood of survival and complications is influenced by the age of the baby, birth weight, administration of maternal medications prior to premature birth (such as steroids and magnesium sulfate), and the circumstances into which the preterm baby is born. Complications of premature birth may include the following health concerns.

Breathing concerns

A premature baby may have trouble breathing due to an immature respiratory system. In some cases, breathing difficulties can prevent other immature organs in the body from receiving enough oxygen. If the baby's lungs lack a substance that allows the lungs to expand, called surfactant, the baby may develop respiratory distress syndrome (see page 35). This condition primarily affects

TRANSPORTING YOUR CHILD

In some cases, a premature baby might need to be moved to a hospital that can provide specialized care. A member of your baby's medical team will explain the situation to you and make the arrangements. Depending on your baby's health and the travel distance involved, your baby might be moved by ambulance, helicopter or airplane. A transport team from one of the hospitals will accompany your baby on the trip. Your baby will likely travel inside a transport incubator, which will provide warmth and allow for any needed medical attention.

Being separated from your baby can be stressful and pose some challenges. Be sure to ask how you will be able to check on your child's condition after the move. If your baby is moved to a hospital that's far away, consider asking a hospital discharge planner or social worker to help you find affordable nearby lodging so that you can spend time with your baby. Ask your baby's medical team about when your baby might be able to return to a hospital near your home and how you can receive regular updates on your baby's care.

infants born before 35 weeks. It's also common for preemies to have pauses in their breathing called apnea.

To detect and treat breathing problems, your baby's medical team may monitor your preemie's breathing and heart rate. To treat breathing problems, your baby may be given oxygen or support through a ventilator or a breathing assistance technique called continuous positive airway pressure (CPAP).

Preterm babies, especially those born between 23 and 32 weeks, may develop chronic lung disease of prematurity, also known as bronchopulmonary dysplasia (BPD). Preemies who develop moderate or severe BPD may need supplemental oxygen at home for the first 6 to 12 months. If this is the case, they will be monitored closely by a healthcare professional who has special training in managing lung problems in children (pediatric pulmonologist).

Heart concerns

The most common heart problems premature babies experience are patent ductus arteriosus (PDA) and low blood pressure. A PDA is an opening between two major blood vessels leading from the heart. This heart defect often closes on its own. But without treatment it can lead to too much blood flowing to the lungs and cause heart failure, when the heart can't pump blood as well as it should. The NICU team will make an individualized recommendation for your baby in the monitoring and treatment of the PDA. If treatment for low blood pressure is needed, your baby may be given additional fluid or intravenous medication.

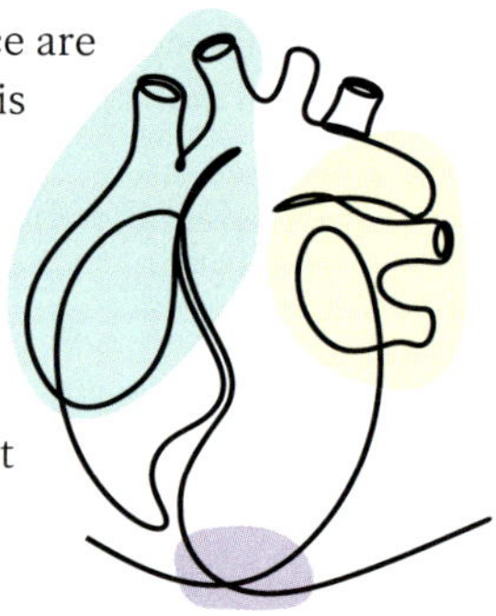

Brain concerns

Babies born before 30 weeks or weighing less than 2 pounds, 12 ounces are at risk of bleeding inside the brain. This is called a germinal matrix or an intraventricular hemorrhage. Most hemorrhages are mild and resolve with little short-term impact. Some babies may eventually develop fluid accumulation in the brain (hydrocephalus) or neurological problems, such as cerebral palsy, autism or a learning disability. Preemies who develop hydrocephalus may need surgery. If muscle tone is a problem, your baby may need to work with a physical therapist.

Gastrointestinal concerns

Preemies are likely to have immature gastrointestinal systems. The earlier a baby is born, the greater the risk of developing necrotizing enterocolitis (NEC). This condition, in which the cells lining the bowel wall are injured, can happen in premature babies after they start feeding. Premature babies who receive only breast milk have a much lower risk of developing NEC. Measures such as antibiotics, intravenous feedings and resting the intestine by withholding feedings for a short period help most babies recover from NEC. Sometimes surgery is needed.

Infant gastroesophageal reflux (GER), a condition that occurs when stomach acid or bile flows back into the food pipe (esophagus), also is very common in premature babies. It can cause a baby to spit up multiple times a day and disrupt weight gain. Most babies outgrow the condition as they reach their original due dates, though reflux remains pretty common. Frequent feedings in small amounts can help. For more information on reflux, see page 449.

Preemies are also at risk of hernias, which happen when a loop of intestine pushes through a weakened muscle or an unusual opening inside the body. While most umbilical hernias heal on their own by the toddler years, inguinal hernias may require surgery. For more information on hernias, see page 38.

Blood concerns

Preemies are at risk of blood problems such as anemia and jaundice. Anemia is a common condition in which the body doesn't make enough red blood cells. With anemia, the body doesn't have enough red blood cells. While all newborns experience a slow drop in red blood cell count during the first months of life, the decrease may be greater in preemies. More severe anemia may occur if your baby has a lot of blood taken for lab tests. Infants without symptoms may not need treatment. However, babies who have symptoms — such as low blood pressure, a fast heart rate, weak pulse, pale color and breathing problems — may need blood transfusions. For more information on anemia, see page 415.

Neonatal jaundice is a yellow discoloration in a newborn baby's skin and eyes. This happens because the baby's blood contains an excess of bilirubin, a yellow-colored pigment of red blood cells. Jaundice is common in babies born before 38 weeks. Most babies who need treatment respond well to light therapy, also called phototherapy. Although complications are rare, all newborns are assessed for jaundice during the first weeks of life. This is because severe infant jaundice can cause permanent deafness and brain damage. For more information on jaundice, see page 36.

Metabolic concerns

Premature babies often have problems with metabolism. That's the process by which the body changes food and drink into energy. Some preemies may develop a low level of blood sugar called hypoglycemia (see page 34). This can happen because preemies typically have smaller amounts of stored blood sugar than do full-term babies. This is because preemies' immature livers have trouble producing blood sugar. Diabetes before or during pregnancy also can increase a baby's risk for hypoglycemia. Additionally, medications given during pregnancy to help control high blood pressure can sometimes contribute to hypoglycemia in a preemie. If your baby is at risk of hypoglycemia, a blood sample may be taken from the baby's heel and tested. Treatment usually consists of feeding the baby breast milk or formula, or giving the baby sugar called dextrose intravenously.

Vision concerns

Preemies born before 30 weeks may develop retinopathy of prematurity (ROP). This is a condition that develops when blood vessels swell and overgrow in the light-sensitive layer of nerves at the back of the eye, called the retina. Sometimes these overgrown vessels slowly scar the retina and pull it out of place. When the retina is pulled away from the back of the eye, it's called retinal detachment. Without treatment, this can harm vision and cause blindness. Screening for ROP can help a medical professional find and treat eye disease before retinal detachment happens.

Premature babies are also at risk of developing other vision problems, such as nearsightedness or a misalignment of the eyes called strabismus.

If your baby is born before 30 weeks or weighs less than 3 pounds, 5 ounces, an ophthalmologist will likely do an eye exam starting when baby is about 4 to 6 weeks old. Generally, preemies need eye exams every couple of weeks or so until the retina has fully developed. Regardless of whether your child has ROP, your baby's medical professional may recommend that your child be periodically examined by an ophthalmologist during the preschool years.

Hearing concerns

Premature babies have a higher risk of losing some hearing. Your baby will likely be given a newborn hearing screening before reaching a corrected age of 1 month (see "Corrected age," below) or before leaving the NICU. If screening results indicate a problem, your baby will likely have follow-up testing with a specialist. Early diagnosis is crucial. The sooner treatment begins, the better your child's chances are of developing age-appropriate language and communication skills. If your child has hearing loss, treatment may involve wearing hearing aids or a cochlear implant.

Dental concerns

Preemies who have been critically ill are at increased risk of developing dental problems, such as delayed tooth eruption, tooth discoloration and improperly aligned teeth.

CORRECTED AGE

Corrected age is your baby's age in weeks since birth or chronological age minus the number of weeks baby was premature. It's used for the first two years to adjust a premature baby's chronological age so that it more accurately reflects the developmental stage.

For example, if your baby is 6 months old but was born eight weeks early, the corrected age is actually closer to 4 months (6 months minus eight weeks). This means that you can expect your baby to be achieving the skills of a 4-month-old, such as holding the head steady and smiling at you. By age 2, most preemies have caught up to full-term babies in terms of typical developmental milestones.

SIDS

Premature babies are at increased risk of sudden infant death syndrome (SIDS). When your baby is home from the hospital, always place your baby on the back to sleep. In the NICU, babies may be placed on the stomach if they have respiratory problems or on the side if they have infant gastroesophageal reflux. In these cases, the medical team will begin placing the baby on the back prior to discharge. For more information on SIDS, see page 126.

Future issues

For some premature babies, difficulties may not appear until later in childhood or even adulthood. Children who were born prematurely may experience developmental delays, learning disabilities, difficulty smoothly controlling their muscles, and behavioral, psychological or other chronic health problems. Preterm babies who have a very low birth weight may also be at increased risk of autism. Research suggests that some premature babies, especially those with severe intrauterine growth restriction, may face an increased risk of type 2 diabetes and high blood pressure as adults.

Take heart. It's natural to be concerned about your baby's health, especially if your baby has spent time in the NICU. But most babies who spend time in the NICU don't have significant disabilities. And many premature babies catch up and become typically developing children.

Keep in mind that the way you and your family care for, interact with and stimulate your baby in the coming months also will have a major impact on baby's development.

TAKING CARE OF YOURSELF

At this point in time, all your attention may be concentrated on helping your child thrive. But remember that you have special needs, too. Taking good care of yourself will help you take the best care of your new baby.

Allow time to heal

You might need more time to recover from the rigors of childbirth than you imagined. Eat a healthy diet and get as much rest as you can. When your medical professional gives you the OK, you can start exercising.

Acknowledge your emotions

Expect to feel joy, anger, fear, powerlessness and a sense of loss. Some parents report feeling strange about getting to know their newborns in the busy NICU. You might celebrate successes one day only to experience setbacks the next.

Give yourself permission to take it one day at a time. Remember that you and your partner might react to stress and anxiety differently, but you both want what's best for your baby. Keep talking and supporting each other during this stressful time.

INTERMEDIATE CARE

While some babies go home after spending time in the NICU, many are transferred to a unit that provides intermediate care before discharge. This unit, which may be located within the NICU or nearby, typically provides care for babies who need less intensive treatment and monitoring. Talk to your baby's medical professional about the type of treatment your baby will receive in the new unit and how you can be involved.

Take a break

If you leave the hospital before your baby, use your time at home to prepare for baby's arrival and get some rest. Your baby needs you, but it's important to balance time at the hospital with time for yourself and your family.

Be honest with siblings

If you have other children, try to answer their questions about the new baby simply. You might explain that the baby is sick and you're worried. Reassure your children that the baby's illness isn't their fault. Ask if you can bring your other children to the NICU to visit your baby. If your children aren't able to see the baby in the NICU, show them pictures.

Seek and accept help

Allow friends and loved ones to care for older children, prepare food, clean the house or run errands. Let them know what would be most helpful. Surround yourself with understanding friends and loved ones. Talk with other NICU parents. Consider joining a local support group for parents of preemies, or check out online communities. Seek professional help if you're feeling depressed or you're finding it difficult to cope with your new responsibilities. Find more information on caring for yourself and your mental health in Chapters 36 and 37.

BRINGING BABY HOME

As your baby's condition begins to improve, you may wonder when you finally can bring baby home. The criteria vary, but generally hospital staff will consider allowing this when your baby:

- Can breathe on their own
- Has a stable heart rate
- Is able to maintain a stable body temperature
- Can breastfeed or bottle-feed
- Is gaining weight steadily

In some cases, a child may be allowed to go home before meeting one of these requirements — as long as the baby's medical team and family agree on a plan for home care and monitoring.

When it's time to bring your baby home, you might feel relieved, excited — and anxious. After days, weeks or months in the hospital, it can be daunting to leave the support of the medical team behind. As you spend more time with your baby, you'll better understand how to meet your baby's needs and your relationship will grow stronger. In the meantime, consider ways to prepare for your child's hospital discharge.

Understand care requirements

Before you leave the hospital, take a course in infant CPR. Ask your baby's medical team any questions you might have and take notes. Make sure you're comfortable caring for your baby, especially if you'll need to administer medications, use special equipment, or give your baby supplemental oxygen or other treatments. Ask if any members of the hospital medical team do home visits, which can be helpful during your baby's first week home.

You'll likely be asked to provide contact information for your baby's medical professional so that a member of the hospital medical team can share details about your baby's medical condition. Discuss what symptoms — such as breathing or feeding problems — should cause you to call your baby's medical professional. Note your baby's need for follow-up visits or referrals, and find out whom to call if you have questions or concerns.

REHOSPITALIZATION

Premature babies' health problems can sometimes make it necessary for them to be readmitted to the hospital. Preterm babies are twice as likely as full-term infants to be readmitted to the hospital in the first year. This risk increases the earlier a baby is born before the due date. Common causes of rehospitalization include infections, respiratory problems, feeding problems and surgical complications.

If your preemie needs to go back to the hospital for treatment, don't get discouraged or blame yourself. You may want to reconnect with some of the support people who helped you through the last hospital stay. For longer hospital stays or more frequent rehospitalizations, some families find it helpful to share their baby's progress online so that they don't have to continuously call family members and well-wishers with updates. Ask the hospital medical team any questions you might have about your baby's condition and find out what you need to know to provide care in the future.

Discuss feedings

Ask the medical team about your baby's need for supplementation in the form of breast milk fortifiers or preterm infant formula. Keep in mind that premature babies usually eat smaller amounts and may need to be fed more often than full-term babies. Preemies also tend to be sleepier than full-term babies and to sleep through feedings (see page 63). Find out how much and how often your baby should be eating.

Make travel arrangements

Because sitting semi-reclined in a car seat can increase the risk of breathing problems or a slow heartbeat, your baby might need to be monitored in a car seat before leaving the hospital. When you have the OK to use a car seat, use it only during travel. Talk with your baby's medical professionals if you may need to take an airplane flight with your newborn. Your baby's lungs may be sensitive to the effects of altitude changes during flight. Also, don't place your preemie in an infant sling, a backpack or other upright positioning devices until you talk to your baby's professional. These devices may make it harder for your baby to breathe.

Protect against illness

Premature babies are more susceptible than are other newborns to serious infections. Try to minimize your preemie's exposure to crowded places, and make sure people who come into contact with your child wash their hands first. Parents of babies at high risk of developing respiratory complications, such as babies who require oxygen at home, should minimize their babies' contact with young children. During the child's first year, or at least first winter, it may be best to avoid child care centers, if it is possible to arrange other care.

It's important for all children to receive immunizations and vaccinations on the recommended schedule. The same is true for premature babies. It's recommended that immunizations be given to medically stable premature babies according to chronological age (on the same schedule as full-term babies) to protect them from vaccine-preventable diseases. Work with your baby's medical professional to stay on schedule for your baby's immunizations. It's also very important for family members and others around your baby to receive their recommended vaccinations each year. Vaccines including the annual flu shot and others can reduce the chance of spreading viruses to your child.

BABY'S CHECKUPS

Depending on your baby's age, weight and health, you'll likely need to schedule a first visit to a medical professional within several days after leaving the hospital. The medical professional may review your baby's stay in the NICU, current medications and treatments. In addition, the medical professional will likely discuss your child's growth, nutrition, vaccinations and specific medical problems and evaluate your baby's progress since leaving the hospital. Tell the medical professional about any concerns you might have. In addition, discuss your baby's need for future appointments with the medical professional and any specialists. Your preemie may initially need to be seen every week or two so that baby's growth and care can be monitored.

Your baby's medical professional also will monitor your baby for developmental delays and disabilities in the coming months. Babies who are identified as being at risk may receive further evaluation and be referred to early intervention services, such as physical therapy for infants. See Chapter 45 for more information on delayed development.

Extremely preterm infants and other babies who experience complications in the NICU are commonly seen in a NICU developmental follow-up clinic. This clinic specializes in monitoring and optimizing the growth and development of preterm infants and those who required critical care after birth. Oftentimes the clinic is staffed by a team of specialists that includes a neonatologist, a neurologist, a dietitian, and physical, occupational and speech therapists. Your child may be followed in this clinic until about age 3 years.

Work with your baby's care team to understand any health problems your baby might experience and what you can do to promote your preemie's health and well-being.

CHAPTER 45

Delayed development

Throughout childhood, your child's medical professional will monitor your child's growth and development to make sure it's progressing steadily and falls within the range of typical development. Monitoring occurs at each well-child visit and can include completion of questionnaires as well as asking questions about what your child is learning. You might be asked whether your child is learning to hold up the head, roll over, sit, crawl, stand, run and jump; make eye contact, smile, coo, laugh, babble and talk; reach for objects, hold toys or a crayon, scribble and draw.

Sometimes a child's abilities will fall below the range of milestones achieved by peers. This isn't always a cause for alarm because children tend to develop at highly individual rates. They may fall behind in one area, such as language, while focusing intently on mastering another area, such as crawling or walking. Soon after they acquire the skill they're pursuing, they move on to achieve other milestones that have been lagging.

But if your child is slower to achieve certain milestones or if you're concerned about your child's development, you and your child's medical professional can take steps to detect any potential problems. The earlier a problem is identified, the sooner you can take measures to help your child achieve the maximum developmental potential. If an underlying condition or disease is present, treatment may help prevent further problems.

WHAT IS DELAYED DEVELOPMENT?

Delayed development is when your child doesn't reach developmental milestones within the same time frame as other children of the same age. When a child is delayed in two or more important areas of development, medical experts refer to this as global developmental delay. Milestones are usually grouped into these categories:

- Gross motor skills — rolling over, sitting, crawling, walking, running, jumping
- Fine motor skills — picking up small objects, self-feeding with hands or utensils, scribbling or drawing, dressing
- Language and communication — recognizing sounds, cooing, imitating speech, babbling, pointing, speaking in words and sentences
- Thinking and reasoning — beginning to understand cause and effect, object permanence, following directions, problem-solving
- Personal and social skills — exploring, smiling, laughing, interacting with others, communicating needs to caregivers

Part 3 of this book discusses typical growth and development for the first three years of your child's life. If you're concerned that your child isn't meeting certain milestones or isn't developing typically, talk to your child's medical professional. Your child's medical professional can reassure you about what's considered typical and offer advice on further testing.

HOW IS A DELAY IDENTIFIED?

Usually a developmental problem is identified over time rather than at a single medical visit. Screening tests are performed as a part of well child care. If you or your child's medical professional has concerns, additional testing may be recommended to see if your child may be at risk for a developmental disorder.

The screening tests are usually brief and inexpensive. Your child's medical professional may ask your child to play a game or perform certain activities, such as playing with a doll or picking up a small object. You may be asked to fill out a questionnaire. Based on the screening test results, the medical professional may recommend a wait-and-see approach to give your child a little more

WILL MY CHILD GROW OUT OF A DEVELOPMENTAL DELAY?

Some premature infants appear delayed based on chronological age. However, the apparent delay may disappear when the baby's corrected age is taken into account. Among children who have true developmental delays in the preschool years — meaning they consistently lag behind in screening tests — most continue to be delayed even as they grow older. This is why early identification is so important. If you're waiting for your child to grow out of a developmental delay, you may be missing out on early opportunities to help your child.

time to develop, or refer you to a childhood development expert for further evaluation.

A developmental evaluation is a more complex procedure carried out by a professional who is specially trained to administer these tests. The evaluation is designed to identify specific developmental disorders that may be affecting the child. Along with the developmental evaluation, a medical diagnostic evaluation can identify any possible underlying conditions that may be affecting development.

If your child is at high risk for a developmental disorder, your child's medical professional or a specialist may refer you to early intervention services. This includes an assessment that can lead to other assistance to support development, even before the diagnostic process is completed.

POSSIBLE CAUSES

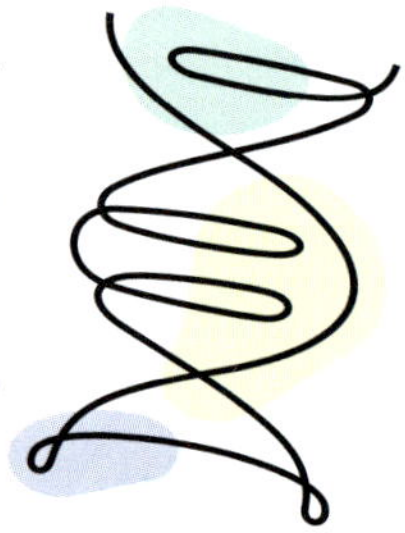

There are many conditions that may contribute to delayed development — for example, genetic disorders, medical conditions, infections and toxin exposure. But most often, the exact cause is hard to identify.

Sometimes during a pregnancy, a fever or infection in the pregnant person will create immune reactions that can harm the development of the baby's brain. Fetal exposure to alcohol or drugs during pregnancy also can damage a baby's developing nervous system. Premature birth or difficulties during labor that impair circulation may lead to developmental problems.

A baby's brain continues to develop even after birth. Excessive exposure to toxins, such as high levels of lead, can harm the body's nervous system and lead to mental deficits. In cases of severe neglect, in which the brain isn't being appropriately stimulated or nourished, delayed development can result. Some babies have a chromosomal abnormality or an inherited disorder that interferes with growth and development. Others have a metabolic disorder, such as an underactive thyroid, that can cause impaired growth and development and slower intellectual function. Newborn screening is recommended to help identify these genetic and metabolic conditions (see page 43).

DIAGNOSING A DEVELOPMENTAL DELAY

To try to determine what may be causing your child to lag in achieving developmental milestones, your child's medical professional likely will do a comprehensive physical exam. This exam also can be done by a developmental pediatrician or a pediatric neurologist or geneticist. Your child also may undergo a variety of tests. The tests may include vision and hearing exams, genetic tests to look for a possible genetic abnormality, imaging tests of the brain to look for a problem or injury, and metabolic and thyroid tests.

Usually the tests aren't done all at once but are carried out in a stepwise fashion. Depending on the results of one examination or test, the medical professional will make recommendations about additional testing.

WHAT CAN BE DONE?

Some causes of developmental delay are treatable, but more often, the condition causing developmental delay isn't curable or even known. Early identification of a problem — whether an underlying cause is discovered or not — will allow your child to be treated when it's most helpful.

Early intervention services are available for children with special needs. Anyone can refer a child to early intervention services. This may be done by your child's medical professional, a child care provider, or even family members who know the child and are concerned about the child's development. A referral can be made at any time, even before a developmental delay is formally diagnosed. Once a referral is submitted, your child is assessed for eligibility for services. Not all children who are referred are eligible to receive early intervention services. If a child is eligible, a caseworker is assigned to your family to coordinate the services that meet your child's specific needs. Together with the caseworker and therapists, you create a written plan called the individualized family service plan (IFSP). This plan outlines the services your child needs and how they will be provided.

The earlier these services are started, the better it is for your child. Therapists may come directly to your home to work with you and your child, but you may also visit a center or clinic for some parts of your plan. Common services offered by an early intervention program typically include:

- Physical therapy to work on gross and fine motor skills
- Speech therapy to work on language and communication skills
- Occupational therapy to work on personal and social skills
- Family training and counseling to help you work with your child at home
- Transportation and assistive technology services if your child needs special equipment to get around
- Nutrition counseling if your child has trouble feeding
- Coordination of services from physicians and other agencies

Early intervention programs are funded mostly by each state but also receive support from the federal government and local resources. In a few cases, a state program will charge a small family fee. Your caseworker can discuss the cost of these services with you and may coordinate with your health insurance provider. But the ability to pay is not needed for eligibility. In general, families pay little to no out-of-pocket costs for these services.

Once your child reaches 3 years of age, services may be available through the public school system. Most kids with special needs start kindergarten on time or the following year. Most attend schools that serve a variety of students, not just children with disabilities.

Your child should continue to receive special services as needed throughout kindergarten, elementary and high school. Periodic reevaluations are done to update your child's needs. Different states have different policies regarding when state-sponsored programs end. Your child's caseworker or school aide or other local resources can help you find out what applies in your state and help you answer any questions you may have.

GET SUPPORT

Determining whether your child has a developmental disability — and if so, what can be done to help your child — can take time. It may require making trips to various specialists, watching your child undergo different tests and waiting for results in between tests. It's not always easy dealing with the uncertainty and anxiety involved. Your medical professional or caseworker, if you've been assigned one by an early intervention program, may be able to help you navigate the various procedures and coordinate the services you need.

In the meantime, it's important to get support — not only through meeting with specialists and reading information but also through meeting other parents in similar circumstances. These are the people most likely to know what you're going through. They may be able to offer valuable information you can't get elsewhere, such as a great dentist for kids with special needs, the best shoes for a child who needs supportive leg bracing, or which kind of sippy cup works best for toddlers with challenges learning how to use a cup. And sometimes a friendly chat with another parent about the ups and downs of your day is just what you need to feel a little more ready to face the next day.

Here again, your medical professional or caseworker may be able to connect you to a local parent group that fits your needs. Or you can check the internet for local chapters or online communities of national organizations for specific disabilities. For information on resources, including websites, books and other sources that may be useful to you, see "Additional resources" beginning on page 575.

CHAPTER 46

Autism spectrum disorder

If you're like most parents, there have probably been times when you've wondered whether your child is developing "on schedule." Shouldn't the baby be starting to smile by now? Why isn't the baby talking yet? Is it a problem that the baby doesn't look up when called?

When it comes to hitting the major infant and toddler milestones, there's a range of what's typical. Each child develops at a unique pace. Most of the time, the differences parents see in their children are well within the typical range. But some parents have an instinct that something isn't quite right. Their baby seems to always be behind in language and social development. Or their toddler appears to be losing communication skills instead of gaining new ones. These parents aren't sure what the problem is — or if there even is a problem — but they worry it could be autism.

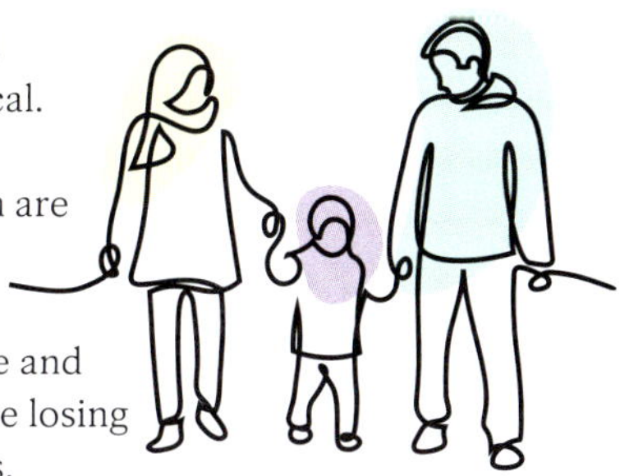

This chapter will walk you through the early signs of autism spectrum disorder. You'll also learn how autism is diagnosed and addressed in early childhood, and how to support a child on the autism spectrum. The good news is that intensive early treatment has a major, lasting impact on many children with autism, allowing them to grow and thrive in their own way.

UNDERSTANDING AUTISM

Autism spectrum disorder is a condition related to brain development that impacts how a person perceives and socializes with others, causing problems in

EARLY WARNING SIGNS

The list below is only a guide, not a way to diagnose your child. Many children exhibit a few of these behaviors even if they don't have autism. Some of these behaviors can also be a sign of other developmental issues. On the other hand, a child may have autism spectrum disorder without showing all these signs. If you're concerned about your child's behavior, bring it up with your child's medical professional. A medical professional can help you determine if further evaluation is necessary.

By age	A child with autism might not . . .
12 months	Babble or coo Respond when called React to back-and-forth interactions, such as waving or peekaboo Look at objects that another person is pointing to
16 months	Say single words
18 to 24 months	Engage in pretend play (make-believe)
24 months	Say meaningful two-word phrases Show an interest in objects by pointing at them
At any age, a child with autism may . . .	Lose language skills or social skills (developmental regression) Avoid eye contact Prefer to look at objects rather than people Show a strong preference to be alone Have extreme difficulty with small changes in daily routines or surroundings Repeat words or phrases without meaning Engage in repetitive movements such as rocking, spinning or hand flapping Show intense interest in an object over time, such as fascination with garage doors going up and down, that is in excess of normal curiosity Show a high sensitivity to sounds, tastes, texture, lights or colors Not seem to be sensitive to pain or temperature Show little or no desire to be picked up or held Show little interest in toys or repeatedly focus on one aspect of a toy, such as how it feels or how one part moves

social interaction and communication. The disorder also leads to fixed and repetitive patterns of behavior, interests or activities. These symptoms can limit or harm everyday functioning.

Not every child diagnosed with autism has the exact same symptoms or shows every sign. That's why the term *spectrum* is included in the name of the disorder. Some children with autism may experience fewer symptoms, while others face more difficult challenges in their day-to-day lives. No two children show signs in the same way.

Autism spectrum disorder includes conditions that were previously considered separate — autism, Asperger's syndrome, childhood disintegrative disorder and an unspecified form of pervasive developmental disorder. Some people still use the term Asperger's syndrome, which was generally thought to be at the mild end of autism spectrum disorder.

What causes autism?

Autism spectrum disorder has no single known cause. In most cases, the disorder likely occurs due to the child's genes, and it's possible that environmental, or at least inherited, effects influence autism. Genetic causes may affect early brain development. Research continues in this field, and there may be other causes that have yet to be discovered.

Over the years, many people have speculated about possible causes. For example, some people have claimed that a parent's child-rearing style is somehow to blame. But there's absolutely no evidence to support this.

One of the biggest controversies centers on whether a link exists between the disorder and childhood vaccines. Scientists have investigated the question extensively. Despite hundreds of studies, there's no evidence that vaccines cause autism. In fact, the original study that ignited the debate years ago was retracted due to poor design and questionable research methods, and the author lost his medical license. More recently, a 2019 nationwide study in Denmark involving over 650,000 children compared autism rates in children who were vaccinated

CAN A CHILD OUTGROW AUTISM?

For the majority of children diagnosed with autism, the disorder is a lifelong condition. Even so, symptoms can improve significantly with treatment and time. In a small percentage of children, symptoms improve so much that the children no longer meet the criteria for autism spectrum disorder. In general, these children tend to receive intensive treatment for the disorder at a young age, have mild symptoms and are of average intelligence. While these children are no longer considered to have autism, they commonly have some remaining social, language, learning and behavioral difficulties. They are also more likely to experience attention and mood disorders.

for measles, mumps and rubella (MMR) with children who weren't vaccinated. The large number of children involved gave the study enough power to look at other risk factors as well. The study found that MMR vaccination did not increase the risk of autism and also found it did not increase the risk for siblings of children with autism. In girls, receiving the MMR vaccine was actually associated with a lower, or reduced, chance of autism.

On the other hand, not vaccinating increases your child's risk of catching and spreading serious diseases such as measles, mumps and rubella — which are unfortunately becoming more common. (For more information about vaccinations, see Chapter 14.)

How common is autism?

Over the past several decades, the rate of diagnosis of autism in children has increased dramatically. Researchers think this is largely due to a rise in the overall awareness of the disorder and a broadening of the diagnostic criteria for autism. But more investigation is needed to rule out other factors.

The Centers for Disease Control and Prevention prevalence estimates have risen by 175% over the past two decades, making autism highly prevalent. Overall, autism is thought to occur in over 2% of the population. The disorder is about four times more common in boys than in girls and occurs among all racial and ethnic groups.

EARLY SIGNS OF AUTISM

Many children with autism spectrum disorder show hints of the disorder within the first year of life. Other children appear to develop typically but then suddenly — or gradually — become withdrawn and lose language skills that they already had. Most children with autism show clear signs before 2 or 3 years of age. However, some kids on the mild end of the spectrum might not be identified as having autism until later in childhood or even adolescence.

Parents of infants and toddlers on the autism spectrum may notice that their child doesn't communicate or interact with adults and children the way that other kids the same age do. Initially, they might assume the problem lies with their child's vision or hearing rather than a delay in their child's development.

Young children who are later diagnosed with autism often show signs of the disorder at early stages of their development. Below are some possible signs in the first years of life.

IDENTIFYING AUTISM IN EARLY CHILDHOOD

If you're at all concerned about your child's development or behavior, don't keep it to yourself. Bring those concerns to your child's medical professional. While autism is most commonly identified in children who are 3 years or older, it's possible to screen for and diagnose the disorder in toddlers. Children who are diagnosed in the toddler and preschool years greatly benefit from early intensive intervention. Research shows that early treatment for the disorder allows many children to function better in life, do better in school and manage their condition more successfully.

Screening for autism

Your child's medical professional will look for signs of developmental delays at regular checkups. If your child's medical professional observes signs of autism — or if you express a particular concern — your child will likely be screened for the disorder. The American Academy of Pediatrics recommends that children be routinely screened for autism at 18 and 24 months. If your child has a sibling with autism, the medical professional may do additional screenings.

During the screening for autism, your child's medical professional will typically ask you a series of questions about your child. Your intimate knowledge of your child's day-to-day life, particularly details related to social and communication skills and behavior, can help in evaluating your child. In some cases, the medical professional might engage your child in a short play session to observe how your child interacts, talks and behaves.

The most common screening for autism is the Modified Checklist for Autism in Toddlers, Revised (M-CHAT-R). This series of questions assesses the risk of the disorder in children between the ages of 16 and 30 months. If you have concerns about autism earlier in your child's life, your child's medical professional may use the Infant-Toddler Checklist. Although this set of questions wasn't designed specifically to screen for autism, it can be used to identify a potential risk of the disorder in infants as young as 9 or 12 months.

Diagnosing autism

If your child's initial screening identifies a risk of autism spectrum disorder, you'll likely be referred to a team of medical professionals who specialize in diagnosing and treating children with autism spectrum disorder. This team will evaluate your child to determine an autism diagnosis.

CAN MY CHILD RECEIVE EARLY INTERVENTION SERVICES WITHOUT A DIAGNOSIS?

If your child shows signs of developmental delays but hasn't received an autism diagnosis, early intervention services may still be available. Ask your child's medical professional for a referral or contact your state's early intervention services office directly. Ask that your child be evaluated under Part C of the Individuals with Disabilities Education Act (IDEA). Depending on the outcome of this free evaluation, your child may be eligible to receive some early intervention services.

Diagnosing autism is often a complex process. The diagnosis is most often made by watching how the child behaves and listening to a parent or caregiver's description of how the child behaves. The child's age, level of development, thinking skills and language ability are also considered.

Because behavior can vary considerably depending on time of day, location, familiarity with medical staff and many other factors, it's important that your child undergo several different observations before a final diagnosis is made.

Typically, these observations are made by different specialists. You and your child might talk with a developmental pediatrician, pediatric neurologist, medical geneticist, neuropsychologist, psychiatrist, speech and language pathologist, occupational or physical therapist, and medical social worker. However, your child may not need to see all these specialists.

To be diagnosed with autism, a child must show consistent difficulties in two key areas:

- ***Social communication.*** This includes a child's ability to react to social cues, such as eye contact or smiling, and engage in back-and-forth interactions, such as waving or pointing. A lack of interest in family members or other children also falls under this category.
- ***Restricted, repetitive behaviors.*** These behaviors can include repetitive movements, a strong need for rigid routines, an intense preoccupation with a particular sensory experience, and an unusually high sensitivity to taste, textures, lights or sound.

UNPROVEN TREATMENTS

Since a cure has yet to be found for autism, many parents seek unproven complementary and alternative therapies for their children. Specialized diets, such as a gluten-free or casein-free diet, are one of the most common therapies that parents try. It has been proposed that these diets may help curb symptoms. But researchers have found no convincing evidence to support this claim. Other popular claims refer to the use of vitamin supplements, probiotics or hyperbaric oxygen chambers. Again, there's little evidence that these products are beneficial for autism symptoms, and they can be expensive.

Some alternative treatments are not only unproven but potentially dangerous. Chelation therapy, which is said to remove mercury and other heavy metals from the body, can be very harmful or even deadly. Another potentially harmful and unproven treatment involves intravenous immunoglobulin (IVIg) infusions.

If you're considering a particular therapy for your child, don't hesitate to talk with your child's medical professional about the scientific evidence behind it, as well as the potential risks and benefits.

To make the diagnosis, medical professionals use a comprehensive list of criteria from the *Diagnostic and Statistical Manual of Mental Disorders* (*DSM*-5), published by the American Psychiatric Association. Your child's medical team can help you understand the criteria as they apply to your child. Some children may not be diagnosed until they're older, when the demands on their social skills become more challenging and difficulties become more apparent.

WHAT HAPPENS AFTER A DIAGNOSIS

In the United States, children under 3 with autism are referred to their local early intervention program, which can provide therapies to improve symptoms. A referral to early intervention can occur before a diagnosis of autism is confirmed.

Early intervention services available to your child will vary depending on the state in which you live. Navigating your options may seem overwhelming at times. A social worker can be another valuable resource as you begin to explore the assistance available to your child through local and state government

THE IMPORTANCE OF OUTSIDE SUPPORT

When it comes to parenting a child with autism, consistent, reliable support can make a big difference. As much as possible, lean on support in these three areas:

- *Extended family and close friends.* In families where grandparents, aunts, uncles, mothers, fathers, brothers, sisters and friends live nearby and are willing to help out, parents of the child with autism report feeling a greater sense of parenting satisfaction and improved family interactions.
- *Professionals.* Lean into any professional support available to you, your child and your family. This can include medical professionals, early intervention specialists, social workers and therapists. Families that take advantage of professional help report that they have a better sense of well-being. They also have an improved understanding of autism and its symptoms and an increased level of confidence in their own abilities as caregivers.
- *Support groups.* Consider seeking out support groups for parents and families affected by autism in your area. You may find that support group meetings become a touchstone in your life, a place where you can truly be yourself and know that group members will understand what you're going through. Fellow members may also be a source of emotional support, providing valuable insight into addressing challenging situations or ideas for coping with stress.

agencies. A social worker can guide families who might be in need of financial assistance through the process of applying for Social Security aid.

Also visit the Center for Parent Information and Resources website. It offers a search function for finding a parent center in your state or territory. These agencies provide support and services to families of children with disabilities and can give you specific state information and guidance on how to navigate your state's early intervention program. Another helpful resource is the Autism Response Team information line run by the organization Autism Speaks. Trained team members may be able to answer questions and help you find autism services and support in your community.

Early intervention services

No cure exists for autism spectrum disorder, and there is no one-size-fits-all treatment. The goal of early intervention services is to help your child gain developmental skills and help your family learn ways to meet your child's needs. Such services may help improve your child's physical, thinking, communication, social and emotional skills.

Once you qualify for early intervention services, one of the first steps is to create an individualized family service plan (IFSP). The IFSP is a personalized plan for children who have not yet turned 3. It helps you identify how to meet your child's needs and your family's needs. To create this plan, you'll typically partner with your assigned service coordinator as well as early intervention specialists or therapists.

With an IFSP in place, your child can begin receiving early intervention services. These services often occur at home but may also take place in a center or through other outpatient programs. Many early intervention services for autism address the range of social, language and behavioral difficulties associated with autism spectrum disorder. They're commonly based on the principles of applied behavior analysis, a method used for helping children with autism and their families. Some therapies provide structured learning opportunities that break down complex skills into small, teachable steps. Therapy may also be

SEEING BEYOND AUTISM

Parenting a child with autism is similar in many ways to parenting any child. Every child needs love, attention, supervision and a safe home. While parenting a child with autism can bring additional challenges, try not to let the disorder take over your child's life or your own. Work on uncovering and celebrating your child's many strengths and interests. Instead of focusing on what your child can't do, take the time to notice what your child can do. Instead of comparing your child with other children, work on accepting your child.

incorporated into play sessions and other everyday activities. As a parent, you'll play a vital role in your child's progress and may receive training on how to support and work with your child.

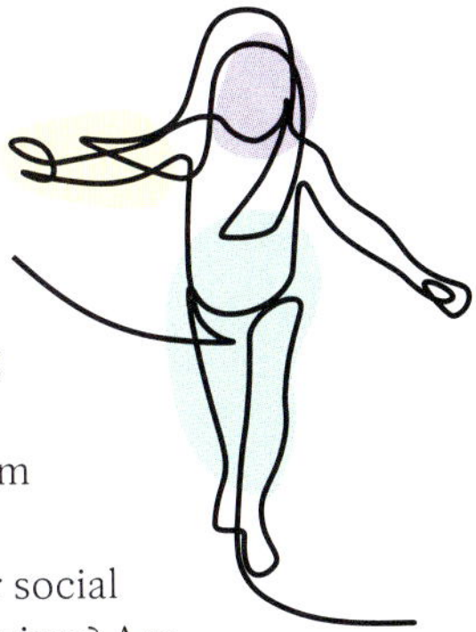

Supporting your child

The care you give as a parent is just as important to your child's overall growth as is the care that any specialist provides. Your child knows you and trusts you to provide care. Your patient and consistent guidance is key to helping your child learn behavior management.

There are many ways you can help your child with autism succeed at home and in social or community settings.

- *Become an expert on your child.* Do specific sensory or social experiences trigger tantrums or other challenging behaviors? Are certain routines or behaviors soothing, comforting or pleasing to your young child? When you're aware of what stresses, calms and entertains your child, you'll be better equipped to head off or manage behavioral problems.
- *Manage tantrums with empathy.* Tantrums are a part of life with a toddler, and even more so when that child has autism. Try to understand and address what triggered the tantrum. Ignore negative behaviors that don't cause self-injury or harm to others (see page 156).
- *Praise positive behaviors.* Instead of continually trying to correct negative behaviors, focus on your child's positive behaviors. Model and explain to your child how to behave appropriately in different situations. When your child shows positive behaviors, be quick to offer praise.
- *Maintain a consistent schedule.* Your toddler will do best with a consistent schedule and routines. Many children with autism do not adapt well to changes. Challenging behaviors tend to happen more often when your child is out of the routine.
- *Provide social experiences.* Get your child out and about when possible to practice encountering new people and places. Arrange play dates and interactions with other children under your supervision. Be sure your child is rested and ready to go. Start with small groups of two or three other children and provide close supervision. Be prepared to leave when your child shows signs of having had enough.
- *Encourage adequate sleep.* Many children with autism have sleep problems. It can help to use a relaxing bedtime routine lasting 30 minutes or less, and stick with a set time for going to bed and waking up. Avoid the use of digital devices — including television, video games and tablets — in the hour or so before bedtime. It may also help to keep your child's bedroom cool and dark for sleep.
- *Promote good nutrition.* Your child has the same nutritional needs as any other child. However, it's common for children with autism to be picky eaters. To help your child toward a balanced diet, have a regular meal and snack schedule, and offer new foods many times. If you have concerns about your child's limited diet or growth, talk to your child's medical professional.

- *Take care of yourself.* It may seem counterintuitive, but one of the best ways you can care for your child is to make time for self-care. When you're refreshed, you have more energy for the challenges of parenting. Try to establish a regular routine that allows you to rest and regain your energy, even if it's just for a few minutes to sit and read your favorite magazine or do a quick exercise session. If you have a partner, take turns getting out of the house to do something that you enjoy on your own. When possible, schedule times when you hire a sitter or have a family member watch your child while you and your partner spend quality time together.

BEYOND THE FIRST YEARS

At age 3 your child will transition from an early intervention program to special education services.

Under Part B of IDEA, these services are offered through your local public school district. They are typically available for children and young adults between the ages of 3 and 21, or until the completion of high school.

In addition to academic instruction, special education services aim to improve your child's communication and social, behavioral and daily living skills. These services may take place at a dedicated school or center, but they can also be integrated into mainstream schools.

As your child grows, the challenges of autism may not go away, but neither will the rewards. You may discover added richness and unexpected joy in your family life. You may see your child achieve milestones you didn't think were possible. Through it all, let your child know that you'll be there, offering love and support, no matter what challenges are ahead.

Additional resources

If you're looking for additional information on a particular topic, you may find the following resources helpful.

American Academy of Pediatrics
www.aap.org
News and research on parenting, helpful tips, and more.

American Red Cross
www.redcross.org
Search tool for local classes on pediatric first aid and CPR.

Bright Futures Family-Centered Care
https://www.aap.org/en/practice-management/bright-futures
Includes resources for families to promote children's health and be active partners in family-centered health care.

Center for Parent Information and Resources
www.parentcenterhub.org
Information and support for parents of children with disabilities.

Centers for Disease Control and Prevention
www.cdc.gov
Resources including developmental milestones, immunization charts and more.

Child Care Aware

www.childcareaware.org

Search tool for quality local child care.

Child Mind Institute

www.childmind.org

Information on the child brain, behavior and emotions.

Consumer Product Safety Commission

www.cpsc.gov

News and recalls on consumer products.

Family Equality

https://familyequality.org

A wealth of information and resources to support LGBTQ+ parents.

Food and Drug Administration

www.fda.gov

Information on food, drugs and medical devices used in the United States

HealthyChildren.org from the American Academy of Pediatrics

www.healthychildren.org

Expert information on children's nutrition, safety, behavior and wellness. Includes the Family Media Plan interactive tool.

La Leche League International

https://llli.org

Tips, research and support for nursing parents, including information for adoptive, transgender and nonbinary parents.

Maternal & New Parent Mental Health | NAMI

www.nami.org/your-journey/maternal-new-parent-mental-health

Resources for all new parents, including non-birthing parents, to understand and care for your mental health.

Mayo Clinic

www.MayoClinic.org

Comprehensive health information, including on babies and toddlers.

Multiples of America

www.multiplesofamerica.org

Information and support for multiple birth families.

National Center for Fathering

www.fathers.com

Research and articles to engage and empower fathers.

National Center on Birth Defects and Developmental Disabilities

www.cdc.gov/ncbddd

Information on childhood disabilities.

National Council for Adoption

www.adoptioncouncil.org

Resources for adoptive families, adopted individuals and birth parents.

National Highway Traffic Safety Administration

www.nhtsa.gov/equipment/car-seats-and-booster-seats

Interactive guide to car seat selection and installation.

National Safety Council

www.nsc.org/home-safety

Information on safety in the home.

Office on Women's Health

www.womenshealth.gov

Basics of breastfeeding and pumping, postpartum mental health, and more.

Parenting, Kids & Teens - Mayo Clinic Press

https://mcpress.mayoclinic.org/parenting

Articles, podcasts and books offering expert insights and practical guidance on a wide range of health topics for kids and parents.

Pathways.org

www.pathways.org

Resources to help understand and track milestones from infancy to preschool.

Poison Help

www.poisonhelp.org

Online help for a possible poisoning;
call 800-222-1222 in the United States to talk to someone directly.

Safe to Sleep

https://safetosleep.nichd.nih.gov

Basics of safe infant sleep.

BIRTH TO 36 MONTHS: GIRLS

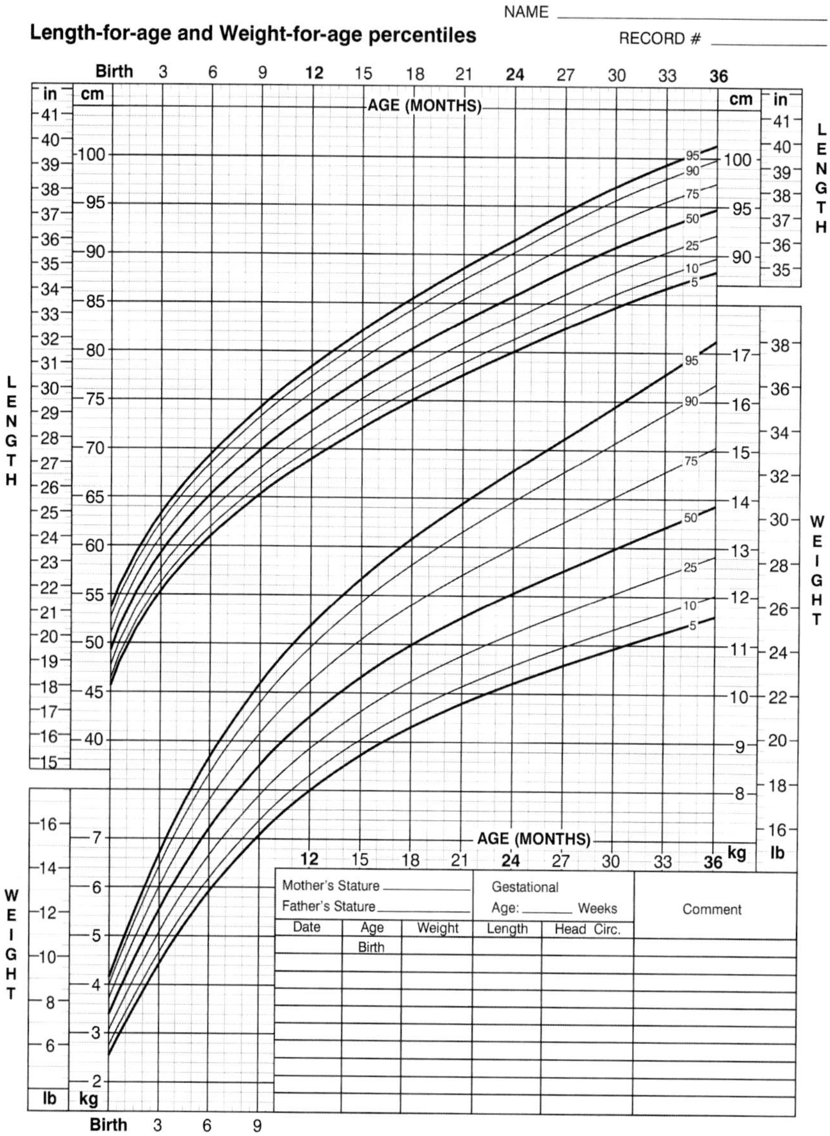

Source: Centers for Disease Control and Prevention

BIRTH TO 36 MONTHS: BOYS

NAME ______________________

Length-for-age and Weight-for-age percentiles

RECORD # ____________

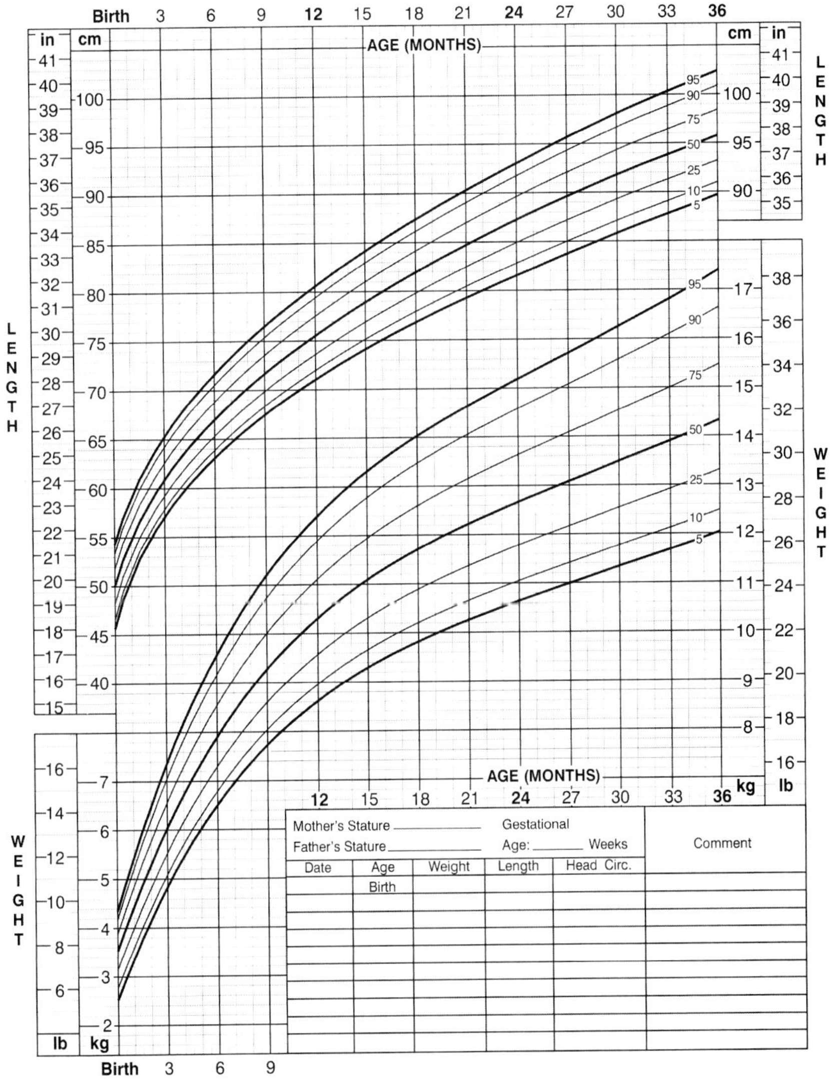

Source: Centers for Disease Control and Prevention

PAIN RELIEVER DOSAGE BY WEIGHT

Acetaminophen (Tylenol, others) — For children over 2 months

	Dose				
Weight	**Infants' or children's oral suspension, 160 mg per 5 mL**	**Children's chewable tablet, 80 mg**	**Junior-strength chewable tablet, 160 mg**	**Adult tablet, 325 mg**	**Adult extra-strength tablet, 500 mg**
6 to 11 lbs	1.25 mL (40 mg)	—	—	—	—
12 to 17 lbs	2.5 mL (80 mg)	—	—	—	—
18 to 23 lbs	3.75 mL (120 mg)	—	—	—	—
24 to 35 lbs	5 mL (160 mg)	2 tablets (160 mg)	1 tablet (160 mg)	—	—
36 to 47 lbs	7.5 mL (240 mg)	3 tablets (240 mg)	1½ tablets (240 mg)	—	—
48 to 59 lbs	10 mL (320 mg)	4 tablets (320 mg)	2 tablets (320 mg)	1 tablet (325 mg)	—
60 to 71 lbs	12.5 mL (400 mg)	5 tablets (400 mg)	2½ tablets (400 mg)	1 tablet (325 mg)	—
72 to 95 lbs	15 mL (480 mg)	6 tablets (480 mg)	3 tablets (480 mg)	1½ tablets (487.5 mg)	1 tablet (500 mg)
96 to 146 lbs	—	—	4 tablets (640 mg)	2 tablets (650 mg)	1 tablet (500 mg)

Source: Mayo Clinic

For a child who is younger than 2 months old, ask your child's medical provider before giving acetaminophen.

Use only the enclosed medication dispenser that comes with the product. (Kitchen teaspoons are not accurate measures for medication.)

Dose may be given every 4 hours. Do not use the medication more than 5 times in 24 hours.

The following abbreviations are used on this dosage chart: milligram (mg), milliliter (mL), pounds (lbs.).

— Not applicable. This form of medication should not be given to a child of this weight.

PAIN RELIEVER DOSAGE BY WEIGHT

Ibuprofen (Advil, Motrin, others) — For children over 6 months

	Dose				
Weight	**Infants' oral suspension drops, 50 mg per 1.25 mL**	**Children's oral suspension, 100 mg per 5 mL**	**Children's chewable tablet, 50 mg**	**Junior-strength caplet or chewable tablet, 100 mg**	**Adult tablet, 200 mg**
12 to 17 lbs	1.25 mL (50 mg)	—	—	—	—
18 to 23 lbs	1.875 mL (75 mg)	—	—	—	—
24 to 35 lbs	—	5 mL (100 mg)	2 tablets (100 mg)	1 tablet (100 mg)	—
36 to 47 lbs	—	7.5 mL (150 mg)	3 tablets (150 mg)	1½ tablets (150 mg)	—
48 to 59 lbs	—	10 mL (200 mg)	4 tablets (200 mg)	2 tablets (200 mg)	1 tablet (200 mg)
60 to 71 lbs	—	12.5 mL (250 mg)	5 tablets (250 mg)	2½ tablets (250 mg)	1 tablet (200 mg)
72 to 95 lbs	—	15 mL (300 mg)	6 tablets (300 mg)	3 tablets (300 mg)	1½ tablets (300 mg)
Greater than 95 lbs	—	20 mL (400 mg)	8 tablets (400 mg)	4 tablets (400 mg)	2 tablets (400 mg)

Source: Mayo Clinic

For a child who is younger than 6 months old, ask your child's medical provider before giving ibuprofen.

If giving less than 100 mg, use infants' drops.

Use only the enclosed medication dispenser that comes with the product. (Kitchen teaspoons are not accurate measures for medication.)

Dose may be given every 6 to 8 hours. Do not use the medication more than 4 times in 24 hours.

The following abbreviations are used on this dosage chart: milligram (mg), milliliter (mL), pounds (lbs.).

-- Not applicable. This form of medication should not be given to a child of this weight.

Index

B

C

D

E

F

G

N

O

P

R

S

T

U

V

W

Y

Image credits

All photographs and illustrations are copyright of Mayo Foundation for Medical Education and Research (MFMER), except for the following:
COVER (front and back), p. 1, 35, 43, 61, 65, 74, 80, 88, 112, 113, 129, 167, 174, 180, 184, 210, 220, 265, 274, 275, 374, 398, 412, 417, 423, 424, 438, 459, 465, 476, 483, 497, 500, 515, 519, 530, 537, 539, 557, 562, CREDIT: Alexander Ryabintsev/iStock/Getty Images Plus; p. 5, CREDIT: timonko/iStock/Getty Images Plus; p. 24, CREDIT: Toltemara/iStock/Getty Images Plus; p. 26, 141, 255, 260, 504, CREDIT: Olga Shevchenko/iStock/Getty Images Plus; p. 47, 296, 413 (utensils), CREDIT: MegaShabanov/iStock/Getty Images Plus; p. 50, 154, CREDIT: Maneeta Chauyrod/iStock/Getty Images Plus; p. 85, 224, 250, 356, CREDIT: Celia Tam/iStock/Getty Images Plus; p. 97, 124, 127, 134, 259, 268, 278, 283, 288, 292, 298, 307, 315, 324, 333, 341, 349, 359, 368, 377, 388, 396, 402, 404, 409, 524, CREDIT: Tyas drawing/iStock/Getty Images Plus; p. 105, 381, CREDIT: Dina Petrova/iStock/Getty Images Plus; p. 106, CREDIT: LuckyStep48/iStock/Getty Images Plus; p. 121 (drool rash), CREDIT: Emilija Manevska/Moment; p. 132, 168, 216, 222, 334, 376, CREDIT: Olga Ubirailo/iStock/Getty Images Plus; p. 147, 470, CREDIT: Yulia Sutyagina/iStock/Getty Images Plus; p. 149, 302, 316, 320, 326, 339, 342, 365, 371, 475, 488, 565, 573, CREDIT: Tetiana Garkusha/iStock/Getty Images Plus; p.158, 526, CREDIT: Vdant/iStock/Getty Images Plus; p. 163, 478, CREDIT: sergeichekman/iStock/Getty Images Plus; p. 172, CREDIT: Gwens Graphic Studio/iStock/Getty Images Plus; p. 190, CREDIT: Julia Ustugova/iStock/Getty Images Plus; p. 201, CREDIT: Thirteen-Fifty/iStock/Getty Images Plus; p. 204, 232, 310, CREDIT: cnythzl/DigitalVision Vectors; p. 223, 235, 245, 401, 434, CREDIT: danang setyo nugroho/iStock/Getty Images Plus; p. 240, CREDIT: Laorue Kammalatbucha/iStock/Getty Images Plus; p. 272, CREDIT: Alina Ivanova/iStock/Getty Images Plus; p. 290, CREDIT: Veronika Oliinyk/iStock/Getty Images Plus; p. 312, 346, 382, 510, CREDIT: Kamila Baimukasheva/iStock/Getty Images Plus; p. 351, CREDIT: ByM/DigitalVision Vectors; p. 366, CREDIT: anna42f/iStock/Getty Images Plus; p. 390, CREDIT: Elena Pimukova/iStock/Getty Images Plus; p. 407, CREDIT: Natalie_/iStock/Getty Images Plus; p. 413 (washing hands), CREDIT: ngupakarti/iStock/Getty Images Plus; p. 413 (using tissue), CREDIT: HearttoHeart0225/iStock/Getty Images Plus; p. 413 (home), 413 (lips), CREDIT: Vitalii Barida/iStock/Getty Images Plus; p. 413 (spray bottle), CREDIT: Aliaksandr Trafimovich/iStock/Getty Images Plus; p. 430, 544, CREDIT: Caramel/DigitalVision Vectors; p. 443, CREDIT: Liubov/iStock/Getty Images Plus; p. 449, CREDIT: budi priyanto/iStock/Getty Images Plus; p. 453, CREDIT: Tetiana Lazunova/iStock/Getty Images Plus; p. 485, CREDIT: naqiewei/DigitalVision Vectors; p. 490, CREDIT: juliawhite/iStock/Getty Images Plus; p. 493, CREDIT: Tanya Shulga/iStock/Getty Images Plus; p. 511, CREDIT: Daria Pilshchikova/iStock/Getty Images Plus; p. 543, CREDIT: Olga Ubirailo/iStock/Getty Images Plus; p. 549, CREDIT: azzurri/DigitalVision Vectors; p. 552, CREDIT: IssaraJarukitjaroon/iStock/Getty Images Plus